D1709430

STROKE
in Children and
Young Adults

STROKE
in Children and Young Adults

SECOND EDITION

José Biller, MD, FACP, FAAN, FAHA
Professor and Chairman
Department of Neurology
Loyola University Chicago
Stritch School of Medicine
Maywood, Illinois

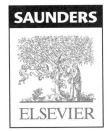

SAUNDERS

ELSEVIER

SAUNDERS
ELSEVIER

1600 John F. Kennedy Blvd.
Ste 1800
Philadelphia, PA 19103-2899

STROKE IN CHILDREN AND YOUNG ADULTS   ISBN: 978-0-7506-7418-8

Notice

Knowledge and best practice in this field are constantly changing. As new research and experience broaden our knowledge, changes in practice, treatment, and drug therapy may become necessary or appropriate. Readers are advised to check the most current information provided (i) on procedures featured or (ii) by the manufacturer of each product to be administered, to verify the recommended dose or formula, the method and duration of administration, and contraindications. It is the responsibility of the practitioner, relying on his or her experience and knowledge of the patient, to make diagnoses, to determine dosages and the best treatment for each individual patient, and to take all appropriate safety precautions. To the fullest extent of the law, neither the Publisher nor the Author assumes any liability for any injury and/or damage to persons or property arising out of or related to any use of the material contained in this book.

The Publisher

Library of Congress Cataloging-in-Publication Data

Biller, José.
Stroke in children and young adults / José Biller. -- 2nd ed.
      p. ; cm.
   Includes bibliographical references and index.
   ISBN-13: 978-0-7506-7418-8
   ISBN-10: 0-7506-7418-0
      1. Cerebrovascular disease in children. 2. Cerebrovascular disease. I. Title.
   [DNLM: 1. Stroke. 2. Adolescent. 3. Child. 4. Infant. 5. Young Adult. WL 355 B597s 2009]
   RJ496.C45S77 2009
   618.92'81--dc22

                                                                        2008054235

Acquisitions Editor: Adrianne Brigido
Developmental Editor: Joan Ryan
Publishing Services Manager: Hemamalini Rajendrababu
Project Manager: Jagannathan Varadarajan

Printed in USA

Last digit is the print number: 9 8 7 6 5 4 3 2 1

This book is dedicated to the memory of Dr. William DeMyer. Known and loved by many as preeminent neuroanatomist, erudite teacher, tireless advisor, compassionate caregiver, gregarious sportsman, and consummate family man. He will be missed by those whom he touched with any facet of his multidimensional life.

CONTRIBUTORS

Thomas J. Altstadt, MD
Neurological Surgery, Medford Neurological and Spine Center, Medford, Oregon

José Biller, MD, FACP, FAAN, FAHA
Professor and Chairman, Department of Neurology, Loyola University Chicago, Stritch School of Medicine, Maywood, Illinois

Rima M. Dafer, MD, MPH
Associate Professor, Department of Neurology, Loyola University Chicago, Stritch School of Medicine, Maywood, Illinois

William E. DeMyer, MD
Professor Emeritus of Child Neurology, Indiana University; Riley Hospital for Children, Indianapolis, Indiana

Meredith R. Golomb, MD, MSc
Assistant Professor, Department of Neurology, Division of Pediatric Neurology, Indiana University School of Medicine; Riley Hospital for Children, Indianapolis, Indiana

Lotfi Hacein-Bey, MD
Professor, Departments of Radiology and Neurosurgery and Director, Neuroradiology and Interventional Neuroradiology, Loyola University Medical Center, Chicago, Illinois

Betsy B. Love, MD
Adjunct Clinical Associate Professor, Department of Neurology, Loyola University Chicago, Stritch School of Medicine, Maywood, Illinois

James F. Meschia, MD
Professor and Director, Cerebrovascular Division, Department of Neurology, Mayo Clinic, Jacksonville, Florida

Thomas C. Origitano, MD, PhD, FACS
Professor and Chair, Department of Neurological Surgery, Co-Director, The Center for Cranial Base Surgery, Director, Loyola Neuroscience Service Line, Loyola University Medical Center, Maywood, Illinois

Hema Patel, MD
Associate Professor, Department of Neurology, Section of Pediatric Neurology, Indiana University School of Medicine; Associate Professor, Department of

Neurology, Section of Pediatric Neurology, Clarian Health Partners – James Whitcomb Riley Hospital for Children, Indianapolis, Indiana

Michael B. Pritz, MD, PhD
Professor, Department of Neurological Surgery and Director, Cerebrovascular and Skull Base Surgery, Indiana University School of Medicine; Attending Neurosurgeon, University Hospitals, Indianapolis, Indiana

Richard B. Rodgers, MD
Assistant Professor, Department of Neurological Surgery, Indiana University School of Medicine, Indianapolis, Indiana

Michael J. Schneck, MD
Associate Professor of Neurology and Neurosurgery, Department of Neurology, Loyola University Chicago, Stritch School of Medicine, Maywood, Illinois

Eugene R. Schnitzler, MD
Associate Professor of Neurology and Pediatrics and Chief, Division of Pediatric Neurology, Loyola University Chicago, Stritch School of Medicine; Department of Neurology and Pediatrics, Loyola University Medical Center, Maywood, Illinois

Mitesh V. Shah, MD, FACS
Associate Professor and Co-Director, Skull Base Surgery, Department of Neurosurgery, Indiana University, Indianapolis, Indiana

Deborah K. Sokol, MD, PhD
Associate Professor of Clinical Neurology, Section of Pediatrics, Indiana University School of Medicine; Pediatric Neurologist, Riley Hospital for Children, Indianapolis, Indiana

Marc G. Weiss, MD
Associate Professor, Department of Pediatrics and Director, Division of Neonatology, Loyola University Chicago, Stritch School of Medicine; Medical Director, Neonatal Intensive Care Unit, Ronald McDonald Children's Hospital of Loyola University Medical Center, Maywood, Illinois

FOREWORD

To write a foreword to a second edition is in many ways much easier than for a first. One responds to success rather than predicting it. Fourteen years ago, Professor James Toole pointed out in the "foreword" the need for and the potential importance of this book, *Stroke in Children and Young Adults*. He concluded with the statement that "Professor Biller and his colleagues have authored a text that will stand the test of time." Obviously he was correct. The success of the first edition established the need for and importance of the publication and, for 14 years, it stood the test of time. He also predicted that the new generation of clinical neuroscientists specializing in the prevention of and therapy for stroke would carry on to new heights of accomplishment. Again, he proved to be correct. Since 1994, this new generation has added so much to our understanding of stroke in children and young adults that this new edition is a necessity.

Professor Biller and his colleagues responded to this challenge and extensively revised and added to the material originally published bringing this document up to date and including information published in the early part of 2008. This has resulted in extensive rewriting of the original 14 chapters and the addition of three new chapters.

This is indeed a state-of-the-art publication. For example, most of the references are published after 1994. As one reviews the galleys, one is struck by how much has been added to our knowledge during this time. In addition to many of the original contributors, others have been added and have continued the high quality of work produced in the first edition.

The additional three chapters extend and add information to that included in the first edition. In particular, the chapter, *Applied Anatomy of the Brain Arteries*, by William DeMyer should serve as an invaluable addition for any understanding of vascular supply and clinical syndromes related to the brain arteries and for a reference in the future. It is unlikely that someone not working primarily in stroke would keep all of these details constantly in mind. As this book was in the final editing process, Dr. DeMyer died at the age of 84 years. Although physically incapacitated during his final few months, he continued to work and contribute in many areas of Neurology and completed his final book, *Taking the Clinical History: Eliciting Symptoms, Ethical Foundations*, a few days before his death. The dedication of this book to him, expresses the high regard that Biller, his colleagues, and all who know of his many contributions and his work ethic have for him. It is also a reflection of Professor Biller's good judgment in selecting outstanding contributors for inclusion in this volume.

Let us hope that the continued rapid acquisition of knowledge makes it necessary for a third edition long before 14 years. In the meantime, this updated volume will serve as the state-of-the-art source for understanding of *Stroke in Children and Young Adults*.

Mark L. Dyken, M.D.
Professor Emeritus of Neurology
Department of Neurology
Indiana University School of Medicine
Indianapolis, Indiana

PREFACE TO THE FIRST EDITION

Cerebrovascular disease in children and young adults represents a challenge to clinical neurologists. Cerebrovascular disease spans all medical specialties, and most clinicians are familiar with the catastrophic consequences of these disorders.

This book addresses the practical needs of house officers, neurologists, neurosurgeons, as well as those of specialists in pediatrics, internal medicine, and family practice who care for a wide variety of young patients with ischemic and hemorrhagic cerebrovascular disease. *Stroke in Children and Young Adults* provides a framework of clinical decision making and management of both commonly and rarely encountered cerebrovascular disorders in the young population.

After an overview of stroke types, risk factors, prognosis, and diagnostic strategies in neonates, children, and young adults, the ischemic stroke subtypes are discussed separately to familiarize the reader with relevant issues in atherosclerotic cerebral infarction, non-atherosclerotic cerebral vasculopathies, cardiac disorders, and disorders of hemostasis. Additionally, a thorough discourse of miscellaneous topics—migraine and stroke, stroke and pregnancy, rare genetic disorders associated with stroke, and cerebral venous thrombosis—is included. The final sections contain further insight into the practical and clinical information relative to intracerebral and subarachnoid hemorrhage.

We hope our readers find this book useful and that it enhances their ability to optimize care for the young stroke patient.

Acknowledgments

I owe a special debt to my family for their support during this project. In particular, I wish to express endless gratitude to my wife Célika for her unfailing patience and her assistance in organizing and preparing this book for publication.

PREFACE

Cerebrovascular disease in children and young adults accounts for 5% to 10% of all stroke cases and remains one of the top ten causes of childhood death, encompassing a broad range of causes and risk factors. This often represents a diagnostic and therapeutic challenge to clinicians with an average recognition time of 35.7 hours for the younger patients. Considerable progress has been made in our understanding of the incidence, etiology, diagnosis, and treatment of stroke in children and young adults. Even with this progress, however, clinicians, parents, patients, and caregivers can sometimes become disappointed or frustrated because the cause of the disease may remain undetermined in a considerable percentage of patients and a uniform approach to treatment is often lacking. Cerebrovascular disease occurring in this age category spans multiple medical specialties. Clinicians caring for young stroke victims are becoming increasingly familiar with the catastrophic consequences of these disorders which include not only a dramatic decline in the quality of life among survivors but potential socioeconomic consequences as well. This edition serves to provide an updated and more expansive resource that will be instrumental to clinical practices focusing on cerebrovascular disease in young people. It continues to address the practical needs of house officers, neurologists, and neurosurgeons as well as the needs of specialists in the fields of pediatrics, internal medicine, family practice, emergency medicine, nursing and other allied health professionals who care for a wide variety of young patients with ischemic and hemorrhagic cerebrovascular disease.

Just as in the First Edition, the book begins with an overview of stroke types, risk factors, prognosis, and diagnostic strategies in neonates, children and young adults. This is followed by a new, highly detailed and thoroughly illustrated chapter on the applied anatomy of brain arteries, which is presented in order to familiarize the reader with the relevant neuroanatomical correlation of symptoms and signs pertaining to important stroke syndromes. Chapters 3 and 4 contain an expanded discussion on the epidemiology, clinical presentation, evaluation, and treatments of stroke during the first 18 years of life and the individualized approach to neonates, children and young adults. The next three chapters provide a detailed discussion on atherosclerotic cerebral infarction, non-atherosclerotic vasculopathies, and cardiac disorders and strokes occurring in children and young adults. There are separate and fully updated chapters pertaining to cerebral infarction and migraines, as well as hemostatic disorders presenting as stroke. Since pregnancy-associated stroke remains a major cause of serious morbidity and mortality, a comprehensive review of pregnancy associated ischemic and hemorrhagic strokes is discussed independently. Similarly, as rare genetic disorders can lead to stroke, and diagnosis of these inherited conditions have important implications for the patient regarding stroke and his family, a concise review of rare genetic disorders that are associated with stroke is contained in Chapter 11. Cerebral venous thrombosis represents less than 1% to 2% of all stroke cases and although patients often present later in the course of their disease, it is more easily diagnosed with the advent of modern neuroimaging. Chapter 12 covers the epidemiology, clinical presentation, diagnosis, and management of thrombosis of the cerebral veins and sinuses along with the various etiologies which contribute to its development. Subsequent chapters contain further insights into neonatal intracranial hemorrhage (a significant problem in neonatal intensive care units), spontaneous intracerebral hemorrhage (which accounts for about 15% of all strokes), and subarachnoid hemorrhage in young adults. Finally, there are two new chapters—one of which focuses on pediatric central nervous system (CNS) vascular malformations (a common cause of non-traumatic intracerebral hemorrhage in this age group), and the other on the various types of spinal cord vascular malformations in children and young adults.

We hope the readers of Stroke in Children and Young Adults, Second Edition, will find it to be current and clinically beneficial. In addition, we hope that the knowledge about the disorders covered in this book will be utilized to benefit the patients who have helped us increase our understanding of stroke within this age group.

Jose Biller, MD

CONTENTS

CHAPTER 1

Stroke in Children and Young Adults: Overview, Risk Factors, and Prognosis

Betsy B. Love • José Biller

KEY TERMS

CADASIL	cerebral autosomal dominant arteriopathy with subcortical infarcts and leukoencephalopathy
CNS	central nervous system
CSVT	cerebral sinovenous thrombosis
FMD	fibromuscular dysplasia
HDL	high-density lipoprotein
HIV	human immunodeficiency virus
MELAS	mitochondrial encephalomyopathy, lactic acidosis, and strokelike symptoms
SAH	subarachnoid hemorrhage
TIA	transient ischemic attack

Cerebrovascular disease is the cause of death in more than 3000 individuals younger than 45 years annually and is one of the top 10 causes of childhood death.[1] Children and adults younger than 45 years account for 5% to 10% of all stroke cases.[2-4] In developing countries, the proportion is even higher, with 19% to 30% of strokes occurring in individuals younger than 45 years.[5,6] The impact of strokes in this age group is devastating to children and young adults, their families, and society.[7]

There are notable differences in incidence, presentation, risk factors, and prognosis in stroke occurring in individuals younger than 45 years compared with individuals older than 45 years. Also, there are significant differences in these parameters within the broad age groups from neonates to childhood to young adults. Where appropriate and where data exist, these differences are addressed in this chapter. Although neonatal/perinatal stroke is an important area of clinical study, this age group is addressed only briefly.

Stroke Incidence

There are worldwide fluctuations in the incidence rates of stroke in young individuals. The peak rate of stroke in this population occurs in the perinatal period, with 26.4 strokes per 100,000 live births in infants less than 30 days old (6.7 for hemorrhagic stroke and 17.8 for ischemic stroke).[8] The incidence of stroke in children in the United States was stable over the 10-year period from 1988 to 1999.[7] The incidence of all strokes in children younger than 15 years was 6.4 per 100,000 in 1999; this figure was not significantly increased compared with statistics from 1988.[7] Conservative estimates in 2004 indicated that approximately 3000 children and adults younger than 20 years would experience a stroke per year in the United States.[9] After 30 to 35 years of age, the rates of ischemic stroke at least doubled in some series to an incidence of 2.7 to 9 per 100,000.[5,10]

Racial differences in the incidence of ischemic stroke exist. The incidence in young black men and women was twice the rate of non-Hispanic whites in data from Baltimore.[6] More recently, data from northern Manhattan showed a higher rate not only in blacks, but also in Hispanics with an incidence of 8 per 100,000.[11]

The age-specific rate of intracerebral hemorrhage in individuals younger than 45 years may be 7 per 100,000 population, and 14 per 100,000 in young black males.[6,10] Generally, the rates are higher for males than females. Blacks and Hispanics have a higher rate than non-Hispanic whites.[11]

The incidence rates of subarachnoid hemorrhage (SAH) are elevated significantly among Swedish and Finn men and women 25 to 44 years old compared with other regions at 20 per 100,000.[12] In central Italy, the rates per 100,000 are seen to increase progressively from 0.41 at 0 to 14 years, to 0.96 at 15 to 24 years, 2.74 at 25 to 34 years, and 5.94 at 35 to 44 years.[13] In a study comparing different ethnic groups in northern Manhattan, the rate per 100,000 was 3 for non-Hispanic whites, 6 for blacks and 6 for Hispanics.[11]

Stroke Presentation in Young Individuals

The presentation of stroke differs in neonates and children compared with older age groups. Perinatal ischemic stroke is defined as "a cerebrovascular event occurring during fetal or neonatal life, before 28 days, with pathological or radiological evidence of focal arterial infarction of brain."[14] Signs in this age group may be nonspecific, including hypotonia, apnea, or neonatal seizures.[14] There may be no detectable focal neurologic signs evident at the onset, but focal neurologic signs may appear during the first year after the stroke as motor skills develop.[15] Strokes may manifest during the first year as pathologic early hand preference, new-onset seizures, or failure to reach developmental milestones.[14,15]

In children with stroke, there is often a considerable delay between the onset of symptoms and presentation to a health care facility. This delay may be attributable to an insidious or stuttering type of onset.[16] After onset of symptoms of stroke, diagnosis may be significantly delayed.[17] Cerebral venous occlusions tend to be diagnosed more promptly, probably because of the presence of seizures.

Older children with strokes typically present with sudden hemiparesis, often associated with seizures.[18] Seizures at the onset or shortly after stroke are more common in young children, particularly children younger than 3 or 4 years.[19] Newborns with neonatal seizures as a manifestation of ischemic stroke may be clinically normal between seizures, or they may have other signs of encephalopathy, such as abnormalities of tone or feeding, or depressed level of alertness.[20] Children with stroke resulting in aphasia may present with loss of speech, paraphasia, and dysgraphia.[9,21,22]

Fever or infection at the time of an acute stroke is much more common in children compared with older populations with stroke.[23] Approximately 50% to 55% of children presenting with cerebral infarction have fever or evidence of infection, often upper respiratory in nature.[24,25] Possible mechanisms of stroke in these children include dehydration as a result of fever, vasculitis, or a thrombotic process.[26] Stroke is a sequela of severe meningitis in children, especially infection secondary to *Haemophilus influenzae*, *Streptococcus pneumoniae*, and *Mycobacterium tuberculosis*. Other infections that are associated with stroke in children include varicella-zoster, human immunodeficiency virus (HIV), cat-scratch fever, and mycoplasma.

The mode of onset of neurologic symptoms strongly correlates with the underlying cause of stroke in children 6 months to 18 years old according to one more recent study.[16] The mode of onset was nonabrupt in 68% of children with arteriopathic stroke compared with an abrupt onset in 72% of children with stroke due to nonarteriopathic causes.[16]

There may be a history of head trauma, sometimes slight, before the onset of stroke in children.[27] Several authors have found a history of mild head trauma, without loss of consciousness or epilepsy, and associated infarction localized in the basal ganglia.[27,28]

Strokes in the distribution of the vertebrobasilar circulation are less common than strokes in the carotid territories and are not as well characterized in children. Most children with posterior circulation stroke are boys with vertebrobasilar arterial abnormalities, more than half of which are dissections.[29] Postulated reasons for a male predominance that have been observed in several studies include an increased potential for trauma and an increase in cervical spinal abnormalities in boys.[29,30] Another unique feature associated with posterior circulation strokes is that most children were previously healthy compared with children with strokes in the anterior circulation, of which half had a preexisting medical condition.[29]

Stroke Causes

Although it is important to review the most common causes of ischemic stroke in the various age groups, direct comparison between various studies can be challenging. Published studies of stroke in children and young adults have yielded variable results regarding what is the most common subtype of stroke because this depends on the population studied, the time period of study, the classification system used, and the extent of investigation. Atherosclerosis and small vessel disease play a minor role before age 35 in most individuals, and there is a preponderance of strokes of nontraditional etiologies (i.e., prothrombotic disorders, cervicocephalic arterial dissections, moyamoya disease, vasculitis), and strokes of unknown

etiologies (idiopathic). The one notable exception to this generalization is the etiologies in blacks, which are discussed subsequently. Cardioembolism from congenital or acquired heart disease continues to play a role, but it does not seem to be the most common cause in some more recent studies of children and young adults.[11,31,32]

Stroke causes and risk factors have not been studied as well in infants with perinatal stroke as in older age groups with stroke. Several studies have identified prothrombotic risk factors in 68% of infants with perinatal stroke compared with 24% of controls.[33] One study showed elevated lipoprotein (a) in 20% of patients, whereas another found 24% of patients had factor V Leiden mutation.[34]

At present, there is no stroke classification system specifically tailored to the multiple risk factors and etiologies in children and young adults. Several studies that have used a validated classification system, the Trial of ORG-10172 in Acute Stroke Therapy (TOAST) subtyping, are reviewed here.[35] In a study comparing the subtypes of stroke in patients 1 year to younger than 15 years old, 48% were classified as "other etiologies," 38% as unknown etiology, and 14% as cardioembolic; no cases were attributed to atherothrombosis or small vessel arterial disease.[36] In patients 15 to 18 years old, 55% were of other etiology, 18% were of unknown etiology, and 27% were cardioembolic. Although this group was small (11 patients), investigators observed that the causes of stroke in this group were more similar to those in young adults than in children. In the group older than 18 to 45 years old, there were 44% with other etiologies, 23% with unknown etiologies, 16% atherothrombotic, 14% cardioembolic, and 3% small vessel disease. Applying the TOAST subtyping for other series of childhood stroke, the results show 0% to 5% atherothrombosis, 3% to 65% cardioembolism, 0% to 2% small vessel, 0% to 46% other etiologies, and 33% to 94% unknown etiologies.[36]

In a more recent study of patients 18 to 45 years old using the TOAST classification, the most common causes were other than traditional causes in 26.4%, cardioembolism in 22.4%, and idiopathic strokes in 20.7%.[37] It also is notable that fewer younger patients (51.9%) had a cause of stroke established with high probability compared with older patients (70%). Using the TOAST subtypes for other studies of this age group, cardio-embolic stroke occurred in 24% to 34%, other etiologies occurred in 19% to 65%, and idiopathic stroke occurred in 24% to 33%.[38-40]

The causes of stroke in young blacks are different than in non-blacks. In individuals 15 to 44 years, the causes were atherosclerotic vasculopathy in 9%, nonatherosclerotic vasculopathy in 4%, lacunar infarcts in 21%, cardioembolism in 20%, hematologic in 14%, drug-related in 6%, and undetermined in 26%.[41,42] This greater number of lacunar infarctions is likely due to a higher prevalence of arterial hypertension among young blacks.[41]

Stroke is more common in boys 18 years and younger than in girls, regardless of stroke etiologic subtypes.[43] The male predominance is 61% for underlying cardiac disease; 59% for vasculopathy; 61% for underlying chronic disease, such as prothrombotic states, sickle cell anemia, and hematologic malignancies; and 66% for head and neck disease, such as otitis media, pharyngitis, and head and neck trauma.

Although ischemic strokes are more common than hemorrhages, hemorrhages account for a disproportionate number of strokes in younger patients.[4] In adults, ischemic stroke occurs in 80% of cases, and hemorrhages account for approximately 20% of strokes. In children, the distribution of hemorrhages is greater, with ischemic strokes accounting for 55% and hemorrhages accounting for 45% of strokes.[4,44] Hemorrhagic stroke is the most common form of stroke among young adults in some series.[45] Stroke patients younger than 45 years have a disproportionate percentage of SAH and intracranial hemorrhage (42.7%) compared with older patients (15.7%), predominantly attributable to aneurysms and arteriovenous malformations.[13]

Risk Factors for Ischemic Stroke in Young Individuals

General

There are multiple risk factors for ischemic stroke in children and young adults, including more than 100 different risk factors in

children alone, and are discussed at length in subsequent chapters (see Tables 3-1, 6-2, 6-3, 7-3, 9-1, and 10-1). Only the more common risk factors are reviewed here.

Perinatal stroke is unique because maternal and fetal risk factors must be considered. Factors such as maternal infertility, oligohydramnios, preeclampsia, prolonged rupture of membranes, umbilical cord abnormality, chorioamnionitis, and primiparity seem to be important as risk factors for arterial stroke in newborns.[46,47] Infection plays a more significant role in this age group. In addition, the neonatal coagulation system is immature and more susceptible to clot formation.[47] Factor V Leiden and prothrombin gene (G20210A) mutation can cause arterial stroke in the perinatal/neonatal period, whereas these are more associated with venous thromboembolism in adults.[47]

There are ethnic disparities in the risk of stroke in children and young adults. Black children have a higher risk of stroke, with a relative risk of 2.59 for ischemic stroke.[42] Hispanic children have a lower risk of ischemic stroke (0.76), whereas Asian children have a similar risk as whites. Among individuals 20 to 44 years, Hispanics and blacks have a higher risk of stroke than non-Hispanic whites.[11]

Ischemic stroke is more common in boys, regardless of stroke subtype, age, or etiology.[48] In a more recent large, national study, ischemic stroke was 2.62 times more likely to occur in boys than girls 16 to 20 years old, and 1.17 times more likely in boys than girls 0 to 5 years old.[48] In terms of risk, the odds are 50% higher for a boy to have an ischemic stroke.

A family history of ischemic stroke is a risk factor for stroke, but the role that this plays in strokes in young individuals is uncertain. The Framingham Heart Study reported a positive association between verified maternal and paternal history of transient ischemic attack (TIA) and stroke and an increased risk of stroke in the offspring.[49] There is a fivefold increase in stroke prevalence among monozygotic twins compared with dizygotic twins.[50,51]

Tobacco use is a significant risk factor for stroke in young individuals. Approximately 4000 children 12 to 17 years old start smoking every day in the United States, and 1140 become daily cigarette smokers.[52] Cigarette smoking increases the risk of stroke in young adults twofold.[53] Smoking in 25- to 37-year-olds is the most consistent predictor of carotid intima-media thickness, a marker of subclinical atherosclerosis.[54] The presence of other risk factors with tobacco use can act synergistically to increase stroke risk in young adults. One study showed that the presence of apolipoprotein E polymorphisms in combination with smoking can increase the risk of stroke in young adults.[55] Smoking cessation reduces the risk of stroke to that of a nonsmoker within 2 years after cessation.[56]

There is an association between very recent alcohol intake, particularly drinking for intoxication, and the onset of ischemic cerebral infarction in young adults 16 to 40 years old with no other known etiology for stroke.[57] This association is concerning in light of the fact that the average age of a child's first drink is now 12, and nearly 20 percent of 12- to 20-year-olds are considered binge drinkers.[58]

Drug use increases the risk of stroke by 6.5 times that of non–drug users.[59] Among patients younger than 35 years, one series showed that drug abuse was the most commonly encountered risk factor for stroke, present in 47%, with an overall relative risk for stroke of 11.7.[59] A more recent study showed that 14 percent of hemorrhagic strokes and 14 percent of ischemic strokes in individuals 18 to 44 years were caused by drug abuse, including amphetamines, cocaine, cannabis (marijuana), and tobacco.[60] In many regions of the United States, use of methamphetamine is increasing dramatically among young people. Amphetamine abuse is associated with a fivefold increased risk of hemorrhagic stroke in individuals 18 to 44 years.[60] Cocaine users have double the risk of ischemic and hemorrhagic stroke.[60] Strokes with use of marijuana have been the subject of case reports, and this association has been confirmed in a large population-based study.[60,61] There also have been reports of episodic marijuana use as a risk factor for stroke in childhood, particularly in the posterior circulation.[60,62] Strokes with the use of stimulants are thought to be related to vasospasm, vasculitis, or increased blood pressure.

Obesity is now the most prevalent disease in children and young adults. The latest statistics indicate that 17% of children 2 to 19 years old are overweight.[63] This percentage represents an increase in prevalence of overweight children and adolescents during the period 1999 to 2004. The prevalence was even greater for non-Hispanic blacks (20%) and Mexican-Americans (19.2%). These overweight children are at risk of becoming overweight young adults with a greater risk of hypercholesterolemia, hypertension, diabetes, heart disease, and stroke.

Atherosclerotic Risk Factors

Atherosclerosis is uncommon as a cause of stroke in individuals younger than 30 to 35 years.[64,65] Only 2% of patients 16 to 30 years old in one series had atherosclerosis as a causative factor for stroke.[64] In the same series, the percentage of patients 31 to 45 years with atherosclerosis as a cause of infarction was 7%. Most of these patients have classic risk factors, such as arterial hypertension, diabetes mellitus, cigarette smoking, and hyperlipidemia. Other factors that increase the risk of atherosclerosis in children and young adults include genetic metabolic disorders such as familial hyperlipidemias and hypercholesterolemias, progeria, familial hypoalphalipoproteinemia, Tangier disease, and high-density lipoprotein (HDL) deficiency states. As previously mentioned, atherosclerotic etiologies are more common in young adult blacks.

Hypertension is the most powerful risk factor for ischemic stroke and intraparenchymal hemorrhage. In a case-control study, arterial hypertension was present in approximately 31% of patients younger than 50 years with stroke, and this was statistically significant compared with the control group.[66] Small artery disease associated with stroke was the most likely cause of ischemic infarction in only 2%, however, of patients 31 to 45 years and did not account for any strokes in patients 16 to 30 years.[64] Stroke in 15- to 44-year-old blacks is more frequently associated with arterial hypertension compared with non-blacks, yielding a higher percentage of lacunar infarctions in this population.[41,42] Some rare, inherited enzyme deficiencies, such as 11β-hydroxylase deficiency, 11β-ketoreductase deficiency, and 17α-hydroxylase deficiency, are associated with arterial hypertension and, rarely, with hypertensive strokes. These syndromes may manifest in children and young adults if the enzyme defect is severe.

Diabetes is a prominent risk factor for ischemic stroke and is reported by some investigators to be second only to hypertension as a risk factor for stroke.[56] Diabetes in combination with other risk factors, such as hypertension, hyperlipidemia, alcohol use, and tobacco use, can greatly increase the risk of stroke.[67] With the epidemic of obesity among children, this risk factor is likely to play more of a role in the young adult population in the future.

The significance of disorders of cholesterol and lipids and the risks of tobacco use have previously been discussed as risk factors for ischemic stroke in young individuals.

Other Risk Factors

Risk factors in the category of "other" are extensive, diverse, and increasingly recognized as causes for stroke in children. Some of these risk factors are discussed, including arterial dissection, fibromuscular dysplasia (FMD), vasculitis, postvaricella arteriopathy, moyamoya disease, sickle cell disease, and metabolic and genetic disorders.

Spontaneous or traumatic cervicocephalic arterial dissections are described in 20% to 25% of cases of stroke in young adults.[64,68] The mean age for stroke caused by cervicocephalic arterial dissection is approximately 40 years.[64] A male predominance that is unexplained by trauma is noted in children.[30] Spontaneous carotid circulation dissections are most commonly intracranial, whereas post-traumatic anterior circulation dissections are more commonly extracranial in location in children.[30]

Cervicocephalic FMD is an angiopathy of unknown etiology involving medium-sized arteries that is more common in young adults and women. In the Lausanne Stroke Registry, cervicocephalic FMD was the cause of stroke in 4% of patients 16 to 30 years old and 1% of patients 31 to 45 years.[64] Although

this condition usually manifests in adults, it has been described in children.[69] FMD has been associated with cervicocephalic arterial dissections, intracranial aneurysms, and carotid cavernous fistulas and moyamoya disease.[70,71]

Vasculitis manifesting in childhood can be noninfectious or infectious. Noninfectious causes include many connective tissue diseases, polyarteritis nodosa, Wegener granulomatosis, central nervous system (CNS) granulomatous angiitis, lymphomatoid granulomatosis, and Takayasu arteritis. Infectious causes include many types of bacterial, fungal, and viral meningitis or meningoencephalitis.

Varicella infection within the preceding year is an important risk factor for stroke. Ischemic stroke is a complication of varicella in 1 in 15,000 cases.[72] In children 6 months to 10 years old with acute ischemic stroke, there is a threefold increase in preceding varicella infection.[72] Most of these strokes occur within 6 months of infection. Some notable characteristics include a likelihood of basal ganglionic infarction, anterior circulation stenotic vasculopathy, and recurrent stroke or TIA in two thirds of patients.[72] The exact mechanism by which varicella causes stroke is unknown, but intraneuronal migration of varicella from the trigeminal ganglion along the trigeminal nerve to the cerebral arteries, causing arteritis and vasospasm, is likely.

Moyamoya disease is a noninflammatory vasculopathy of uncertain etiology that produces progressive narrowing and obliteration of the distal internal carotid arteries and their branches, often bilaterally and with involvement of the circle of Willis. Extensive collateral networks form at the base of the brain, producing an angiographic pattern resembling a puff of smoke. This condition is uncommon but increasingly recognized in children and young adults in North America. It is one of the major causes of stroke in Japanese children.[73] The condition may be congenital in some patients, and it may be familial in 7% to 12% of patients.[73] Neurologic disorders in childhood include ischemic strokes, seizures, headaches, and movement disorders. Patients older than 30 years may develop cerebral hemorrhages. There is a female preponderance.[74] Moyamoya syndrome has been associated with many other systemic conditions, including sickle cell disease and neurofibromatosis 1.

In early studies, migraine was implicated as a cause of stroke in 1.7% of cases of stroke in children and in 10% to 15% of strokes in young adults.[59,75,76] More recent studies have confirmed migraine with visual aura as a risk for ischemic stroke in women 15 to 49 years old.[77] Concurrent smoking and the use of oral contraceptives increases the risk of stroke substantially. It is important to evaluate this population fully for other causes for stroke, especially because of the possible association of migraine with patent foramen ovale and hemostatic abnormalities.[78] Certain metabolic abnormalities, resulting from inborn errors of metabolism, are associated with an increased risk of stroke. Classic homocystinuria is due to cystathionine β-synthase deficiency and causes premature cardiovascular disease and venous thrombosis at a young age. Moderate hyperhomocysteinemia, owing to a defect in the methylenetetrahydrofolate reductase gene, is a risk factor for ischemic stroke, causing a fourfold increased risk for ischemic stroke in children and a similar risk in adults.[79,80] Other rare conditions resulting from inborn errors of metabolism that increase the risk of stroke include Fabry's disease, organic acid disorders, ornithine transcarbamylase deficiency, carbohydrate-deficient glycoprotein syndrome, and mitochondrial encephalomyopathy, lactic acidosis, and strokelike symptoms (MELAS).

Genetic disorders such as cerebral autosomal dominant arteriopathy with subcortical infarcts and leukoencephalopathy (CADASIL), cerebral autosomal recessive arteriopathy with subcortical infarcts and leukoencephalopathy (CARASIL), and hereditary endotheliopathy, retinopathy, nephropathy, and strokes (HERNS) are rare causes of ischemic stroke in young adults. Genetic causes of stroke in children and young adults are discussed in Chapter 11.

Cardiac Disorders

Approximately 15% to 20% of ischemic strokes in individuals 1 month to 18 years old are attributed to cardiac disorders.[36,81] In children

younger than age 15, the most common cardiac sources of stroke are congenital heart defects. Children with cyanotic congenital heart disease are at risk for stroke owing to many factors, including intracardiac shunts, infective endocarditis, polycythemia, anemia, hemoglobinopathies, coagulation disturbances, preexisting brain malformations, perioperative hypoxemia and low cardiac output states, catheterization procedures, sequelae of cardiopulmonary bypass, deep hypothermic circulatory arrest, and postoperative arrhythmias.[82,83] The use of cardiopulmonary bypass has a risk of gaseous and particulate microembolization, macroembolization, and hypoperfusion.[84] Hypothermic bypass techniques can cause stroke because of decreased perfusion.[84] In children and young adults older than age 15, the most common cardiac risk factors are patent foramen ovale, atrial septal defect, noninfectious valvular disease, left atrial or left ventricular thrombus, cardiomyopathy, and atrial fibrillation.

Hematologic Risk Factors

Coagulation abnormalities are increasingly recognized as important causes of stroke in young individuals. Prothrombotic abnormalities have been identified in 20% to 50% of children with ischemic stroke.[85] Some of these conditions are inherited disorders, which may predispose to either thrombosis or hemorrhage. Prothrombotic disorders, such as antithrombin deficiency, protein C and protein S deficiencies, and factor V Leiden, are causes of stroke in young individuals. In one study, most infants with neonatal/perinatal stroke had at least one thrombophilia marker.[86] Anticardiolipin antibodies and lupus anticoagulant have been associated with an increased risk of ischemic stroke and cerebral venous thrombosis in young adults.[87,88] In children, case-control studies have reported an association between anticardiolipin antibodies or lupus anticoagulant and first stroke, but not for recurrent stroke.[89,90]

Sickle cell disease is a risk factor for thrombotic and hemorrhagic infarcts. Approximately 60% to 80% of patients with sickle cell disease who eventually have a stroke have it before age 10 years, with a mean age for first-time stroke of slightly older than 6 years.[91-93] The Cooperative Study of Sickle Cell Disease showed that 25% of patients with homozygous sickle cell anemia and 10% of patients with hemoglobin sickle cell disease had a stroke by age 45 years.[94] There also are reports of the presence of "silent" infarctions in 23% of children with homozygous sickle cell anemia.[95]

Oral contraceptive use is infrequently the cause of stroke. A meta-analysis of studies indicates that it is a risk factor with a relative risk of 1.93 for low-estrogen preparations in population-based studies that controlled for tobacco use and arterial hypertension.[96]

Pregnancy is a risk factor for stroke, particularly in women older than 35 years and in black women.[97] The highest risk for stroke is in the peripartum period and up to 6 weeks after delivery.[98-100] Numerous factors contribute to this risk and are reviewed elsewhere.[97]

Multiple Risk Factors

Two more recent studies have emphasized the view that ischemic stroke in children is a multifactorial process.[31,32] The presence of multiple risk factors has been described in 25% of children with ischemic stroke, and their presence is associated with a higher risk of stroke recurrence.[32]

Stroke of Uncertain Etiology

In approximately one third of children and young adults with stroke, no cause is found after a complete workup.[8,36] It is important to perform comprehensive evaluations in children and young adults and to consider uncommon prothrombotic disorders, antiphospholipid antibodies, and genetic disorders as causes for stroke in this population. In one study of ischemic stroke in children in which most patients (87%) underwent a cerebral arterial imaging study (either cerebral angiography or magnetic resonance angiography), and in which there was aggressive evaluation for modifiable risk factors, such as anemia and hyperhomocysteinemia, the proportion of children with stroke of uncertain etiology was very low (1.9%).[31]

Cerebral Sinovenous Thrombosis

Cerebral sinovenous thrombosis (CSVT) most commonly affects children and young adults. It is being diagnosed with increasing frequency as a result of increased awareness of the disorder and increased detection with more sensitive neuroimaging techniques. The Canadian Pediatric Stroke Survey, a population-based study, found an incidence of 0.67 per 100,000 children 0 to 18 years of age per year.[101] Neonates accounted for 43% of the cases, and 54% of cases were in infants younger than 1 year old. Stroke resulting from CSVT is more common in boys (63%) than in girls 0 to 18 years.[43] In adults, 75% of cases occur in women.[102] One study showed that 61% of women with CSVT were 20 to 35 years old.[103] Pregnancy and oral contraceptive use may contribute to this finding.

Risk factors for CSVT are numerous (see Table 12-3), and this topic is discussed further in Chapter 12. Despite extensive evaluation, no cause is found in approximately 25% of children.[104] In approximately 75% of children, a risk factor is identified, and multiple risk factors may be identified in 65% of children.[105,106]

Clinical features of CSVT in childhood can be subtle. Neonates may present with fever, lethargy, irritability, seizures, and respiratory distress. Older children may have fever, lethargy, and signs of increased intracranial pressure. Approximately half of children present with focal abnormalities or seizures.[8] Young adults with CSVT may present with signs of intracranial hypertension (headache and papilledema) if the superior sagittal sinus is affected, as occurs in 70% to 80% of cases. Impaired consciousness, focal signs, or seizures may be present with cortical vein involvement and associated venous infarction.

Brain Hemorrhage

Hemorrhagic stroke accounts for 20% of all strokes, but it accounts for at least half of events in children and young adults in some series.[45] Stroke patients younger than 45 years have a disproportionate percentage of SAH and intracerebral hemorrhage (42.7%)

compared with older patients (15.7%), predominantly attributable to aneurysms and arteriovenous malformations.[13]

There is a higher risk for brain hemorrhages in boys. The odds are 37% higher for a boy to have a hemorrhagic stroke.[48] Black children have a higher risk of stroke, with a relative risk of 1.59 for SAH and 1.66 for intracerebral hemorrhage.[42]

Causes for hemorrhagic stroke are listed in Tables 14-1 and 15-1. There are numerous causes for hemorrhagic strokes in children. Among children younger than 20 years, 46% of hemorrhages are due to structural abnormalities (79% arteriovenous malformation, 37% cavernous malformation, 33% aneurysm, and 7% tumor).[107] Other causes are trauma in 24%, idiopathic in 19%, and medical in 10%. In adults younger than 49 years old, 33% have arterial hypertension; 41% have intracranial aneurysms, arteriovenous malformations, or other vasculopathies; and 20% abuse drugs.[108] In another review of risk factors for intraparenchymal hemorrhage in 68 children, the most common risk factors were vascular malformation/fistula in 32%, hematologic causes in 17.6%, coagulopathies in 14.7%, and brain tumor in 13.2%; no risk factors were found in 10.3%. Aneurysms accounted for 5.9%; cavernous malformation, 2%; hemorrhagic infarct, 8.8%; and spontaneous arterial dissection, 2.9%.[109] In blacks 15 to 44 years old, the most common causes of intracerebral hemorrhage are hypertensive vasculopathy in 64.2%; undetermined, 22.4%; aneurysm, 4.5%; arteriovenous malformation, 4.5%; and thrombolysis/anticoagulation, 3%.[41] For SAH, the distribution in blacks is aneurysm in 69.4%, undetermined in 21%, and arteriovenous malformation in 10.5%.[41]

Alcohol and drug abuse contribute to the risk for brain hemorrhage. There is a dose-dependent increased risk for subarachnoid and intracerebral hemorrhage associated with alcohol abuse that is probably secondary to chronic elevation of blood pressure.[110-112] Individuals with heavy alcohol consumption have a 1.9 times higher risk for hemorrhagic stroke compared with individuals who do not consume alcohol.[113] The risk of SAH with alcohol use is dose-dependent, increasing to 1.5 in individuals drinking 1 to 2 drinks per day and 3.8 times in individuals drinking more than 2 drinks per day compared with nondrinkers.[114]

In a study of women 15 to 44 years old, the use of amphetamines and cocaine was associated with a 9.6 times higher risk for intracranial hemorrhage than in women with no drug abuse.[115] The primary mechanism of cocaine-induced intracranial hemorrhage is probably acute elevation of blood pressure, with or without an underlying cerebrovascular malformation.

Risk of Stroke Recurrence

Clinically apparent and clinically silent recurrent ischemic stroke are common after an initial ischemic stroke in children.[116] One study showed a high rate of recurrent stroke, with nearly 40% of children experiencing a recurrence 1 day to 11.5 years later (median 267 days).[116] Another more recent study showed a more modest rate of recurrence, with 1 in 10 children having a recurrence within 5 years despite standard treatment.[117] Clinically silent infarctions occurred in 19% of 103 children in one study, who remained asymptomatic after their initial infarction.[116] So-called silent infarctions may have effects on cognitive function in children, however.

Some studies have shown that the presence of multiple risk factors is associated with a higher risk of recurrence.[31,32] Risk factors that have been associated with recurrence include previous TIA; bilateral infarction; leukocytosis; and the presence of a medical diagnosis before the stroke (especially immunodeficiency), such as elevated lipoprotein (a), protein C deficiency and stroke of vascular origin, and moyamoya disease.[116,117] The risk factors for recurrence of CSVT are not well studied. It is suggested that individuals with chronic medical conditions, such as anemia or congenital nephrotic syndrome, are at risk of CSVT recurrence.[118] The risk of recurrent hemorrhagic stroke in children is 10% within 5 years, with a higher risk of recurrence acutely for children with medical etiologies and a more prolonged and high risk for recurrence with structural lesions.[107]

Prognosis

Figure 1-1 shows the incidence of deaths from cerebrovascular disease in children and young adults.[119] The peaks for deaths are in infants younger than 1 year and in adults 35 to 44 years. The mortality rate from stroke has declined 58% over the period from 1979 to 1998.[120] Estimates of the death rate from recurrent stroke are 15% to 20%.[117] The mortality rate is higher for patients having a recurrent stroke (40%) compared with a single stroke (16%).[121] There is a higher risk for death with hemorrhage and with stupor or coma at presentation.[122] One study showed no ethnic differences in stroke severity or case-fatality rate, but boys have a higher case-fatality rate for stroke.[120]

One study indicated that children with subcortical strokes have a better outcome than children with cortical strokes.[123] Although 86% of children with subcortical stroke had good outcomes, only 38% with cortical strokes had similar outcomes.[123]

Children surviving an initial ischemic stroke may have varying degrees of hemiparesis, learning disabilities, attention-deficit/hyperactivity disorder, mental retardation, seizures and movement disorders.[124,125] Certain clinical features or risk factors are associated with a poorer outcome. Children who present with seizures tend to have a worse prognosis for intellectual development and a higher incidence of recurrent seizures compared with children who do not have seizures during the acute phase.[24]

One study of young adults with acute ischemic cerebral infarction had a 30-day mortality of 6.6%, which is less than mortality reported with older adults.[126] Patients with a cardiac source of stroke had the greatest mortality.[126] After a stroke in a young adult, the prognosis is slightly better for patients 16 to 30 years old compared with patients 31 to 45 years. Approximately 60% of the younger group had either no or minor disability compared with 51% of the older group.[64] After rehabilitation, approximately 80% of young adult patients resume their previous jobs within 6 months after discharge.[127]

There have been few studies of the long-term prognosis of CVST in children. Data from the Canadian Pediatric Stroke Survey in children (0 to 18 years) found that 8% of 160 patients died.[129] Death occurred in 5 of 42 children in another study and was associated with coma at presentation.[118] Predictors of a good cognitive outcome included older age, lack of parenchymal abnormality, anticoagulation, and lateral or sigmoid sinus (or both) involvement.[118] Complications of CSVT that can persist include pseudotumor cerebri, cognitive and behavioral disabilities, epilepsy, and persistent focal neurologic abnormalities.[118] In a small study of 17 children with CVST, children who survived had a fair prognosis, with most showing normal cognitive and physical development.[128]

In a study of 56 children with hemorrhagic stroke over a mean follow-up of 10.3 years, death occurred in 23% as a result of the initial hemorrhage; rebleeding occurred in 16%, which resulted in death in 33%; and seizures developed in 11%.[129] Although most surviving children functioned independently, only 25% of these children were free of physical or cognitive deficits.

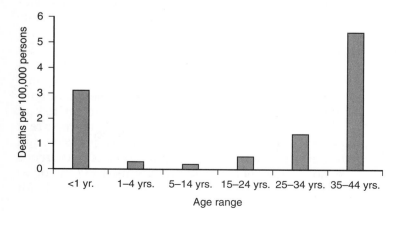

FIGURE 1-1   Deaths from cerebrovascular disease in children and young adults. (Data from Kung HC, Hoyert DL, Xu JQ, Murphy SL. Deaths: final data for 2005. In National Vital Statistics Reports, vol 56, no 10. Hyattsville, MD: National Center for Health Statistics, 2008.)

Conclusion

Stroke in children and young adults is notably different in regard to incidence, presentation, risk factors, and prognosis compared with stroke in older age groups. Risk factors are extensive and diverse in this population. This is an exciting area of ongoing study in which there is high motivation for finding ways to prevent stroke and to improve outcome.[130]

REFERENCES

1. Kung HC, Hoyert DL, Xu J, Murphy SL. Deaths: preliminary data for 2005. In National Vital Statistics Reports, vol 56, no 10. Hyatsville, MD: National Center for Health Statistics, 2008.
2. Hart R, Sherman D, Miller V, Easton JD. Diagnosis and management of ischemic stroke: selected controversies. Curr Probl Cardiol 1983;8:43.
3. Bogousslavsky J, Van Melle G, Regli F. The Lausanne Stroke Registry: analysis of 1000 consecutive patients with first stroke. Stroke 1988;19:1083.
4. Neucini P, Inzitari D, Baraffi MC, et al. Incidence of stroke in young adults in Florence, Italy. Stroke 1988;19:977.
5. Radhakrishan K, Ashok FP, Sridharan R, et al. Stroke in the young: incidence and pattern in Benghazi, Libya. Acta Neurol Scand 1986;73:434.
6. Kittner SJ, McCarter RJ, Sherwin RW, et al. Black-white difference in stroke risk among young adults. Stroke 1993;24(suppl I)I-13.
7. Rosamond W, Flegal K, Furie K, et al. Heart disease and stroke statistics 2008 update: a report from the American Heart Association Statistics Committee and Stroke Statistics Subcommittee. Circulation 2008;117:e25.
8. Lynch JK, Hirtz DG, deVeber G, Nelson KB. Report of the National Institute of Neurological Disorders and Stroke workshop on perinatal and childhood stroke. Pediatrics 2002;109:116.
9. Kleindorfer D, Khoury J, Kissela B, et al. Temporal trends in the incidence and case fatality of stroke in children and adolescents. J Child Neurol 2006;21:415.
10. Mettinger KL, Soderstrom CE, Allander E. Epidemiology of acute cerebrovascular disease before the age of 55 in the Stockholm County 1973-1977, I: incidence and mortality rates. Stroke 1984;15:795.
11. Jacobs BS, Boden-Albala B, Lin I-F, Sacco RL: Stroke in the young in the Northern Manhattan Stroke Study. Stroke 2002;33:2789.
12. Terent A. Increasing incidence of stroke among Swedish women. Stroke 1988;19:598.
13. Marini C, Totaro R, De Santis F, et al. Stroke in young adults in the community-based L'Aquila registry: incidence and prognosis. Stroke 2001;32:52.
14. Nelson KB. Perinatal ischemic stroke. Stroke 2007;38(part 2):742.
15. Lanska MJ, Lanska DJ, Horwitz SJ, Aram DM. Presentation, clinical course, and outcome of childhood stroke. Pediatr Neurol 1991;7:333.
16. Braun KPJ, Rafay MF, Uiterwaal CSPM, et al. Mode of onset predicts etiological diagnosis of arterial ischemic stroke in children. Stroke 2007;38:298.
17. Gabis LV, Yangala R, Lenn NJ. Time lag to diagnosis of stroke in children. Pediatrics 2002;110:924.
18. Lanska MJ, Lanska DJ, Horowitz SJ, Aram DM. Presentation, clinical course, and outcome of childhood stroke. Pediatr Neurol 1991;7:333.
19. Dusser A, Goutieres F, Aicardi J. Ischemic strokes in children. J Child Neurol 1986;1:131.
20. Nelson KB, Cowan F, Rutherford M, et al. Origin and timing of brain lesion in term infants with neonatal encephalopathy. Lancet 2003;361:735.
21. Van Dongen HR, Loonen CB, Van Dongen KJ. Anatomical basis for acquired fluent aphasia in children. Ann Neurol 1985;17:306.
22. Granberg LD, Filley CM, Hart EJ, Alexander MP. Acquired aphasia in childhood: clinical and CT investigation. Neurology 1987;37:1165.
23. Hutchinson JS, Ichord R, Guerguerian A-M, deVeber G. Cerebrovascular disorders. Semin Pediatr Neurol 2004;11:139.
24. Trescher WH. Ischemic stroke syndromes in childhood. Pediatr Ann 1992;21:374.
25. Eeg-Olofsson O, Ringheim Y. Stroke in children: clinical characteristics and prognosis. Acta Pediatr Scand 1983;72:391.
26. Raybaud CA, Livet MO, Jiddane M, Pinsard N. Radiology of ischemic stroke in children. Neuroradiology 1985;27:567.
27. Satoh S, Sirane R, Yoshimoto T. Clinical survey of ischemic cerebrovascular disease in children in a district of Japan. Stroke 1991;22:586.
28. Giroud M, Lemesle M, Gouyon JB, et al. Cerebrovascular disease in children under 16 years of age in the city of Dijon, France: a study of incidence and clinical features from 1985 to 1993. J Clin Epidemiol. 1995;48:1343.
29. Ganesan V, Chong WK, Cox TC, et al. Posterior circulation stroke in childhood: risk factors and recurrence. Neurology 2002;59:1552.
30. Fullerton HJ, Johnston SC, Smith WS. Arterial dissection and stroke in children. Neurology 2001;57:1155.
31. Ganesan V, Prengler M, McShane MA, et al. Investigation of risk factors in children with arterial ischemic stroke. Ann Neurol 2003;53:167.
32. Lanthier S, Carmant L, David M, et al. Stroke in children: The coexistence of multiple risk factors predicts poor outcome. Neurology 2000;54:371.
33. Gunther G, Junker R, Strater et al, for the Childhood Stroke Study Group. Symptomatic ischemic stroke in full-term neonates: role of acquired and genetic prothrombotic risk factors. Stroke 2000;31:2437.
34. Nelson KB, Mercuri E, Cowan F, Gupte G, et al. Prothrombotic disorders and abnormal neurodevelopmental outcome in infants with neonatal cerebral infarction. Pediatrics 2001;107:1400.
35. Gordon DL, Bendixen BH, Adams HP Jr, et al. Interphysician agreement in the diagnosis of subtypes of acute ischemic stroke: implications for clinical trials. The TOAST investigators. Neurology 1993;43:1021.

36. Williams LS, Garg BP, Cohen M, et al. Subtypes of ischemic stroke in children and young adults. Neurology 1997;49:1541.

37. Telman G, Kouperberg E, Sprecher E, Yarnitsky D. Distribution of etiologies in patients above and below age 45 with first-ever ischemic stroke. Acta Neurol Scand 2007;117(5):311.

38. Cerrato P, Grasso M, Imperiale D, et al. Stroke in young patients: etiopathogenesis and risk factors in different age classes. Cerebrovasc Dis 2004;18:154.

39. Lee TH, Hsu WC, Chen CJ, Chen ST. Etiologic study of young ischemic stroke in Taiwan. Stroke 2002;33:1950.

40. Kwon SU, Kim JS, Lee JH, Lee MC. Ischemic stroke in Korean young adults. Acta Neurol Scand 2000;101:19.

41. Qureshi A, Safdar K, Patel M, et al. Stroke in young black patients: risk factors, subtypes, and prognosis. Stroke 1995;26:1995.

42. Fullerton HJ, Wu YW, Zhao S, Johnson SC. Risk of stroke in children: ethnic and gender disparities. Neurology 2003;61:189.

43. Golomb M, Fullerton H, deVeber G; and members of International Paediatric Stroke Study. Childhood ischemic stroke is more common in boys. The International Paediatric Stroke Study. Stroke 2008;39:546.

44. Daniels SR, Bates R, Lukin RR, et al. Cerebrovascular arteriopathy (arteriosclerosis) and ischemic childhood stroke. Stroke 1982;13:360.

45. Reiner AP, Schwartz SM, Frank M, et al. Polymorphisms of coagulation factor XIII subunit A and risk of nonfatal hemorrhagic stroke in young white women. Stroke 2001;32:2580.

46. Lee J, Croen LA, Backstrand KH, et al. Maternal and infant characteristics associated with perinatal arterial stroke in the newborn. JAMA 2005;293:723.

47. Nelson K, Lynch J. Stroke in newborn infants. Lancet Neurol 2004;3:150.

48. Lo W, Hayes J, Stephens JA, Fernandez J. Pediatric stroke in the United States. Stroke 2008;39:644.

49. Kiely DK, Wolf PA, Cupples LA, et al. Familial aggregation of stroke. The Framingham Study. Stroke 1993;24:1366.

50. Brass LM, Isaacsohn JL, Merikangas KR, Robinette CD. A study of twins and stroke. Stroke 1992;23:221.

51. Hrubec Z, Robinette CD. The study of human twins in medical research. N Engl J Med 1984;310:435.

52. Substance Abuse and Mental Health Services Administration. Results from the 2005 National Survey on Drug Use and Health (PDF-1.41MB). Rockville, MD: Office of Applied Studies, NSDUH Series H-27, DHHS Publication No. SMA 05-4061, 2005. Available at: http://oas.samhsa.gov/nsduh/2k5nsduh/2k5results.pdf. Accessed March 1, 2008.

53. Love BB, Biller J, Jones MP, et al. Cigarette smoking as a risk factor for stroke in young adults. Arch Neurol 1990;47:693.

54. Johnson HM, Douglas PS, Srinivasan SR, et al. Predictors of carotid intima-media thickness progression in young adults. Stroke 2007;38:900.

55. Pezzini A, Grassi M, Del Zotto E, et al. Synergistic effect of apolipoprotein E polymorphisms and cigarette smoking on risk of ischemic stroke in young adults. Stroke 2004;35:438.

56. Wolf PA, D'Agostino RB, Kannel WB, et al. Cigarette smoking as a risk factor for stroke: the Framingham study. JAMA 1988;259:1025.

57. Hillbom M, Haapaniemi H, Juvela S, et al. Recent alcohol consumption, cigarette smoking, and cerebral infarction in young adults. Stroke 1995;26:40.

58. Brain damage risks: AMA report on alcohol's adverse effects on the brains of children, adolescents and college students. Available at: www.ama-assn.org/ama/pub/category/9416.html. Accessed March 1, 2008.

59. Barlow CF. Headaches and migraine in child hood. Clin Dev Med 1984;91:138.

60. Westover AN, McBride S, Haley RW. Stroke in young adults who abuse amphetamines or cocaine: a population-based study of hospitalized patients. Arch Gen Psychiatry 2007;64:495.

61. Mateo I, Pinedo A, Gomez-Beldarrain M, et al. Recurrent stroke associated with cannabis use. Journal of Neurology Neurosurgery and Psychiatry 2005;76:435.

62. Geller T, Loftis L, Brink DS. Cerebellar infarction in adolescent males associated with acute marijuana use. Pediatrics 2004;113:e365.

63. Ogden CL, Carrol MD, Curtin LR, et al. Prevalence of overweight and obesity in the United States, 1999-2004. JAMA 2006;295:1549.

64. Bogousslavsky J, Pierre P. Ischemic stroke in patients under age 45. Neurol Clin 1992;10:113.

65. Bendixen B, Posner J, Lango R. Stroke in young adults and children. Curr Neurol Neurosci 2001;1:54.

66. Matias-Guiu J, Alvarez J, Insa R, et al. Ischemic stroke in young adults, II: analysis of risk factors in the etiological subgroups. Acta Neurol Scand 1990;81:314.

67. Lindegard B, Hilibom M. Associations between brain infarction, diabetes, and alcoholism: observations from the Gothenburg population cohort study. Acta Neurol Scand 1987;75:195.

68. Gautier JC, Pradat-Diehi P, Loron P, et al. Accidents vasculaires cerébraux des sujets jeunes: une étude de 133 patients ages de 9 a 45 ans. Rev Neurol 1989;145:437.

69. Shields WD, Ziter FA, Osborn AG, Allen J. Fibromuscular dysplasia as a cause of stroke in infancy and childhood. Pediatrics 1977;59:899.

70. Schievink WI: Spontaneous dissections of cervicocephalic arteries in childhood and adolescence. Neurology 1994;44:1607.

71. Leary MC, Finley A, Caplan LR. Cerebrovascular complications of fibromuscular dysplasia. Curr Treat Options Cardiovasc Med 2004;6:237.

72. Askalan R, Laughlin S, Mayank S, et al. Chickenpox and stroke in childhood: a study of frequency and causation. Stroke 2001;32:1257.

73. Kurokawa T, Chen YJ, Tomita S. Cerebrovascular occlusive disease with and without the moyamoya vascular network in children. Neuropediatrics 1985;16:29.

74. Numaguchi Y, Gonzalez CF, Davis PC, et al. Moya-moya disease in the United States. Clin Neurol Neurosurg. 1997;99(suppl 2):S26.

75. Bogousslavsky J, Despland PA, Regli F. Spontaneous carotid dissection with acute stroke. Arch Neurol 1987;44:137.

76. Sacquegna T, Andreoli A, Baidrati A, et al. Ischemic stroke in young adults: the relevance of migrainous infarction. Cephalalgia 1989;9:255.

77. MacClellan LR, Giles W, Cole J, et al. Probable migraine with visual aura and risk of ischemic stroke. The Stroke Prevention in Young Women Study. Stroke 2007;38:2438.

78. Schwerzmann M, Nedeltchev K, Lagger F, et al. Prevalence and size of directly detected patent foramen ovale in migraine with aura. Neurology 2005;65:1415.

79. van Beynum IM, Smeitink J, den Heijer M, et al. Hyperhomocysteinemia: a risk factor for ischemic stroke in children. Circulation 1999;99:2070.

80. Boushey CJ, Beresford SAA, Omenn GS, Motulsky AG. A quantitative assessment of plasma homocysteine as a risk factor for vascular disease. JAMA 1995;274:1049.

81. Lanthier S, Carmant L, David M, et al. Stroke in children: the coexistence of multiple risk factors predicts poor outcome. Neurology 2000;54:371.

82. Andropoulos DB, Stayer SA, Diaz LK, Ramamoorthy CR. Neurological monitoring for congenital heart surgery. Anesth Analg 2004;99:1365.

83. Caldwell RL. Stroke and congenital heart disease in infants and children. Semin Cerebrovasc Dis Stroke 2003;3:200.

84. Newburger JW, Bellinger DC. Brain injury in congenital heart disease. Circulation 2006;113:183.

85. Barnes C, deVeber G. Prothrombotic abnormalities in childhood ischaemic stroke. Thromb Res 2006;118:67.

86. Kenet G, Sadetzki S, Murad H, et al. Factor V Leiden and antiphospholipid antibodies are significant risk factors for ischemic stroke in children. Stroke 2000;31:1283.

87. Brey RL, Stallworth CL, McGlasson DL, et al. Antiphospholipid antibodies and stroke in young women. Stroke 2002;33:2396.

88. Rosendaal FR. Thrombosis in the young: epidemiology and risk factors: a focus on venous thrombosis. Thromb Haemost 1997;78:1.

89. Angelini L, Ravelli A, Caporali R, et al. High prevalence of antiphospholipid antibodies in children with idiopathic cerebral ischemia. Pediatrics 1994;94:500.

90. Lanthier S, Kirkham FJ, Mitchell LG, et al. Increased anticardiolipin antibody IgG titers do not predict recurrent stroke or TIA in children. Neurology 2004;62:194.

91. Earley CJ, Kittner SJ, Feeser BR, et al. Stroke in children and sickle-cell disease. Neurology 1998;51:169.

92. Ohene-Frempony K. Stroke in sickle cell disease: demographic, clinical, and therapeutic considerations. Semin Hematol 1991;28:213.

93. Balkaran B, Char G, Morris JS, et al. Stroke in a cohort of patients with homozygous sickle cell disease. J Pediatr 1992;120:360.

94. Ohene-Frempony K, Weiner SJ, Sleeper LS, et al. Cerebrovascular accidents in sickle cell disease: rates and risk factors. Blood 1998;91:288.

95. Miller ST, Macklin EA, Pegelow CH, et al; and the Cooperative Study of Sickle Cell Disease. Silent infarction as a risk factor for overt stroke in children with sickle cell anemia: a report from the Cooperative Study of Sickle Cell Disease. J Pediatr 2001;139:385.

96. Gillum LA, Mamidipudi SK, Johnston SC. Ischemic stroke risk with oral contraceptives: a meta-analysis. JAMA 2000;284:72.

97. Davie C, O'Brien P. Stroke in pregnancy. Journal of Neurology Neurosurgery and Psychiatry 2008;79:240.

98. Salonen Ros H, Lichtenstein P, Bellocco R, et al. Increased risks of circulatory diseases in late pregnancy and puerperium. Epidemiology 2001;12:456.

99. Kittner SJ, Stern BJ, Feeser BR, et al. Pregnancy and the risk of stroke. N Engl J Med 1996;335:768.

100. James AH, Bushnell CD, Jamison MG, Myers ER. Incidence and risk factors for stroke in pregnancy and the puerperium. Obstet Gynecol 2005;106:509.

101. de Veber G, Adams C, Bjornson B, et al, for the Canadian Pediatric Ischemic Stroke Study Group. Cerebral sinovenous thrombosis in children. N Engl J Med 2001;345:417.

102. Stam J. Thrombosis of the cerebral veins and sinuses. N Engl J Med 2005;352:1791.

103. Ameri A, Bousser MG. Cerebral venous thrombosis. Neurol Clin 1992;10:87.

104. Carvalho KS, Garg BP. Cerebral venous thrombosis and venous malformations in children. Neurol Clin 2002;20:1061.

105. Carvalho KS, Bodensteiner JB, Connolly PJ, et al. Cerebral venous thrombosis in children. J Child Neurol 2001;16:574.

106. deVeber G, Andrew M, Adams M, et al. Treatment of pediatric sinovenous thrombosis with low molecular weight heparin. Ann Neurol 1995;38(suppl):S32.

107. Fullerton HJ, Wu YW, Sidney S, Johnston SC. Recurrent hemorrhagic stroke in children: a population-based cohort study. Stroke 2007;38:2658.

108. Hoffman M, Malek A. Intracranial hemorrhage in young people is mostly due to vascular abnormality or drug abuse and mortality rate is low (abstract). Stroke 2006;37:725.

109. Al-Jarallah M, Al-Rifai T, Riela AR, et al. Spontaneous intraparenchymal hemorrhage in children: a study of 68 patients. J Child Neurol 2000;15:284.

110. O'Connor AD, Rusyniak DE, Bruno A. Cerebrovascular and cardiovascular complications of alcohol and sympathomimetic drug abuse. Med Clin North Am 2005;89:1343.

111. Thrift AG, Donnan GA, McNeil JJ. Heavy drinking, but not moderate or intermediate drinking, increases the risk of intracerebral hemorrhage. Epidemiology 1999;10:307.

112. Gillman MW, Cook NR, Evans DA, et al: Relationship of alcohol intake with blood pressure in young adults. Hypertension 1995;25:1106.

113. Klatsky AL, Armstrong MA, Friedman GD, et al: Alcohol drinking and risk of hemorrhagic stroke. Neuroepidemiology 2002;21:115.

114. Longstreth WT Jr, Nelson LM, Koepsell TD, et al: Cigarette smoking, alcohol use, and subarachnoid hemorrhage. Stroke 1992;23:1242.

115. Petitti DB, Sidney S, Quesenberry C, et al: Stroke and cocaine or amphetamine use. Epidemiology 1998;9:596.

116. Ganesan V, Prengler M, Wade A, Kirkham FJ. Clinical and radiological recurrence after childhood arterial ischemic stroke. Circulation 2006;114:2170.

117. Strater R, Becker S, von Eckardstein A, et al. Prospective assessment of risk factors for recurrent stroke during childhood: a 5-year follow-up study. Lancet 2002;360:1540.

118. Sebire G, Tabarki B, Saunders DE, et al. Cerebral venous sinus thrombosis in children: risk factors, presentation, diagnosis and outcome. Brain 2005;128:477.

119. Kung HC, Hoyert DL, Xu JQ, Murphy SL. Deaths: final data for 2005. In National Vital Statistics Reports, vol 56, no 10. Hyattsville, MD: National Center for Health Statistics, 2008.

120. Fullerton HJ, Chetkovich DM, Wu YW, et al. Deaths from stroke in US children, 1979-1998. Neurology 2002;59:6.

121. Chabrier S, Husson B, Lasjunias P, et al. Stroke in childhood: outcome and recurrence risk by mechanism in 59 patients. J Child Neurol 2000;15:290.

122. Higgins JJ, Kammerman LA, Fitz CR. Predictors of survival and characteristics of childhood stroke. Neuropediatrics 1991;22:190.

123. Abram HS, Knepper LE, Warty VS, Painter MJ. Natural history, prognosis, and lipid abnormalities of idiopathic ischemic childhood stroke. J Child Neurol 1996;11:276.

124. Schoenberg BS, Mellinger JF, Schoenberg DG. Cerebrovascular disease in infants and children: a study of incidence, clinical features, and survival. Neurology 1978;28:763.

125. Max JE, Mathews K, Manes F, et al. Attention deficit hyperactivity disorder and neurocognitive correlates after childhood stroke. Journal of the International Neuropsychological Society 2003;9:815.

126. Biller J, Adams Jr HP, Bruno A, et al. Mortality in acute cerebral infarction in young adults: a ten-year experience. Angiology 1991;42:224.

127. Adunsky A, Hershkowitz M, Rabbi R, et al. Functional recovery in young stroke patients. Arch Phys Med Rehabil 1992;73:859.

128. De Schryver E, Blom I, Braun K, et al. Long-term prognosis of cerebral venous sinus thrombosis in childhood. Dev Med Child Neurol 2004;46:514.

129. Blom I, DeSchryver E, Kappelle LJ, et al. Prognosis of haemorrhagic stroke in childhood: a long-term follow-up study. Dev Med Child Neurol 2003;45:233.

130. Roach ES, Golomb MR, Adams R, et al. Management of stroke in infants and children. A Scientific Statement from the Special Writing Group of the American Heart Association Stroke Council and the Council on Cardiovascular Disease in the Young. Stroke 2008;39:2644–2691.

CHAPTER 2

Applied Anatomy of the Brain Arteries

William DeMyer

Four Major Arteries to the Brain and Formation of the Circle of Willis

Origin of the Brain Arteries

Four major arteries, the two internal carotid arteries (ICAs) and the two vertebral arteries (VAs), irrigate the brain. They arise directly or indirectly from the aortic arch (Fig. 2-1). In succession, the aortic arch gives off the brachiocephalic (innominate) artery, the left common carotid artery (LCCA), and the left subclavian artery (see Fig. 2-1).

The brachiocephalic artery divides into the right common carotid artery (RCCA) and the right subclavian artery. The RCCA divides into the external carotid artery (ECA) for the face, and the ICA for the forebrain. The right VA originates from the right subclavian artery.

The LCCA arises directly from the aortic arch and likewise divides into an ECA and ICA (see Fig. 2-1). Because it arises directly from the aortic arch, the LCCA is 4 to 5 cm longer than the RCCA. The left subclavian artery arises from the aortic arch distal to the LCCA. The left VA arises from the left subclavian artery.

Mechanical compression of the four major arteries in their course through the

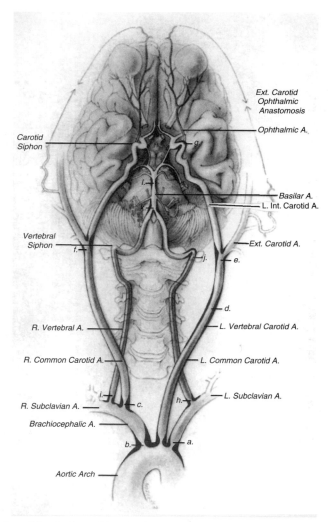

FIGURE 2-1 **Ventral drawing of the brain and its arteries.** Two carotid arteries and two vertebral arteries convey blood from the aortic arch to the brain. *a-j* show predilection sites for narrowing by arteriosclerosis. L, left; R, right. (Reprinted with permission and relabeled from Hoyt WF. Some neuro-ophthalmologic considerations in vascular insufficiency. Arch Ophthalmol 1959;62:260.)

neck or dissections of their wall may cause strokes in children and adults.[1,2] The ICAs enter the cranium at the foramen lacerum, located in the floor of the middle fossa. The VAs enter through the foramen magnum, located in the posterior fossa. These arteries all emerge into the subarachnoid space on the ventral aspect of the brain.

Siphons of the Four Major Brain Arteries

Although running a fairly straight extracranial course through the neck, all four major arteries display an S-shaped configuration, or "siphon," before reaching the brain. The ICA siphon is in the parasellar region. The VA siphon is at C1 (see Fig. 2-1). The siphons may act to dampen arterial pressure or absorb the force of the pulse bolus.

The subclavian steal syndrome refers to stenosis of the left subclavian artery at its origin, which results in diversion of blood from the brainstem when the individual exercises the left arm, causing brainstem signs including vertigo and syncope (Fig. 2-2).

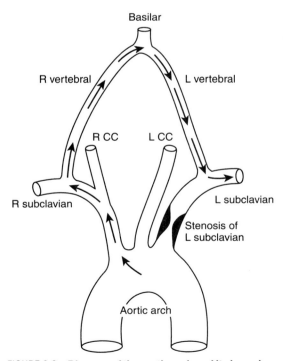

FIGURE 2-2 **Diagram of the aortic arch and its branches.** *Arrows* show how stenosis of the left subclavian artery can "steal" blood from the basilar artery and brainstem. CC, common carotid; L, left; R, right.

Structural Differences in the Walls of Extracranial and Intracranial Arteries

Intracranial arteries lack the vasa vasorum of the larger extracranial arteries. The vasa vasorum stop shortly after the VAs enter the intracranial cavity from their siphons. In a jaundiced patient, the yellowish discoloration of the extracranial vessel walls stops where the vasa vasorum stop, part of the way up the VA.

For the caliber of their lumen, the internal elastic membrane of intracranial arteries is relatively thick, but they have a thinner adventitia and media than extracranial arteries of similar diameter. The media contains fewer muscle fibers. The lack of muscle fibers where the arteries branch may explain the tendency for aneurysms to form at these sites.

Because central nervous system (CNS) arterioles have fewer muscle fibers than systemic arterioles, they consist essentially of endothelial-lined tubes. The endothelial cells form tight junctions. Astrocytic end feet cover the intraparenchymal surfaces of the neuraxial vessels. These anatomic peculiarities constitute the blood-CNS barrier that keeps the CNS a metabolically and, in certain ways, an immunologically privileged site.

Anastomotic Circle of Willis

The large arteries on the ventral surface of the brain form a major anastomotic circle of Willis anteriorly. It consists of the ICAs, the anterior cerebral arteries (ACAs), the anterior communicating artery (AcomA), the posterior communicating arteries (PcomAs), and the proximal segments of the posterior cerebral artery (PCA) at the bifurcation of the basilar artery (BA).

Because these arteries vary considerably in size and symmetry, a "normal" circle occurs only about half of the time.[3,4] The VAs and the ventral spinal arteries (VspAs) form a diamond-shaped minor anastomotic circle caudally (Fig. 2-3).

Because the four major arteries approach the brain ventrally, their branches must run dorsally to reach the brain. They reach the brain either directly by deep perforating

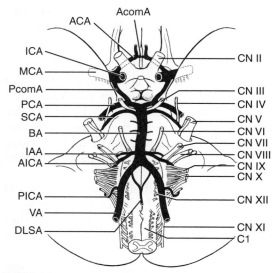

FIGURE 2-3 Diagram of the arterial pattern on the ventral surface of the brain. See Key Terms for abbreviations.

arteries or by encircling its external surface as superficial, short, and long circumferential arteries before penetrating the brain. The BA and VAs and the arteries of the circle of Willis originate as perforators and short and long circumferential arteries.

Groups of Perforating Arteries and Their Origin

Four groups of perforating arteries arise from the circle of Willis (Fig. 2-4). The medial striate arteries (MstrAs = anterior

striate arteries) arise from the ACAs. The lateral striate arteries (LstrAs = lenticulostriate arteries) arise from the MCAs. The thalamo-perforant arteries (TPAs) arise from the proximal part of the PCAs at the BA bifurcation. Hypothalamic perforating arteries (not shown in Fig. 2-4) arise from the arterial ring formed by the circle of Willis around the hypothalamus. A fifth group of perforators, brainstem perforators, arise along the BA and intracranial part of the VAs.

Master Plan for the Distribution of the Arteries from the Ventral Surface of the Brain

The four large arteries that irrigate the brain all approach it from its ventral surface, and from there all arteries must run dorsally to penetrate the brain from its external surface. There are four patterns of distribution of the ventral neuraxial arteries to the brain. Median or paramedian perforating arteries arise from the VAs, the BA, the circle of Willis, and the proximal part of the named long circumferential arteries (Fig. 2-5). Short circumferential arteries end in between paramedian and posterolateral sectors of the brain. Long circumferential arteries encircle the brain surface. Dorsolateral spinal arteries (DLspAs) irrigate the dorsal aspect of the medulla and spinal cord (see Figs. 2-5, 2-37, and 2-38).

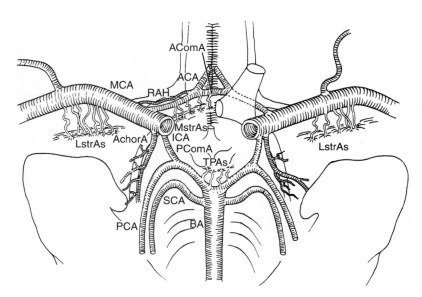

FIGURE 2-4 The circle of Willis and its branches in situ on the basal forebrain. See Key Terms for abbreviations. (From DeMyer W. Neuroanatomy, 2nd ed. Baltimore: Williams & Wilkins, 1998.)

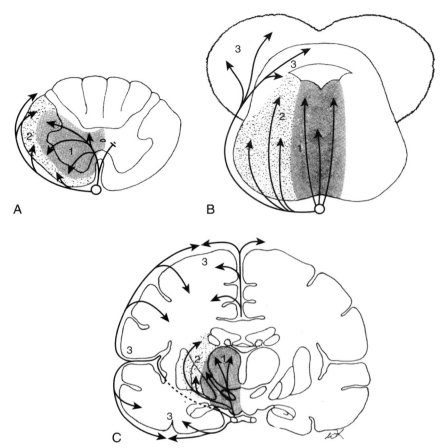

FIGURE 2-5 **A-C,** Transverse sections of spinal cord (**A**), brainstem (**B**), and cerebrum (**C**). Arteries located on the ventral surface of the neuraxis send deep perforating branches to (*1*) a median-paramedian zone, (*2*) an intermediate zone, and (*3*) long superficial branches that encircle the brain. (From DeMyer W. Neuroanatomy, 2nd ed. Baltimore: Williams & Wilkins, 1998.)

Long Circumferential Arteries of the Brain

The carotid system originates four pairs of long circumferential arteries: the ACAs, MCAs, the PCAs, and the anterior choroidal arteries (AchorAs) (Figs. 2-6 and 2-7; see Figs. 2-4 and 2-5). Each artery gives off perforating branches proximally, before encircling the cerebrum to irrigate specific regions (see Figs. 2-5, 2-6, and 2-7).

Similarly, three pairs of long circumferential arteries—the superior cerebellar arteries (SCAs), the anterior inferior cerebellar arteries (AICAs), and the posterior inferior cerebellar arteries (PICAs)—arise from the vertebrobasilar system. While encircling the brainstem, and before reaching the cerebellum, each artery gives off perforating branches proximally (Fig. 2-8; see Figs. 2-3, and 2-37 through 2-40).

The long circumferential arteries of the cerebrum follow the contours of the cerebral

fissures (sylvian, interhemispheric, transverse, and choroid), but do not closely match the sulci. The vessels already have developed and covered the cerebral surface during the lissencephalic stage of the cerebrum, long before cerebral sulcation begins at 16 weeks (see Fig. 2-16).

As they ramify over the brain surface, branches from the ACA, MCA, and PCA penetrate it by sending right-angled short arteries limited to the cortex, short medullary arteries to the subcortical white matter, and long medullary arteries that penetrate the centrum semiovale to the lateral angle of the ventricles (Fig. 2-9).[5-9] Combinations of hemodynamic factors and hypoxia may restrict lesions to one or more of these anatomic distributions or may affect all of them.

At their junctions, the cerebral arteries end in networks of small vessels. Anastomoses occur in many terminal arterial fields, but they are generally insufficient to maintain

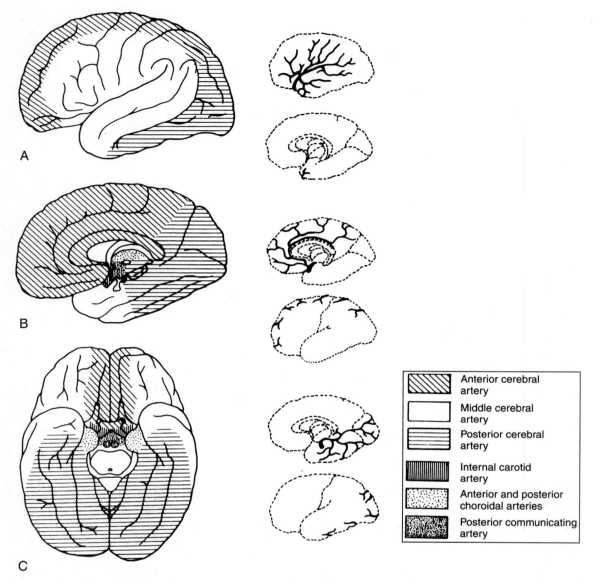

FIGURE 2-6   Surface distribution of the superficial branches of the long circumferential arteries. **A,** Lateral view of the left cerebral hemisphere. **B,** Medial view of the right cerebral hemisphere. **C,** Ventral view of the cerebrum. (From DeMyer W. Neuroanatomy, 2nd ed. Baltimore: Williams & Wilkins, 1998.)

Legend:
- Anterior cerebral artery
- Middle cerebral artery
- Posterior cerebral artery
- Internal carotid artery
- Anterior and posterior choroidal arteries
- Posterior communicating artery

circulation after acute occlusion of the larger trunks. Gradual occlusions may result in enlarged, functioning anastomoses.

Internal Carotid Arteries

Course of Internal Carotid Arteries

After arising from the brachiocephalic and subclavian arteries, the common carotid artery and ICAs course rostrally through the neck. The ICAs enter the carotid canal in the petrous bone at the base of the skull, just anterior to the jugular foramen. They exit from the carotid canal through the foramen lacerum, traverse the cavernous sinus, pierce the dura, and enter the subarachnoid space lateral to the sella turcica. Each ICA produces extradural, interdural, and intradural branches.

Extradural Branches

Extradural branches of the ICA arise in the carotid canal before the ICA enters the cavernous sinus:

- Caroticotympanic artery to the tympanic membrane

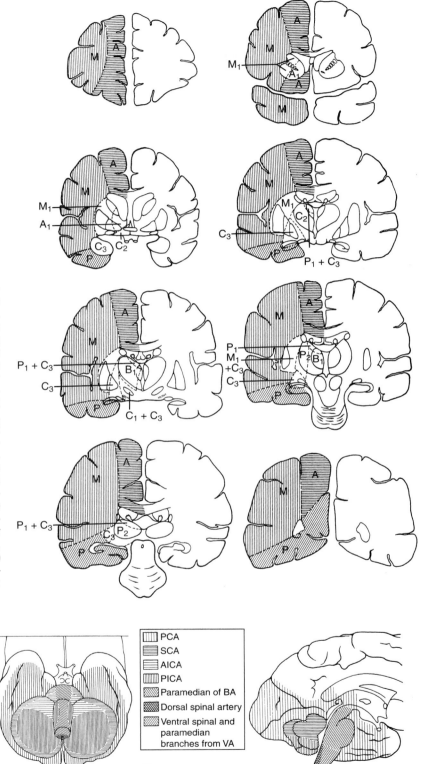

FIGURE 2-7 **Anterior to posterior coronal sections of the cerebrum and diencephalon.** The *shaded areas* show the internal distribution of the long circumferential arteries. The clear areas in the cerebrum show the distribution of their perforating branches. A, anterior cerebral artery; A_1, medial striate arteries from ACA; B_1, paramedian thalamoperforant arteries from PCA; C_1, paramedian perforators from PCA; C_2, TTA perforators from the PcomA; C_3, anterior choroidal artery from ICA; M, middle cerebral artery; M_1, lateral striate perforators from MCA; P, posterior cerebral artery; P_1, posterior choroidal artery from PCA; P_2, thalamogeniculate artery from PCA. (From DeMyer W. Neuroanatomy, 2nd ed. Baltimore: Williams & Wilkins, 1998.)

FIGURE 2-8 **Distribution of brain arteries. A,** Ventral view of the brain showing the surface distribution of arteries of the vertebrobasilar system. **B,** Sagittal section of the brain showing the surface distribution of the posterior cerebral artery and the internal distribution of the vertebrobasilar system arteries. See Key Terms for abbreviations. (From DeMyer W. Neuroanatomy, 2nd ed. Baltimore: Williams & Wilkins, 1998.)

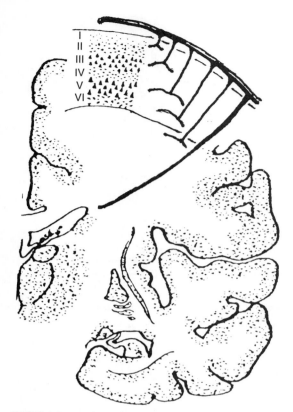

FIGURE 2-9 Pattern of internal branching of the superficial long circumferential arteries of the cerebrum into cortical, subcortical, and medullary arteries. The enlarged section shows the branches to the six layers of the cerebral cortex. A long artery that may extend as deep as the lateral angle of the ventricle is called a medullary artery (comparable to an arteria nutricia that supplies the medulla [marrow] of a long bone).

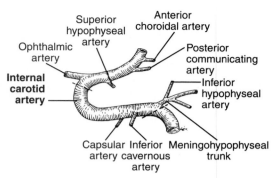

FIGURE 2-10 Lateral view of the left internal carotid artery siphon in the parasellar region. The *dashed line* on the lower right shows where the artery enters the cavernous sinus, and the *dashed line* on the upper left shows where the artery exits into the subarachnoid space.

meningohypophyseal trunk (see Fig. 2-10) are as follows:

- Inferior hypophyseal artery sends branches to the neurohypophysis
- Dorsal meningeal artery (also supplies CN VI as it runs through Dorello canal at the tip of the petrous bone)
- Tentorial artery (also sends minute branches to CNs III and IV)
- Inferior cavernous sinus artery sends branches to CNs III, IV, and VI; the trigeminal ganglion; and branches that anastomose with the middle meningeal arteries

Segments of the ICA are related to its siphon. To facilitate description on frontal and lateral angiograms, Fischer-Brügge[11] numbered the cavernous region of the ICA, MCA, and ACA (Fig. 2-11).

Intradural Branches

The ICA pierces the dural wall of the cavernous sinus to enter the subarachnoid space just lateral to the optic chiasm Now intradural, the ICA originates in sequence:

- OphtA (see Fig. 2-10)—runs forward through the optic foramen to the retina, accompanied by the optic nerve and ophthalmic vein
- Superior hypophyseal artery—supplies the portal system through which blood-borne messengers from the hypothalamus control the release of adenohypophysial hormones

- Pterygoid artery to the pterygoid canal, in company with the vidian (pterygopalatine = sphenopalatine) nerve

Interdural or Intracavernous Branches

Because the cavernous sinus is a cleft between two dural layers, the next arteries arise interdurally (inter = existing within or between) (Fig. 2-10).[10] Cavernous branches of the ICA extend to the surrounding dura, and cranial nerves (CNs) III, IV, V, and VI, all of which run along the cavernous sinus. Branches anastomose with the middle meningeal arteries, with the meningeal rami of the ophthalmic arteries (OphtAs), and openly with each other across the midline. The branches and distribution of the

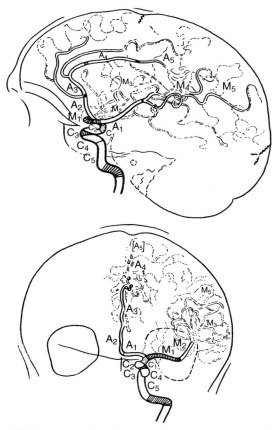

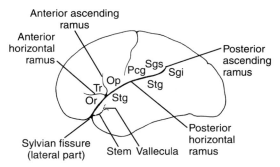

FIGURE 2-12 **Lateral diagram of the left cerebral hemisphere.** Notice the medial origin of the sylvian (lateral) fissure at the vallecula (see Fig. 2-22) and its subdivisions into a stem and rami. Or, Tr, and Op, pars orbitalis, pars triangularis, and pars opercularis of the inferior frontal gyrus; Pcg, postcentral gyrus; Sgs, supramarginal gyrus, superior part; Sgi, supramarginal gyrus, inferior part; Stg superior temporal gyrus. (From DeMyer W. Neuroanatomy, 2nd ed. Baltimore: Williams & Wilkins, 1998.)

Syndromes of Insufficiency or Occlusion of the Internal Carotid Artery

Clinical deficits reflect the distribution of the ophthalmic, diencephalic, or cerebral branches of the carotid arteries. The symptoms and signs include neck pain and headache, ipsilateral amaurosis fugax, contralateral hemiparesis, focal seizures or involuntary movements that imitate seizures, hemianopsia, contralateral numbness and tingling, and aphasia with left hemisphere lesions or left-sided hemineglect with right hemisphere lesions. Symptoms and signs may be intermittent and precipitated by exercise or changes in head position that alter blood flow through the carotid or vertebral arteries.[12,13]

Clues to a carotid lesion are a localized bruit over the affected carotid artery, an ipsilateral peripheral type of Horner syndrome, transitory amaurosis of the ipsilateral eye from OphtA insufficiency, and contralateral motor and sensory signs from involvement of the ipsilateral cerebral hemisphere. Hemispheric infarctions, if large, may cause obtundation or loss of consciousness along with hemiplegia and hemisensory loss. Obtundation of consciousness occurs with about equal frequency in acute ischemic infarcts of either the right or the left hemisphere.[14]

A large hemispheric infarct can cause the telodiencephalic ischemic syndrome of

FIGURE 2-11 Alphabetic-numerical segments of the internal carotid, middle, and anterior cerebral arteries. *Top*, Lateral angiogram. *Bottom*, Frontal angiogram. Notice that A_1, C_1, and M_1 are adjacent. See similar subdivisions of the posterior cerebral artery in Figure 2-19. A_{1-5}, anterior cerebral artery; C_{1-5}, internal carotid artery; M_{1-5}, middle cerebral artery. (Reprinted with permission from Fischer-Brügge E. Die Langeabweichungen der vordern Hirnarterie im Gefässbild. Zentalbl Neurochir 1938;3:300.)

- PcomA (see Fig. 2-4)
- AchorA (see Fig. 2-4)

The ICA terminates by bifurcating into the ACA and MCA in the vallecula, which is the origin of the sylvian fissure. The vallecula is a cistern in the subarachnoid space. The vallecula is roofed by the anterior perforated substance and bounded medially by the optic chiasm and posterolaterally by the uncus (Fig. 2-12; see Figs. 2-4 and 2-22). The first numerical segments of the ICA, MCA, and ACA—C1, M1, and A1—begin at the vallecula (see Fig. 2-12).

Schiffter.[15] The infarct includes the standard MCA territory (see Fig. 12-7), but also extends into the hypothalamus. Interruption of the hypothalamospinal sympathetic tract causes a central type of Horner syndrome and thermoregulatory hemianhidrosis ipsilateral to the lesion, whereas the major signs, such as hemiplegia or hemianesthesia, are contralateral. Horner syndrome in vascular disease may arise from lesions of CNS pathways and peripherally, along the carotid artery system.

Anterior Cerebral Artery

Origin and Distribution

Starting at the vallecula, the A1 segment of ACA runs anteromedially. It then angles sharply upward to enter the interhemispheric fissure and ramify over the flat medial surface of the cerebrum (Figs. 2-13 and 2-14; see Figs. 2-4 and 2-11). Its first branches are deep perforators, the MstrAs (see Fig. 2-4). See Basal Forebrain Arteries. The medial striate arteries: origin, distribution and syndromes of occlusion, for distribution of the deep perforators. Figures 2-13 and 2-14 show the superficial branches of the ACA,[16,17] which consist of the following:

- Medial orbitofrontal artery (reciprocates with the lateral orbitofrontal branch from MCA)
- Frontopolar artery

- Callosomarginal artery and its named branches (see Fig. 2-13B, and see numbers 5-10 in legend for Fig. 2-13)
- Anterior internal frontal artery
- Middle internal frontal artery
- Posterior internal frontal artery
- Paracentral artery (to paracentral lobule of Ecker)
- Superior and inferior parietal arteries
- Pericallosal artery—this artery ends by anastomosing at the splenium of the corpus callosum with splenial branches of PCA (see Figs. 2-13 and 2-20 [#9]).

Functional-Anatomic Regions Irrigated by the Anterior Cerebral Artery

The MstrAs, the deep perforators from the ACA, irrigate the medial part of the basal forebrain and septal region up to the genu of the corpus callosum (see Basal Forebrain Arteries. The medial striate arteries: origin, distribution and syndromes of occlusion and Figs. 2-23 and 24). The above-listed superficial, named branches irrigate the medial part of the orbital surface of the frontal lobe, the frontal pole, the rim of the frontoparietal cortex adjacent to MCA territory, the whole medial aspect of the frontal lobe, and the subjacent white matter (see Figs. 2-6, 2-7, and 2-13).

Medially, the superficial branches of the ACA serve in anterior-posterior order the frontal pole; medial prefrontal cortex

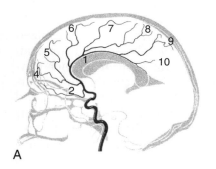

A

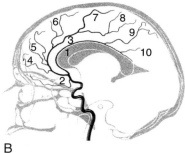

B

FIGURE 2-13 Lateral diagram of angiogram showing two branching patterns of the anterior cerebral artery, superimposed on a sagittal section of the head and corpus callosum. **A,** Note the branches of the pericallosal artery, #1, in the absence of a callosomarginal branch, #3. **B,** Note the branches of the callosomarginal artery, #3. *1,* pericallosal artery; *2,* fronto-orbital artery; *3,* callosomarginal artery; *4,* frontopolar artery; *5,* anterior internal frontal artery; *6,* middle internal frontal artery; *7,* posterior internal frontal artery; *8,* paracentral artery; *9,* superior internal parietal artery; *10,* internal inferior parietal artery. (From Huber P. Krayenbuhl/Yasargil Cerebral Angiography. New York: Georg Thieme Verlag, 1982.)

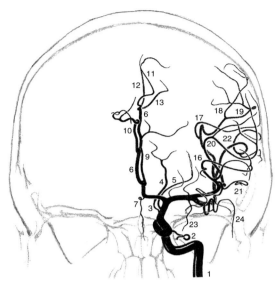

FIGURE 2-14 Frontal angiogram showing the anterior cerebral artery along the midline and the middle cerebral artery laterally. *1,* Internal carotid artery; *2,* ophthalmic artery; *3,* posterior communicating artery; *4,* posterior cerebral artery; *5,* anterior choroid artery; *6,* pericallosal artery; *7,* fronto-orbital artery; *8,* omitted; *9,* frontopolar artery; *10,* anterior internal frontal artery; *11,* middle internal frontal artery; *12,* posterior internal frontal artery; *13,* superior internal parietal artery; *14,* omitted (see Fig. 2-15); *15,* orbitofrontal artery; *16,* prefrontal artery; *17,* prerolandic artery; *18,* anterior parietal artery; *19,* posterior parietal artery; *20,* angular artery; *21,* middle temporal artery; *22,* posterior temporal artery; *23,* temporal polar artery; *24,* anterior temporal artery; *25,* temporo-occipital artery. (From Huber P. Krayenbuhl/Yasargil Cerebral Angiography. New York: Georg Thieme Verlag, 1982.)

superior to the genu of the corpus callosum, which is a micturition center[18-20]; the supplementary motor cortex; and the paracentral lobule of Ecker. The lobule sends pyramidal tract fibers to the lumbosacral region and receives the lumbosacral somatosensory fibers. The ACA irrigates the entire corpus callosum back to the splenium, where the PCA takes over.

Syndromes of Occlusion of the Superficial Branches of the Anterior Cerebral Artery

Mental and Speech Dysfunctions

The patient displays abulia or apathy and loss of frontal lobe executive functions. Severe emotional lability and mood swings are uncommon. Amnesia implies infarction of the deep perforators or bilateral infarcts (see Basal Forebrain Arteries. The medial striate

arteries: origin, distribution and syndromes of occlusion, 3). Left-sided lesions may result in mutism, hypophonia, and transcortical motor aphasia, implicating the supplementary motor cortex. Right-sided lesions may lead to left-sided hemineglect and underuse of the left arm. Interruption of the corpus callosum may cause ideomotor apraxia.[13,16,21]

Motor Dysfunctions

Because the ACA irrigates the paracentral lobule, the classic syndrome of unilateral ACA occlusion is contralateral leg monoplegia, with mild upper extremity involvement, mainly in the shoulder, or leg monoplegia combined with arm ataxia.[16,22] Because of the infrequency of ACA infarction, hemiparesis predominating in the leg actually occurs more often after discrete infarcts of the pyramidal tract in the deep cerebral white matter or brainstem, rather than after ACA infarction.[23] Some patients have a complete faciobrachiocrural hemiplegia, which causes confusion with MCA infarcts.[21] Other motor abnormalities of the arm include a grasp reflex, forced grasping, paratonia, gegenhalten, micrographia, left arm apraxia or the "alien hand,"[24] and motor perseveration with the hand.[16] Damage to the supplementary motor cortex causes some of the foregoing motor deficits of the hand including underuse and lack of spontaneous movements.[16,25] Urinary incontinence may occur after bilateral lesions or large unilateral ACA infarctions.[18,20,26]

Sensory Dysfunctions

The patient loses superficial and deep sensation, generally paralleling the distribution of the motor involvement.[26]

Bilateral Anterior Cerebral Artery Occlusion

Bilateral ACA occlusion results in impaired consciousness; sometimes akinetic mutism; paraplegia; incontinence; and severe frontal lobe signs of abulia, indifference to stimuli, and loss of executive functions.[16] A patient with an azygous ACA had gait apraxia from bilateral infarction of the supplementary motor area.[27]

Middle Cerebral Artery

Origin and Distribution

The M1 segment of the MCA begins at the vallecula. After the ICA gives off the PcomA and AchorA, it splits into the MCA and ACA (Fig. 2-15; see Figs. 2-4, 2-11, 2-12, and 2-14). The M1 (sphenoidal) segment runs directly laterally through the stem of the sylvian fissure where it first gives off its deep perforators, the LstrAs (see Figs. 2-3, 2-4, 2-14, 2-25, and 2-26). While in the stem of the sylvian fissure and approaching the limen insulae, the MCA bifurcates in 78% of individuals, trifurcates in 12%, and divides into multiple trunks in 10%.[28]

The first superficial branch of the MCA, the temporopolar artery (#23 in Figs. 2-14 and 2-15), arises opposite the LstrAs or slightly more distally. Other early branches distal to the LstrAs are the lateral orbitofrontal artery and anterior/middle temporal arteries (#15, #21, and #24 in Fig. 2-15).

At the limen insulae, the major trunks of the MCA curve sharply backward and upward over the insula, forming a genu that marks the transition between M1 and M2. The M2 (insular) segment continues backward on the insula and in the plane of the posterior horizontal ramus of the sylvian fissure (see Fig. 2-11). M2 irrigates the insula and gives off the M3 branches that ultimately reach the cortical convexity.

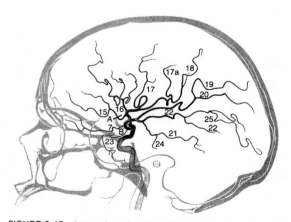

FIGURE 2-15   Lateral angiogram showing the branches of the middle cerebral artery. **A**, Upper trunk of the middle cerebral artery. **B**, Lower trunk of the middle cerebral artery. See legend for Figure 2-14 for explanation of numbers. (From Huber P. Krayenbuhl/Yasargil Cerebral Angiography. New York: Georg Thieme Verlag, 1982.)

Figure 2-16 shows how frontoparietal and temporal opercula cover the insula during development, burying the MCA in the sylvian fissure. The M3 (opercular) segment begins at the circular sulcus that bounds the insula and marks the transition from M2 to M3. The M3 segments loop downward on the medial surface of the frontoparietal operculum and irrigate their inner side and then exit from the sylvian fissure. The buried M3 and M4 arteries loop under the lips of the frontoparietal operculum or over the temporal operculum to escape from the hidden insular surface onto the exposed lateral surface of the cerebrum where they become the M5 segments (see Fig. 2-11).[28-30]

Sylvian Triangle and the Insula

A line tangential to the upper, frontoparietal loops of the MCA delimits the upper side of the sylvian triangle (Fig. 2-17A). A line drawn along the main MCA trunk in the posterior horizontal ramus of the sylvian fissure delimits the lower side of the sylvian triangle. A line from the anterior aspect of the MCA to the most anterior branch of the prefrontal artery delimits the anterior side (see arrow in Fig. 2-17B).

The most posterior and medial of the upper lying loops as seen on frontal and horizontal angiograms is at the apex of the sylvian triangle; this is called the sylvian point (Fig. 2-18 [see arrows]). The angular branch of the MCA emerges at the sylvian point at the posterior end of the posterior horizontal ramus of the sylvian fissure (M5; see Fig. 2-11). The angular branch of the MCA then runs posteriorly and crosses the supramarginal and angular gyri on the lateral, exposed surface of the cerebrum (see Fig. 2-15). The MCA forms a junction with the PCA in front of the occipital pole (see Fig. 2-6A). The posterior horizontal ramus of the sylvian fissure and the MCA branches it contains are more vertical in the immature cerebrum of fetuses and infants and are bowed upward, as if the temporal lobe were swollen.

Sequential Branches of the Middle Cerebral Artery

The sequential branches of the MCA (see Figs. 2-14 and 2-15) are as follows.

FIGURE 2-16   **A,** Lateral view of the right cerebral hemisphere in a fetus before growth of the opercula to cover the insula. **B** and **C,** Coronal sections at the level of the *dashed line* in **A,** showing two stages in opercularization. The middle cerebral arteries become enfolded as opercula grow over the insula. The arteries then form loops around the lips of the opercula. (From DeMyer W. Neuroanatomy, 2nd ed. Baltimore: Williams & Wilkins, 1998.)

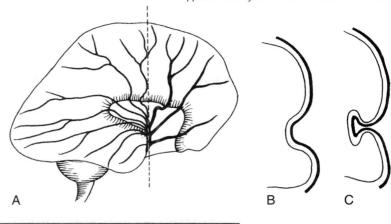

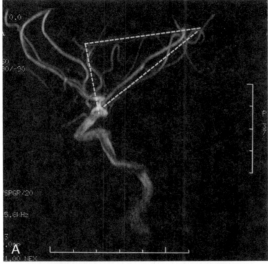

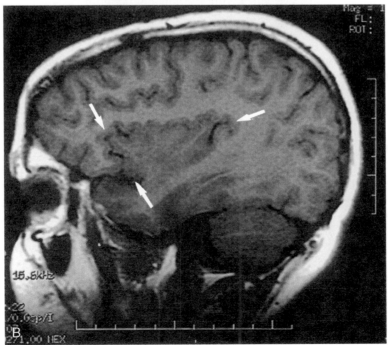

FIGURE 2-17   **Sylvian triangle. A,** Lateral view of magnetic resonance angiogram. The *dashed lines* demarcate the sylvian triangle. See text for description. **B,** Parasagittal T1-weighted magnetic resonance image of the cerebrum. Notice the correspondence of the angiographic sylvian triangle to the extent of the insular cortex (*arrows*).

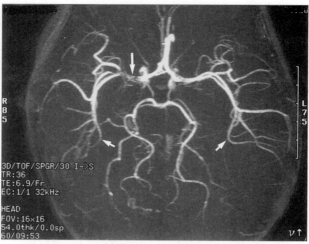

FIGURE 2-18   Horizontal view of magnetic resonance angiogram showing the sylvian point (*posterior arrows*). This point corresponds to the last loop formed by the posteriormost artery to exit from the insular region at the apex of the sylvian triangle. It continues on the surface as the angular branch of the middle cerebral artery. The stem of the right middle cerebral artery is occluded (*anterior arrow*).

Main Stem

- LstrAs (see Fig. 2-4, see Basal Forebrain Arteries. The lateral striate (lenticulostriate) arteries: origin, distribution and syndromes of occlusion and Figs. 2-25 and 26)
- The temporopolar artery (may arise opposite the LstrAs, Figure 2-14).

Upper Trunk

- Lateral frontobasilar or orbitofrontal artery
- Prefrontal artery (candelabra, operculofrontal) artery
- Precentral artery (prerolandic artery)
- Central artery (rolandic artery)[31]

Either Trunk of the Middle Cerebral Artery

- Anterior parietal artery
- Posterior parietal artery
- Angular artery

Lower Trunk

- Temporopolar artery
- Anterior temporal artery
- Middle temporal artery
- Posterior temporal artery
- Temporo-occipital artery

Functional-Anatomic Regions Irrigated by the Middle Cerebral Arteries

The deep perforators of the MCA, the LstrAs, irrigate the basal forebrain, corpus striatum, and internal capsule (see Basal Forebrain Arteries. The lateral striate (lenticulostriate) arteries: origin, distribution and syndromes of occlusion and see Basal Forebrain Arteries. The lateral striate (lenticulostriate) arteries: origin, distribution and syndromes of occlusion and; Summary of the distribution of the arteries of the basal forebrain and deep gray matter). The superficial branches of the MCA irrigate the lateral part of the orbitofrontal region, the temporal pole, the superior and middle temporal gyri, the insula, and the lateral convexity of the frontoparieto-occipital region (see Figs. 2-6, 2-7, and 2-8).[9,29]

The branches of the superior trunk of the MCA irrigate in anterior-posterior sequence the prefrontal cortex; area 8 (the frontal eye fields); areas 44 and 45 (Broca's area); area 6 (the premotor cortex); area 4 (the motor cortex of the precentral gyrus); areas 3, 1, and 2 (the somatosensory cortex of the parietal lobe); the vestibular receptive area in the inferior-anterior parietal lobule; much of the lateral aspect of the parietal lobe; the adjacent temporal cortex; and the supramarginal and angular gyri (see Figs. 2-6, 2-7, and 2-8). The branches of the inferior trunk of the

MCA irrigate the superior and middle temporal gyri of the temporal lobe, including the primary auditory receptive cortex in the transverse temporal gyri and on the left the surrounding auditory word association cortex and planum temporale.

Posteriorly, the MCA forms a junction with the PCA on the lateral aspect of the occipital lobe (see Figs. 2-6, 2-7, and 2-8) to irrigate the visual word association area. Deep, medullary branches of the superficial arteries of the MCA extend through the centrum semiovale to the lateral angle of the lateral ventricle (see Fig. 2-9) and geniculocalcarine tract, but do not reach the corpus striatum and internal capsule per se, which are irrigated by deep perforators of the basal forebrain (see The basal forebrain arteries: Origin, distribution and syndromes of occlusion).

Syndromes of Occlusion of the Superficial Middle Cerebral Artery Branches Distal to the Lateral Striate Arteries

Some deficits are common to a lesion of the MCA territory of either hemisphere, and some characterize right or left hemisphere lesions. Common to lesions of either hemisphere are contralateral hemiplegia and hemisensory deficits, dysarthria, and dysphagia.[32]

Mental Dysfunctions

Impaired consciousness of some degree affects 73% of patients with acute ischemic stroke and occurs equally with right or left hemisphere lesions.[14] Enduring amnesia and dementia is unusual, but poststroke depression is common.[33]

Motor and Speech Dysfunctions

Although faciobrachiocrural hemiplegia is usual, the topographic representation of the body parts in the paracentral region, centrum semiovale, and internal capsule allows restricted forms of upper motoneuron (UMN) paralysis or sensory loss limited to the face, arm, or leg.[34] Infarction limited to the "knob" of the precentral gyrus causes paralysis only of the contralateral fingers that may suggest a lower motoneuron (LMN) or median nerve

palsy rather than an UMN lesion,[35-37] or it may cause ataxia[38] or dysarthria.[39] Similarly, small lesions of the postcentral cortex can cause restricted sensory findings in proximal or distal distributions,[40] as can lateral medullary infarction.[41]

Infarction limited to area 6, the premotor cortex, causes a unique syndrome characterized by paresis of abduction and elevation of the arm and paresis of all hip movements, sparing the distal muscles of the limbs. Limb-kinetic apraxia occurs during tasks that require coordination between the arms and legs.[42]

Centrum semiovale or capsular lesions may cause pure motor or pure sensory symptoms. The medullary penetrating arteries of the superficial branches of the MCA irrigate most of the centrum semiovale (see Figs. 2-7, 2-8, and 2-9). The motor deficits may include ataxic hemiplegia, relatively pure dysarthria,[39] or dysarthria–clumsy hand syndrome.[43] Infarcts of the basis pontis may cause similar signs (see The vertebrobasilar arteries: origin, distribution, and syndromes of occlusion. The pons: syndromes of basilar artery occlusion).

In the acute phase of right-sided or left-sided MCA infarcts, the head and eyes deviate to the side of the lesion. Normally, each hemisphere produces a vector that tends to turn the eyes and head contralaterally. The vectors balance out, and the eyes and head tend to remain centered. The lesion abolishes the head and eye–centering vector from one hemisphere, allowing the opposite vector to predominate, turning the head to the side of the lesion, contralateral to the intact hemisphere.[32]

Left-sided MCA occlusions regularly cause aphasia and ideomotor apraxia. Anterior infarcts in Broca's area in the posterior inferior frontal region cause expressive (nonfluent) aphasia, whereas infarcts that are more posterior, in the posterior parasylvian area, cause receptive aphasia and may not be accompanied by hemiplegia. Infarcts in the angular gyrus region tend to cause Gerstmann syndrome of right-left disorientation, finger agnosia, dyscalculia, and dysgraphia.[44] Infarcts in the posterior distribution of the MCA, at its junction with the PCA, cause dyslexia.

Sensory Dysfunctions

Contralateral loss of superficial and deep sensation is usual after infarction of the postcentral gyrus or pathways to it. Right-sided infarctions regularly cause neglect of the left side, along with left hemiplegia, constructional apraxia for the left half of figures, and lack of awareness of the neurologic deficits (anosognosia).[9] Extension of the lesion into the geniculocalcarine tract as it sweeps around the temporal horn and trigone of the lateral ventricle causes contralateral visual field defects that are usually congruent.

The Foix-Chavany-Marie syndrome (anterior operculum syndrome = perisylvian syndrome) is caused by bilateral infarction of the opercula and insula, causing a faciopharyngolaryngoglossomasticatory supranuclear palsy. The lesion destroys the cortex located in the frontal operculum of the posterior inferior frontal gyrus that contains the supranuclear neurons for the bulbar muscles. The patient drools constantly, but cannot suck or swallow, leading to aspiration pneumonia. Palatal paralysis and restricted tongue and laryngeal movements preclude speech. The facial diplegia extends to the orbicularis oculi and imitates a peripheral seventh nerve palsy. The jaw jerk is brisk. Despite paresis of volitional movements, emotional or automatic movements of the bulbar muscles are preserved (e.g., the patient can blink automatically, but cannot close the eyes voluntarily, or may yawn automatically but cannot open the jaw voluntarily). An operculum syndrome may follow CNS infections and status epilepticus. Absence of pathologic laughter and crying in Foix-Chavany-Marie syndrome, a cortical type of supranuclear palsy, differs from the pseudobulbar palsy caused by lesions that interrupt the pyramidal tract in the deep white matter or brainstem, from which the patient has pseudobulbar effect, with pathologic laughing and crying.[45-47] Selective unilateral infarction of the right insular cortex causes a neglect syndrome,[48] but on the left, impairment of verbal memory.[49]

Worster-Drought syndrome is a congenital suprabulbar palsy, but with minimal motor deficits of the extremities.[50-52] The clinical features duplicate features of acquired Foix-Chavany-Marie syndrome. The child has behavioral and cognitive dysfunctions and may have seizures. The causes of Worster-Drought syndrome include prenatal brain hypoxia or ischemia or perisylvian pachygyria (the Oekonomakis malformation). (This Worster-Drought syndrome in children is distinct from the adult Worster-Drought syndrome of familial presenile dementia and spastic paraplegia, related to amyloid deposition.)

Posterior Cerebral Artery

Origin of the Posterior Cerebral Artery, the Basilar Communicating Artery, and the True Junction of the Carotid and Vertebrobasilar Arterial Systems

In most adult brains, the PCAs look like terminal bifurcations of the BA (see Fig. 2-4), but embryologically they arise from the carotid system as an extension of the PcomAs. Initially, the bifurcations consist of tiny anastomoses that connect the BA with the PcomAs, completing the circle of Willis. These tiny anastomoses usually enlarge to form the P1 segments of the PCAs and usually become their main source of blood. Percheron (1982) named the P1 segments the basilar communicating arteries (BcomAs) (Fig. 2-19). In about 20% of normal adult angiograms, the PCA still fills after carotid injection (fetal pattern), not from the vertebrobasilar route.

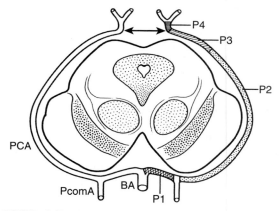

FIGURE 2-19 Cross section of the rostral midbrain showing the segments, P1-P4, of the posterior cerebral artery. The P1 segment = the basilar communicating artery of Percheron.[113] Figure 2-11 shows similar segments of the anterior and middle cerebral arteries.

Sympathetic nerve fibers innervate the PCA by traveling along the carotid plexus and the PcomA.[53] The sympathetic fibers of the vertebrobasilar plexus stop where the BcomA anastomoses with the PcomA and PCA. The site of this anastomosis between the BcomA and the PcomA marks the true junction of the carotid and vertebrobasilar systems. Further anastomoses between the anterior and posterior circulations are provided by the splenial branch of the PCA with the pericallosal branch of the ACA and of the AchorAs with the PchorAs.

Distribution of the Superficial Branches of the Posterior Cerebral Artery

The PCA sends branches to the choroid plexus of the third and lateral ventricles, deep perforators or circumflex arteries to the midbrain and thalamus, and superficial branches distally to the medial and inferior temporo-parieto-occipital region. See The thalamic arteries: Origin, distribution, and syndromes of occlusion. The thalamogeniculate artery: origin, distribution and syndromes of occlusion—Lateral posterior choroidal artery, E-I describes the deep, proximal branches of the PCA. The superficial cerebral branches that arise distally from the P2 and P3 segments of the PCA are as follows (Fig. 2-20):[54]

- Posterior pericallosal artery (courses around the splenium)

- Anterior temporal artery
- Posterior temporal artery (= occipito-temporal artery[32])
- Parieto-occipital artery
- Calcarine artery

To reach the cerebral surface, the PCA crosses the free edge of the tentorium. Transtentorial herniation of the parahippo-campal gyrus may stretch the PCA across the firm tentorial edge, resulting in infarction of the medial temporo-occipital region, including the calcarine cortex (Fig. 2-21).

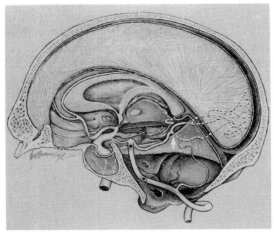

FIGURE 2-21   Sagittal diagram of the head showing the posterior cerebral artery crossing the free edge of the tentorium (*arrow*), where it is subject to compression in transtentorial herniation of the cerebrum. (Reprinted with permission from Ecker A. The Normal Cerebral Angiogram. Springfield, IL, Charles C Thomas, 1951.)

FIGURE 2-20 **Branches of the posterior cerebral artery. A,** Lateral view. **B,** Inferior view. *1,* internal carotid artery; *2,* posterior communicating artery; *3,* basilar artery; *4,* anterior thalamoperforant artery; *5,* posterior thalamoperforant artery; *6,* posterior cerebral artery; *7,* medial posterior choroidal artery; *8,* lateral posterior choroidal artery; *9,* posterior pericallosal artery; *10,* parieto-occipital artery; *11,* calcarine artery; *12,* posterior temporal artery; *13,* anterior temporal artery. (From Huber P. Krayenbuhl/Yasargil Cerebral Angiography. New York: Georg Thieme Verlag, 1982.)

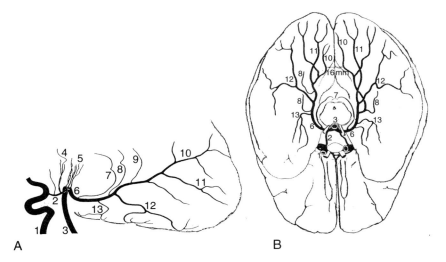

Syndromes of Occlusion of the Superficial Branches of the Posterior Cerebral Artery

Mental Dysfunctions

Unilateral infarction of the PCA territory in the ventromedial part of the temporal lobe, which includes the hippocampal formation, may cause transitory amnesia, whereas bilateral infarction causes enduring amnesia.

Motor Dysfunction

Hemiplegia is not present unless proximal PCA occlusion causes infarction of the pyramidal tract in the PCA distribution in the midbrain basis, when it can imitate MCA occlusion.[55] Hemisensory loss owing to PCA occlusion indicates extension to the territory of the thalamogeniculate or lateral posterior choroidal arteries (see The thalamic arteries: Origin, distribution, and syndromes of occlusion. The thalamogeniculate artery: origin, distribution and syndromes of occlusion and Lateral Posterior Choroidal Artery).[56]

Sensory Dysfunctions

Contralateral homonymous visual field defects are characteristic of PCA infarction. When an infarct destroys all but the posterior end of the primary visual cortex along the calcarine fissure, macular vision is preserved. If it destroys all but the anteriormost end of the visual cortex, the only vision left is a preserved temporal crescent.[57]

Contralateral superior quadrantanopia is caused by infarction of the inferior fibers of the geniculocalcarine tract or inferior bank of the calcarine fissure. Contralateral inferior quadrantanopia is caused by infarction of the superior part of the geniculocalcarine tract.

Bilateral lesions limited to either the upper or the lower banks of the calcarine fissure may cause corresponding superior or inferior altitudinal visual field defects. The patient may experience various formed and unformed visual hallucinations, color agnosias, and anomias.[58] The patient may have dyslexia with or without dysgraphia with restricted lesions of the lateral aspect of the occipital lobe.

Prosopagnosia

With prosopagnosia, the patient fails to identify the face of a person by sight, but identifies the person by voice if the person speaks.[59] The lesion usually involves the medial inferior temporo-occipital region bilaterally in the posterior temporal artery region (the posterior lingual gyrus and its transition to the occipital lobe). Unilateral lesions of this site, usually on the right, also may cause prosopagnosia. Right hemisphere lesions also impair the recognition of facial affect, such as smiling and sadness, more than left hemisphere lesions.

Anton Syndrome of Anosognosia for Cortical Blindness

After bioccipital lesions of area 17 that cause cortical blindness, the patient may deny loss of vision. The patient may confabulate vision or offer plausible rationalizations, such as "It's too dim in here to see." Acute unilateral occipital lobe infarction may cause temporary complete cortical blindness until the accompanying diaschisis of the intact occipital lobe resolves.

Balint Syndrome

Balint syndrome follows bilateral parieto-occipital lesions, at the junction zone of the MCA and PCA.[60,61] The patient fails to attend to the periphery of the visual fields and cannot voluntarily direct the eyes to a peripheral target or to scan the peripheral fields; this form of optic apraxia is called psychic paralysis of fixation. Although unable to attend to the periphery of a visual field, the patient attends to nonvisual stimuli from the side.

The patient fails to touch or grasp precisely an object seen—a failure of visual guidance of movements called optic ataxia. The patient also may fail to synthesize the parts of the visual scene into a coherent whole, or to recognize more than one visual object at a time (simultanagnosia), although he or she recognizes individual objects in the field. Elements of Anton syndrome and Balint syndrome may coexist.

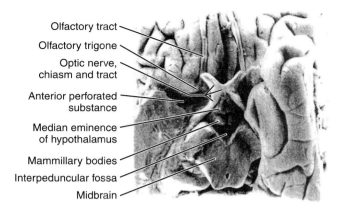

Olfactory tract
Olfactory trigone
Optic nerve, chiasm and tract
Anterior perforated substance
Median eminence of hypothalamus
Mammillary bodies
Interpeduncular fossa
Midbrain

FIGURE 2-22 Photograph of the basal forebrain, a block of tissue based on the anterior perforated substance, optic chiasm, and hypothalamus. See text for description of the three-dimensional boundaries of the block.

Basal Forebrain Arteries

Definition of the Basal Forebrain

As seen on the ventral surface of the brain, the basal forebrain centers on the optic chiasm. The subarachnoid space, which admits a fingertip just lateral to the X of the chiasm, is the vallecula. It continues laterally as the stem of the sylvian fissure (see Fig. 2-8). The adjacent structures include the base of the olfactory tract and the olfactory trigone, the anterior perforated substance, the diagonal band of Broca, the uncus, the median eminence, and the mammillary bodies (Fig. 2-22).

These structures underlie a block of tissue that extends in the anteroposterior plane from the lateral part of the anterior perforated substance to the diencephalic-mesencephalic junction; in the lateral plane from external capsule to external capsule; and in the vertical plane up to the superolateral angle of the lateral ventricle. This overlying block includes the lamina terminals and the septal region up to the genu of the corpus callosum, the anterior pillars of the fornix and anterior commissure, the corpus striatum, the internal capsule, and the entire diencephalon. This block of tissue is the recipient of all three groups of perforating arteries—medial, lateral, and posterior or TPAs.

Origin and Anatomic Features of Perforating Arteries of the Basal Forebrain

Perforators for the basal forebrain branch from all of the arteries of the circle of Willis—ICA, ACA, AcomA, PcomA, and BcomA (P1 segment

of PCA). Some also arise from the AchorA (see Figs. 2-4 and 2-28B).

The perforators consist of leashes of several tiny vessels (see Fig. 2-3 and 2-4). The three forebrain leashes are the MstrAs, LstrAs, and the posterior group, the TPAs (see Fig. 2-4). The whole leash of vessels is named as if it were a single vessel (e.g., the thalamotuberal artery [TTA]). A few leashes that arise from a single branch of the circle of Willis receive a special name (e.g., the recurrent artery of Heubner [RAH] of the medial striate group) (see Fig. 2-4).

The individual perforating vessels arise at right angles to the axis of the parent vessels and after crossing the subarachnoid space perforate the brain at right angles to its surface. After piercing the basal forebrain, the perforators generally take an undulating or curving course.

Within the brain, the leashes irrigate exclusive territories and show little effective anastomotic interchange at their junctions. On radiographs or at autopsy, characteristic patterns of infarction identify the responsible vessels. The distribution of infarcts in children matches that of adults.[62,63] The adjacent groups of perforating leashes show reciprocity in the size of their irrigation territories. Enlargement of the territory of one leash means reciprocal reduction in the territory of the adjacent leash.

All of the vessels of a leash may be occluded or only individual branches. An infarct less than 1.5 cm in diameter is defined as a lacune. A lacune can be restricted to any part of the internal capsule or adjacent gray matter. A small or isolated lacune may be clinically silent, unless it involves a discrete nucleus or sensory or motor pathway, such as the pyramidal tract. If multiple, lacunes can cause serious neurologic and mental deficits. Larger infarcts in the territory of the deep perforators of the forebrain tend to cause syndromes similar to ipsilateral cortical lesions—dysarthria and aphasia with deep left-sided infarcts[64] and deficits of attention and spatial orientation with deep right-sided infarcts.[65]

Perforating arteries, particularly the LstrAs, tend to rupture in hypertensive patients. Challa and colleagues[66] showed that the so-called Charcot-Bouchard aneurysms of these vessels actually consist of tiny vascular coils. The hemorrhage occurs along the intra-axial course of the perforator,[67] and may or may not dissect into the ventricles.

Medial Striate Arteries

Subdivision of the Medial Striate Arteries

The MstrAs arise all along the A1 segment, the proximal most part of the A2 segment of the ACAs, and the AcomA. They penetrate the forebrain through the anterior perforated substance, the septal region, and the suprachiasmatic region of the hypothalamus (see Fig. 2-4).[68-71]

Differences in the distribution of the MstrAs allow at least two syndromes of occlusion: one from infarction in the median-paramedian MstrAs, which consist of hypothalamic perforators and the subcallosal artery arising from the AcomA. The second syndrome comes from infarction in the distribution of the RAH, which serves a zone lateral to the median-paramedian arteries. Although perforators arise from the proximal part of A1, near its carotid origin,[71,72] no specific clinical syndrome is recognized after their occlusion.

Origin and Distribution of the Median-Paramedian Group of Medial Striate Arteries

Figure 2-23 shows the territory of the median-paramedian group of MstrAs (the hypothalamic and subcallosal arteries) that arise from the AcomA.[69,73-76] The territory consists of the following:

- Medial part of the anterior perforated substance, septal end of the diagonal band of Broca, and the optic chiasm
- Anterior hypothalamus and medial forebrain bundle
- Lamina terminalis and the midline fibers of the anterior commissure, stria terminalis, and interbulbar connections between the olfactory bulbs
- Parolfactory gyrus, and septal region up to the inferior half of the genu of the corpus callosum—the territory may extend to the anterior cingulate gyrus[69]
- Anterior pillars of the fornix and anterior part of the septum pellucidum

A subcallosal artery that irrigates the inferior half of the genu (see Fig. 2-23) exists in about 50% of brains. If this median artery

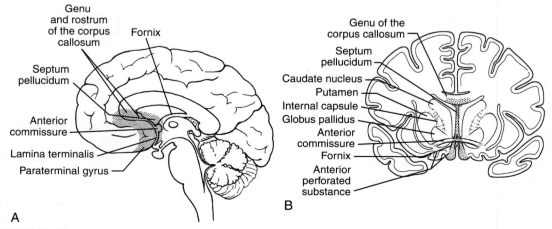

FIGURE 2-23 The *shaded area* shows the distribution of the median-paramedian group of medial striate (medial perforating) arteries that arise from the AcomA. Compare with the distribution of the lateral group of medial striate arteries (recurrent artery of Heubner) in Figure 2-24. **A,** Sagittal section of the cerebrum. **B,** Coronal section of the cerebrum.

extends around the genu to the body (or even splenium), as it does in 30%, it is called the median callosal artery.[76]

Clinical Syndrome of Occlusion of the Median-Paramedian Group of Medial Striate Arteries

The patient experiences the sudden onset of anterograde amnesia that may be accompanied by confabulation.[73-75] Infarction in the territory of these MstrAs apparently causes the amnesia related to aneurysms of the AcomA.[77] No dementia, hemiparesis, aphasia, or other hard neurologic signs are present.[75,77,78]

Sites other than the basal forebrain at which discrete infarctions or other lesions may cause relatively pure amnesia include the medial quadrant of the temporal lobes, nucleus medialis dorsalis of the thalamus, fornices, mammillary bodies, and retrosplenial cortex.[77,79] The role of lesions of the nucleus accumbens in amnesia is controversial.[79]

Origin and Distribution of the Recurrent Artery of Heubner (Artery Centralis Media)

The RAH arises in close relation to the AcomA. It arises from the A2 segment of the ACA just distal to the AcomA, at the level of the AcomA, or, less frequently (in 8% to 14% of hemispheres), just proximal to the AcomA.[68-70,80,81] At about 0.8 mm in diameter, the MstrA stem is larger than most other MstrAs. Although the RAH arises medially, it runs laterally and conveys blood laterally (recurrently) (see Fig. 2-4). The RAH irrigates the zone just lateral to the zone of the paramedian MstrA, as follows (Fig. 2-24):

- Anterior perforated substance, inferomedial third of the head of the caudate nucleus, and anteroinferior third of the putamen, essentially the caudate-putamen bridge formed by the nucleus accumbens[80,82]
- Inferior part of the anterior limb of the internal capsule, interposed between the caudate and putamen—RAH branches may extend back as far as the genu of the internal capsule and sometimes into the adjacent anteromedial edge of the globus pallidus

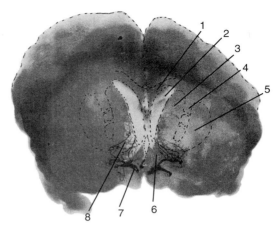

FIGURE 2-24 Radiograph of coronal slice of the cerebrum after injection of the recurrent artery of Heubner, showing its distribution to the inferomedial part of the corpus striatum (nucleus accumbens septi) and anterior limb of the internal capsule. The recurrent artery of Heubner does not extend medially into the median-paramedian zone served by branches from the AcomA. Compare with Figures 2-4 and 2-23B. *1,* corpus callosum; *2,* lateral ventricle; *3,* head of caudate nucleus; *4,* internal capsule; *5,* putamen; *6,* septal area; *7,* anterior cerebral artery; *8,* rami of the recurrent artery of Heubner. (Reprinted with permission from Kaplan H, Ford D. The Brain Vascular System. New York: Elsevier, 1966.)

Although the RAH arises medially, it courses laterally (recurrently) to irrigate the territory of the basal forebrain lateral to the median-paramedian MstrAs. The clinical syndromes of infarction of the two regions differ. See the distributions in Figures 2-23, 2-24, and 2-27.

Clinical Syndrome of Recurrent Artery of Heubner Occlusion

Mild faciobrachial monoplegia without sensory disturbance occurs. The patient may have transitory, mild contralateral hemiparesis, but with faciobrachial predilection. A combination of occlusion in the RAH distribution and in the superficial branches of ACA to the paracentral region causes a faciobrachiocrural hemiplegia.[82]

Apathy and decreased drive are present, presumably resulting from infarction of the nucleus accumbens (the limbic striatum), but no coma. Transitory amnesia occurs. If small, the infarct may be clinically silent, without causing strokelike signs, but it appears on radiographs.

Lateral Striate (Lenticulostriate) Arteries

Origin

The LstrAs arise from the M1 segment of the MCA in 85% of individuals (see Fig. 2-4) and from secondary trunks in the stem of the sylvian fissure in the remaining 15%. They arise as a medial group of smaller, shorter perforators and a larger, longer group of lateral perforators (Figs. 2-25 and 2-26).[83,84]

Distribution

LstrAs enter the cerebrum through the lateral two thirds of the anterior perforated substance[85,86] and distribute to the following:

- Anterior perforated substance
- Lateral thirds of the anterior commissure
- Lateral part of the globus pallidus. The medial group of LstrAs supplies the lateral pallidum and some of the adjacent

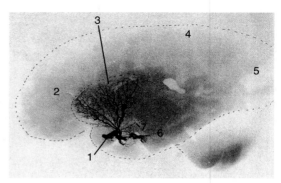

FIGURE 2-26   Lateral radiograph of a sagittal slice of the cerebrum after injection of the lateral striate branches of the middle cerebral artery. The branches spare the thalamus and hypothalamus. *1,* middle cerebral artery; *2,* frontal lobe; *3,* rami to striatum; *4,* parietal lobe; *5,* occipital lobe; *6,* temporal lobe; *7,* caudate nucleus, tail. (Reprinted with permission from Kaplan H, Ford D. The Brain Vascular System. New York: Elsevier, 1966.)

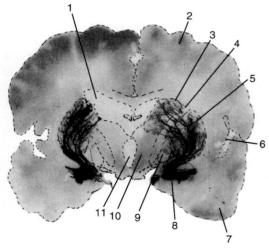

FIGURE 2-25   Radiograph of coronal slice of the cerebrum after injection of the lateral striate (lenticulostriate) branches of the middle cerebral artery. The arteries arch around and spare the medial structures, the medial part of the pallidum, the lower part of the internal capsule, and the thalamus. *1,* lateral ventricle; *2,* frontal lobe; *3,* body of caudate nucleus; *4,* internal capsule; *5,* putamen and lateral pallidum; *6,* insula; *7,* middle cerebral artery; *8,* pallidum, medial part; *9,* thalamus; *10,* third ventricle; *11,* temporal lobe. (Reprinted with permission from Kaplan H, Ford D. The Brain Vascular System. New York: Elsevier, 1966.)

putamen. The AchorA or RAH irrigates the medial pallidum.

- Superolateral two thirds of the head and all of the body of the caudate nucleus and most of the putamen out to and including the external capsule.[86] The RAH irrigates the inferomedial third of the head of the caudate and putamen (the nucleus accumbens) and intervening inferior part of the anterior limb of the internal capsule, back to the genu (Figs. 2-27 and 2-28; see Fig. 2-24).
- Superior part of entire anterior limb and superior part of the posterior limb of the internal capsule (see Figs. 2-25 and 2-26)
- Periventricular white matter (corona radiata) at the angle of the lateral ventricle (see Fig. 2-25). This is a junction site for the LstrAs (see Fig. 2-25), the long medullary arteries (see Fig. 2-9), and the AchorA (see Figs. 2-27 and 2-28B)

Comparison of Medial Striate Artery and Lenticulostriate Artery Territories

The MstrAs, RAH, and the LstrAs fan out into the basal forebrain from their bases on their parent arteries, as do perforators from the AchorA (see Figs. 2-24, 2-25, and 2-26). The LstrA branches run superiorly, arching around and over the territory of the RAH,

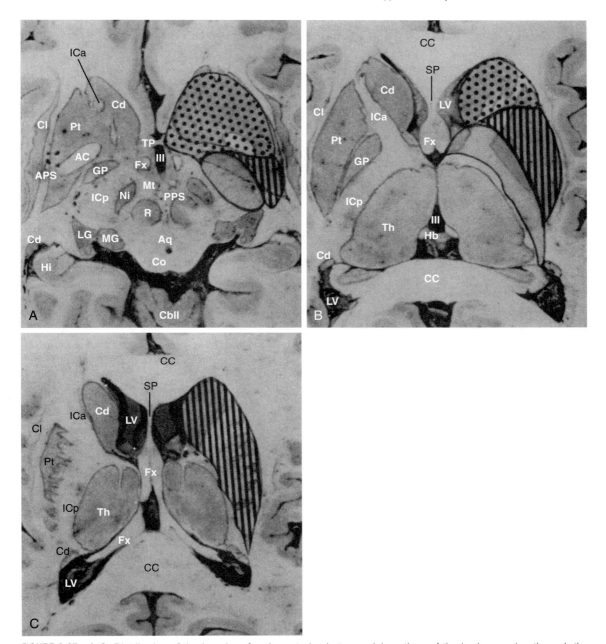

FIGURE 2-27   **A-C,** Distribution of the basal perforating arteries in transaxial sections of the brain, passing through the anterior commissure (**A**), foramen of Monro (**B**), and uppermost aspect of the putamen (**C**). The diagrams show the areas supplied by the RAH and MSA (⬚), LSA (▥), and anterior choroidal artery (⬚). AC, anterior commissure; APS, perforations of the anterior perforated substance; Aq, aqueduct of Sylvius; Cbll, cerebellum; CC, corpus callosum; Cd, caudate nucleus; Cl, claustrum; Co, quadrigeminal body; Fx, fornix; GP, globus pallidus; Hb, habenula; Hi, hippo-campus; ICa, anterior limb of the internal capsule; ICp, posterior limb of the internal capsule; LG, lateral geniculate body; LV, lateral ventricle; MG, medial geniculate body; Mt, mammillothalamic tract; Ni, substantia nigra; PPS, perforations of the posterior perforated substance; Pt, putamen; R, red nucleus; SP, septum pellucidum; Th, thalamus; TP, terminal plate; III, third ventricle. (From Takahashi S, Goto K, Fukasawa H, et al. Computed tomography of cerebral infarction along the distribution of the basal perforating arteries, part I: striate arterial group. Radiology 1985;155:107.)

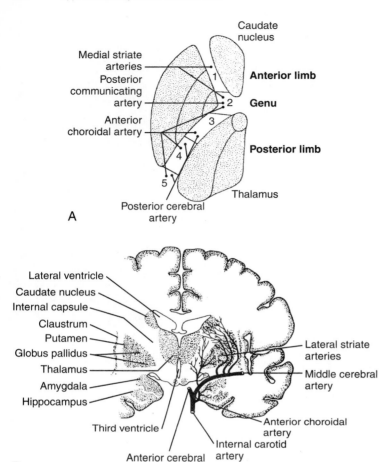

FIGURE 2-28   A and **B,** Arterial irrigation of the superior and inferior levels of the internal capsule. **A,** Horizontal section through an inferior level of the internal capsule. **B,** Coronal section through the thalamus showing irrigation of the superior part of the internal capsule by the lateral striate arteries (lenticulostriate) arteries and the inferior part of the posterior limb by the anterior choroidal artery. (From DeMyer W. Neuroanatomy, 2nd ed. Baltimore: Williams & Wilkins, 1998.)

the AchorA, and the thalamic arteries (see Figs. 2-25 and 2-28). The LstrAs irrigate the superior parts of the anterior and posterior limbs of the internal capsule up to the corona radiata at the lateral angle of the lateral ventricle. The AchorA mainly and PCA branches minimally irrigate the rest of the posterior limb. These distributions (i.e., with the LstrAs above and the RAH, PcomA, and AchorA below) illustrate the characteristic two-tiered superior-inferior irrigation pattern of the whole basal forebrain block.

Feekes and colleagues[83,84] state that the territories of the RAH, medial and lateral groups of the lenticulostriate arteries, and the AchorA are distinct with little overlap or anastomosis. The lateral group of lenticulostriate arteries supply the sensorimotor zone of the striatum, the medial group of lenticulostriate arteries supply the associative zone, and the RAH supplies the limbic zone.[84] These zones correlate with the well-known corticostriatothalamocortical loops and may explain specific symptoms based on striatal circuitry.

Sometimes the LstrAs supply the entire corpus striatum, taking over the MstrA territory, but the MstrA group does not take over the entire LstrA territory. The insular branches of the MCA, not the LstrAs, irrigate the insular cortex, extreme capsule, and claustrum. The lateralmost of the LstrAs irrigate the putamen and the external capsule, which marks the dividing line between the superficial and deep distributions of the MCA.[86]

Clinical Syndromes of Large Lateral Striate Artery (Striatocapsular) Infarcts

Infarcts larger than 1.5 cm that encroach on the internal capsule and adjacent putamen and caudate nucleus are called striatocapsular infarcts. Large striatocapsular infarcts may involve the entire LstrA distribution. Best seen 1 to 6 weeks after onset, they have a characteristic teardrop or comma shape in horizontal scans (see the vertical stripes in Fig. 2-27C).[86-89]

Mental Dysfunctions

The patient retains consciousness and memory, but exhibits abulia and loss of executive abilities without overt dementia. Mood changes may occur.[90] Dysphasia and reduced voice volume (hypophonia) may accompany left-sided lesions,[91] whereas left-sided visual and sensory neglect may accompany right-sided lesions. Weiller and associates[89] and Godefroy and colleagues[92] suggest that associated cortical ischemia accounts for these "cortical-type" deficits, but the issue remains open.[86] Interruption of the well-known frontostriatothalamocortical loops also could be responsible.[84]

Motor Dysfunctions

Contralateral, often severe hemiparesis is virtually constant. The arm is usually paralyzed, with the face and leg less affected.

Sensory Dysfunction

Only about half of patients lose sensation.

Clinical Syndromes of Restricted Infarcts of the Lateral Lenticulostriate Arteries

Restricted corona radiata infarcts can occur near the lateral angle of the lateral ventricles. This site is vulnerable because it is at the junction of the lateral lenticulostriate artery perforators with the long medullary penetrating arteries from the superficial MCA and the superior limit posteriorly of the distribution of the AchorA in the posterior limb of the internal capsule. The syndrome may variously consist of pure hemiplegia, sensory loss in the face and arm, dysarthria–clumsy hand syndrome of the AchorA, and dysphasia or hemineglect.[86,93]

Restricted anterior limb infarcts of the internal capsule, completely sparing the adjacent striatum, corona radiata, and posterior limb, are rare. Single lacunes may be silent, but may cause pure dysarthria or sometimes mild frontal lobe signs or weakness of proximal movements.[86]

Restricted caudate infarction may cause behavioral and cognitive deficits consisting of abulia, restlessness, agitation, disinhibition, and mood changes, sometimes associated with dysarthria and movement disorders.[88] Restricted putaminal infarction may cause amnesia; falling to one side; and hemidystonia, chorea, or facial palsy. Language dysfunction with micrographia and expressive aphasia may follow left-sided lesions,[86] and hemineglect may follow right-sided lesions.[94]

Restricted pallidal infarction causes acute memory loss, abulia, loss of drive, reduced emotional expression, and reduced spontaneity in some patients, and disinhibition and obsessive-compulsive symptoms in others.[94] Medial pallidal infarction also may cause contralateral dystonia.[95] Dystonia may arise from lesions at several different sites in the basal ganglia and thalamus.

Syndrome of Restricted Unilateral Infarction at a Superior Level of the Genu of the Internal Capsule

The patient has contralateral partial hemiparesis involving the faciolingual-masseter-pharyngeal and laryngeal muscles with dysarthria and dysphagia. The faciolingual syndrome is highly suggestive of a capsular genu lesion.[96] In contrast, except for the lower facial muscles, Willoughby and Anderson[97] found that unilateral paralysis of bulbar muscles was infrequent from most strokes that cause hemiplegia.

Frequently, the hand is paretic, but the sternocleidomastoid muscle is spared.[96] Sparing of the sternocleidomastoid muscle in this syndrome underscores the uncertainty about the location of the UMN pathway for this muscle because it is regularly paralyzed ipsilateral to the lesion in large, acute hemispheric lesions.

Syndrome of Restricted Unilateral Infarction at the Inferior Level of the Genu of the Internal Capsule

Tatemichi and associates[98] indicated that the genu syndrome differs depending on whether the lesion affects the genu at superior or inferior levels. The LstrAs supply the dorsal tier of the capsule; the candidate arteries for the inferior genu are the RAH, AchorA, and PcomA. The clinical features are as follows:

- Fluctuating alertness
- Amnesia, abulia, apathy, inattention, and often an enduring dementia. Right-sided lesions may cause impairment of visuospatial functions, and left-sided lesions may impair language functions. Tatemichi and associates[98] emphasized that these mental changes result from lesions limited to white matter, particularly left-sided lesions, and pointed out the difficulty in differentiating the capsular genu syndrome from the syndrome of TTA and TPA occlusion. The extensive mental changes are attributed to interruption of thalamofrontal connections and frontal diaschisis.[98,99] (See the anterior thalamic peduncle in Fig. 2-29.)
- Mild, transitory hemiparesis, mainly faciolingual with dysarthria. Chukwudelunzu and coworkers[99] reported frontal release signs, but their patient also had extensive periventricular lesions.

Location of the Pyramidal Tract in Relation to the Genu

The pyramidal tract appears as a rectangular area of hypointensity in horizontal T1-weighted magnetic resonance images of the posterior limb of the internal capsule by 4 years of age. It is hyperintense in T2-weighted images of children older than 9 years of age and thereafter for life.[100] The pyramidal tract also is visualized by tensor diffusion-weighted imaging and during wallerian degeneration.[101] Because of the restricted location of the pyramidal tract in the internal capsule, a small lacune can cause a pure contralateral hemiplegia, sparing the somatosensory pathways.

Anterior limb

1. Anterior thalamic peduncle
2. Frontopontine tract

Genu

Posterior limb

Lenticulothalamic part
3. Superior thalamic peduncle
4. Pyramidal tract

Sublenticular part
5. Ansa peduncularis
6. Thalamotemporal radiations
7. Auditory radiations
8. Optic radiations (geniculocalcarine tract)

Retrolenticular part
9. Posterior thalamic peduncle
10. Temporoparietopontine tract
11. Corticotectotegmental tract

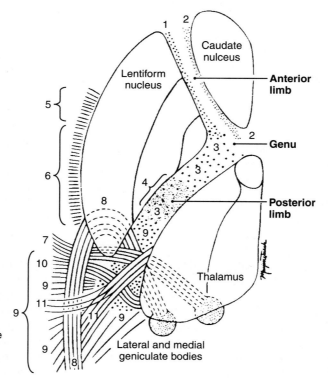

FIGURE 2-29 Horizontal section of the internal capsule showing the pathways that run through it. (From DeMyer W. Neuroanatomy, 2nd ed. Baltimore: Williams & Wilkins, 1998.)

Internal capsule

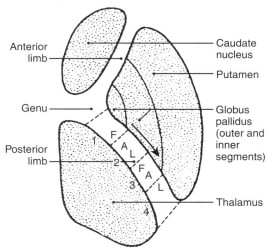

FIGURE 2-30 Horizontal section of the internal capsule showing the migration of the pyramidal tract from a forward location in the posterior limb of the capsule at a superior level to a more posterior location at lower levels. (From DeMyer W. Neuroanatomy, 2nd ed. Baltimore: Williams & Wilkins, 1998.)

Older texts depict the corticobulbar fibers of the pyramidal tract at the genu and the corticospinal fibers just behind. This anterior position holds only for the superior part of the capsule. As the pyramidal tract descends through the internal capsule, the fibers migrate toward the posterior part of the posterior limb before entering the midbrain basis (Fig. 2-30).[102,103] A lesion high in the internal capsule at the level of the genu causes a more severe faciolingual hemiparesis than an inferior level lesion.

Clinical Syndromes of Infarction of the Posterior Limb

Clinical syndromes of infarction of the posterior limb include partial or complete hemianesthesia-hemiplegia and pure hemianesthesia.[98,104,105]

Partial or Complete Hemianesthesia-Hemiplegia

Lacunes may cause pure hemiplegia or ataxic hemiparesis. Sometimes restricted UMN paralysis of the face, arm, or leg occurs, rather than the usual faciobrachiocrural hemiparesis.

Pure Hemianesthesia

Neglect occurs with right-sided lesions, and aphasia occurs with left-sided lesions.[106,107] Infarcts of the posterior limb of the capsule do not cause the profound mental changes that characterize the inferior capsular genu syndrome, which are attributed to interruption of the anterior and inferior thalamic peduncles.[98] Left-sided putaminal infarction may cause aphasia and dysgraphia.[108]

Anterior Choroidal Arteries

Origin and Distribution

The AchorA usually arises from the supraclinoid segment of the ICA just distal to the origin of the PcomA (see Fig. 2-4).[109] It arises from the MCA in about 4% of brains. Its distribution borders on most of the other groups of basal forebrain arteries. It anastomoses freely with the PchorA of the PCA. It has lesser anastomoses with the PcomA and the MCA (Fig. 2-31).

In anteroposterior sequence, the AchorA irrigates:

- Medial part of anterior perforated substance
- Optic tract
- Mesial temporal lobe: uncus, piriform cortex, and posterior part of the amygdala. After the AchorA enters the choroid fissure, it irrigates the hippocampal formation and choroid plexus, supplemented by anastomoses with the lateral posterior choroidal artery (LPchorA), often in the form of arcades.[110]
- Medial part of globus pallidus
- Posterior limb of the internal capsule posterior to the genu and inferior to the LstrAs. The AchorA may irrigate the genu or even anterior limb if the PcomA is small. Hupperts and colleagues[8,111] concluded that the AchorA territory extends superiorly from the posterior limb of the internal capsule to the posterior paraventricular corona radiata, but the issue is still in some doubt.[112]
- Retrolenticular part of the internal capsule (see Fig. 2-29)
- Portions of the thalamus (anastomoses with the LPchorA)

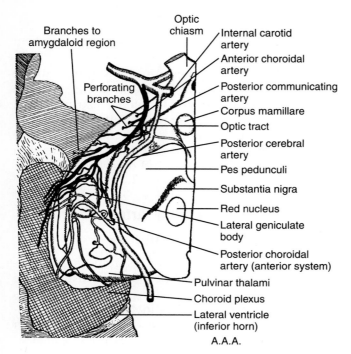

Optic
chiasm
Branches to
amygdaloid region
Perforating
branches
Internal carotid
artery
Anterior choroidal
artery
Posterior communicating
artery
Corpus mamillare
Optic tract
Posterior cerebral
artery
Pes pedunculi
Substantia nigra
Red nucleus
Lateral geniculate
body
Posterior choroidal
artery (anterior system)
Pulvinar thalami
Choroid plexus
Lateral ventricle
(inferior horn)
A.A.A.

FIGURE 2-31 Ventral diagram of the basal forebrain showing the anterior choroidal artery. (Reprinted with permission from Abbie AA: The clinical significance of the anterior choroidal artery. Brain 1933;56:233.)

- Wings of the lateral geniculate body and origin of geniculocalcarine radiation
- Medial geniculate body and origin of the auditory radiation
- Posterior part of the reticular nucleus of the thalamus
- Pulvinar (minimal)
- Nucleus ventralis posterolateralis (variably but minimally)
- Lateroventral branch to the thalamus. Percheron[113] denied a lateroventral branch to the thalamus as described by Plets and coworkers.[114] Hupperts and colleagues[111] indicated occasional minimal supply from the AchorA to the ventral-anterior region of the thalamus.
- Most of the subthalamic nucleus, reaching to field H2 of Forel and the zona incerta

Sometimes the AchorA irrigates the middle third of the midbrain basis, substantia nigra, and part of the red nucleus, in reciprocity with peduncular branches of PCA.

Syndrome of Anterior Choroidal Artery Occlusion

The classic syndrome of occlusion consists of contralateral hemiplegia, hemisensory loss, and a hemideficit of the visual field. The clinician can suspect the diagnosis, but radiographic confirmation is required.[112,115]

Mental Dysfunctions

Left-sided lesions frequently cause mild deficiencies in memory and oral word association, dysarthria, and slight aphasia. Right-sided lesions may cause mild dysfunctions of visual perception and visual memory for designs, anosognosia, and other right parietal signs. No amnesia or dementia occurs.

Motor Dysfunctions

Contralateral hemiparesis may include pure hemiparesis,[116] ataxic hemiparesis, or dysarthria–clumsy hand syndrome. Dysarthria is common. Rarely, the patient has fits of severe pathologic crying.[117] Contralateral dystonia from infarction of the medial pallidum occurs.[95]

Sensory Dysfunctions

The patient may experience headache and nausea at onset. Contralateral paresthesias and loss of light touch and pinprick may occur, but proprioception and vibration may be preserved.

A few patients may have contralateral visual field defects. The defect may vary from homonymous hemianopia, to upper quadrantanopia, to a relatively pathognomonic homonymous upper and lower quadrantic sectoranopia, with a wedge-shaped area of preserved macular vision straddling the horizontal meridian. The LPchorA irrigates the preserved macular sector of the lateral geniculate body.[13,118]

Thalamic Arteries

Where the Thalamic Arteries Do Not Come From

The ACA and the RAH do not supply the thalamus. The MCA contributes only if the AchorA happens to arise from the MCA (4%) instead of from the supraclinoid part of the ICA. No LstrAs reach the thalamus.[113] In Figures 2-25 and 2-28B, the LstrAs arch around and over the thalamus, without branching to it. No thalamic arteries arise from the trunk per se of the BA and its brainstem and cerebellar branches. The TPAs arise as a group, however, with the midbrain perforators at the distal tip of the BA where it bifurcates into the BcomAs (see Figs. 2-4 and 2-34).

Where the Thalamic Arteries Do Come From

Table 2-1 presents the thalamic arteries and their origins.

Location and Characteristics of Thalamic Infarcts

Figures 2-32 and 2-33 show the thalamic artery distributions.[119] Because most thalamic nuclei receive blood from more than one artery, the infarction syndromes reflect destruction of thalamic regions, rather than single nuclei. Percheron[113] and Pullicino[120] detail the arterial supply of the individual thalamic nuclei. Infarctions involve the territory of the thalamogeniculate artery (TGA) about 45% of the time; the TPA, 35%; the TTA, about 12%; and the PchorA, 8%.

Determinants of the Size and Distribution of Thalamic Infarcts

The size and distribution of thalamic infarcts are determined by the following:

- Reciprocities in the size of thalamic arteries (e.g., with hypoplasia or absence of the TTA, the TPAs may extend to the anterior pole of the thalamus)
- Size of the parent vessels of the circle of Willis and the pattern of anastomosis
- Site and extent of the occlusion in the parent vessels, and proximity of the ostia of perforators to the occlusion site

Because the TGA and the PchorAs arise close together from the PCA, the same thrombus or embolus frequently occludes all three vessels. Hypoplasia of the PcomA on the affected side favors extension of the lesion to PCA zones beyond the thalamus.

TABLE 2-1 **Six Thalamic Arteries and Their Origins***

Thalamic Arteries	Origin
Thalamotuberal artery (TTA) = thalamopolar artery	Posterior communicating artery from the internal carotid artery
Thalamoperforant artery (TPA)	Basilar artery bifurcation = basilar communicating artery of Percheron = P1 segment of posterior cerebral artery
Thalamogeniculate artery (TGA)	Posterior cerebral artery, P2 segment
Anterior choroidal artery (AchorA)	Internal carotid artery
Medial and lateral posterior choroidal arteries (MPchorA and LPchorA)	Posterior cerebral artery, P1, P2, or P3 segments

*Although named as single arteries, the thalamic arteries consist of leashes of perforators.

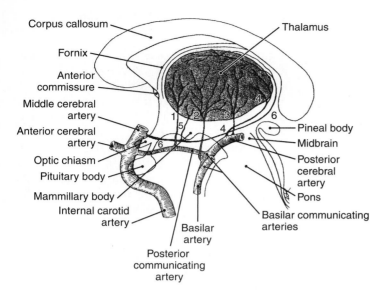

FIGURE 2-32 Sagittal drawing of the distribution of the thalamic arteries. *1,* thalamotuberal artery; *2,* thalamoperforant artery; *3,* thalamogeniculate artery; *4,* posterior choroidal artery; *5,* lateroventral artery; *6,* anterior choroidal artery. (Modified from Plets C, De Reuck J, Vander Eecken H, et al. The vascularization of the human thalamus. Acta Neurol Belg 1970;70:687.)

Because the TPAs and rostral paramedian midbrain perforators from the BA and BcomAs form a continuous leash, paramedian thalamic infarcts may extend into the rostral midbrain. Bilateral infarction of the thalamus and midbrain with extension of the infarct into the temporo-occipital region irrigated by the PCA completes the rostral or top of the basilar syndrome (see Rostral basilar artery syndrome (top of the basilar syndrome), later).[121]

The distribution of thalamic infarcts in children matches that of adults,[2,63] but hypertension is much less frequently the cause.[62] Even isolated lacunes can cause significant changes in executive functions and memory, particularly by interrupting the mammillothalamic tract[122] or intralaminar nuclei.[123]

Thalamotuberal Artery (= Thalamic Polar Artery = Premammillary Artery = Anterior Thalamosubthalamic Paramedian Artery = Anterior Thalamoperforating Artery)

Origin and Distribution

The TTA arises from the PcomA (see Fig. 2-32).[124] The PcomA also originates hypothalamic perforators, about six in all, which extend to the tuberal region of the hypothalamus and to the anterior part of the mammillary bodies. Because the TTA does not give off tuberal branches, Percheron[113]

named it the thalamic polar artery. The TTA passes through Forel fields to reach the nucleus ventralis anterior, the anterior intralaminar nuclei, and the mammillothalamic tract,[33,120,125] but reportedly does not extend superiorly to the nucleus anterior.[113] Presumably, the LPchorA irrigates the nucleus anterior, but see the discussion in Medial posterior choroidal artery: origin, distribution, and syndromes of occlusion and Lateral Posterior Choroidal Artery, later.

Syndrome of Thalamotuberal Artery Occlusion

Infarction of the ventral anterior thalamus results in neuropsychological deficits, with only minimal or transitory motor and sensory deficits, if any.[126-128] Ghika-Schmid and Bogousslavsky[125] described the acute onset of severe perseveration apparent in speech, memory, and executive tasks; increased sensitivity to interference; mixing of mental activities ordinarily processed separately (labeled palipsychism); anterograde memory impairment; word-finding difficulties; and abulia and apathy. Remaining as outstanding chronic deficits are amnesia, word-finding difficulties, and apathy.

Left-sided TTA infarcts may cause severe and wide-ranging deficits in language (thalamic aphasia, dysprosody, dysarthria, and hypophonia).[129,130] The patient also has deficits in orientation, memory, visual

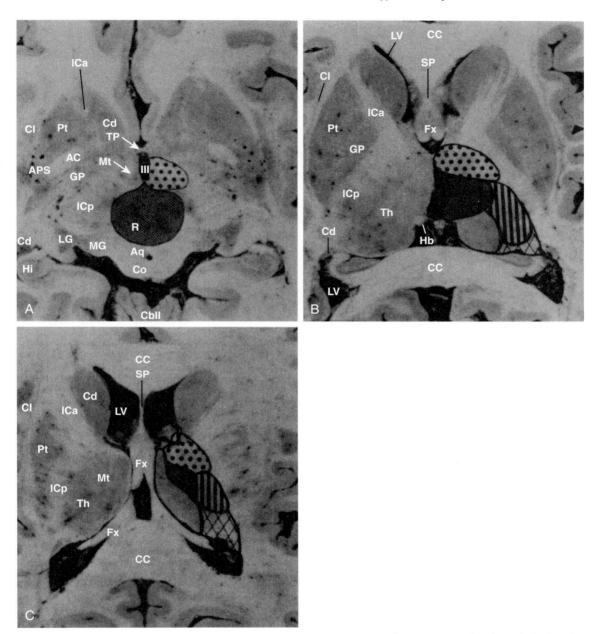

FIGURE 2-33   **A-C,** Distribution of the thalamic arteries on transaxial sections of the brain, passing through the junction of the midbrain and diencephalon (**A**), midthalamus (**B**), and dorsal portion of the thalamus (**C**). The diagrams show the areas supplied by the TTA (⬚), TPA (⬚), TGA (⬚), MPChA (⬚), and LPChA (⬚). AC, anterior commissure; APS, perforations of the anterior perforated substance; Aq, aqueduct of Sylvius; Cbll, cerebellum; CC, corpus callosum; Cd, caudate nucleus; Cl, claustrum; Co, quadrigeminal body; Fx, fornix; GP, globus pallidus; Hb, habenula; Hi, hippocampus; ICa, anterior limb of the internal capsule; ICp, posterior limb of the internal capsule; LG, lateral geniculate body; LV, lateral ventricle; MG, medial geniculate body; Mt, mammillothalamic tract; Pt, putamen; R, red nucleus; SP, septum pellucidum; Th, thalamus; TP, terminal plate; III, third ventricle. (Reprinted from Takahashi S, Goto KL, Fukasawa H, et al. Computed tomography of cerebral infarction along the distribution of the basal perforating arteries, part II: thalamic arterial group. Radiology 1985;155:119.)

perception, and constructional praxis.[131,132] Right-sided TTA infarcts cause deficits of nonverbal intellect, visuoperceptual performance, constructional praxis, and visual memory for designs, but verbal functions are preserved.

Some patients with only unilateral TTA territory infarction may have severe dementia or amnesia.[133] Even unilateral interruption of the left mammillothalamic tract may cause acute dysphasia and persistent selective episodic memory impairment for verbal material, but with preservation of visual memory.[122]

Thalamogeniculate Artery

Origin and Distribution

The TGA originates as several stems from the ambient or P2 segment of the PCA (Fig. 2-34; see Fig. 2-32). The TGA perforates between the geniculate bodies and distributes to the nucleus ventralis posterolateralis, the nucleus ventralis lateralis, and sometimes the posterior part of the nucleus ventralis anterior, the inferolateral part of the pulvinar, the nucleus lateralis posterior, the

nucleus lateralis dorsalis, and the lateral part of centrum medianum.[113,120]

Syndrome of Thalamogeniculate Artery Occlusion

Mental Deficits

Usually, the patient has no major deficits in mental function, but left-sided lesions may cause aphasia.[134]

Motor Deficits

Transient contralateral hemiplegia occurs, with late evolving ataxia, after the hemiparesis improves. Involuntary movements occur contralaterally, including mild choreiform unrest of the hand and fingers,[135,136] or larger choreiform movements superimposed on volitional movements, and sometimes dystonia.[137] The onset of the movement disorder may be delayed. Isolated hemiataxia-hypesthesia syndrome may occur.[138] Sometimes there is loss of emotional facial expression.

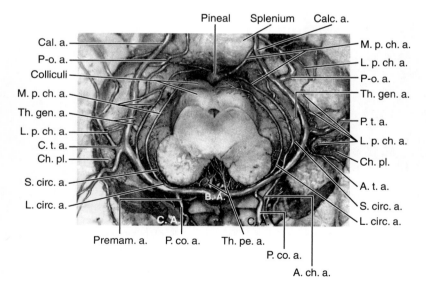

FIGURE 2-34 Photograph of the bifurcation of the basilar artery into the posterior cerebral artery and the midbrain-diencephalic junction. A.Ch.A., anterior choroidal artery; A.T.A., anterior temporal artery; B.A., basilar artery; C.A., carotid artery; Calc.A., calcarine artery; C.T.A., common temporal artery; Ch. Pl., choroid plexus; L.Circ.A., long circumflex artery = quadrigeminal artery; L.P.Ch.A., lateral posterior choroidal artery; M.P.Ch.A., medial posterior choroidal artery; P.Co.A., posterior communicating artery; P-O.A., parieto-occipital artery; Premam.A., premammillary artery = thalamotuberal artery; P.T.A., posterior temporal artery; S.Circ.A., short circumflex artery; Th.Gen.A., thalamogeniculate artery; Th.Pe.A., thalamoperforant artery. (From Zeal AA, Rhoton AL. Microsurgical anatomy of the posterior cerebral artery. J Neurosurg 1978;48:534.)

Sensory Deficits

There is contralateral elevation of the sensory thresholds with hemihypesthesia or hyperesthesias, and often a severe, disagreeable response to various cutaneous stimuli (allodynia), or much less commonly a feeling of extreme pleasure. The pain or the movement disorders may occur weeks to months after the stroke. Poststroke pain may result from lesions at various sites along the central pain pathways besides the thalamus.[40,122]

Deep modalities generally are severely impaired,[139] in contrast to AchorA infarction involving the posterior limb of the internal capsule. Facial sensation is frequently spared because of the more medial location of the nucleus ventralis posteromedialis. Usually, the infarct spares the geniculate bodies, but some patients may have contralateral visual field defects. Pure sensory stroke of thalamic origin results from an infarct limited to the nucleus ventralis posterior alone, rather than the entire TGA territory.[140]

The Dejerine-Roussy syndrome[141] consists of mild or transient hemiparesis; mild hemichorea; hemiathetosis or tremor; hemisensory loss of superficial and deep sensation including astereognosis, hemianesthesia, or hyperesthesia; and very disagreeable poststroke pain.[13]

Paramedian Posterior Thalamoperforant Arteries (= Superior Paramedian Branches of Basilar Communicating Artery = Paramedian Peduncular Artery = Postmammillary Artery)

Origin

This leash of perforators arises from the BcomA (P1 segment of PCA) and the bifurcation of the BA at its tip (see Figs. 2-4, 2-32, and 2-34).[142] The BcomA originates arteries to four destinations:[113] the posterior hypothalamus, paramedian zone of the diencephalon, paramedian zone of the midbrain at its junction with the diencephalon, and the circumferential mesencephalic arteries that extend to the superior quadrigeminal bodies (quadrigeminal artery) (see Figs. 2-4 and 2-34).

Course and Distribution

The TPAs run through the interpeduncular fossa to enter the thalamus and midbrain through the posterior perforated substance and anterior foramen caecum. Within the neuraxis, the TPAs irrigate rostral midbrain, subthalamic, and thalamic territories (see Figs. 2-33 and 2-34).[113,120]

The peduncular distribution variously includes the medial parts of the midbrain basis, substantia nigra, and red nucleus; the interpeduncular region; the oculomotor nucleus; and the ventral part of the periaqueductal gray matter (see Fig. 2-38E). The P1 territory may include the pyramidal tract in the midzone of the basis pedunculi.

The subthalamic distribution includes part of the subthalamic nucleus, field H of Forel, and the zona incerta. The thalamic distribution includes the nucleus medialis dorsalis, medial and anterior part of the nucleus centrum medianum, the parafascicular nucleus, and, in part, the nucleus ventralis lateralis. Because paramedian infarcts do not usually reach laterally to include the nucleus ventralis posterior; they cause little or no enduring sensory loss.[113,120]

Laterality of Infarction in the Thalamoperforant Artery Territory

Whether a paramedian thalamic infarct is unilateral or bilateral may depend on how the TPAs originate from the BcomA.[113,143-145] Unilateral occlusion of the BcomA when it originates the TPAs as the stem of a Y causes bilateral thalamic infarction (Fig. 2-35).

Bilateral infarcts usually involve the maximum extent of the TPA irrigation area and typically extend into the rostral midbrain. The thalamic syndrome then overlaps with the syndrome of occlusion of the paramedian perforators to the midbrain (see Rostral basilar artery syndrome (top of the basilar syndrome), infra). In the 28 autopsied cases of Castaigne and coworkers,[143] 4 had unilateral paramedian thalamic infarcts, 5 bilateral paramedian thalamic infarcts, and 19 had paramedian thalamic plus midbrain infarcts.

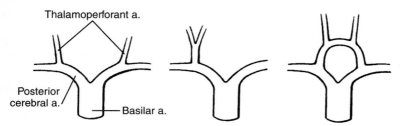

FIGURE 2-35   Diagram of the parallel, Y, and goalpost (cross-bar) patterns of the thalamoperforant arteries. Figure 2-34 shows the parallel pattern. When the TPAs of each side come off a common stem (Y pattern), unilateral occlusion of the BcomA that originates the stem causes bilateral infarction.

Clinical Syndromes of Paramedian Thalamic Infarction (Thalamoperforant Artery Territory)

Infarcts limited to the TPA zone cause impairment of mentation and consciousness without the frank motor and sensory defects of infarction in the TGA zone.[128,143] Midbrain extension may add motor signs, such as vertical gaze and convergence palsy, but the neuropsychologic features may occur alone.[146]

Unilateral Paramedian Thalamic Infarcts

The patient experiences mood and behavioral changes. Agitation, aggression, disorientation, and amnesia occur. There usually is no coma, motor signs, or sensory deficits. There is no or mild aphasia with left-sided lesions. Left-sided infarcts generally cause more severe impairment than right-sided infarcts.

Bilateral Paramedian Thalamic Infarcts

Cardinal features consist of impairment of consciousness, mood, and memory; paresis of upward gaze; and sometimes cerebellar signs.[147] No sensory loss occurs. The patient has abrupt, transient, fluctuating disturbances of consciousness up to brief coma or hypersomnolence alternating with periods of verbal communication.[148,149] Sometimes no disturbance of consciousness occurs at onset.[150]

Other features are as follows:

- Dysphoria, mood lability, apathy, indifference, and lack of initiative and insight[151]
- Inattentiveness and inability to monitor, but the patient may display "utilization behavior" (i.e., exhibit exaggerated responses to objects and environmental stimuli)[152]
- Korsakoff-like amnestic-confabulatory syndrome with severe, persistent amnesia
- Visual spatial defects

Medial Posterior Choroidal Artery
Origin and Distribution

The medial posterior choroidal artery (MPchorA) and LPchorA usually arise from the P1-P3 segments of the PCA (see Fig. 2-34), or they may arise from TGAs or cortical branches of the PCA.[113,153,154] After origination from the P1 or proximal P2 segment, the MPchorA curves around the midbrain in the perimesencephalic cistern (see Fig. 2-34). It irrigates the pretectal area, superior quadrigeminal body, and rostral part of the midbrain tegmentum habenula, pineal body, and pulvinar.[120] The MPchorA then extends forward medial to the pulvinar and irrigates medial and lateral territories on the dorsum of the thalamus (Figs. 2-36 and 2-37).[114]

The medial branches of the MPchorA supply the choroid plexus and roof of the third ventricle (the floor of the cavum velli interpositi) up to the foramen of Monro (see Fig. 2-36). The lateral branches of the MPchorA supply the superomedial aspect of the pulvinar and parts of the nucleus medialis dorsalis adjacent to the paramedian zone. The territory extends anteriorly along the thalamus adjacent to and lateral to the attachment of the roof of the third ventricle to the stria medullaris thalami (see Fig. 2-36). It reaches the nucleus anterior,[113,114,120] but nucleus anterior infarction is not seen in radiographs of MPchorA or LPchorA occlusion.[118] The pulvinar receives blood from the MPchorA, LPchorA, and TGA.

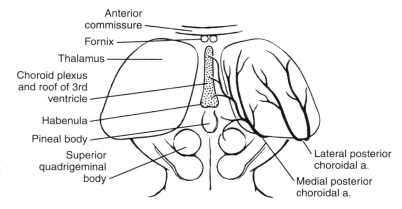

FIGURE 2-36 Dorsal view of the thalamus and rostral midbrain, showing the distribution of the medial and lateral posterior choroidal arteries.

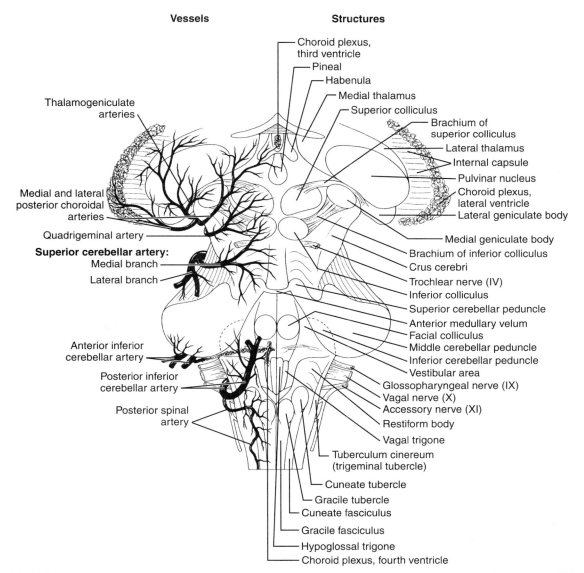

FIGURE 2-37 Dorsal drawing of the brainstem showing the successive arteries that irrigate the tectum. (From Haines DE. Neuroanatomy: An Atlas of Structures, Sections, and Systems, 5th ed. Baltimore: Lippincott Williams & Wilkins, 2000.)

Clinical Syndrome of Medial Posterior Choroidal Artery Occlusion

Because of the rarity of pure MPchorA occlusion, no distinctive syndrome is defined. Pretectal signs predominate. The patient may have upgaze and horizontal gaze paralysis, miosis, or, uncommonly, midbrain tegmental signs.[118] Infarction of the medial part of the pulvinar and nucleus medialis dorsalis nucleus may be silent, but it is usually combined with infarction in the LPchorA territory, midbrain, and geniculate body.[118]

Lateral Posterior Choroidal Artery

Origin and Distribution

The LPchorA arises from the PCA distal to the MPchorA, usually as multiple branches and often from the early cortical trunks of the PCA. The presence of multiple sites of origin and anastomoses with the AchorA may explain the infrequency of isolated infarction in LPchorA territory (see Figs. 2-31, 2-34, and 2-36).

Branches extend laterally and forward to anastomose with the AchorA, which has followed the optic tract to the lateral geniculate body. Plets and colleagues[114] and Percheron[113] concluded that AchorA and LPchorA anastomose so freely that they lose their identity, obviating claims that the AchorA ends at the lateral geniculate body, but Percheron[113] also stated that when the AchorA extends over the thalamus (see Fig. 2-32), it gives only choroidal branches.

The amalgamated AchorAs-LPchorAs irrigate the hippocampal formation, often in the form of arcades[110] and the parahippocampal gyrus. They supply the choroid plexus of the temporal horn, the glomus, and the body of the lateral ventricle up to the level of the foramen of Monro. At this point, where the choroid plexus reflects back as the roof of the third ventricle, the MPchorA takes over the irrigation of the choroid plexus (see Fig. 2-36).[114,155] Branches run to the crus, commissure, body, and part of the anterior columns of the fimbria-fornix adjacent to the choroid plexus. Some choroid branches extend into the thinned tail of the caudate nucleus, but not into the periventricular white matter. The capsular branches may reach this white matter (see the discussion in The basal forebrain arteries: origin, distribution, and syndromes of occlusion. The lateral striate (lenticulostriate) arteries: origin, distribution and syndromes of occlusion. Distribution of LstrAs).

The thalamic branches of the LPchorA supply the posterior part of the nucleus lateralis dorsalis, the superoposterior part of the pulvinar, and the central wedge of the lateral geniculate body that mediates macular vision.[154] Branches do not reach the nucleus anterior, but sometimes extend posteriorly into the rostral part of the midbrain (see Fig. 2-37).[118,155]

Clinical Syndrome of Lateral Posterior Choroid Artery Occlusion

Mental Deficits

The patient has mild neuropsychologic dysfunction, such as aphasia with left-sided lesions and memory loss.

Motor Deficits

The patient may have faciobrachial paresis, hemiparesis, and involuntary movements, sometimes of delayed onset.[118]

Sensory Deficits

Visual field defects and blurred vision are the most common findings. A variety of visual field defects may ensue; although uncommon, a horizontal wedge-shaped sectoranopia involving the macular field is virtually pathognomonic of the lesion site.[13,112,118] The visual defect may be transient.[154] Uncommonly, the patient may have hemihypesthesia and the delayed onset of a thalamic pain syndrome.[9]

Neighborhood Signs Not Found

There is no loss of consciousness and no disturbance of eye movements with LPchorA occlusion, unless the infarction also involves other branches of the PCA.

Rostral Basilar Artery Syndrome (Top of the Basilar Syndrome)

Occlusion of the distal BA at its bifurcation may cause limited or extensive infarction. Extensive infarction may involve the entire distribution of the PCA—the thalamus, subthalamus, rostral midbrain, and inferomedial temporoparieto-occipital region.[55,121,156,157]

Origin and Distribution of Paramedian Perforators of the Midbrain

Paramedian midbrain perforators to the rostral midbrain exit from the distal tip of the BA and from the BcomA along with TPAs.[142] They enter the midbrain through the posterior perforated space of the interpeduncular fossa to irrigate the median-paramedian zone of the midbrain (see Fig. 2-38E). The midbrain distribution includes branches to the basis and tegmentum, as follows:

- Medial part of the basis pedunculi, pars compacta of the substantia nigra, and interpeduncular nucleus
- Fasciculus retroflexus of Meynert (habenulointerpeduncular tract)
- Medial part of the red nucleus and dentatothalamic tract, the region dorsomedial to red nucleus, and the ascending pathways from nucleus locus coeruleus (norepinephrine) and the raphe nuclei (serotonin)
- Rostral interstitial nucleus of the MLF
- Nucleus of CN III[158]
- Ventral part of the periaqueductal gray matter

These paramedian perforators do not reach the midbrain tectum. The tectum receives its blood through the long circumflex (quadrigeminal) branch of the PCA and SCA (see Figs. 2-34 and 2-37).

Clinical Features of Rostral Basilar Artery Syndrome

Mental Deficits

The patient may display confusion, disorientation, peduncular hallucinosis, abulia, coma, akinetic mutism, or hypersomnolence.[159-161] If the patient survives, significant cognitive impairment consisting of deficits in attention span, orientation, memory, intellect, and visual perception persist, but language may be preserved.[162] Any of the findings described under occlusion of the superficial branches of PCA also may be present (see The posterior cerebral artery: origin distribution, and syndromes of occlusion. Syndromes of occlusion of the superficial branches of the posterior cerebral artery).

Abnormal Eye Movements

The patient may have selective paralysis of conjugate downward eye movements if the lesion selectively involves the region dorsomedial to the red nucleus. (See also the vertebrobasilar arteries: origin, distribution, and syndromes of occlusion. The midbrain: syndromes of basilar and posterior cerebral artery occlusion. The rostral-dorsal midbrain or pretectal syndrome for pretectal signs.)

Pupillary Changes

Pupillary changes include cormiosis, corectasia, or corectopia. The patient may have esotropia without pupillary changes.[163]

Motor Deficits

Motor deficits include decerebrate rigidity and central neurogenic hyperventilation. Infarction of the midbrain basis causes hemiplegia or double hemiplegia. Sometimes convulsive jerks occur.[164] A patient who regains consciousness may show movement disorders varying from ataxia and tremor to ballismus.

Lemniscal Sensory Deficits

Brainstem signs not present include vertical nystagmus, conjugate horizontal nystagmus, and ocular bobbing.

Combined Paramedian Thalamic and Midbrain Infarcts (Paramedian Thalamopeduncular Infarcts)

The patient has a more restricted lesion of the midbrain-diencephalic junction, rather than the full top of the rostral BA syndrome.[143,165]

Comparison of Thalamic Artery and Middle Cerebral Artery Infarcts

Infarcts limited to the MCA distribution, whether deep, superficial, or both, spare the thalamus. Infarcts in the distribution of the superficial branches of the MCA may extend from the cortex through the centrum semiovale to the lateral angle of the ventricle where they border on the LstrA and AchorA territory (see Figs. 2-7 and 2-25). Even a combined MCA and thalamic infarct may spare the internal capsule, presumably because of greater resistance of the white matter and overlapping blood supply from the AchorA, PcomA, and PCA branches.

The insular cortex, extreme capsule, and claustrum receive their blood supply from insular branches of the MCA, not the LstrAs. The junction zone between the cortical branches of the MCA and the LstrAs is at the external capsule.[86] Thalamic arteries do not extend laterally to these regions.

Summary of the Distribution of the Arteries of the Basal Forebrain and Deep Gray Matter

The corpus striatum, the thalamus, and the internal capsule up to the angle of the lateral ventricle—the block of tissue anchored on the basal forebrain (see Fig. 2-22)—receive arterial blood in two tiers, a superior and an inferior, as listed subsequently, in anteroposterior order.

Striatum

See Figure 2-27.

- Inferior block of striatum (nucleus accumbens and inferior third of the head of the caudate and adjacent putamen) and intervening inferior fibers of the anterior limb of the internal capsule: RAH
- Superior block of striatum (superior two thirds of the caudate, putamen, and intervening superior fibers of the anterior limb of the internal capsule: LstrAs

Lentiform nucleus

See Figure 2-28B.

- Inferomedial block, the pallidum
- Medial part of pallidum: AchorA
- Lateral part of pallidum: medial group of LstrAs

- Superolateral block of the putamen: lateral group of LstrAs[84]

Thalamus Dorsalis

See Figures 2-32 and 2-33.

- Inferior block of thalamus
- TTA (= polar artery)
- TPA
- TGA
- Choroidal arteries to metathalamus (medial and lateral geniculate bodies)
- Superior cap of the thalamus: PchorAs and AchorA

Internal Capsule

See Figure 2-28.

- Anterior limb
- Inferior part: RAH
- Superior part: LstrAs
- Genu and most anterior part of the posterior limb
- Inferior part: RAH in reciprocity with the PcomA and the AchorA
- Superior part: LstrAs
- Posterior limb of the internal capsule
- Inferior part
- AchorA: starts to supply the posterior limb inferiorly; behind the genu of the capsule, the zone of the AchorA expands posteriorly
- TTA and TGA supply the capsule slightly, if at all; mild, brief hemiparesis may accompany infarction in their territories
- Other PCA perforators supply the corticofugal systems of the capsule after they exit the basal forebrain into the basis pedunculi[156,157]
- Superior part (see Figs. 2-25 and 28)
- LstrAs irrigate the superior part of the anterior limb and genu and the superior part of the posterior limb

Behind and inferior to the LstrAs, the AchorA expands to irrigate the posterior limb. Its posterior and superior expansion reaches superiorly to the periventricular white matter of the centrum semiovale at the superior angle of the body of the lateral ventricle. See the AchorA distribution in Figures 2-27 and 2-28B.

The blood supply of the internal capsule and the transition of the corticofugal fibers to the midbrain basis involves major contributions from the RAH, LstrAs, AchorA, and

PcomAs (see Figs. 2-24 to 2-28). The PCA contributes to the posterior limb to the degree that it anastomoses with the AchorA, or that the TGA may minimally supply the posterior limb. (See the Dejerine-Roussy Syndrome in The Thalamic arteries: origin, distribution, and syndromes of occlusion, earlier.)

Vertebrobasilar Arteries

Vertebral Arteries: Origin and Branches

The VAs arise from the subclavian arteries (see Fig. 2-1) and ascend through foramina in the transverse process of the cervical vertebrae beginning with C6. After the siphon at C1, the VAs pierce the dura and enter the intracranial space through the foramen magnum. The left VA is usually longer and larger than the right.

The VAs angle medially and join at the pontomedullary sulcus to form the BA (see Fig. 2-3). Before joining, they give off the following arteries:

- Paired PICAs
- Median and paramedian perforating vessels
- Paired branches from the VAs join to form the VspAs (see Fig. 2-3). The two VAs and two branches to the VspA form a small, rhomboid-shaped posterior anastomotic circle.
- DLspAs that arise either from the VAs or PICA irrigate the dorsum of the caudal levels of the medulla and continue on into the spinal cord (see Fig. 2-37).

Basilar Artery: Origin and Branches

The two VAs (see Fig. 2-3) unite at the pontomedullary sulcus to form the BA. It extends precisely the length of the pons and ends at the pontomesencephalic sulcus by bifurcating into right and left BcomAs that continue as PCAs.

Along its way, the BA gives off numerous unnamed median and paramedian perforating branches and pairs of named long circumferential arteries, which themselves give off perforators. In rostrocaudal order, these long circumferential arteries are the PCAs via the BcomAs, SCAs, and AICAs (see Fig. 2-3). In a few brains, the internal auditory artery (IAA) arises directly from the BA, just rostral to the AICA (see Fig. 2-41).

The PCA supplies paramedian and peduncular perforators, short and long circumferential arteries, and PchorAs (see Figs. 2-20, 2-34, and 2-37). These arteries, especially the quadrigeminal arteries, irrigate the rostral wafer of the midbrain, whereas SCAs irrigate the caudal midbrain wafer, including its laterodorsal quadrant (see Fig. 2-37 and the arteries of the cerebellum and medulla oblongata: origin, distribution, and syndromes of occlusion, later).

Embryologically, arteries reach the brainstem with each branchial cranial nerve. Sometimes these primitive branchial arteries remain (e.g., a persistent trigeminal artery), but most atrophy. Minor arteries also travel along the roots of the somite CNs, III, IV, VI, and XII.

Internal Distribution of the Vertebrobasilar Branches

Duvernoy[166] recognized four brainstem irrigation zones, named by where the artery penetrates the circumference (Fig. 2-38):

- Anteromedial zone—irrigated by median-paramedian perforators off the vertebrobasilar trunks; these arteries do not extend into the tectum, which is served by long circumferential arteries
- Anterolateral zone—irrigated by paramedian and short circumferential perforators
- Lateral zone—irrigated by short circumflex and medial branches of the long circumferential arteries (SCA and AICA)
- Posterior zone—irrigated by medial branches of the long circumferential arteries (PCA, SCA, and AICA)

Midbrain: Syndromes of Basilar Artery and Posterior Cerebral Artery Occlusion

The clinical features of syndromes of basilar artery and posterior cerebral artery occlusion depend on the extent and level of the infarct. The infarct may involve medial or lateral zones of the midbrain basis, tegmentum, or tectum at rostral or caudal levels.[167] It may extend from the brainstem to thalamic or cortical zones of the PCA or cerebellar zones of the SCA. Infarcts also may be limited to junction zones between larger territories.[167]

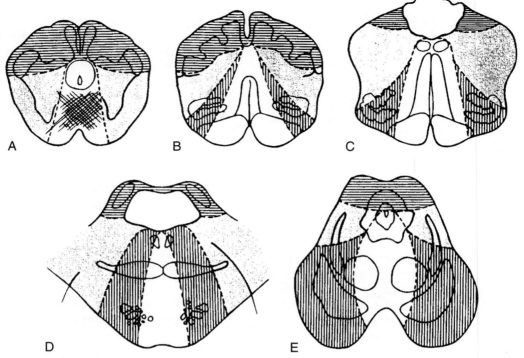

FIGURE 2-38 **Transverse drawings of the brainstem showing the internal irrigation zones of the vertebrobasilar arteries. A,** Medullocervical junction. **B,** Medulla oblongata, caudal level. **C,** Medulla oblongata, middle level. **D,** Pons, middle level. **E,** Midbrain, rostral level. *White area* = paramedian arteries (anteromedial group). *Vertical lines* = short circumferential arteries, intermediate group (anterolateral group). *Shading* = short circumferential arteries, lateral group. *Transverse lines* = long circumferential arteries or in the caudal medulla the dorsolateral spinal arteries (posterior group). (From DeMyer W. Neuroanatomy, 2nd ed. Baltimore: Williams & Wilkins, 1998.)

Rostral-Dorsal Midbrain or Pretectal Syndrome (= Dorsal Midbrain Syndrome, Sylvian Aqueduct Syndrome = Koerber-Salus-Elschnig Syndrome)

Eye signs predominate. Core signs consist of upward gaze palsy (volitional and reflex), disjunctive vertical or horizontal eye positions, skew deviation, head tilt, lid retraction (Collier sign, reptilian stare, lid lag, and convergence-retraction nystagmus).[168,169] Some patients show forced down gaze or combined palsy of upward and downward gaze. Convergence spasm may cause pseudo–abducens palsy. Pupillary changes consist of anisocoria, corectasia, corectopia, absence of constriction to light, or dissociated reactions to light and accommodation. Pure downward gaze palsy is a midbrain tegmental sign from a lesion dorsomedial to the red nuclei, not a pretectal sign.[170]

Other Neuro-ophthalmologic Syndromes of Midbrain Infarction

Occlusion of individual median-paramedian arteries can cause discrete infarcts, a few millimeters in diameter, limited to small regions such as the oculomotor nuclei or fascicles of the third nerve,[158] or, in the basis, pure hemiplegia.[171] Larger infarcts cause multiple deficits related to the control of vertical eye movements, the third nerve, rostral interstitial nuclei of the medial longitudinal fasciculus (riMLF), dentatorubrothalamic tracts, reticular formation of the tegmentum, and pyramidal and corticopontine tracts of the basis.

Syndromes of Benedikt, Claude, and Nothnagel

For these and other classic eponymic syndromes see Table 2-2, and Liu and colleagues,[172] Seo and colleagues,[173] and Shah and Biller.[174]

TABLE 2-2 **Clinical Syndromes of Midbrain Infarction**

Syndrome	Site of Lesion	Clinical Features
Top of the basilar	Medial-inferior temporo-occipital area, posterior thalamus, rostral midbrain	See The thalamic arteries: origin, distribution, and syndromes of occlusion. Rostral basilar artery syndrome (top of the basilar syndrome)
Pretectal	Junction of mesencephalic tectum and diencephalon	See The vertebrobasilar arteries: origin, distribution, and syndromes of occlusion. The midbrain: syndromes of basilar and posterior cerebral artery occlusion. The rostral-dorsal midbrain or pretectal syndrome
Parinaud	Superior colliculus-pretectum-riMLF	Paralysis of upward gaze, often with pupillary paralysis
Benedikt	Mesencephalic tegmentum, affecting CN III, brachium conjunctivum–red nucleus region	Ipsilateral third nerve palsy and contralateral movement disorder: intention tremor, hemichorea, and hemiathetosis
Nothnagel	Tectum—extending to third nerve nucleus	Bilateral third nerve palsies, varying in degree and symmetry, gait ataxia[171]
Foville	Interruption of horizontal gaze fibers in cerebral peduncle	Paralysis of horizontal conjugate gaze to the opposite side
Claude	Brachium conjunctivum just caudal and medial to the red nucleus	Ipsilateral third nerve palsy, often partial, with pupillary sparing and contralateral cerebellar signs[171,172]
Weber	Midbrain basis plus intra-axial course of CN III	Ipsilateral third nerve palsy, and contralateral hemiplegia
Locked-in	Complete bilateral interruption of the pyramidal tracts at the capsular, midbrain, or much more commonly in the pontine basis	See Table 2-3

Locked-in Syndrome

Complete bilateral interruption of the pyramidal tracts in the brainstem basis, sparing the tegmentum and reticular activating system, may cause a locked-in syndrome (see Pons: Syndromes of Basilar Artery Occlusion, later).

Top of the Basilar Syndrome

For a description of the full syndrome, see The thalamic arteries: origin, distribution, and syndromes of occlusion. Rostral basilar artery syndrome (top of the basilar syndrome), earlier.

Pons: Syndromes of Basilar Artery Occlusion

Arterial Distribution Pattern

Median-paramedian perforators from the BA irrigate the medial part of the basis pontis and tegmentum. Short circumferential branches irrigate lateral parts of the basis and middle cerebellar peduncle. Long circumferentials, the SCA and AICA (see The arteries of the cerebellum and medulla oblongata: origin distribution, and syndromes of occlusion, later), irrigate the lateral parts of the middle cerebellar peduncle, lateral part of the tegmentum, and the tectum (see Fig. 2-37).

Alternating Long Tract Signs and Cranial Nerve Palsies

Because of the proximity of motor and sensory nuclei and pathways, pontine infarcts cause multiple clinical signs. These signs result from involvement of CN V rostrally or the motor nuclei or intra-axial course of CNs VI and VII caudally; the conjugate gaze center in the paramedian pontine reticular formation; the MLF, medial and trigeminal lemnisci, superior olivary nuclei, and lateral lemnisci; the central tegmental tract; the cerebellar peduncles; and the pyramidal

TABLE 2-3 **Clinical Syndromes of Pontine Infarction**

Syndrome	Site of Lesion	Clinical Features
Basis Pontis Only		
Locked-in syndrome = de-efferented state	Large bilateral infarction of basis pontis completely interrupts both pyramidal tracts	Complete double hemiplegia, including the face, with aphonia-aphagia, but sparing of consciousness and vertical eye movements
Pure hemiplegia	Restricted to pyramidal tract	Hemiplegia without other signs
Ataxic-hemiparesis	Unilateral infarction, usually in caudal basis pontis	Hemiparesis worse in leg, ataxia of the arm
Dysarthria-clumsy hand	Unilateral infarction in rostral part of basis pontis	Dysarthria, dysphagia, contralateral UMN facial palsy, and ataxic paresis of the hand
Raymond	Unilateral infarction in caudal basis pontis	Ipsilateral palsy of CN VI and contralateral hemiplegia
Millard-Gubler	Unilateral infarction in caudal basis pontis	Ipsilateral palsy of CNs VI and VII and contralateral hemiplegia
Basis Pontis plus Tegmentum		
Foville	Caudal tegmentum, paramedian reticular formation, and basis pontis	Ipsilateral peripheral palsy of CN VII, paralysis of conjugate gaze ipsilaterally, contralateral hemiplegia, facial sparing
Marie-Foix	Lateral, in brachium pontis, basis, and tegmentum	Ipsilateral ataxia, contralateral hemiparesis and sensory loss
Raymond-Cestain-Chenais	Rostral tegmentum, lemnisci, brachium conjunctivum; may extend into cerebellum and basis	Ipsilateral ataxia with coarse, "rubral" tremor at rest and during movement, paralysis of conjugate lateral eye movements, contralateral reduction of somatic sensory modalities, may have contralateral hemiparesis
Pontine Tegmentum		
Internuclear ophthalmoplegia (MLF syndrome)	Selective infarction of MLF	Ipsilateral paralysis of adducting eye on volitional lateral gaze, with monocular nystagmus of abducting eye
One-and-a-half syndrome	Infarction of paramedian pontine reticular formation	Paralysis of ipsilateral conjugate lateral gaze and preserved abduction of opposite eye on attempted contralateral gaze

tracts. Classic pontine syndromes with a cranial nerve palsy on one side and a long tract sign on the other are uncommon, but strongly localizing (Table 2-3).

Combinations of Hemiparesis, Ataxia, and Dysarthria

Unilateral ventromedial and ventrolateral infarcts of the basis pontis cause combinations of hemiparesis, ataxic hemiparesis, dysarthria,[39] dysarthria–clumsy hand syndrome, and dysarthria–facial palsy.[175] Interruption of the pyramidal tract at levels higher than the pons, including the corona radiata, may cause similar combinations of motor signs. The hemiparesis may differentially affect the proximal or distal muscles and sometimes the leg more than the arm. Dysarthria is more common with left-sided pontine lesions, as with left-sided cerebellar lesions.

Tegmental plus Basis Pontis Infarction

Tegmental infarction accompanies infarction of the pontine basis about three fourths of the time. These tegmental lesions add lemniscal sensory deficits; LMN palsies of CNs V, VI, or VII; internuclear ophthalmoplegia; conjugate gaze paralysis; and the one-and-a-half syndrome (see Table 2-3). Isolated, tiny tegmental lesions may affect only the MLF,[176] but Bassetti and colleagues[175] did not find isolated medial tegmental or extreme lateral tegmental infarcts without extensive vertebrobasilar occlusion.

Locked-in Syndrome

Bilateral infarction of the basis pontis completely interrupts both pyramidal tracts.[13] The patient is completely paralyzed except for vertical eye movements and sometimes eye blinking, but remains conscious.[149] Communication can be established by the patient using upward eye movements as a "Yes" answer. Bilateral infarction of pyramidal tracts at midbrain and the internal capsular levels also may cause a locked-in syndrome.[177]

Palatal Tremor (Myoclonus)

Lesions in the Mollaret triangle between the dentate nucleus, red nucleus, and inferior olivary nucleus may cause palatal tremor at about 60 to 180 beats/min. The triangle consists of the dentatorubral tract to the red nucleus, the central tegmental tract to the inferior olivary nucleus, and the olivocerebellar tract back to the cerebellum.

Miscellaneous Clinical Features

Bassetti and coworkers[175] found that about one third of patients with infarcts confined to the pons had spontaneous laughing and crying spells (*fou rire prodromique*) and tonic limb spasms preceding the onset of hemiparesis. Dissociated emotional and volitional UMN facial palsy also can occur. Warning signs of impending BA occlusion may precede by weeks the onset of severe infarction, and the infarct itself may evolve slowly rather than abruptly.[178] In contrast, pontine gliomas may manifest with an ictal onset because of hemorrhage, rather than a slow progression of signs and symptoms. Magnetic resonance imaging is necessary for correct differential diagnosis.

Arteries of the Cerebellum and Medulla Oblongata

Three long circumferential arteries irrigate the brainstem and cerebellum: the SCA, the AICA, and the PICA. Cerebellar infarctions can affect the irrigation zones of one cerebellar artery, of more than one, or their junction zones.[179,180]

Each of the three cerebellar arteries has a brainstem distribution and a cerebellar distribution. The clinical deficits differ with the artery involved, and whether the infarct affects the brainstem or cerebellar distribution or both. Cardinal deficits common to acute cerebellar lesions are headache, vertigo, vomiting, dysarthria, nystagmus, ataxia, hypotonia, gait imbalance, and loss of verticality (Table 2-4).[13]

The most common and often the major symptom is vertigo.[13,181] Gait examination, especially tandem walking, is the best clinical test for most cerebellar lesions. A completely normal gait argues against any sizable cerebellar infarct,[32] even though silent cerebellar infarctions do occur.[182] Because the specific cerebellar signs appear during volitional movements or volitionally sustained postures, the presence of coma, hemiplegia, or quadriplegia may preclude clinical recognition of the cerebellar infarct.

The selective gait dystaxia from degeneration of the rostral vermis in adult alcoholics[32] does not appear as such in children, but infarcts affecting the vermis cause prominent truncal and gait dystaxia and dysequilibrium. In the postsurgical posterior vermal split syndrome, a disturbance of tandem walking rather than the regular gait or limb dystaxia is the outstanding deficit,[183] whereas hemispheric lesions are expressed by ipsilateral extremity dystaxia.

Initial obtundation and trunk and limb ataxia are more common with infarcts in the SCA zone than in the AICA or PICA zones,[184] but life-threatening delayed obtundation from swelling is more common after PICA infarcts or combined arterial infarcts. Mass effects of swelling from cerebellar infarction or hemorrhage cause upward or downward cerebellar herniation, obstructive hydrocephalus, cardiorespiratory complications, and death, particularly when combined with brainstem infarcts.[13] Surgical decompression of the posterior fossa then becomes lifesaving.[185] Clinical differentiation of cerebellar hemorrhage and infarction requires radiographic imaging.[179] Cerebellar infarcts occur in low-birth-weight infants[186,187] and in children and young adults.

Superior Cerebellar Artery

Origin and Distribution

The SCAs arise symmetrically from the BA just before its terminal bifurcation into the PCAs. CNs III and IV run between the PCA and SCA (see Fig. 2-3). As it encircles the midbrain, the SCA divides into medial (SCAm or mSCA) and lateral (SCAl or lSCA) trunks, or these trunks may arise separately from the BA (Figs. 2-39 and 2-40). The SCA trunks run dorsally superior to and often in contact with the sensory root

TABLE 2-4 **Clinical Syndromes of Cerebellar Infarction**

Cerebellar artery	Site of Lesion	Clinical Syndrome
Acute, large infarct	Dorsolateral brainstem quadrant and cerebellum	Headache, vertigo, vomiting, unsteady gait, dystaxia, dysarthria, nystagmus, saccadic inaccuracy, hypotonia, and crossed sensory loss
	Dorsolateral tegmental area of the caudal midbrain/rostral pons	Ipsilateral Horner syndrome, contralateral pain and temperature loss and sixth nerve palsy with diplopia, sometimes hearing loss
Superior cerebellar artery (SCA)	Cerebellum, superior half	Dysarthria, ipsilateral dysmetria/ataxia, nystagmus, saccadic errors
Medial SCA zone (mSCA)	Predominantly vermis	Dysarthria, ataxia
Lateral SCA zone (lSCA)	Paravermian region	Relatively pure gait/truncal dystaxia
	Lateral part of hemisphere	May cause isolated dysarthria, particularly with left-sided lesion
		Ipsilateral ataxia and lateropulsion, nystagmus, and dysarthria; no brainstem signs or sensory loss
Anterior inferior cerebellar artery (AICA)	Cerebellopontine junction	Vertigo, vomiting, tinnitus, ipsilateral deafness and facial palsy; sometimes isolated vertigo if just IAA affected
	Caudolateral area of the pontine tegmentum	Ipsilateral Horner syndrome, trigeminal sensory loss; may have ipsilateral conjugate gaze palsy, somnolence; contralateral pain and temperature pain loss
	Middle peduncle/cerebellum	Ataxia, dysarthria; patient may have only cerebellar signs if lesion restricted
Posterior inferior cerebellar artery (PICA)	Dorsolateral medullary wedge	Vertigo, headache, vomiting, and ataxia, crossed sensory loss
Medial PICA zone (mPICA)	Cerebellum	Wallenberg syndrome; see Table 2-5
Lateral PICA zone (lPICA)	Lateral part of cerebellar hemisphere	Isolated vertigo or vertigo with dysmetria and ipsilateral lateropulsion and ataxia
		Ipsilateral limb ataxia and gait unsteadiness without vertigo or dysarthria[126]

Note: Large cerebellar infarcts, particularly in PICA or combined distributions, may cause cerebellar swelling and delayed coma (pseudotumoral form). Surgical decompression or ventriculostomy is lifesaving.

of CN V. Microvascular decompression at this site of contact is one method of treating trigeminal neuralgia.

At the brainstem, the SCA supplants, in rostrocaudal order, the quadrigeminal artery from the PCA (see Fig. 2-37). The quadrigeminal artery irrigates the rostralmost transverse wafer of the mesencephalon, at the level of the superior quadrigeminal body (see Fig. 2-37). The SCA irrigates the transverse wafer extending from the level of the inferior quadrigeminal body into the rostral pons. Included in the dorsolateral quadrant of this sector of the caudal midbrain and rostral pons are the superior cerebellar peduncle (see Fig. 2-37), the ipsilateral fourth CN nucleus (with contralateral superior oblique palsy), the lemnisci, and the descending sympathetic pupillodilator pathway. After clearing the brainstem, the SCA irrigates the half of the cerebellum above the plane of the great horizontal fissure (see Figs. 2-39 and 2-40).

The lateral branch of the SCA (lSCA), also called the marginal branch, enters the horizontal fissure of the cerebellum and irrigates the margin around the periphery of a cerebellar hemisphere. The medial or vermian branch (mSCA) continues medially along the superior edge of the cerebellum. It gives off one or more intermediate hemispheric branches for the part of the cerebellum between the lSCA and the vermis (see Fig. 2-39). Near the midline, the mSCA turns sharply back over the vermis. It anastomoses with the opposite vermian

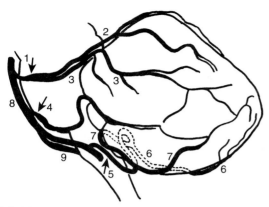

FIGURE 2-39 Lateral drawing of the brainstem and cerebellum showing the superior, anterior inferior, and posterior inferior cerebellar arteries. 1, SCA; 2, medial branch of SCA; 3, lateral branch of SCA; 4, AICA; 5, PICA; 6, medial branch of PICA; 7, lateral branch of PICA; 8, basilar artery; 9, vertebral artery. (From Amarenco P. Cerebellar stroke syndromes. In Bogousslavsky J, Caplan L, eds. Stroke Syndromes, 2nd ed. New York: Cambridge University Press, 2001.)

branch and with the vermian branch of the PICA. The internal branches of the SCA extend through the deep white matter to reach the interpositus and fastigial nuclei and most of the dentate nucleus. The PICA irrigates the remainder of the dentate nucleus.

Syndromes of Superior Cerebellar Artery Occlusion

Although the classic or complete SCA syndrome includes brainstem and cerebellar signs, cerebellar signs are much more prominent than brainstem signs in SCA occlusions. The classic syndrome consists of ipsilateral limb dysmetria, ipsilateral Horner syndrome, contralateral pain and temperature loss, and contralateral superior oblique palsy (Table 2-5).[188] Less commonly, the patient experiences loss of hearing, presumably from interruption of the lateral lemniscus; sleep disturbances from destruction of the locus coeruleus; and sometimes undulating tremor.

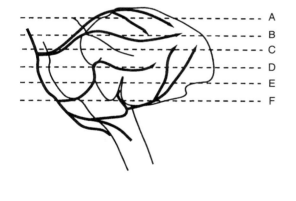

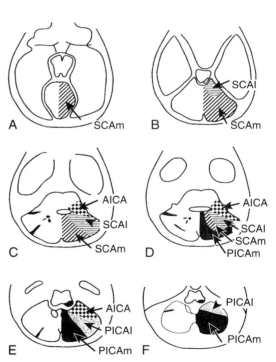

FIGURE 2-40 **A-F,** Templates of the distribution of the cerebellar arteries. *Left,* Lateral view of the cerebellum and brainstem showing the levels depicted on the right. *Right,* Axial views of the brainstem and cerebellum. AICA, anterior inferior cerebellar artery territory; PICAl and PICAm, lateral and medial posterior inferior cerebellar artery territory; SCAl and SCAm, lateral and medial superior cerebellar artery territory. (From Hommel M, Besson G. Brainstem and cerebellar infarcts. In Ginsburg MD, Bogousslavsky J, eds. Cerebrovascular Disease: Pathophysiology, Diagnosis, and Management, Vol II. Malden, MA: Blackwell Science, 1998.)

TABLE 2-5   **Neuroanatomic Correlation of Symptoms and Signs of the Lateral Medullary Wedge Syndrome of Wallenberg***

Symptom or Sign	Structure Involved
Ipsilateral	
Facial pain, dysesthesia or anesthesia, reduced corneal reflex	Descending root of CN V
Dysphagia and dysarthria	CN IX or X, or nucleus ambiguus
Paralysis of palatal elevation, pharyngeal constrictors, and vocal cord	
Ataxia, dysmetria, intention tremor, hypotonia	Spinocerebellar tracts and cerebellar hemisphere
Horner syndrome of miosis and anhidrosis of the face	Descending sympathetic tract in lateral reticular formation
Nystagmus	Vestibular pathways
Ipsilesional lateropulsion tract	Vestibulospinal or dorsal spinocerebellar
Contralateral	
Loss of pain and temperature	Lateral spinothalamic tract
Nonlateralized symptoms	
Nausea, vomiting, vertigo, and hiccoughing	Reticular formation and vestibular nuclei

*See also Figure 2-42.

Isolated cerebellar infarcts that cause dysarthria are in the SCA territory, usually on the left, whereas extracerebellar infarcts that cause dysarthria involve the corticobulbar tract.[39] Occlusion of the mSCA with infarction of the vermis may lead mainly to gait ataxia in keeping with other vermian lesions. Infarction in the PCA distribution often accompanies SCA infarction.

Anterior Inferior Cerebellar Artery

Origin

The AICA arises from the BA, just rostral to the union of the VAs to form the BA. The AICA runs laterally, just caudal to CN VI. It shows two common variations:

- Equal right and left origins from the BA, with a major anastomosis between the AICA and the PICA (Fig. 2-41)
- AICA dominant on the left and PICA dominant on the right. With a left dominant AICA, the ipsilateral VA and PICA are usually hypoplastic (see Fig. 2-41).[189]

Course and Distribution

The AICA runs laterally to irrigate the ventrolateral pons, essentially the caudal part of the middle cerebellar peduncle, which is its core distribution; the spinothalamic tract; the trigeminal, facial, vestibular, and cochlear nuclei; the roots of CN VII and VIII; and the ventral parts of the cerebellum, including the flocculus. Typically, the AICA

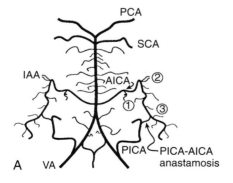

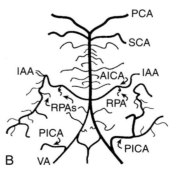

FIGURE 2-41 Variations of the anterior inferior cerebellar arteries and posterior inferior cerebellar arteries. **A,** PICA anastomoses with IAA, and both irrigate the inferior surface of the cerebellum. **B,** PICA has no anastomosis with IAA, but IAA irrigates much of PICA's territory on one side (viewer's left). RPA, recurrent penetrating arteries. For other abbreviations, see Key Terms. (From Oas JG, Baloh RW. Vertigo and the anterior inferior cerebellar artery syndrome. Neurology 1992;42:2274.)

also gives rise to an IAA that enters the internal acoustic meatus (see internal auditory artery (IAA), infra). The AICA acts as the artery of the cerebellopontine angle.[190]

As seen ventrally, the AICA irrigates a triangle with its base toward the midline, where it abuts on the paramedian zone irrigated by perforators from the BA and VA (see Fig. 2-8A). Its cerebellar territory borders on and is reciprocal in size with the territories of the SCA and PICA. When the PICA is missing, the territory of the AICA includes the territory of the PICA (see Fig. 2-41). The AICA also may reciprocate with SCA.

Comparison of Anterior Inferior Cerebellar Artery and Superior Cerebellar Artery Infarcts

AICA infarcts most consistently involve the lateral pons and the middle cerebellar peduncle,[191] often sparing the cerebellum itself, in contrast to SCA infarction, which predominantly affects the cerebellum, sparing the brainstem.

Syndrome of Anterior Inferior Cerebellar Artery Occlusion

The findings reflect involvement of the peripheral nervous system and CNS structures at the cerebellopontine angle. Usual symptoms are nausea, vertigo, tinnitus, and hearing loss.[189,192,193] Other features include vomiting, ipsilateral facial numbness, facial palsy, Horner syndrome, and contralateral loss of pain and temperature. Ipsilateral conjugate gaze palsy may reflect infarction of the flocculus (see Table 2-5).

Internal Auditory Artery

Origin

The IAA usually originates from the AICA, but may arise from the BA rostral to AICA (see Fig. 2-41).

Course, Distribution, and Syndromes of Occlusion

The IAA enters the internal acoustic meatus with CNs VII and VIII, which it irrigates. Because the IAA irrigates the middle ear

without collaterals, AICA or IAA occlusion or insufficiency causes vertigo and deafness (see Table 2-5).[194] Occasionally, isolated vertigo occurs if the IAA territory alone is affected. VA insufficiency may cause attacks of vertigo, tinnitus, and ataxia.[195]

Posterior Inferior Cerebellar Artery

Origin

The two PICAs may arise symmetrically from the VAs, or one may arise from the AICA, combining the territories of the AICA and the PICA (see Figs. 2-3, 2-39, and 2-41).

Course and Distribution

The PICA takes a redundant, looping course on the lateral aspect of the medulla. The caudal loop (#5 in Fig. 2-39) may dip down through the foramen magnum. The PICA usually irrigates the half of the cerebellum below the plane of the great horizontal fissure. A few direct branches may irrigate the dorsolateral region of the medulla (the lateral medullary wedge). PICA infarcts can affect the cerebellum or the lateral medullary wedge or both. Infarction of both areas causes the full Wallenberg syndrome (see later).

On reaching the dorsum of the medulla, the PICA divides into two main branches: the vermian or medial branch and the tonsillar-hemispheric or lateral branch (see Fig. 2-40). The PICA also supplies the dorsal part of the medulla via the posterior spinal or DLspA (see Figs. 2-37 and 2-38A).

The vermian or medial branch of the PICA supplies the inferior part of the vermis, including the nodule, the adjacent paramedian parts of the cerebellar hemispheres, and the choroid plexus of the fourth ventricle. The artery curves upward over the pyramid of vermis, sometimes as far as the declive, and anastomoses with the mSCA. Infarcts of the medial branch of the PICA can result in isolated vertigo, which can be confused with IAA insufficiency or labyrinthitis.[179,181] One PICA may supply the territory of both medial PICAs.[196]

The lateral, tonsillar-hemispheric branch of the PICA descends on the posteromedial aspect of the tonsil and divides into its tonsillar and hemispheric branches. The hemispheric rami proceed posterolaterally to supply the parts of the cerebellar hemisphere below (ventral to) the plane of the horizontal fissure (see Fig. 2-40).[126,179] Occlusion of only the lateral branch territory of the PICA does not cause dysarthria or impair eye movements.[182]

Wallenberg Syndrome or Lateral Medullary Wedge Syndrome

Branches from the VA or, less commonly, the PICA irrigate the lateral medullary wedge (Fig. 2-42; see Table 2-5). The PICA also may send branches to the dorsum of the medulla that correspond to the DLspAs that irrigate the dorsal part of the spinal cord (see Figs. 2-5, 2-37, and 2-38). Involvement of the ipsilateral DLSAs that arise from the VA or PICA may account for ipsilateral sensory loss from infarction of the ipsilateral dorsal column nuclei[41] as a component of the lateral medullary wedge syndrome. Likewise, an ipsilateral hemiplegia may occur because of infarction of the pyramidal tract at or just after its decussation.[197]

Ipsilesional lateropulsion is often prominent and disabling in PICA infarction.[198] Occasionally, patients with a lateral medullary wedge infarct have wild, flinging movements of the extremities during volitional movements.[199]

Median-Paramedian Arteries of the Medulla and the Medial Medullary Syndromes of Dejerine, Babinski-Nageotte, and Opalski

In the classic unilateral medial medullary syndrome of Dejerine, in the caudalmost medulla, the VspAs give off paramedian arteries for the pyramidal tracts, but more rostrally, the VAs give off the paramedian branches. The usual site of occlusion or stenosis is the distal VA, just before joining to form the BA.[200] The paramedian arteries irrigate the pyramidal tract and overlying medial lemniscus, which is vertical in the medulla, and the MLF, which caps the medial lemniscus (see Fig. 2-38A-C). CN XII runs along the margin of the paramedian zone (see Fig. 2-42A).

The clinical features of the medial medullary syndrome of Dejerine are contralateral, initially flaccid, but then spastic hemiparesis and sensory loss of dorsal column type in the arms and legs[201] and often severe dysphagia. Correct management of dysphagia

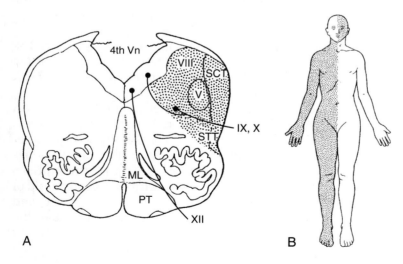

A   B

FIGURE 2-42 **Wallenberg syndrome showing the cruciate face-body areas of sensory loss after medullary lesions. A,** Transverse section of the medulla showing the lesion site (*dots*) for Wallenberg lateral medullary wedge syndrome. **B,** Interruption of the descending root of CN V causes ipsilateral loss of pain and temperature on the face. Interruption of the spinothalamic tract (STT) causes contralateral loss of pain and temperature sensation. See Table 2-5 for a summary of the syndrome. ML, medial lemniscus; PT, pyramidal tract; SCT, spinocerebellar tracts; STT, spinothalamic tract; Vn, ventricle; V, descending nucleus and root of CN V; VIII, vestibular nuclei; IX, X, nucleus ambiguus for CNs IX and X; XII, CN XII. (From DeMyer W. Technique of the Neurologic Examination: A Programmed Text, 5th ed. New York: McGraw-Hill, 2004.)

depends on differentiating medial medullary infarction from lateral medullary infarction.[202] Because the leg fibers run in the ventral part of the medial lemniscus, just dorsal to the pyramidal tract, sensory loss in the leg may be more severe than in the arm. The hemiparesis usually excludes the face, but facial palsy may occur in patients whose UMN fibers for the face swing down into the medulla and recurve rostrally onto the pons to reach the seventh nerve nucleus.[200,203] Sometimes ipsilateral LMN tongue weakness occurs because of the paramedian intra-axial course of CN XII and its conjunction with the lateral edge of the pyramidal tract (see Fig. 2-42). UMN tongue paralysis also may occur with medial medullary infarction.[204] Isolated bilateral tongue paralysis may be the only manifestation of medial medullary infarction.[205] Some patients have vertical nystagmus[201] or other eye movement disorders.[206] Bilateral medial medullary infarction leads to double hemiplegia[207] and often respiratory failure and death.

The Babinski-Nageotte syndrome is caused by hemimedullary infarction and combines the medial medullary and the lateral medullary syndromes. The submedullary syndrome of Opalski is caused by VA occlusion with extensive infarction of the cervicomedullary junction. The patient has the lateral medullary wedge syndrome plus ipsilateral hemiplegia because of infarction of the pyramidal tract after its decussation.[197] The lesion also may affect the ipsilateral dorsal column nuclei. In hemiplegia cruciata, the patient has contralateral paresis of the arm and ipsilateral paresis of the leg from involvement of one set of corticospinal fibers before crossing and the other after crossing at the cervicomedullary junction.[208]

The syndromes listed here under: The median-paramedian arteries of the medulla and the medial medullary syndromes of Dejerine, Babinski-Nageotte and Opalski are very rare.

REFERENCES

1. Garg P, Edwards-Brown MK. Vertebral artery compression due to head rotation in thalamic stroke. Pediatr Neurol 1995;12:162.
2. Garg BP, Durocher A, Biller J. Strokes in children and young adults. In Ginsburg MD, Bogousslavsky J, eds. Cerebrovascular Disease: Pathophysiology, Diagnosis, and Management, Vol II. Malden, MA: Blackwell Science, 1998.
3. McCormick W. Vascular diseases of nervous tissue: anomalies, malformations, and aneurysms. In Bourne G, ed. The Structure and Function of Nervous Tissue, Vol 3. New York: Academic Press, 1970.
4. Riggs HE, Rupp C. Variation in form of the circle of Willis: the relation of the variations to collateral circulation: anatomic analysis. Arch Neurol 1963;8:24.
5. Bogousslavsky J, Regli F. Centrum semiovale infarcts: subcortical infarction in the superficial territory of the middle cerebral artery. Neurology 1992;42:1992.
6. Donnan G, Norrving B, Bamford J, et al, eds. Subcortical Stroke, 2nd ed. New York: Oxford University Press, 2002.
7. Duvernoy HM, Delon S, Vannson JL. Cortical blood vessels of the human brain. Brain Res Bull 1981;7:519.
8. Hupperts RMM, Lodder J. Anterior choroidal artery territory infarcts. In Ginsberg M, Bogousslavsky J, eds. Cerebrovascular Disease: Pathophysiology, Diagnosis, and Management, Vol II. Malden, MA: Blackwell Science, 1998.
9. Neu J-P, Bogousslavsky J. Centrum semiovale infarcts: subcortical infarction in the superficial territory of the middle cerebral artery. In Bogousslavsky J, Caplan L, eds. Stroke Syndromes, 2nd ed. New York: Cambridge University Press, 2001.
10. Parkinson D. Collateral circulation of cavernous carotid artery: anatomy. Can J Surg 1964;7:251.
11. Fischer-Brügge E. Die Lageabweichungen der vordern Hirnarterie im Gefässbild. Zentalbl Neurochir 1938;3:300.
12. Bogousslavsky J, Caplan L, eds. Stroke Syndromes, 2nd ed. New York: Cambridge University Press, 2001.
13. Brazis PW, Masdeu JC, Biller J. Localization in Clinical Neurology, 5th ed. Philadelphia: Lippincott Williams & Wilkins, 2007.
14. Cucchiara B, Kasner SE, Wolk DA, et al. Lack of hemispheric dominance for consciousness in acute ischemic stroke. J Neurol Neurosurg Psychiatry 2003;74:889.
15. Schiffter R. Telodiencephalic ischemic syndrome. Arch Neurol 1987;44:1218.
16. Brust JCM, Sawada T, Kazui S. Anterior cerebral artery. In Bogousslavsky J, Caplan L, eds. Stroke Syndromes, 2nd ed. New York: Cambridge University Press, 2001.
17. Perlmutter D, Rhoton AL. Microsurgical anatomy of the distal anterior cerebral artery. J Neurosurg 1978;49:204.
18. Andrew J, Nathan PW, Spanos NC. Disturbances of micturition and defaecation due to aneurysms of anterior communicating or anterior cerebral arteries. Brain 1965;88:1.
19. Kuntzer T, Waeber B. Muscle, peripheral nerve and autonomic changes. In Bogousslavsky J,

Caplan L, eds. Stroke Syndromes, 2nd ed. New York: Cambridge University Press, 2001.

20. Sakakibara R, Hattori T, Yasuda K, et al. Micturitional disturbance after acute hemispheric stroke: analysis of the lesion site by CT and MRI. J Neurol Scie 1996;137:47.

21. Klatka LA, Depper MH, AM Marini. Infarction in the territory of the anterior cerebral artery. Neurology 1998;51:620.

22. Bogousslavsky J, Martin R, Moulin T. Homolateral ataxia and crural paresis: a syndrome of anterior cerebral artery territory infarction. J Neurol Neurosurg Psychiatry 1992;55:1146.

23. Schneider R, Gautier JC. Leg weakness due to stroke: site of lesions, weakness patterns, and causes. Brain 1994;117:347.

24. McNabb AW, Carroll WM, Mastaglia FL. "Alien hand" and loss of bimanual coordination after dominant anterior cerebral artery infarction. J Neurol Neurosurg Psychiatry 1988;51:218.

25. Krainik A, Lehéricy S, Duffau H, et al. Role of the supplementary motor area in motor deficit following medial frontal lobe surgery. Neurology 2001;57:871.

26. Bogousslavsky J, Regli F. Anterior cerebral artery territory infarction in the Lausanne stroke registry: clinical and etiologic patterns. Arch Neurol 1990;47:144.

27. Della Sala S, Francescani A, Spinnler H. Gait apraxia after bilateral supplementary motor area lesions. J Neurol Neurosurg Psychiatry 2002;72:77.

28. Gibo H, Carver CC, Rhoton AL, et al. Microsurgical anatomy of the middle cerebral artery. J Neurosurg 1981;54:151.

29. Saver JL, Biller J. Superficial middle cerebral artery. In Bogousslavsky J, Caplan LR, eds. Stroke Syndromes. New York: Cambridge University Press, 1995.

30. Osborn AG. Diagnostic Cerebral Angiography, 2nd ed. St. Louis: Mosby, 1999.

31. Huber P. Krayenbuhl/Yasargil Cerebral Angiography, 2nd ed. New York: Georg Thieme Verlag, 1982.

32. DeMyer W. Technique of the Neurologic Examination: A Programmed Text, 5th ed. New York: McGraw-Hill, 2004.

33. Ghika-Schmid F, Bogousslavsky J. Disorders of mood behaviour. In Bogousslavsky J, Caplan L, eds. Stroke Syndromes, 2nd ed. New York: Cambridge University Press, 2001.

34. de Freitas GR, Devuyst G, van Melle G, et al. Motor strokes sparing the leg: different lesions and causes. Arch Neurol 2000;57:513.

35. Gass A, Szabo K, Behrens S, et al. A diffusion-weighted MRI study of acute ischemic distal arm paresis. Neurology 2001;57:1589.

36. Kim JS, Chung JP, Ha SW. Isolated weakness of index finger due to small cortical infarction. Neurology 2002;59:985.

37. Takahashi N, Kawamura M, Araki S. Isolated hand palsy due to cortical infarction: localization of the motor hand area. Neurology 2002;58:1412.

38. Noda K, Miwa H, Miyashita N, et al. Monoataxia of upper extremity in motor cortical infarction. Neurology 2001;56:1418.

39. Urban PP, Wicht S, Vukurevic G, et al. Dysarthria in acute ischemic stroke: lesion topography, clinicoradiologic correlation, and etiology. Neurology 2001;56:1021.

40. Kim JS. Sensory abnormality. In Bogousslavsky J, Caplan L, eds. Stroke Syndromes. New York: Cambridge University Press, 2001.

41. Kim JS. Sensory symptoms in ipsilateral limbs/body due to lateral medullary infarction. Neurology 2001;57:1230.

42. Freund H-J, Hummelsheim H. Lesions of the premotor cortex in man. Brain 1985;108:697.

43. Golomb MR, Ibrahim S, deVeber G. A 15 year old boy with central nervous system vasculopathy presenting with dysarthria-clumsy hand syndrome. J Child Neurol 2002;17:241.

44. Heimberger R, DeMyer W, Reitan R. Implications of Gerstmann's syndrome. J Neurol Neurosurg Psychiatry 1964;27:52.

45. Besson G, Bogousslavsky J, Regli F, et al. Acute pseudobulbar or suprabulbar palsy. Arch Neurol 1991;48:501.

46. Grattan-Smith PJ, Hopkins IJ, Boldt DW. Acute pseudobulbar palsy due to bilateral focal cortical damage: the opercular syndrome of Foix-Chavagny-Marie. J Child Neurol 1989;4:131.

47. Mao C-C, Coull BM, Golper LAC, et al. Anterior opercular syndrome. Neurology 1989;39:1169.

48. Manes F, Paradiso S, Springer JA, et al. Neglect after right insular cortex infarction. Stroke 1999;30:946.

49. Manes F, Springer J, Jorge R, et al. Verbal memory impairment after left insular cortex infarction. J Neurol Neurosurg Psychiatry 1999;67:532.

50. Christen H-J, Hanefeld F, Kruse E, et al. Foix-Chavany-Marie (anterior operculum) syndrome in childhood: a reappraisal of Worster-Drought syndrome. Dev Med Child Neurol 2000;42:122.

51. Gordon N. Worster-Drought and congenital bilateral perisylvian syndromes. Dev Med Child Neurol 2002;44:201.

52. Worster-Drought C. Suprabulbar paresis: congenital suprabulbar paresis and its differential diagnosis, with special reference to acquired suprabulbar paresis. Dev Med Child Neurol 1974;16(suppl 30):1-33.

53. Williams DJ. The origin of the posterior cerebral artery. Brain 1936;59:175.

54. Margolis MT, Newton TH, Hoyt WF. The posterior cerebral artery, Section II: gross and roengtenographic anatomy. In Newton TH, Potts DG, eds. Radiology of the Skull and Brain: Angiography. St. Louis: CV Mosby, 1974.

55. Chambers B, Brooder R, Donnan G. Proximal posterior cerebral artery occlusion simulating middle cerebral artery occlusion. Neurology 1991;41:385.

56. Georgiadis AL, Yamamoto Y, Kwan ES, et al. Anatomy of sensory findings in patients with posterior cerebral artery territory infarction. Arch Neurol 1999;56:835.

57. Lepore FE. The preserved temporal crescent: the clinical implications of an "endangered" finding. Neurology 2001;57:1918.

58. Cole M. When the left brain is not the right brain may be left: report of personal experience of occipital hemianopia. J Neurol Neurosurg Psychiatry 1999;67:169.

59. Wada Y, Yamamoto T. Selective impairment of facial recognition due to a hematoma restricted to the right fusiform and lateral occipital region. J Neurol Neurosurg Psychiatry 2001;71:254.

60. Gillen JA, Dutton GN. Balint's syndrome in a 10-year old male. Dev Med Child Neurol 2003;45:349.

61. Rizzo M, Vecera SP. Psychoanatomical substrates of Balint's syndrome. J Neurol Neurosurg Psychiatry 2002;72:162.

62. Brower MC, Rollins N, Roach ES. Basal ganglia and thalamic infarction in children: cause and clinical features. Arch Neurol 1996;53:1252.

63. Garg BP, DeMyer WE. Ischemic thalamic infarction in children: clinical presentation, etiology, and outcome. Pediatr Neurol 1995;13:46.

64. Wallesch C-W, Kornhuber HH, Brunner RJ, et al. Lesions of the basal ganglia, thalamus, and deep white matter: differential effects on language function. Brain Language 1983;20:286.

65. Frimm B, Zahn R, Mull M, et al. Asymmetries of visual attention after circumscribed subcortical vascular lesions. J Neurol Neurosurg Psychiatry 2001;71:652.

66. Challa VR, Moody DM, Bell MA. The Charcôt-Bouchard aneurysm controversy: impact of a new histologic technique. J Neuropathol Exp Neurol 1992;51:264.

67. Fisher CM. Hypertensive cerebral hemorrhage: demonstration of the source of bleeding. J Neurol Neurosurg Psychiatry 2003;62:104.

68. Avci EW, Fossett D, Aslan M, et al. Branches of the anterior cerebral artery near the anterior communicating artery complex: an anatomic study and surgical perspective. Neurol Med Chir (Tokyo) 2003;43:329.

69. Dunker PO, Harris AB. Surgical anatomy of the proximal anterior cerebral artery. J Neurosurg 1976;44:359.

70. Perlmutter D, Rhoton AL. Microsurgical anatomy of the anterior cerebral–anterior communicating–recurrent artery complex. J Neurosurg 1976;45:259.

71. Vasquez-Loayza M, Dujovny M, Agner C, et al. Microsurgical anatomy of the short central artery. Neurol Res 1998;20:209.

72. Grand W, Hopkins LN. Vasculature of the Brain and Cranial Base: Variations in Clinical Anatomy. New York: Thieme, 1999.

73. Alexander MP, Freedman M. Amnesia after anterior communicating artery aneurysm rupture. Neurology 1984;34:752.

74. Hashimoto R, Tanaka Y, Nakano I. Amnesic confabulatory syndrome after focal basal forebrain damage. Neurology 2000;54:978.

75. Moudgil SS, Azzouz M, Al-Azzaz A, et al. Amnesia due to fornix infarction. Stroke 2000;31:1418.

76. Türe U, Yaşargil Krist AF. The arteries of the corpus callosum: a microsurgical anatomic study. Neurosurgery 1996;39:1075.

77. Abe K, Inokawa M, Kashiwagi A, et al. Amnesia after a discrete basal forebrain lesion. J Neurol Neurosurg Psychiatry 1998;65:126.

78. Park SA, Hahn JH, Kim JI, et al. Memory deficits after bilateral anterior fornix infarction. Neurology 2000;54:1379.

79. Goldenberg C, Schuri U, Grömminger O, et al. Basal forebrain amnesia: Does the nucleus accumbens contribute to human memory? J Neurol Neurosurg Psychiatry 1999;67:163.

80. Gomes F, Dujovny M, Umansky F, et al. Microsurgical anatomy of the recurrent artery of Heubner. J Neurosurg 1984;60:130.

81. Loukas M, Louis RG, Childs RS. Anatomical examination of the recurrent artery of Heubner. Clin Anat 2006;19:25.

82. Takahashi S, Goto K, Fukasawa H, et al. Computed tomography of cerebral infarction along the distribution of the basal perforating arteries, part I: striate arterial group. Radiology 1985;155:107.

83. Feekes JA, Hsu S-W, Chaloupka JC, et al. Tertiary microvascular territories define lacunar infarcts in the basal ganglia. Ann Neurol 2005;58:18.

84. Feekes JA, Cassell MD. The vascular supply of the functional compartments of the human striatum. Brain 2006;129:2189.

85. Marinkovic SV, Milisavljevic MM, Kovacevic MS. Perforating branches of the middle cerebral artery: microanatomy, and clinical significance of their intracerebral segments. Stroke 1985;16:1022.

86. Pullicino P. Lenticulostriate arteries. In Bogousslavsky J, Caplan L, eds. Stroke Syndromes, 2nd ed. New York: Cambridge University Press, 2001.

87. Bladin PF, Berkovic SF. Striatocapsular infarction: large infarcts in the lenticulostriate arterial territory. Neurology 1984;34:1423.

88. Chung C-S, Lee H-S, Caplin LR. Caudate infarcts and hemorrhage. In Bogousslavsky J, Caplan L, eds. Stroke Syndromes, 2nd ed. New York: Cambridge University Press, 2001.

89. Weiller C, Willmes K, Reiche W, et al. The cause of aphasia or neglect after striatocapsular infarction. Brain 1993;116:1509.

90. Starkstein SE, Robinson RG, Berthier ML, et al. Differential mood changes following basal ganglia vs thalamic lesions. Arch Neurol 1988;45:725.

91. Mega MS, Alexander MP. Subcortical aphasia: the core profile of capsulostriatal infarction. Neurology 1994;44:1824.

92. Godefroy O, Rousseaux M, Pruvo JP, et al. Neuropsychological changes related to unilateral lenticulostriate infarcts. J Neurol Neurosurg Psychiatry 1994;57:480.

93. Russmann H, Vingerhoets F, Ghika J, et al. Acute infarction limited to the lenticular nucleus: clinical, etiologic, and topographic features. Arch Neurol 2003;60:351.

94. Giroud M, Lemesle M, Madinier G, et al. Unilateral lenticular infarcts: radiological and clinical syndromes, aetiology, and prognosis. J Neurol Neurosurg Psychiatry 1997;63:611.

95. Münchau A, Mathen D, Cox T, et al. Unilateral lesions of the globus pallidus: report of four patients presenting with focal or segmental

dystonia. J Neurol Neurosurg Psychiatry 2000;69: 494.

96. Bogousslavsky J, Regli F. Capsular genu syndrome. Neurology 1990;40:1499.

97. Willoughby EW, Anderson NE. Lower cranial nerve motor function in unilateral vascular lesions of the cerebral hemisphere. BMJ 1984;289:791.

98. Tatemichi TK, Desmond DW, Prohovnik I, et al. Confusion and memory loss from capsular genu infarction: a thalamocortical disconnection syndrome? Neurology 1992;42:1966.

99. Chukwudelunzu FE, Meschia JF, Graff-Radford NR, et al. Extensive metabolic and neuropsychological abnormalities associated with discrete infarction of the genu of the internal capsule. J Neurol Neurosurg Psychiatry 2001;71:658.

100. Yoshimura K, Kurashige T. Age-related changes in the posterior limb of the internal capsule revealed by magnetic resonance imaging. Brain Dev 2000;22:118.

101. Werring DJ, Toosy AT, Clark CA, et al. Diffusion tensor imaging can detect and quantify corticospinal tract degeneration after stroke. J Neurol Neurosurg Psychiatry 2000;69:269.

102. Englander R, Netsky M, Adelman L. Location of the pyramidal tract in the internal capsule: anatomic evidence. Neurology 1975;25:823.

103. Ross E. Localization of the pyramidal tract in the internal capsule by whole brain dissection. Neurology 1980;30:59.

104. Fisher CM. Lacunar strokes and infarcts: a review. Neurology 1982;32:871.

105. Kashihara M, Matsumoto D. Acute capsular infarction: Location of the lesions and the clinical features. Neuroradiology 1985;27:248.

106. Ferro JM. Neurobehavioral aspects of deep hemispheric stroke. In Bogousslavsky J, Caplan L, eds. Stroke Syndromes, 2nd ed. New York: Cambridge University Press, 2001.

107. Watson RT, Valenstein E, Heilman KM. Thalamic neglect: possible role of the medial thalamus and nucleus reticularis in behavior. Arch Neurol 1981;38:501.

108. Tanridag O, Kirshner HS. Aphasia and agraphia in lesions of the posterior internal capsule and putamen. Neurology 1985;35:1797.

109. Rhoton A, Kyotaka F, Fradd B. Microsurgical anatomy of the anterior choroidal artery. Surg Neurol 1979;12:171.

110. Muller J, Shaw L. Arterial vascularization of the human hippocampus. Arch Neurol 1965;13:45.

111. Hupperts RMM, Lodder J, Heuts-van Raak EP, et al. Infarcts in the anterior choroidal artery territory: anatomical distribution, clinical syndromes, presumed pathogenesis and early outcome. Brain 1994;117:825.

112. Vuadens P, Bogousslavsky J. Anterior choroidal artery territory infarcts. In Bogousslavsky J, Caplan L, eds. Stroke Syndromes, 2nd ed. New York: Cambridge University Press, 2001.

113. Percheron G. Arterial supply of thalamus. In Schaltenbrand G, Walker AE, eds. Stereotaxy of the Human Brain. New York: Georg Thieme Verlag, 1982.

114. Plets C, De Reuck J, Vander Eecken H, et al. The vascularization of the human thalamus. Acta Neurol Belg 1970;70:687.

115. Takahashi S, Ishii K, Matsumoto K, et al. The anterior choroidal artery syndrome, II: CT and/or MR in angiographically verified cases. Neuroradiology 1994;36:340.

116. Helgason C, Caplan LR, Goodwin J, et al. Anterior choroidal artery-territory infarction: report of cases and review. Arch Neurol 1986;43:681.

117. Derex L, Ostrowsky K, Nighoghossian N, et al. Severe pathologic crying after left anterior choroidal artery infarct: reversibility with paroxetine treatment. Stroke 1997;28:1464.

118. Neu J-P, Bogousslavsky J. The syndrome of posterior choroidal artery territory infarction. Ann Neurol 1996;39:779.

119. Takahashi S, Goto KL, Fukasawa H, et al. Computed tomography of cerebral infarction along the distribution of the basal perforating arteries, part II: thalamic arterial group. Radiology 1985;155:119.

120. Pullicino PM. Diagrams of perforating artery territories in axial, coronal and sagittal planes. In Pullicino PM, Caplan LR, eds. Advances in Neurology, Vol 62. New York: Raven Press, 1993.

121. Schwarz S, Egelhof T, Schwab S, et al. Basilar artery embolism: clinical syndrome and neuroradiologic patterns in patients without permanent occlusion of the basilar artery. Neurology 1997;49:1346.

122. Schott GD. From thalamic syndrome to central poststroke pain. J Neurol Neurosurg Psychiatry 1995;61:560.

123. Van Der Werf YD, Weerts JGE, Jolles J, et al. Neuropsychological correlates of a right unilateral lacunar thalamic infarction. J Neurosurg Neurol Psychiatry 1999;66:36.

124. Engelborghs S, Marien P, Martin JJ, de Dayn PP. Functional anatomy, vascularization and pathology of the human thalamus. Acta Neurol Belg 1998;98(3):252.

125. Ghika-Schmid F, Bogousslavsky J. The acute behavioral syndrome of anterior thalamic infarction: a prospective study of 12 cases. Ann Neurol 2000;48:220.

126. Barth A, Bogousslavsky J, Regli F. Infarcts in the territory of the lateral branch of the posterior inferior cerebellar artery. J Neurol Neurosurg Psychiatry 1994;57:1073.

127. Biller J, Merchut M, Emanuele M. Nonhemorrhagic infarction of the thalamus. Neurology 1984; 34:1268.

128. Graff-Radford NR, Eslinger PJ, Damasio AR, et al. Nonhemorrhagic infarction of the thalamus: behavioral, anatomic, and physiologic correlates. Neurology 1984;34:14.

129. Bruyn RPM. Thalamic aphasia: a conceptual critique. J Neurol 1989;236:21.

130. Gorelick PB, Hier DB, Benevento L, et al. Aphasia after left thalamic occlusion. Arch Neurol 1984;41:1296.

131. Bogousslavsky J, Regli F, Assal G. The syndrome of unilateral tuberothalamic artery territory infarction. Stroke 1986;17:434.

132. Nadeau SE, Roeltgen DP, Sevush S, et al. Apraxia due to a pathologically documented thalamic infarction. Neurology 1994;44:2133.

133. Malamut BL, Graff-Radford N, Chawluk J, et al. Memory in a case of bilateral thalamic infarction. Neurology 1992;42:163.

134. Weisman D, Hisama FM, Waxman SG, et al. Going deep to cut the link: cortical disconnection syndrome caused by a thalamic lesion. Neurology 2003;60:1865.

135. Caplan LR, Dewitt LD, Pessin MS, et al. Lateral thalamic infarcts. Arch Neurol 1988;45:959.

136. Miwa H, Hatori K, Kondon T, et al. Thalamic tremor. Neurology 1996;46:75.

137. Lehéricy S, Grand S, Pollak P, et al. Clinical characteristics of lesions in movement disorders due to thalamic lesions. Neurology 2001;57:1055.

138. Melo TP, Bogousslavsky J. Hemiataxia-hypesthesia: a thalamic stroke syndrome. J Neurol Neurosurg Psychiatry 1992;55:581.

139. Timmerman L, Ploner M, Freund H-J, et al. Separate representation of static and dynamic touch in human somatosensory thalamus. Neurology 2000;54:2024.

140. Fisher CM. Thalamic pure sensory stoke: a pathologic study. Neurology 1978;28:1141.

141. Dejerine J, Roussy G. Le syndrome thalamique. Rev Neurol 1906;14:521.

142. Saeki N, Rhoton AL. Microsurgical anatomy of the upper basilar artery and the posterior circle of Willis. J Neurosurg 1977;46:563.

143. Castaigne P, Lhermitte F, Bude A, et al. Paramedian thalamic and midbrain infarcts: clinical and neuropathological study. Ann Neurol 1981;10:127.

144. Marinkovic SV, Milisavljevic MM, Kovacevic MS. Anastomoses among the thalamoperforating branches of the posterior cerebral artery. Arch Neurol 1986;43:811.

145. Marinkovic SE, Milisavljevic MM, Marinkovic ZD. Microanatomy and possible clinical significance of anastomoses among hypothalamic arteries. Stroke 1989;20:1341.

146. Charles PD, Fenichel GM. Sneddon and antiphospholipid antibody syndromes causing bilateral thalamic infarction. Pediatr Neurol 1994;10:262.

147. Martinez P-BA, Marti-Masso JF, Carrera N, et al. Variabilidad clinica de los infartos talamicos paramedianos bilaterales. Rev Neurol 1997;25:1353.

148. Bassetti C, Mathis J, Gugger M, et al. Hypersomnia following paramedian thalamic stroke: report of 12 patients. Ann Neurol 1996;39:471.

149. Bassetti C. Disturbances of consciousness and sleep-wake functions. In Bogousslavsky J, Caplan L, eds. Stroke Syndromes, 2nd ed. New York: Cambridge University Press, 2001.

150. Karabelas G, Kalfakis N, Kasvikis I, et al. Unusual features in a case of bilateral paramedian thalamic infarction. J Neurol Neurosurg Psychiatry 1985; 48:186.

151. Meissner I, Sapir S, Kokmen E, et al. The paramedian diencephalic syndrome: a dynamic phenomenon. Stroke 1987;18:380.

152. Eslinger PJ, Warner GC, Gratton LM, et al. 'Frontal lobe' utilization behavior associated with paramedian thalamic infarction. Neurology 1991;41:450.

153. Vinas FC, Lopez F, Dujovny M. Microsurgical anatomy of the posterior choroidal arteries. Neurol Res 1995;17:334.

154. Saeki N, Shimazaki K, Yamaura A. Isolated infarction in the territory of the lateral posterior choroidal arteries. J Neurol Neurosurg Psychiatry 1999;67:413.

155. Zeal AA, Rhoton AL. Microsurgical anatomy of the posterior cerebral artery. J Neurosurg 1978;48:534.

156. Hommel M, Besson G, Pollak P, et al. Hemiplegia in posterior cerebral artery occlusion. Neurology 1990;40:1496.

157. Hommel M, Moreaud O, Besson B, et al. Site of arterial occlusion in the hemiplegic posterior cerebral artery syndrome. Neurology 1991;41:604.

158. Biller J, Shapiro R, Evans LS, et al. Oculomotor nuclear complex infarction. Arch Neurol 1984;41:985.

159. Caplan LR. Syndromes related to large artery thromboembolism within the vertebrobasilar arterial system. In Bogousslavsky J, Caplan LR, eds. Stroke Syndromes, 2nd ed. New York: Cambridge University Press, 2001.

160. Feinberg WM, Rapcsak SZ. "Peduncular hallucinosis" following paramedian thalamic infarction. Neurology 1989;39:1535.

161. Mehler MF. The rostral basilar artery syndrome: diagnosis, etiology, and prognosis. Neurology 1989;39:9.

162. Katz DI, Alexander MP, AM Mandell. Dementia following strokes in the mesencephalon and diencephalon Arch Neurol 1987;44:1127.

163. Gomez CR, Gomez SM, Selhorst JB. Acute thalamic esotropia. Neurology 1988;38:1759.

164. Saposnik G, Caplan LR. Convulsive-like movements in brainstem stroke. Arch Neurol 2001;58: 654.

165. Tatemichi TK, Steinke W, Duncan C, et al. Paramedian thalamopeduncular infarction: clinical syndromes and magnetic resonance imaging. Ann Neurol 1992;32:162.

166. Duvernoy HM. Human Brainstem Vessels: Including the Pineal Gland and Information on Brain Stem Infarction. Berlin: Springer Verlag, 1999.

167. Bogousslavsky J, Maeder P, Regli F, et al. Pure midbrain infarction: clinical syndromes, MRI, and etiologic patterns. Neurology 1994;44:2032.

168. Baloh RW, Furman JM, Yee RD. Dorsal midbrain syndrome: clinical and oculographic findings. Neurology 1985;35:54.

169. Keane JR. The pretectal syndrome. Neurology 1990;40:684.

170. Jacobs L, Herrner RR, Newman RP. Selective paralysis of downward gaze caused by bilateral lesions of the mesencephalic periaqueductal gray matter. Neurology 1985;35:516.

171. Ikeda K, Kuwajima A, Iwasaki Y, et al. Cerebral peduncular infarction. Neurology 2002;59:183.

172. Liu GT, Crenner CW, Logigian EL, et al. Midbrain syndromes of Benedikt, Claude, and Nothnagel: setting the record straight. Neurology 1992;42: 1820.

173. Seo SW, Heo JH, Lee KY, et al. Localization of Claude's syndrome. Neurology 2001;57:2304.
174. Shah MV, Biller J. Rostral brainstem and thalamic infarctions. MedLink Neurology 2003.
175. Bassetti C, Bogousslavsky J, Barth A, et al. Isolated infarcts of the pons. Neurology 1996;46:165.
176. Ross AT, DeMyer WE. Isolated syndrome of the medial longitudinal fasciculus in man: anatomical confirmation. Arch Neurol 1966;15:203.
177. Chia L-G. Locked-in state with internal capsule infarcts. Neurology 1984;34:1365.
178. Von Campe B, Regli F, Bogousslavsky J. Heralding manifestations of basilar artery occlusion with lethal or severe stroke. J Neurol Neurosurg Psychiatry 2003;74:1621.
179. Amarenco P. Cerebellar stroke syndromes. In Bogousslavsky J, Caplan L, eds. Stroke Syndromes, 2nd ed. New York: Cambridge University Press, 2001.
180. Canapale S, Bogousslavsky J. Multiple large and small cerebellar infarcts. J Neurol Neurosurg Psychiatry 1999;66:739.
181. Lee H, Sohn S-I, Chow Y-W, et al. Cerebellar infarction presenting as vertigo: frequency and vascular topographical patterns. Neurology 2006;67:1178.
182. Hommel M, Besson G. Brainstem and cerebellar infarcts. In Ginsberg MD, Bogousslavsky J, eds. Cerebrovascular Disease: Pathophysiology, Diagnosis and Management, Vol II. Malden, MA: Blackwell Science, 1998.
183. Bastian AJ, Mink JW, Kaufman BA, et al. Posterior vermal split syndrome. Ann Neurol 1998;44:601.
184. Tohgi H, Takahashi S, Chiba K, et al. Cerebellar infarction: clinical neuroimaging analysis in 293 patients. Stroke 1993;24:1697.
185. Macdonell RAL, Kalnins RM, Donnan GA. Cerebellar infarction: natural history, prognosis, and pathology. Stroke 1987;16:849.
186. Johnsen SD, Tarby TJ, Lewis KS, et al. Cerebellar infarction: An unrecognized complication of very low birthweight. J Child Neurol 2002;17:320.
187. Johnsen SD, Bodensteiner JB, Lotze TE. Frequency and nature of cerebellar injury in the extremely premature survivor with cerebral palsy. J Child Neurol 2005;20:60.
188. Luhan JA, Pollack SL. Occlusion of the superior cerebellar artery. Neurology 1953;3:77.
189. Oas JG, Baloh RW. Vertigo and the anterior inferior cerebellar artery syndrome. Neurology 1992;42:2274.
190. Martin RG, Grant JL, Peace D, et al. Microsurgical relationships of the anterior inferior cerebellar artery and the facial-vestibulocochlear nerve complex. Neurosurgery 1980;6:483.
191. Amarenco P, Hauw J-J. Cerebellar infarction in the territory of the anterior inferior cerebellar artery: a clinicopathologic study of 20 patients. Brain 1990;113:139.
192. Kim JS, Lopez I, DiPatre PL, et al. Internal auditory artery infarction: clinicopathologic correlation. Neurology 1999;52:40.
193. Lee H, Cho Y-W. Auditory disturbance as a prodrome of anterior inferior cerebellar artery infarction. J Neurol Neurosurg Psychiatry 2003;74:1644.
194. Lee H, Yi HA, Baloh RW. Sudden bilateral simultaneous deafness with vertigo as a sole manifestation of vertebrobasilar insufficiency. J Neurol Neurosurg Psychiatry 2003;74:539.
195. Strupp M, Planck JH, Arbusow V, et al. Rotational vertebral artery occlusion syndrome with vertigo due to "labyrinthine excitation." Neurology 2000;54:1376.
196. Kang DW, Lee SH, Bae HJ, et al. Acute bilateral cerebellar infarcts in the territory of posterior inferior cerebellar artery. Neurology 2000;55:582.
197. Dhamoon SK, Iqbal J, Collins GH. Ipsilateral hemiplegia and the Wallenberg syndrome. Arch Neurol 1984;41:179.
198. Thömke F, Marx JJ, Iannetti GD, et al. A topodiagnostic investigation on body lateropulsion in medullary infarcts. Neurology 2005;64:716.
199. Currier RD, Beben J. A medullary syndrome characterized by wild arm ataxia. Neurology 1999;53:1608.
200. Toyoda K, Imamura T, Saku Y, et al. Medial medullary infarction: analysis of eleven patients. Neurology 1996;47:1141.
201. Bassetti C, Bogousslavsky J, Mattle H, et al. Medial medullary stroke: report of seven patients and review of the literature. Neurology 1997;48:882.
202. Kwon M, Lee JH, Kim JS. Dysphagia in unilateral medullary infarction: lateral versus medial lesions. Neurology 2005;65:714.
203. Terao S, Miura N, Takeda A, et al. Course and distribution of facial corticobulbar tract fibres in the lower brain stem. J Neurol Neurosurg Psychiatry 2000;69:262.
204. Chang D, Cho S-H. Medial medullary infarction with contralateral glossoplegia. J Neurol Neurosurg Psychiatry 2005;76:888.
205. Benito-León J, Alvarez-Cermeno J.C. Isolated total tongue paralysis as a manifestation of bilateral medullary infarction. J Neurol Neurosurg Psychiatry 2003;74:1698.
206. Kim JS, Choi K-D, Oh S-Y, et al. Medial medullary infarction: abnormal eye findings. Neurology 2005;65:1294.
207. Zickler P, Seitz RJ, Hartung H, et al. Bilateral medullary pyramid infarction. Neurology 2005;64:1801.
208. Dickman CA, Hadley MN, Pappas CT, et al. Cruciate paralysis and radiographic analysis of injuries to the cervicomedullary junction. J Neurosurg 1990;73:850.

CHAPTER 3

Stroke in Neonates and Children: Overview

Meredith R. Golomb

This chapter reviews the epidemiology, clinical presentation, etiologies, evaluations, and treatments of stroke during the first 18 years of life. Discussion includes stroke resulting from ischemia owing to arterial or venous occlusion, from hemorrhage, or from metabolic causes such as mitochondrial disease. Sinovenous thrombosis that does not progress to infarction is included in the discussion of childhood stroke. The term "neonate" refers to a child from the time of birth to the 28th day of life.[1] The neurologic issues of premature neonates born before 36 weeks' gestation, including stroke, are not addressed in this chapter. The term "children" includes neonates and children up to age 18 years.

Epidemiology

Estimates of the incidence of stroke in the general population of children vary widely, ranging from 2.5 to 13 cases per 100,000 children per year, with estimates of the incidence of ischemic stroke ranging from 0.6 to 8 per 100,000 children per year, and estimates of the incidence of hemorrhagic stroke ranging from 1.2 to 5 per 100,000 children per year.[2-4] These studies did not agree on whether hemorrhagic or ischemic strokes predominated. Some of this variation is explained by whether or not strokes caused by trauma or meningitis were included, and whether neonates were included. The study by deVeber and colleagues[5] reported the incidence of sinovenous thrombosis as 0.67 per 100,000 children per year. Some groups of children may have an elevated risk of stroke, including neonates; children with blood disorders; children with perfusion abnormalities such as cardiac defects and diseases requiring treatment with extracorporeal membrane oxygenation (ECMO); and children with cerebral vascular malformations, cancer, and certain genetic syndromes.

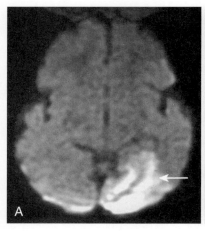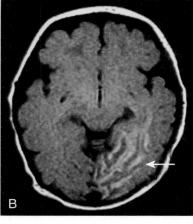

FIGURE 3-1 **Neonatal stroke.** This full-term newborn presented with shaking of both arms and legs on the fifth day of life. **A** and **B,** MRI diffusion-weighted imaging (**A**) and fast spin echo inversion recovery (**B**) showed left occipital infarction (*arrows*).

Several studies suggest that neonates are at a far higher risk for ischemic and hemorrhagic strokes (Fig. 3-1). For arterial ischemic stroke, Estan and Hope[6] in England reported an incidence of 1 in 4000 term births, and Lynch JK and Nelson KB[7] at the National Institutes of Health in the United States reported an incidence of 1 in 5600 term births. Gunther and colleagues[8] in Germany reported an incidence of only 1.35 per 100,000 term births, however. Of the childhood sinovenous thrombosis cases reported by deVeber and colleagues,[5] 43% occurred in neonates, but the incidence per 100,000 term births was not calculated. Gradnitzer and colleagues[9] reported that intracranial hemorrhage affects 1 in 100 full-term neonates. Because so many studies suggest that neonates have a higher risk of stroke than older children, and because the etiologies, clinical presentations, and therapies are different, neonates are discussed separately from older children in subsequent sections.

Children with hematologic disorders affecting coagulation are at increased risk of stroke. Children with sickle cell disease have a particularly high rate of stroke, estimated at 285 per 100,000 children per year.[10] These children develop thrombosis or progressive vascular occlusion or both from sickling, or in rare cases develop fat emboli[11] or aneurysms and resultant hemorrhage.[12,13] Children with hemoglobin SC or S-β thalassemia also may develop stroke, but have a lower risk than children with sickle cell disease.[14] Children with other prothrombotic disorders also have increased rates of stroke, but are often diagnosed only after presenting with stroke or other thrombotic events. The workup does not always reveal the cause of the prothrombotic state (Fig. 3-2). It is unclear how many children with thrombophilic disorders do not present during the childhood years and remain undiagnosed. Children with bleeding disorders are at increased risk for intracranial hemorrhages. Klinge and colleagues[15] reported that 4% of hemophiliacs have intracranial bleeds, 48% of which are intracerebral (see Chapter 14).

Children with illnesses affecting perfusion and blood pressure are at increased risk for stroke, particularly children with cardiac disorders or who are treated with ECMO. Children with cardiac defects, particularly complex congenital heart disease, are at increased risk for cardioembolic stroke (Fig. 3-3). They also may develop local thrombosis, sinovenous thrombosis, or watershed infarcts from decreases in blood pressure during periods of arrhythmia, cardiac failure, or surgery.[16] Surgery and cardiac catheterization seem to be the times of highest risk,[17] and the risk is probably highest in children with the most severe disease. Mayer and colleagues[18] reported cerebrovascular complications in 5 of 77 children (6.5%) who had received heart transplants. Children treated with ECMO have perfusion abnormalities that may be similar to the abnormalities in children with complex congenital heart disease and are at increased risk for embolic ischemic stroke and intracranial hemorrhage. The reported

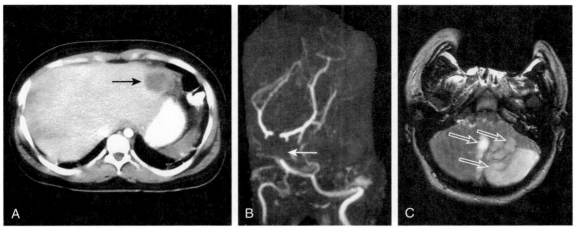

FIGURE 3-2 **Hepatic infarction, followed by basilar thrombosis and cerebellar and brainstem infarction.** This 14-year-old child presented with abdominal pain. **A,** CT imaging of the abdomen showed hepatic (*arrow*) and splenic infarctions. Evaluation for etiology, including prothrombotic workup, was unremarkable. Warfarin sodium (Coumadin) was given for 6 months. After warfarin was discontinued, the child presented with decreased mental status. **B,** MR angiography showed extensive basilar thrombosis (*arrow*). **C,** MRI showed multiple cerebellar and brainstem infarcts (*arrows*), suggesting an ongoing prothrombotic state. The child did not survive.

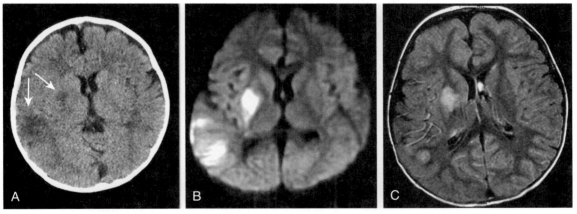

FIGURE 3-3 **Multiple infarcts in a child with complex congenital heart disease.** This 3-year-old child with complex congenital heart disease presented with a left hemiparesis. **A-C,** The lesions are subtle on CT (*arrows* in **A**), but easier to distinguish on diffusion-weighted MRI (**B**) and fast spin echo inversion recovery imaging (**C**).

stroke rates vary from 0%[19] to 26%[20]; in children dying after receiving ECMO, the rate of ischemic infarctions and intracranial hemorrhage may be 50% (see Chapter 7).[21]

Children with cerebrovascular malformations often present with intracranial hemorrhage; it is unclear what percentage of children with cerebrovascular malformations remain asymptomatic. In a Toronto study of children diagnosed with arteriovenous malformations, 80% presented with spontaneous intracranial hemorrhage.[22]

Children with cancer are at increased risk for ischemic infarction and intracranial hemorrhage. Cancer may lead to prothrombotic hematologic abnormalities resulting from the cancer itself, such as leukostasis in leukemia, or resulting from chemotherapy such as asparaginase, which causes decreases in plasminogen, antithrombin, and fibrinogen. Immunosuppression from chemotherapy may lead to bacterial or fungal meningitis with subsequent vascular inflammation and infarction. Radiation may lead to stenotic vasculopathy with subsequent thrombosis. Intracranial surgery may lead to vascular damage and thrombosis. Bone marrow suppression from chemotherapy may lead to platelet counts that predispose to intracranial hemorrhage, and bleeding may occur from metastases to brain.[23,24] Coplin and colleagues[25] looked at 1245 bone marrow transplant patients ranging from 5 to 60 years old and found strokes in almost 3%. Bowers and colleagues[26] reported nonperioperative strokes in 1.6% of 807 pediatric brain tumor patients.

Children with certain genetic syndromes and metabolic diseases are at increased risk for stroke. Children with connective tissue disorders such as Marfan syndrome, Ehlers-Danlos type IV, and pseudoxanthoma elasticum may be at higher risk for arterial dissection with subsequent thrombosis or for aneurysm formation.[27-29] Children with Marfan syndrome may develop mitral valve prolapse or aortic root dilation or both, which may increase their risk of stroke.[30] Disorders that compromise the integrity of the vascular wall may increase the risk of arterial perforation or dissection during angiography.[31]

Children with metabolic disorders that cause endothelial damage, such as homocystinuria,[32] the familial hyperlipidemias,[33]

and Fabry disease,[34] are at risk for intracranial thrombosis and stroke. Patients with Fabry disease usually do not develop cerebrovascular lesions before 23 years of age, but by age 55 years, virtually all patients with Fabry disease have cerebrovascular lesions if they remain untreated[35]; α-galactosidase enzyme replacement decreases cerebrovascular injury.[36]

Children with mitochondrial diseases are at risk for metabolic cerebral infarction, which may be the first manifestation of the disease.[37] Children with neurofibromatosis 1 (NF1) are at increased risk for occlusive vasculopathies, such as moyamoya disease; these vasculopathies are sometimes secondary to radiation, but may occur before the presentation of other symptoms of NF1 (Fig. 3-4).[38-41]

Children with Down syndrome have higher rates of stroke because they have higher rates of risk factors for stroke, including congenital heart disease, leukemia, vasculopathy from moyamoya disease, and vertebral dissection from abnormalities of the cervical spine.[42-46] Children with Down syndrome also have higher rates of obstructive sleep apnea,[47] which may be a risk factor for ischemic stroke.[48,49] Children with Menkes kinky hair syndrome have tortuous intracranial vessels and evidence on magnetic resonance imaging (MRI) of ischemic injury with unclear etiology;

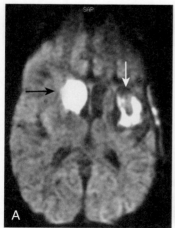 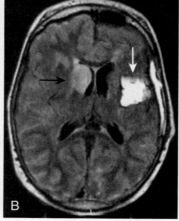 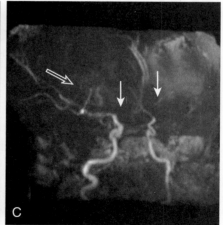

FIGURE 3-4   **Left glioblastoma, right basal ganglia infarction, and moyamoya disease in a child with neurofibromatosis 1.** This 12-year-old girl with neurofibromatosis 1 was undergoing treatment for a left glioblastoma multiforme when she presented with decreased mental status. **A** and **B,** Diffusion-weighted MRI (**A**) and fast spin echo inversion recovery imaging (**B**) showed the old glioblastoma (*white arrow*) and new right basal ganglia infarction (*black arrow*). **C,** MR angiography showed stenosis of the left middle cerebral artery and right A1 segment (*white arrows*) and vessels with moyamoya disease on the left (*black arrow*).

metabolic factors may be contributory.[50] Children with Klippel-Trenaunay-Weber syndrome may develop intracranial angiomas and other vascular malformations that may bleed (see Chapter 16).[51,52]

Clinical Presentation

Neonates

More than half of all neonates with arterial ischemic stroke, intracranial hemorrhage, and sinovenous thrombosis present with seizures.[5,53,54] Other presentations include lethargy, apnea, irritability, jitteriness, bulging fontanelle, and hypotonia.[53-56] Some children remain apparently asymptomatic in the perinatal period and present after 2 months of age with increased tone, pathologic early hand preference (using one hand preferentially before 1 year of age), or seizures.[57-59]

Infants and Children

Clinical presentations of arterial ischemic stroke, sinovenous thrombosis, intracranial hemorrhage, and metabolic infarction from mitochondrial disease may be similar to the presentations seen in adults and may include seizures and focal neurologic signs. Sinovenous thrombosis and intracranial hemorrhage may manifest with headache. Clinical presentations in children may be subtle and initially missed by parents and physicians. Parents may attribute a sudden hemiparesis or aphasia to behavior. Children with multiple infarctions resulting from sickle cell disease or mitochondrial disease may show only developmental delay or learning difficulty. Pegelow and colleagues[60] reported that 21.8% of children with sickle cell disease have clinically silent infarctions; 37% of children with sickle cell disease and Doppler ultrasound–measured elevated cerebral artery blood flow velocity have silent infarcts.[61]

Many parents and physicians do not realize children can have strokes, which contributes to missed clinical signs and delay in diagnosis. Gabis and colleagues[62] reviewed 47 strokes in 41 children; they found that the average time from clinical presentation to physician contact was 28.5 hours, and the average time to diagnosis was 35.7 hours.

Causes

Neonates: Perinatal Factors

Neonates have been exposed to two circulations; the maternal and fetal circulations interact at the placenta. In the period around the time of delivery, the maternal coagulation system becomes more prothrombotic, with increases in the levels of the vitamin K–dependent clotting factors, a decrease in protein S levels, and activation of the endothelium.[63] Maternal hematologic risk factors have been associated with stroke in the placenta and neonate. Preeclampsia may predispose to placental infarction by impairing perfusion,[64,65] and gestational diabetes may predispose to infarction by causing endothelial activation and thrombosis.[66] Placental infarction may lead to fetal cerebral infarction through embolization to the fetus.[67-70] Inflammatory responses against fetal blood components may lead to hemorrhage; fetal/neonatal alloimmune thrombocytopenia may manifest with intracranial hemorrhage (see Chapter 14).[71]

Neonates, Infants, and Children

Cardiac

As discussed earlier in the section on epidemiology, children with complex congenital heart disease and valvular defects are at increased risk for stroke. Abnormalities in blood flow resulting from arrhythmia, abnormal anatomy, or changes in perfusion during surgery may predispose to intracardiac thrombus formation with subsequent embolization to the brain. A temporary prothrombotic state may exist during cardiac surgery.[72,73] Cardiac catheterization and cardiac surgery may contribute to increased risk of stroke because they cause endothelial disruption, predisposing to thrombosis. Children with chronic cardiac disease have chronically impaired perfusion, which may predispose to impaired cerebral perfusion and to polycythemia, which can lead to increased blood viscosity and impaired perfusion. This condition may be more severe in children with iron deficiency because the resulting microcytic cells are less flexible, carry less oxygen, and have a shorter survival time.[74]

Hematologic

Abnormalities of components of the coagulation system may lead to thrombotic or cardioembolic stroke or to intracranial hemorrhage. The list of prothrombotic abnormalities associated with pediatric stroke is long (Table 3-1). Studies vary widely as to how much prothrombotic risk factors are associated with and responsible for childhood stroke. Studies by deVeber and colleagues[75] and Nowak-Gottl and colleagues[76] found prothrombotic risk factors in more than 25% of children with stroke, but Ganesan and colleagues[77] found them in only 12%. Neonates have low levels of the vitamin K–dependent clotting factors and are at risk for intracranial hemorrhage if vitamin K is not administered. The hemophilias may manifest with intracranial hemorrhage (see Chapter 9).

TABLE 3-1   **Prothrombotic Hematologic Abnormalities Associated with Childhood Stroke**

Anemia
Anemia
Sickle cell anemia

Increased Blood Cells Leading to Increased Blood Viscosity
Polycythemia
Leukostasis

Coagulation Factor Deficiencies and Abnormalities
Protein C deficiency
Protein S deficiency
Antithrombin deficiency
Activated protein C resistance
Elevated factor VIII
Low plasminogen
High fibrinogen

Identified Genetic Mutations in Coagulation Factors or Enzymes Affecting Coagulation
Factor V Leiden mutation
Prothrombin gene 20210 A mutation
Methylene tetrahydrofolate reductase mutation C677T
Plasminogen activator promoter polymorphism (PAI 1)

Antiphospholipid Antibodies
Lupus anticoagulant
Anticardiolipin antibody

Lipid Abnormalities
Elevated lipoprotein (a)
Hyperlipidemia

Metabolic

Metabolic disease may cause stroke by contributing to arterial damage or instability of the arterial wall, or by directly causing neuronal damage. Homocystinuria and the C677T methylene tetrahydrofolate reductase (MTHFR) gene mutation lead to elevated levels of plasma homocysteine, which damages the endothelium.[32,78] In Fabry disease, arterial wall damage is caused by accumulation of glycolipids in the endothelium.[79] The familial hyperlipidemias cause atherosclerotic changes in the arteries of children similar to those seen in older adults.[80] In α_1-antitrypsin deficiency, the balance between protease and antiprotease activity is disrupted, predisposing to stenotic changes, dissection, and aneurysm formation.[81,82] By contrast, mitochondrial diseases such as MELAS (mitochondrial encephalomyopathy, lactic acidosis, and strokelike symptoms) are thought to cause infarction by direct cell damage when the cell is subject to oxidative stress. Mitochondrial infarctions are usually not in vascular territories.[83] Mitochondrial disease also may cause cardiomyopathy, however, with resultant cardioembolic stroke.[84]

Migraine and Vasculopathy

There are many reports of childhood stroke after migraine, with infarction thought to be secondary to arterial vasospasm (see Chapter 8).[85-88] Autoimmune inflammatory vasculopathies, such as primary angiitis of the central nervous system, may cause progressive multiple vascular stenoses and lead to death unless treated with aggressive immunotherapy,[89] or may be more benign, requiring only a brief course of steroids[90] or no treatment at all. Some children develop what seems to be a limited vasculopathy after chickenpox (see Chapter 6).[91,92] Vascular malformations may bleed spontaneously, causing hemorrhagic infarction.

Infection

Meningitis may lead to infarction by causing arteritis and disseminated intravascular coagulopathy.[93] Patients with AIDS are at increased risk for the common infectious causes of meningitis, but also may develop

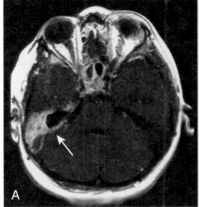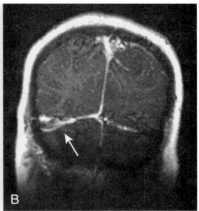

FIGURE 3-5 **Right mastoiditis and right sinovenous thrombosis.** This 8-year-old child developed a severe headache after several days of ear pain and vomiting. **A** and **B,** MRI showed mastoiditis (*arrow* in **A**) and thrombosis of the right transverse sinus (*arrow* in **B**).

an arteriopathy affecting medium and small vessels thought to be due to direct infection.[94] Mastoiditis may contribute to transverse sinus thrombosis on the same side.[95] Dehydration, which often occurs in the setting of infection, also is a risk factor for sinovenous thrombosis (Fig. 3-5).[5,95]

Trauma

Trauma is an important cause of stroke in infants and children. Trauma may cause arterial dissection with resultant thrombosis or vascular tearing. Bony abnormalities of the cervical spine[96,97] and vascular abnormalities[98] may predispose to dissection after minor trauma. Injury to the soft palate, which may occur when a child falls with a popsicle stick or other object in the mouth, may lead to internal carotid dissection.[99] Children with broken bones rarely may develop cerebral infarction owing to fat emboli from the bone marrow.[100] More than 90% of serious intracranial injuries in children younger than 1 year of age are due to nonaccidental trauma (i.e., abuse).[101]

Drugs and Toxins

Stroke risk may be increased by therapeutic and recreational drugs. Asparaginase leads to decreased levels of antithrombin, plasminogen, and fibrinogen, and is a well-known cause of thrombosis in children with leukemia.[102] Phenylpropanolamine has been associated with an increased risk of hemorrhagic stroke and is no longer used in cold medicines in the United States.[103] Cocaine leads to vasospasm and has been associated with stroke in adolescent users[104] and in the infants of mothers who use it during pregnancy.[105,106] Smoking causes endothelial activation and may promote thrombosis.[107,108]

Multiple Risk Factors

Multiple risk factors seem to interact in many cases. Children who have complex congenital heart disease[109] or who are undergoing treatment with asparaginase[110] who also have prothrombotic disorders are at higher risk of stroke than children with those medical problems who do not have prothrombotic risk factors. The presence of multiple risk factors increases the risk of recurrence and poor outcome.[111,112]

Evaluation

Radiology

In neonates, cranial ultrasound has a low sensitivity for detecting arterial ischemic stroke,[113] but is commonly used to detect intracranial hemorrhage.[53] Doppler ultrasound is useful for assessing vascular flow and is used to screen sickle cell anemia patients for stroke risk.[114] Computed tomography can detect ischemic infarction after 24 hours, but may detect hemorrhage immediately. Diffusion-weighted MRI can detect acute infarction within hours, and MR angiography and MR venography can provide detailed pictures of the vascular anatomy with minimal risk. Cerebral angiography is the most sensitive technique for depicting vascular anatomy, but may itself lead to vascular injury and infarction, and is technically difficult in infants.

Serum Studies

The multiple prothrombotic causes of stroke described in the section on causes may be evaluated using serum studies. Factor levels and levels of protein C, protein S, antithrombin, homocysteine, and antiphospholipids can be assayed. The activated protein C resistance screen suggests the presence of the factor V Leiden mutation. Serum amino acids can be used to evaluate for hyperhomocysteinemia or homocystinuria. Elevated serum lactate may be associated with mitochondrial disease. Genetic screens can be performed for known prothrombotic mutations, including the factor V Leiden mutation, prothrombin 20210 mutation, MTHFR, and plasminogen activator promoter polymorphism. and for mitochondrial disease such as MELAS.

Cerebrospinal Fluid

Cerebrospinal fluid (CSF) may reveal an elevated white blood cell count suggestive of vasculitis or infection, or an elevated red blood cell count suggestive of hemorrhage. An elevated CSF lactate supports the diagnosis of mitochondrial disease. CSF cultures are vital in choosing the appropriate therapy for bacterial and fungal meningitis.

Urine Studies

Elevated homocystine in the urine may confirm the diagnosis of homocystinuria.

General Physical Examination

The general physical examination may provide important clues to the etiology of the infarction. Dysmorphic facial features and hyperpigmented or hypopigmented skin lesions may signal a genetic syndrome; unusual skin elasticity or flexible joints or both and long limbs may suggest a collagen abnormality; a heart murmur may suggest a cardiac defect.

The evaluation of young patients with stroke is discussed in more detail in Chapter 4.

Treatment

Acute Therapy

Ischemic Stroke

Although thrombolytic therapies have been widely used in adults, there are few reports of their use in children,[115-120] and they should be used with caution. Neonates may be inappropriate candidates for tissue plasminogen activator because they have lower levels of plasminogen than older children and adults.[121] Intravenous and low-molecular-weight heparin have been used for arterial ischemic stroke and sinovenous thrombosis with few complications when patients are carefully selected and monitored.[122–124] Exchange transfusion is often used to treat acute stroke in patients with sickle cell anemia. Replacement of deficient protein C and antithrombin III has been tried in several case reports and small pilot studies with good results,[125-128] but these factors are not commonly available.

Intracranial Hemorrhage

Children with intracranial hemorrhage resulting from hemophilia require immediate factor replacement and may need blood transfusion. Surgery may be required to remove large hematomas exerting mass effect. Children with a history of trauma or no clear etiology should be systematically evaluated for other areas of injury and for possible abuse.

Long-term Therapy

Aspirin, low-molecular-weight heparin, and warfarin (Coumadin) have been tried for long-term ischemic stroke prophylaxis in children, but there are few large studies. Strater and colleagues[129] followed 135 children with stroke and found that low-dose low-molecular-weight heparin was not superior to aspirin in preventing recurrence, but this was not a double-blinded randomized controlled trial, and the doses were lower than those used by some physicians.[130] Children with sickle cell have a decreased risk of stroke when treated with regular transfusions.[114] In one vasculopathy, moyamoya disease, and in vascular malformations, surgery plays a role in long-term treatment. Therapy of mitochondrial disease with antioxidant vitamins has had variable results, but treatment of Fabry disease with α-galactosidase seems promising. Children with hemophilia may require regular factor transfusions. For children with sickle cell disease, regular transfusions were shown to decrease the rate of recurrent stroke in the STOP study (Stroke Prevention Trial in Sickle Cell Anemia).[114] Therapies and prognoses are described further in Chapters 6 through 17.

Conclusion

Children do have strokes, and some subgroups of children are at high risk for stroke. Neonates usually present with seizures, whereas older children may present with seizures or focal neurologic signs. The causes of stroke include cardiac, hematologic, metabolic, and vascular pathologies; infections; trauma; and therapeutic and recreational drug use. In many cases, the causes may be multifactorial. Multiple therapies have been tried for strokes in children, but there are few large studies. Pediatric stroke is an important area for future research.

REFERENCES

1. Anderson KN, Anderson LE. Mosby's Pocket Dictionary of Medicine, Nursing, and Allied Health. St. Louis: Mosby, 1990.
2. Schoenberg BS, Mellinger JF, Schoenberg DG. Cerebrovascular disease in infants and children: a study of incidence, clinical features, and survival. Neurology 1978;28:763.
3. Broderick J, Talbot GT, Prenger E, et al. Stroke in children within a major metropolitan area: the surprising importance of intracerebral hemorrhage. J Child Neurol 1993;8:250.
4. Giroud M, Lemesle M, Gouyon JB, et al. Cerebrovascular disease in children under 16 years of age in the city of Dijon, France: a study of incidence and clinical features from 1985 to 1993. J Clin Epidemiol 1995;48:1343.
5. deVeber G, Andrew M, Adams C, et al. For the Canadian Pediatric Ischemic Stroke Study Group. Cerebral sinovenous thrombosis in children. N Engl J Med 2001;345:417.
6. Estan J, Hope P. Unilateral neonatal infarction in full term neonates. Arch Dis Child 1997;76:F88.
7. Lynch JK, Nelson KB. Neonatal stroke in the United States: results of the national hospital discharge survey, 1980-1998 (abstract). Neurology 2001;56:A10.
8. Gunther G, Junker R, Strater R, et al; Childhood Stroke Study Group. Symptomatic ischemic stroke in full-term neonates: role of acquired and genetic prothrombotic risk factors. [erratum appears in Stroke 2001 Jan;32(1):279]. Stroke 2000;31:2437.
9. Gradnitzer E, Urlesberger B, Maurer U, et al. [Cerebral hemorrhage in term newborn infants—an analysis of 10 years (1989-1999)]. Wien Med Wochenschr 2002;152:9.
10. Earley CJ, Kittner SJ, Feeser BR, et al. Stroke in children and sickle-cell disease: Baltimore-Washington Cooperative Young Stroke Study. Neurology 1998;51:169.
11. Adams RJ. Stroke prevention and treatment in sickle cell disease. Arch Neurol 2001;58:565.
12. Ohene-Frempong K, Weiner SJ, Sleeper LA, et al. Cerebrovascular accidents in sickle cell disease: rates and risk factors. Blood 1998;91:288.
13. Pegelow CH. Stroke in children with sickle cell anaemia: aetiology and treatment. Paediatr Drugs 2001;3:421.
14. Gill FM, Sleeper LA, Weiner SJ, et al. Clinical events in the first decade in a cohort of infants with sickle cell disease. Cooperative Study of Sickle Cell Disease. Blood 1995;86:776.
15. Klinge J, Auberger K, Auerswald G, et al. Prevalence and outcome of intracranial haemorrhage in haemophiliacs—a survey of the paediatric group of the German Society of Thrombosis and Haemostasis (GTH). Eur J Pediatr 1999;158(suppl 3):S162.
16. Roach ES, Riela AR. Pediatric Cerebrovascular Disorders. Futura, Armonk, NY, 1995.
17. Roach ES. Stroke in children. Curr Treat Options Neurol 2000;2:295.
18. Mayer TO, Biller J, O'Donnell J, et al. Contrasting the neurologic complications of cardiac transplantation in adults and children. J Child Neurol 2002;17:195.
19. Griffin MP, Minifee PK, Landry SH, et al. Neurodevelopmental outcome in neonates after extracorporeal membrane oxygenation: cranial magnetic resonance imaging and ultrasonography correlation. J Pediatr Surg 1992;27:33.
20. Lazar EL, Abramson SJ, Weinstein S, Stolar CJ. Neuroimaging of brain injury in neonates treated with extracorporeal membrane oxygenation: lessons learned from serial examinations. J Pediatr Surg 1994;29:186.
21. Jarjour IT, Ahdab-Barmada M. Cerebrovascular lesions in infants and children dying after extracorporeal membrane oxygenation. Pediatr Neurol 1994;10:13.
22. Humphreys RP, Hoffman HJ, Drake JM, Rutka JT. Choices in the 1990s for the management of pediatric cerebral arteriovenous malformations. Pediatr Neurosurg 1996;25:277.
23. Antunes NL. The spectrum of neurologic disease in children with systemic cancer. Pediatr Neurol 2001;25:227.
24. Arboix A. Enfermedad cerebrovascular en el paciente con cancer. Rev Neurol 2000;31:1250.
25. Coplin WM, Cochran MS, Levine SR, Crawford SW. Stroke after bone marrow transplantation: frequency, aetiology and outcome. Brain 2001;124:1043.

26. Bowers DC, Mulne AF, Reisch JS, et al. Nonperioperative strokes in children with central nervous system tumors. Cancer 2002;94:1094.

27. Schievink WI, Bjornsson J, Piepgras DG. Coexistence of fibromuscular dysplasia and cystic medial necrosis in a patient with Marfan's syndrome and bilateral carotid artery dissections. Stroke 1994;25:2492.

28. Schievink WI. Genetics and aneurysm formation. Neurosurg Clin N Am 1998;9:485.

29. Pieczuro A, Lozza M. [Cerebrovascular disease and pseudoxanthoma elasticum: apropos of a case]. Riv Neurol 1981;51:261.

30. Figueiredo S, Martins E, Lima MR, Alvares S. Cardiovascular manifestations in Marfan syndrome. Rev Port Cardiol 2001;20:1203.

31. Slingenberg EJ. Complications during intravascular diagnostic manipulations in the Ehlers-Danlos syndrome. Neth J Surg 1980;32:56.

32. Kanwar YS, Manaligod JR, Wong PW. Morphologic studies in a patient with homocystinuria due to 5, 10-methylenetetrahydrofolate reductase deficiency. Pediatr Res 1976;10:598.

33. Yamanouchi H, Seki Y, Yanagisawa T, et al. [Two cases of brain infarction associated with hypertriglyceridemia]. No To Hattatsu 1990;22:364.

34. Whybra C, Kampmann C, Willers I, et al. Anderson-Fabry disease: clinical manifestations of disease in female heterozygotes. J Inherit Metab Dis 2001;24:715.

35. Schiffmann R. Natural history of Fabry disease in males: preliminary observations. J Inherit Metab Dis 2001;24(suppl 2):15.

36. Schiffmann R, Kopp JB, Austin HA 3rd, et al. Enzyme replacement therapy in Fabry disease: a randomized controlled trial. JAMA 2001;285:2743.

37. Martinez-Fernandez E, Gil-Peralta A, Garcia-Lozano R, et al. Mitochondrial disease and stroke. Stroke 2001;32:2507.

38. Horikawa M, Utunomiya H, Hirotaka S, et al. Case of von Recklinghausen disease associated with cerebral infarction. J Child Neurol 1997;12:144.

39. Hornstein L, Borchers D. Stroke in an infant prior to the development of manifestations of neurofibromatosis. Neurofibromatosis 1989;2:116.

40. Jamjoom AB, Malabarey T, Jamjoom ZA, et al. Cerebro-vasculopathy and malignancy: catastrophic complications of radiotherapy for optic nerve glioma in a von Recklinghausen neurofibromatosis patient. Neurosurg Rev 1996;19:47.

41. Kwong KL, Wong YC. Moyamoya disease in a child with neurofibromatosis type-1. J Paediatr Child Health 1999;35:108.

42. Baram TZ, Fishman MA. "Top of the basilar" artery stroke in an adolescent with Down's syndrome. Arch Neurol 1985;42:296.

43. Cramer SC, Robertson RL, Dooling EC, Scott RM. Moyamoya and Down syndrome: clinical and radiological features. Stroke 1996;27:2131.

44. Cros T, Linares R, Castro A, et al. [A radiological study of the cervical alterations in Down syndrome: new findings on computerized tomography and three dimensional reconstructions]. Rev Neurol 2000;30:1101.

45. Pueschel SM, Scola FH, Tupper TB, Pezzullo JC. Skeletal anomalies of the upper cervical spine in children with Down syndrome. J Pediatr Orthop 1990;10:607.

46. Pueschel SM, Pueschel JK. Biomedical Concerns in Persons with Down Syndrome. Baltimore: Paul H. Brooks Publishing Company, 1992.

47. Mitchell RB, Call E, Kelly J. Ear, nose and throat disorders in children with Down syndrome. Laryngoscope 2003;113:259.

48. Kirkham FJ, Hewes DK, Prengler M, et al. Nocturnal hypoxaemia and central-nervous-system events in sickle-cell disease. Lancet 2001;357:1656.

49. Young T, Peppard PE, Gottlieb DJ. Epidemiology of obstructive sleep apnea: a population health perspective. Am J Respir Crit Care Med 2002;165:1217.

50. Hsich GE, Robertson RL, Irons M, et al. Cerebral infarction in Menkes' disease. Pediatr Neurol 2000;23:425.

51. Williams DW 3rd, Elster AD. Cranial CT and MR in the Klippel-Trenaunay-Weber syndrome. AJNR Am J Neuroradiol 1992;13:291.

52. Suga T, Yasuda J, Okudaira Y, et al. [A case of Klippel-Trenaunay-Weber syndrome associated with intracranial multiple angiomas]. No To Shinkei 1994;46:889.

53. Volpe JJ. Neurology of the Newborn. Philadelphia: WB Saunders, 2001.

54. Shevell MI, Silver K, O'Gorman AM, et al. Neonatal dural sinus thrombosis. Pediatr Neurol 1989;5:161.

55. Sreenan C, Bhargava R, Robertson CM. Cerebral infarction in the term newborn: clinical presentation and long-term outcome. J Pediatr 2000;137:351.

56. Perlman JM, Rollins NK, Evans D. Neonatal stroke: clinical characteristics and cerebral blood flow velocity measurements. Pediatr Neurol 1994;11:281.

57. Bouza H, Rutherford M, Acolet D, et al. Evolution of early hemiplegic signs in full-term infants with unilateral lesions in the neonatal period: a prospective study. Neuropediatrics 1994;25:201.

58. Uvebrant P. Hemiplegic cerebral palsy: aetiology and outcome. Acta Paediatr Scand Suppl 1988;345:1.

59. Golomb M, MacGregor D, Domi T, et al. Presumed pre- and perinatal stroke: risk factors and outcomes. Ann Neurol 2001;50:163.

60. Pegelow CH, Macklin EA, Moser FG, et al. Longitudinal changes in brain magnetic resonance imaging findings in children with sickle cell disease. Blood 2002;99:3014.

61. Pegelow CH, Wang W, Granger S, et al. Silent infarcts in children with sickle cell anemia and abnormal cerebral artery velocity. Arch Neurol 2001;58:2017.

62. Gabis LV, Yangala R, Lenn NJ. Time lag to diagnosis of stroke in children. Pediatrics 2002;110:924.

63. Clark P, Greer IA, Walker ID. Interaction of the protein C/protein S anticoagulant system, the endothelium and pregnancy. Blood Rev 1999;13:127.

64. Becroft DM, Thompson JM, Mitchell EA. The epidemiology of placental infarction at term. Placenta 2002;23:343.

65. Naeye RL. Placental infarction leading to fetal or neonatal death: a prospective study. Obstet Gynecol 1977;50:583.

66. Naeye RL. The outcome of diabetic pregnancies: a prospective study. Ciba Foundation Symposium 1978, p 227.

67. Redline RW, Wilson-Costello D, Borawski E, et al. Placental lesions associated with neurologic impairment and cerebral palsy in very-low-birth-weight infants. Arch Pathol Lab Med 1998;122:1091.

68. Burke CJ, Tannenberg AE. Prenatal brain damage and placental infarction—an autopsy study. Dev Med Child Neurol 1995;37:555.

69. Kraus FT, Acheen VI. Fetal thrombotic vasculopathy in the placenta: cerebral thrombi and infarcts, coagulopathies, and cerebral palsy. Hum Pathol 1999;30:759.

70. Adams-Chapman I, Vaucher YE, Bejar RF, et al. Maternal floor infarction of the placenta: association with central nervous system injury and adverse neurodevelopmental outcome. J Perinatol 2002;22:236.

71. Kanhai HH, Porcelijn L, van Zoeren D, et al. Antenatal care in pregnancies at risk of alloimmune thrombocytopenia: report of 19 cases in 16 families. Eur J Obstet Gynecol Reprod Biol 1996;68:67.

72. Petaja J, Peltola K, Sairanen H, et al. Fibrinolysis, antithrombin III, and protein C in neonates during cardiac operations. J Thorac Cardiovasc Surg 1996;112:665.

73. Petaja J, Lundstrom U, Sairanen H, et al. Central venous thrombosis after cardiac operations in children. J Thorac Cardiovasc Surg 1996;112:883.

74. Territo MC, Rosove M, Perloff JK. Cyanotic congenital heart disease. In Perloff JK, Child JS, eds. Congenital Heart Disease in Adults. Philadelphia: WB Saunders, 1991.

75. deVeber G, Monagle P, Chan A, et al. Prothrombotic disorders in infants and children with cerebral thromboembolism. Arch Neurol 1998;55:1539.

76. Nowak-Gottl U, Strater R, Heinecke A, et al. Lipoprotein (a) and genetic polymorphisms of clotting factor V, prothrombin, and methylenetetrahydrofolate reductase are risk factors of spontaneous ischemic stroke in childhood. Blood 1999;94:3678.

77. Ganesan V, McShane MA, Liesner R, et al. Inherited prothrombotic states and ischaemic stroke in childhood. J Neurol Neurosurg Psychiatry 1998;65:508.

78. Cardo E, Monros E, Colome C, et al. Children with stroke: polymorphism of the MTHFR gene, mild hyperhomocysteinemia, and vitamin status. J Child Neurol 2000;15:295.

79. Grewal RP. Stroke in Fabry's disease. J Neurol 1994;241:153.

80. Guidelines for the detection of high-risk lipoprotein profiles and the treatment of dyslipoproteinemias. Canadian Lipoprotein Conference Ad Hoc Committee on Guidelines for Dyslipoproteinemias. Can Med Assoc J 1990;142:1371.

81. Schievink WI, Prakash UB, Piepgras DG, Mokri B. Alpha 1-antitrypsin deficiency in intracranial aneurysms and cervical artery dissection. Lancet 1994;343:452.

82. Schievink WI, Puumala MR, Meyer FB, et al. Giant intracranial aneurysm and fibromuscular dysplasia in an adolescent with alpha 1-antitrypsin deficiency. J Neurosurg 1996;85:503.

83. Fosslien E. Mitochondrial medicine—molecular pathology of defective oxidative phosphorylation. Ann Clin Lab Sci 2001;31:25.

84. Ito T, Hattori K, Obayashi T, et al. Mitochondrial DNA mutations in cardiomyopathy. Jpn Circ J 1992;56:1045.

85. Harbaugh RE, Saunders RL, Reeves AG. Pediatric cerebellar infarction: case report and review of the literature. Neurosurgery 1982;10:593.

86. Hilton-Jones D, Warlow CP. The causes of stroke in the young. J Neurol 1985;232:137.

87. Garg BP, DeMyer WE. Ischemic thalamic infarction in children: clinical presentation, etiology, and outcome. Pediatr Neurol 1995;13:46.

88. Dunn DW. Vertebrobasilar occlusive disease and childhood migraine. Pediatr Neurol 1985;1:252.

89. Calabrese LH. Vasculitis of the central nervous system. Rheum Dis Clin North Am 1995;21:1059.

90. Calabrese LH, Gragg LA, Furlan AJ. Benign angiopathy: a distinct subset of angiographically defined primary angiitis of the central nervous system. J Rheumatol 1993;20:2046.

91. Askalan R, Laughlin S, Mayank S, et al. Chickenpox and stroke in childhood: a study of frequency and causation. Stroke 2001;32:1257.

92. Chabrier S, Rodesch G, Lasjaunias P, et al. Transient cerebral arteriopathy: a disorder recognized by serial angiograms in children with stroke. J Child Neurol 1998;13:27.

93. Takeoka M, Takahashi T. Infectious and inflammatory disorders of the circulatory system and stroke in childhood. Curr Opin Neurol 2002;15:159.

94. Joshi VV, Pawel B, Connor E, et al. Arteriopathy in children with acquired immune deficiency syndrome. Pediatr Pathol 1987;7:261.

95. Carvalho KS, Bodensteiner JB, Connolly PJ, Garg BP. Cerebral venous thrombosis in children. J Child Neurol 2001;16:574.

96. Bhatnagar M, Sponseller PD, Carroll C, Tolo VT. Pediatric atlantoaxial instability presenting as cerebral and cerebellar infarcts. J Pediatr Orthop 1991;11:103.

97. Sasaki H, Itoh T, Takei H, Hayashi M. Os odontoideum with cerebellar infarction: a case report. Spine 2000;25:1178.

98. Plaschke M, Auer D, Trapp T, et al. Severe spontaneous carotid artery dissection and multiple aneurysmal dilatations: a case report. Angiology 1996;47:919.

99. Borges G, Bonilha L, Santos SF, et al. Thrombosis of the internal carotid artery secondary to soft palate injury in children and childhood: report of two cases. Pediatr Neurosurg 2000;32:150.

100. Forteza AM, Rabinstein A, Koch S, et al. Endovascular closure of a patent foramen ovale in the fat embolism syndrome: changes in the embolic

patterns as detected by transcranial Doppler. Arch Neurol 2002;59:455.

101. Johnson CF. Abuse and neglect of children. In Jenson H, ed. Nelson Textbook of Pediatrics. Philadelphia: WB Saunders, 2000.

102. Hongo T, Okada S, Ohzeki T, et al. Low plasma levels of hemostatic proteins during the induction phase in children with acute lymphoblastic leukemia: A retrospective study by the JACLS. Japan Association of Childhood Leukemia Study. Pediatr Int 2002;44:293.

103. Kernan WN, Viscoli CM, Brass LM, et al. Phenylpropanolamine and the risk of hemorrhagic stroke. N Engl J Med 2000;343:1826.

104. Kaku DA, Lowenstein DH. Emergence of recreational drug abuse as a major risk factor for stroke in young adults. Ann Intern Med 1990;113:821.

105. Dominguez R, Aguirre Vila-Coro A, Slopis JM, Bohan TP. Brain and ocular abnormalities in infants with in utero exposure to cocaine and other street drugs. Am J Dis Child 1991;145:688.

106. Chasnoff IJ, Bussey ME, Savich R, Stack CM. Perinatal cerebral infarction and maternal cocaine use. J Pediatr 1986;108:456.

107. Celermajer DS, Sorensen KE, Georgakopoulos D, et al. Cigarette smoking is associated with dose-related and potentially reversible impairment of endothelium-dependent dilation in healthy young adults. Circulation 1993;88:2149.

108. Love BB, Biller J, Jones MP, et al. Cigarette smoking: a risk factor for cerebral infarction in young adults. Arch Neurol 1990;47:693.

109. Strater R, Vielhaber H, Kassenbohmer R, et al. Genetic risk factors of thrombophilia in ischaemic childhood stroke of cardiac origin: a prospective ESPED survey. Eur J Pediatr 1999;158(suppl 3):S122.

110. Nowak-Gottl U, Wermes C, Junker R, et al. Prospective evaluation of the thrombotic risk in children with acute lymphoblastic leukemia carrying the MTHFR TT 677 genotype, the prothrombin G20210A variant, and further prothrombotic risk factors. Blood 1999;93:1595.

111. Nowak-Gottl U, Junker R, Kreuz W, et al; Childhood Thrombophilia Study Group. Risk of recurrent venous thrombosis in children with combined prothrombotic risk factors. Blood 2001;97:858.

112. Lanthier S, Carmant L, David M, et al. Stroke in children: the coexistence of multiple risk factors predicts poor outcome. Neurology 2000;54:371.

113. Golomb M, Dick P, MacGregor D, et al. Cranial ultrasonography has a low sensitivity for detecting arterial ischemic stroke in term neonates. J Child Neurol 2003;18:98.

114. Adams RJ. Lessons from the Stroke Prevention Trial in Sickle Cell Anemia (STOP) study. J Child Neurol 2000;15:344.

115. Cannon BC, Kertesz NJ, Friedman RA, Fenrich AL. Use of tissue plasminogen activator in a stroke after radiofrequency ablation of a left-sided accessory pathway. J Cardiovasc Electrophysiol 2001;12:723.

116. Thirumalai SS, Shubin RA. Successful treatment for stroke in a child using recombinant tissue plasminogen activator. J Child Neurol 2000;15:558.

117. Noser EA, Felberg RA, Alexandrov AV. Thrombolytic therapy in an adolescent ischemic stroke. J Child Neurol 2001;16:286.

118. Carlson MD, Leber S, Deveikis J, Silverstein FS. Successful use of rt-PA in pediatric stroke. Neurology 2001;57:157.

119. Gruber A, Nasel C, Lang W, et al. Intra-arterial thrombolysis for the treatment of perioperative childhood cardioembolic stroke. Neurology 2000;54:1684.

120. Golomb MR, Rafay M, Armstrong D, et al. Intra-arterial tissue plasminogen activator for thrombosis complicating cerebral angiography in a 17-year-old girl. J Child Neurol 2003;18(6):420.

121. Andrew M, Brooker L, Leaker M, et al. Fibrin clot lysis by thrombolytic agents is impaired in newborns due to a low plasminogen concentration. Thromb Haemost 1992;68:325.

122. deVeber G, Chan A, Monagle P, et al. Anticoagulation therapy in pediatric patients with sinovenous thrombosis: a cohort study. Arch Neurol 1998;55:1533.

123. Andrew M, Michelson AD, Bovill E, et al. Guidelines for antithrombotic therapy in pediatric patients. J Pediatr 1998;132:575.

124. Andrew M, deVeber G. Pediatric Thromboembolism and Stroke Protocols. Hamilton: BC Decker, 1999.

125. Ettingshausen CE, Veldmann A, Beeg T, et al. Replacement therapy with protein C concentrate in infants and adolescents with meningococcal sepsis and purpura fulminans. Semin Thromb Hemost 1999;25:537.

126. Kreuz WD, Schneider W, Nowak-Gottl U. Treatment of consumption coagulopathy with antithrombin concentrate in children with acquired antithrombin deficiency—a feasibility pilot study. Eur J Pediatr 1999;158(suppl 3):S187.

127. Hossmann V, Heiss WD, Bewermeyer H. Antithrombin III deficiency in ischaemic stroke. Klin Wochenschr 1983;61:617.

128. Ueyama H, Hashimoto Y, Uchino M, et al. Progressing ischemic stroke in a homozygote with variant antithrombin III. Stroke 1989;20:815.

129. Strater R, Kurnik K, Heller C, et al. Aspirin versus low-dose low-molecular-weight heparin: antithrombotic therapy in pediatric ischemic stroke patients: a prospective follow-up study. Stroke 2001;32:2554.

130. deVeber G, Chan A. Aspirin versus low-molecular-weight heparin for ischemic stroke in children: an unanswered question. Stroke 2002;33:1947; author reply 1947.

CHAPTER 4

Diagnostic Strategies in Neonates, Children, and Young Adults with Stroke

Deborah K. Sokol • Hema Patel

The approach to a neonate, child, or young adult with a stroke must be individualized. The age of the child, previous medical history, and intercurrent illnesses should be taken into account. There is often a time lag in the identification of stroke in children compared with stroke in adults, probably as a result of a low index of suspicion of this condition in children. Although there has been increased emphasis to recognize ischemic stroke within 3 hours in adults to initiate thrombolytic therapy, recognition time has been reported as an average of 35.7 hours in children.[1] This time lag should improve with greater awareness that children do have strokes, and that children with specific medical conditions have a higher risk for strokes.

Evaluation of a child presenting with acute focal neurologic signs suggestive of a stroke involves three steps. First, acute medical problems, such as seizures, increased intracranial pressure, and glucose or electrolyte abnormalities, should be addressed. Second, the specific neurologic condition (stroke versus tumor, ischemic versus hemorrhagic stroke) must be diagnosed. Third, the cause of the stroke should be determined.

This chapter outlines the standard evaluation of stroke in neonates, children, and young adults. The term "preterm infant" refers to infants less than 36 weeks' gestational age. "Neonate" refers to an infant from birth to the 28th day of life. "Children" refers to individuals ages 1 to 15. "Young adult" refers to individuals ages 15 to 45.

Clinical Presentation

Preterm Infants

Cerebral hypoperfusion in a premature infant results in periventricular leukomalacia (PVL), or diffuse cerebral white matter necrosis. The most common site for PVL is at the level of the optic radiation at the trigone of the lateral ventricles and at the level of the cerebral white matter around the foramen of Monro. These sites represent border zones between penetrating branches of the middle cerebral artery and the posterior cerebral artery (optic radiations) or the anterior cerebral artery (frontal white matter). More diffuse damage to the white matter results in the formation of cystic encephalomalacia. Most premature neonates who develop PVL or cystic encephalomalacia have experienced cardiorespiratory disturbance requiring artificial ventilation. These infants usually show generalized hypotonia followed by spastic diplegia.[2]

Neonates

Cerebral hypoperfusion in term neonates is associated with widespread cortical/subcortical infarcts in the parasagittal and white matter regions.[3] Term neonates may show fetal bradycardia, reduced respiratory effort, seizures, and coma. A term newborn shows a recognizable progression of clinical features after asphyxia.[2] During the first 12 hours, there is a decreased level of consciousness. Over the next 12 hours, there is "apparent" improvement in consciousness, although the brain impairment is shown clinically by seizures and apnea. Seizures, seen in 50% of cases, usually occur within the first day of life and suggest moderate to severe encephalopathy. Focal or multifocal seizures may indicate

focal or multifocal cerebral infarction. After 3 to 4 days, gradual improvement occurs, lasting into the subsequent weeks. Coma persisting beyond 1 week is associated with poor neurologic prognosis.[2]

Neonates with arterial ischemic stroke may present with focal weakness and focal seizures without significant depression of consciousness.[3] In contrast, some neonates show no clinical signs at birth and present at 6 to 12 months of age with gradual hemiparesis, the predominant use of one hand before hand dominance is usually established (i.e., "pathologic hand dominance"), or seizures.[4]

Seizures are commonly seen in premature infants with intraventricular hemorrhage (IVH) and in neonates with sinovenous thrombosis and intracranial hemorrhage.[2,5] Fever, lethargy, irritability, and respiratory distress are other common signs of sinovenous thrombosis in neonates.[6] Subarachnoid hemorrhage (SAH) in neonates can be heralded by seizures on the second day of life.[2]

Intracranial hemorrhage also can be seen in neonates with vein of Galen malformations (VGM), a unique cerebral vascular anomaly seen in neonates and older infants. VGM often presents in the neonatal period, but can be diagnosed prenatally via Doppler ultrasound. It is commonly associated with high-output congestive heart failure. Neonates and older infants may present with dilated scalp veins, a loud bruit over the head, and heart murmur associated with congestive heart failure or congenital cardiac anomalies, especially aortic coarctation and sinus venosus atrial septal defect.[7]

Children

Seizures and focal neurologic signs are commonly seen in children with arterial ischemic stroke, metabolic infarction from mitochondrial disease, sinovenous thrombosis, and intracranial hemorrhage. Headache or neck pain followed by focal neurologic signs occurring after even trivial trauma[8] suggests cervicocephalic dissection.

Fever and focal neurologic signs can be seen in stroke associated with infective endocarditis. Fever, weight loss, fatigue, renal disease, and skin disease are clinical signs of vasculitis. Patients may present with encephalopathy or focal or multifocal deficits. Fever, meningismus, and focal neurologic deficits suggest stroke associated with meningitis.[9] Arterial or venous stroke has been identified in 5% to 12% of children with meningitis, most commonly caused by *Streptococcus pneumoniae, Haemophilus influenzae,* or *Neisseria meningitidis.*[10] Stroke has been associated with other systemic infections, such as *Mycoplasma pneumoniae,* cat-scratch fever, Rocky Mountain spotted fever, varicella, and human immunodeficiency virus (HIV).[11-13] Children with history of recurrent ear infections may present with fever and mastoiditis, resulting in transverse sinus thrombosis ipsilateral to the mastoiditis.[14]

Headache is commonly seen with sinovenous thrombosis and intracranial hemorrhage. In addition to headache, fever, lethargy, and signs of increased intracranial pressure, such as vomiting, papilledema, and abducens nerve palsy, have been reported in children with sinovenous thrombosis.[6,15] Headache, meningeal signs, increased intracranial pressure, coma, and death can result from the rupture of vascular malformations and aneurysms associated with SAH.[16] Decreased consciousness at presentation of SAH is associated with a worse prognosis.[17]

In contrast to the frequently dramatic presentation of acute stroke in adults, the clinical signs of stroke in children may be subtle and gradual, initially missed by parents and physicians. Children with multiple infarctions resulting from congenital heart disease, sickle cell disease, or mitochondrial abnormality may show only developmental delay or learning disabilities. Primary angiitis of the central nervous system (CNS), an idiopathic small vessel vasculitis confined to the CNS, may cause gradual neurobehavioral impairment and neurologic deficit reflecting multifocal or diffuse brain damage.[18]

Young Adults

Seizures and focal neurologic deficits accompany arterial ischemic stroke, metabolic infarction, sinovenous thrombosis, and intracranial hemorrhage in young adults, as was seen in children. Young adults with migraine, focal neurologic deficits, and family history of migraine may have cerebral autosomal dominant arteriopathy and subcortical infarcts with leukoencephalopathy (CADASIL). These individuals are at higher risk for ischemic stroke and early signs of dementia.[19] Acute headache can be seen with sinovenous thrombosis and intracranial hemorrhage. Young adults using illicit drugs, such as amphetamines, ecstasy, cocaine, phencyclidine (PCP), and glue sniffing, are at risk for cerebral infarct and hemorrhage.[20] Young women taking first-generation oral contraceptives with 50 µg or more of estrogen may present with thromboembolic stroke.[21] Individuals taking appetite suppressants containing phenylpropanolamine may present with hemorrhagic stroke.[22] Women with breast cancer taking tamoxifen, an oral medication used to reduce risk of further breast cancer, are at higher risk for venous and arterial thrombosis.[23,24]

History and Physical Examination in Young Patients with Stroke

Preterm Infants

Clinical evaluation of preterm infants who have experienced cerebral hypoperfusion or IVH relies on a detailed history accounting for complications of the pregnancy, labor and delivery, and the clinical course contributing to cerebral injury. Prematurity alone, especially when associated with ventilator dependence, predisposes to cerebral hypoperfusion, primarily in the form of PVL. Generalized hypotonia followed by spastic diplegia can be seen on examination. IVH usually occurs within the first 3 to 4 postnatal days, with greater than 50% detectable within the first 6 postnatal hours.[25] Premature infants exposed to high fraction of inspired oxygen, early sepsis, pneumothorax, sudden decline in hematocrit,[26] and rapid volume re-expansion[27] are more likely to develop IVH. Examination can show generalized hypotonia and depressed consciousness.

Neonates

Clinical evaluation of neonates includes obtaining information about the pregnancy, the mother's health, the placenta, and the neonatal course. Preeclampsia may predispose to placental infarction via impairment of perfusion.[28,29] Maternal hematologic risk factors have been associated with neonatal stroke and placental infarction.[30] Fetal/neonatal autoimmune thrombocytopenia may manifest with intracranial hemorrhage.[31]

In term neonates presenting with arterial ischemic stroke (intrauterine stroke), the condition of the placenta should be determined. Placental infarction may lead to fetal cerebral infarction through embolization to the fetus.[32,33] It is important to contact the pathologist who has access to the placenta to determine the presence of placental emboli. History of dehydration, often caused by difficulty in breastfeeding, predisposes to sinovenous thrombosis. Family history of bleeding problems should be determined in neonates presenting with hemorrhagic stroke. Evidence of nonaccidental trauma must always be sought in taking the parental history, particularly in cases of intracranial hemorrhage.

Children and Young Adults

Clinical evaluation of a child or young adult presenting with acute stroke involves obtaining a detailed history, including previous medical diagnosis, recent trauma, fever, weight loss, infection including chickenpox, and drug ingestion. Certain diseases are associated with a higher risk for stroke, such as complex congenital heart disease, sickle cell disease, or coagulopathy. Past history of developmental delay or mental retardation suggests an underlying metabolic or genetic condition; history of prolonged bleeding after dental procedures suggests a coagulation defect. A careful family history should be taken, with attention to premature vascular disease, hematologic disease, and mental retardation.

Physical examination should include measurement of head circumference because enlargement may be associated with VGM or neurofibromatosis. Stature and build should be assessed, checking for clinical signs of Marfan or Ehlers-Danlos syndrome, or the thin habitus of homocystinuria. The skin should be examined for birthmarks, rash, signs of trauma, or intravenous drug abuse.

Café au lait spots would implicate neurofibromatosis 1, whereas neurocutaneous telangiectasias may be seen with Wyburn-Mason syndrome and hereditary hemorrhagic telangiectasia. Livedo reticularis would be associated with Sneddon syndrome, and purpuric rash would be associated with Henoch-Schönlein purpura. Homozygous patients with homocystinuria tend to have pale hair and blotchy erythematous skin pigmentation. Trauma is suggested by bruises in unusual locations or of varying ages. Splinter hemorrhages or embolic skin rash may be seen in infective endocarditis.

Funduscopic examination is important in looking for disc elevation or hemorrhage. Retinal hemorrhage in a young child with acute onset of neurologic signs is a sign of trauma. Consideration should be given to obtaining photographs of the fundus in this instance. Changes of chronic hypertension or retinal emboli may be seen in young adults with stroke. Abnormal retinal vasculature is associated with cerebrovascular anomalies.[34] Subhyaloid retinal hemorrhages can be detected in SAH.

Because cardiac disease is a major cause of stroke in children, a detailed cardiovascular examination is necessary. Murmurs and heart sound abnormalities may be identified in patients with underlying structural heart disease or acquired cardiac disease, such as infective endocarditis. Careful examination for bruits in the neck and head should be conducted on all patients, and bruits may be found in patients with atherosclerotic vascular narrowing or arteriovenous malformation (AVM). Hypertension may be the result of stroke or causally related to either ischemic or hemorrhagic stroke.

Neuroimaging

Head Ultrasound

Premature Infants

In a critically ill preterm infant, ultrasound is preferable to magnetic resonance imaging (MRI) because it can be performed at the bedside. Cerebral hypoperfusion injury may be recognized on ultrasound scans as increased parenchymal echogenicity; however, this requires subjective interpretation.[35] Ultrasound shows high reliability in the detection of severe cases of PVL and cystic white matter injury.[36] Because of the difficulty in determining parenchymal echogenicity, however, it has been estimated that 70% of PVL remains undetected by ultrasonography, particularly in less severe cases.[37,38] This deficiency of neonatal ultrasound is important because noncystic white matter injury in the form of PVL is more common than cystic white matter injury.[36]

In premature infants, ultrasound is the technique of choice for diagnosis of the germinal matrix hemorrhage/IVH (Fig. 4-1).[35,38] IVH larger than 5 mm in diameter is detected with a sensitivity approaching 100%.[37,39] IVH can be classified into four grades: (1) germinal matrix hemorrhage, (2) blood within but not distending the ventricle, (3) blood filling and distending the ventricle, and (4) intraparenchymal.[40] Better outcome is associated with grades 1 and 2. Common sequelae of IVH include posthemorrhagic hydrocephalus. When IVH is diagnosed, serial ultrasound scans can be used to follow ventricular size.[41]

Ultrasonography has more limited clinical utility in term newborns. Generalized increased echogenicity may indicate diffuse cerebral hypoperfusion, but echogenicity may be difficult to interpret.[35] Focal ischemic lesions may show up as localized areas of increased echogenicity that over time may develop into a porencephalic cyst.[2] Ultrasound may miss ischemic stroke altogether.[42]

On ultrasound, acute hemorrhage is echo dense or whiter than the surrounding brain. Ultrasound measurement of cisternal SAH in 63 premature infants who went on to autopsy correctly predicted SAH with an accuracy of 75%, sensitivity of 69%, and specificity of 93%.[43] Parenchymal hemorrhage is associated with mass effect and distortion of normal brain anatomy seen on ultrasound. This technique may miss isolated SAH or subdural hematomas, however.[44] MRI should be performed on term infants with intracranial hemorrhage when patients are stable, especially for infants found to have IVH because structural lesions are more often associated with IVH in this age group.

Computed Tomography

Computed tomography (CT) scan can be done quickly (<15 minutes for a noncontrast study). During the scan, the patient can be viewed with easy access in case of an emergency. Although young children often require sedation, older children and sometimes infants can be imaged without sedation. These characteristics make CT a good first study in acutely ill patients. Noncontrast CT scan is the usual first study in an older child or adult with sudden onset of focal neurologic signs. CT detection of early (<6 hours after ictus) ischemic infarct, compared with subsequent MRI, has shown sensitivity ranging from 47% to 85%, with

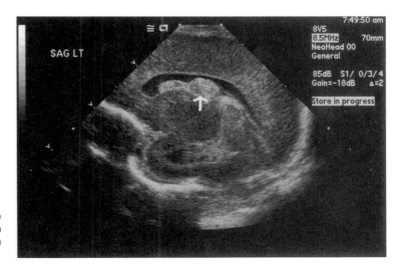

FIGURE 4-1   Ultrasound showing grade 3 intraventricular hemorrhage (*arrow*) in a premature infant who presented with seizures.

excellent specificity.[45,46] Availability of a clinical history indicating that early stroke is suspected significantly improves the sensitivity for detecting strokes on unenhanced CT without reducing specificity.[47]

CT scan may suggest sinovenous thrombosis, but can miss the diagnosis in 10% to 40% of cases.[15,48] A dense triangle sign pertains to opacification of the torcula by freshly thrombosed blood that can be seen on head CT scan without contrast enhancement. An empty delta sign pertains to hypodensity in the torcula correlating with the thrombus in the sinus that can be seen on head CT scan with contrast enhancement.

CT is still the most sensitive technique to detect fresh hemorrhage in most parts of the CNS. Parenchymal, subarachnoid, subdural, and epidural hemorrhage can be easily visualized. Acute hemorrhage appears hyperdense on CT scan in a patient with a normal hematocrit. Over the course of the next 1 to 3 weeks, the resolving blood becomes isodense with brain. Ultimately, an intraparenchymal hemorrhage may leave an area of encephalomalacia, which appears more hypodense than the surrounding tissue.

Perfusion Computed Tomography

In perfusion CT, quantitative determination of cerebral blood flow is derived via injection of intravenous iodinated contrast material followed by sequential acquisition of CT images as the dye passes through the brain. Areas of decreased perfusion appear as a change in color.[49] Serial images are obtained through the level above the confluence of sinuses at the superior sagittal sinus and at the level of the basal ganglia. Similar to conventional CT, the posterior fossa is less well defined via perfusion CT. Measures of cerebral blood flow, cerebral blood volume, and the time to peak maximal level of contrast enhancement in brain parenchyma are obtained. These values predict subsequent infarction. Prediction of acute supratentorial ischemia with 91% to 93% sensitivity has been shown for cerebral blood flow measurement, with infarction ultimately occurring in all patients with cerebral blood flow reduction of more than 70%.[50]

Magnetic Resonance Imaging

Brain MRI is the most sensitive and specific of the imaging techniques in children and adults.[51] It is more specific for ischemic and hemorrhagic lesions than CT or ultrasound. MRI is particularly useful if the symptoms suggest that the lesion is likely to involve the brainstem, the base of the brain, or other posterior fossa structures, areas not well seen on CT scans. MRI is indicated after CT scan has provided initial information about the presence or absence of blood or mass effect or both. Obtaining an MRI study in the acute setting of ischemic stroke or brain hemorrhage provides clinical challenges, however. Brain MRI usually requires 1 hour of imaging time. Children younger than 5 or 6 years almost always require sedation (Table 4-1). Patients with cardiac pacemakers or paramagnetic foreign bodies cannot undergo MRI; vagal nerve stimulators must be turned off. During the study, the patient cannot be seen clearly and must be mechanically monitored.

Premature Infants and Neonates

There is increasing belief that MRI has greater sensitivity and specificity for the detection of perinatal hypoxic-ischemic injury than either ultrasound or CT. Early T2 prolongation on standard MRI within 12 to 18 hours after injury seems to correlate with transient edema, whereas T1 shortening (high signal) after 3 days and T2 shortening (low signal) after 6 to 7 days correlate with permanent brain injury.[35,52] MRI permits a more detailed picture of patterns of cerebral hypoperfusion, including PVL and parasagittal injury.[52] Presently, MRI is considered the optimal neuroimaging modality for detection of perinatal hypoxic-ischemic cerebral injury.[53]

Children and Young Adults

Standard MRI may show ischemic changes (increased signal on T2-weighted and proton density images) 6 to 12 hours after infarction.[54-57] Established infarction is readily identified on MRI as an area of increased signal on T2-weighted and proton density

TABLE 4-1   **Sedation Policy for Magnetic Resonance Imaging/Magnetic Resonance Angiography at Riley Hospital for Children, Indianapolis, Indiana**

Chloral Hydrate	Dosage
Newborns (0-4 wk)	75-100 mg/kg chloral hydrate syrup
≥1 month (≤10 kg)	50-75 mg/kg chloral hydrate syrup
If patient is still not unconscious after 20-30 min, give another 25 mg/kg of chloral hydrate	
Maximum dose of chloral hydrate not to exceed 1000 mg	
Intravenous Sedation	
Midazolam and sodium pentobarbital in patients >10 kg	
Midazolam Dose	
0.05-0.1 mg/kg (if patient is <12 mo, give 0.05 mg/kg of midazolam)	
Sodium Pentobarbital Dose	
2-6 mg/kg	
Push sodium pentobarbital slowly; do not give >50 mg/min; maximum total dose not to exceed 100 mg or 6 mg/kg	
Procedure	
Midazolam is given first; 2 min later, sodium pentobarbital is injected slowly	
Treatment for Overdose and Respiratory Depression	
Intravenous flumazenil 0.01-0.2 mg/kg	

images and decreased signal on T1-weighted images. Normal vessels are seen as a flow void on MRI. Absence of this normal flow void or abnormally increased signal within an artery suggests arterial occlusion or very slow flow.[57] MRI often can distinguish arterial from venous occlusive disease.

MRI is more sensitive than CT in detecting small ischemic lesions. In Kawasaki or sickle cell disease, MRI can detect clinically silent lesions that may identify individuals at increased risk for recurrent strokes.[58,59] In sickle cell disease and childhood migraine, MRI may identify small infarcts in the white matter or basal ganglia that can be missed on CT. MRI may detect a constellation of findings (absence of middle cerebral artery flow void, linear or circular intensities in the basal ganglia representing telangiectatic vessels, and multiple strokes in the carotid circulation) that is suggestive of the diagnosis of moyamoya disease (Fig. 4-2A). Such findings should be followed by an investigation of the cerebral vasculature (Fig. 4-2B).[60]

The ability of MRI to visualize absent flow, the presence of thrombus, "clot" progression, resolution over time, and parenchymal lesions has made it the diagnostic study of choice in sinovenous thrombosis.[61,62] Signs of sinovenous thrombosis on MRI and MR venography include visualization of thrombus and an absence of flow void signal in a given cerebral vein or intracranial venous sinus. Thrombus appears as an increased signal on T1-weighted, proton density, and T2-weighted images in a cerebral vein or sinus.

MRI is more specific than CT in the identification and staging of hemorrhage and clot formation associated with the breakdown of hemoglobin. Blood breaks down quickly, and each stage of degradation is associated with a different MRI appearance. In addition, the appearance of blood on MRI depends on the imaging conditions and the field strength of the instrument used.[63] Generally, acute hemorrhage is isointense on T1-weighted images and dark on T2-weighted images, whereas subacute blood appears hyperintense on T1-weighted and T2-weighted images.[63] MRI may be as sensitive as CT for parenchymal hemorrhages and more sensitive than CT for petechial blood in an area of ischemia.[63] MRI is the procedure of choice for angiographically occult lesions, such as cavernous angiomas. Echo gradient MRI sequence has improved identification of parenchymal blood.[64] MRI is less sensitive, however, than CT for identifying subarachnoid blood.

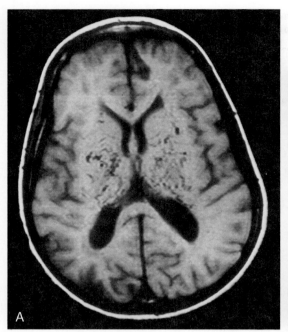
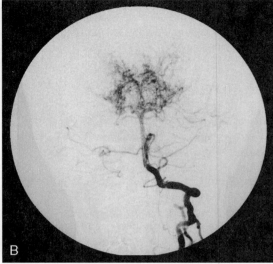

FIGURE 4-2   **A,** T2-weighted MR image showing bilateral thalamic flow voids in a 9-year-old boy with right hemiparesis. He was found to have moyamoya disease. **B,** Angiogram showing near-complete occlusion of both posterior cerebral arteries with hypertrophy of the anterior and posterior thalamoperforate and thalamogeniculate vessels. The patient also had bilateral internal carotid artery stenosis, left greater than right (not shown).

MRI sequences, such as diffusion-weighted imaging (DWI) and perfusion-weighted imaging, can better define damaged cerebral tissue and tissue at risk for stroke progression. These techniques may show abnormality in acute stroke when T1-weighted and T2-weighted MR images appear normal.[65]

Diffusion-weighted Imaging

DWI measures the motion of water diffusion across tissue, which can aid in the determination of acute ischemic stroke. Water would be less likely to diffuse across regions that have sustained ischemic damage owing to cytotoxic edema; this generates a hyperintense signal relative to surrounding tissue and a decreased apparent diffusion coefficient, which is a quantitative measurement of ischemia (Fig. 4-3).[66] Detection of DWI signal abnormality may be age dependent. In infants, DWI abnormality after cerebral hypoperfusion can be seen within 4 days of the ischemic event. DWI then becomes falsely negative (pseudonormalization) 1 week after

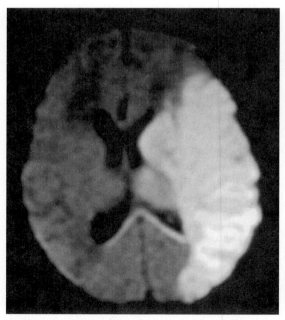

FIGURE 4-3   Diffusion-weighted MRI showing left middle cerebral artery infarct in a newborn who presented with seizures.

the event.[67] In adults, pseudonormalization occurs in 12 to 14 days. DWI has shown high sensitivity (57% to 99.1%) and specificity (78% to 88.5%) for detection of acute ischemic infarction in adults.[68,69]

Perfusion-weighted Imaging

Perfusion-weighted imaging involves uptake of gadolinium contrast material by the penumbra, the area of the brain surrounding the ischemic core. Apparent diffusion coefficient values are obtained for the penumbra. Perfusion-weighted imaging can be used to assess regional blood supply and to delineate a region of decreased perfusion that may or may not proceed to infarction. The extent to which the penumbra volume is larger than the ischemic core is a measure of "mismatch," which may have clinical importance. Initial studies suggest that poorer functional outcome is associated with lesions involving a large penumbra surrounding the ischemic core.[70] A better functional outcome has been associated with perfusion-weighted imaging signs of a penumbra without an ischemic core.[65]

Investigation of Cerebral Vessels

When the diagnosis of cerebral hemorrhage, arterial infarction, or venous infarction has been made, direct examination of the cerebral vessels must be considered. If spontaneous hemorrhage has occurred in the setting of normal coagulation and hematologic studies, angiography is almost always indicated, looking for a surgically resectable AVM, aneurysm, or vasculopathy. The decision about whether or not to perform angiography or some other assessment of the cerebral vasculature, such as MR angiography, must be made on a case-by-case basis. If venous infarction is suspected, MR venography may be used instead of more invasive venography to confirm the diagnosis and define the extent of the thrombosis.

Magnetic Resonance Angiography

MR angiography can be performed at the same time as MRI and adds information about the cerebral arteries. MR angiography can visualize blood flow in the major cerebral arteries at the level of the circle of Willis. It also can image flow in the extracranial carotid and vertebral arteries in the neck, at sites prone to dissection.[70] MR angiography has been used successfully to identify vascular anomalies, such as persistent fetal or atretic vessels in vertebrobasilar stenosis,[71] cerebral aneurysms,[72] and arterial lesions in sickle cell disease.[73] MR angiography cannot show small vessel disease. Abnormalities suggestive of moyamoya disease can be imaged, but the diagnostic basal collateral vessels are not always visible.[71]

MR angiography should be performed in patients with unexplained arterial ischemic infarction, especially if large vessel disease is a plausible cause for the stroke. Identification of a diagnostic abnormality may eliminate the need for angiography. MR angiography has been found to correlate well with conventional angiography in children with ischemic stroke.[70] MR angiography is the study of choice in patients at higher risk for complications from angiography, such as patients with sickle cell disease or renal disease. MR angiography may be a useful way to follow patients with documented lesions and to screen patients at risk for cerebrovascular disease.[73,74]

Magnetic Resonance Venography

MR venography employs the same principles as MR angiography except for the saturation (suppression) of inflowing arterial blood along with brain tissue.[72] MR venography is excellent for visualizing venous thrombosis, and in many departments this technique has supplanted conventional venography.[72] Knowledge of venous thrombosis is important because this condition can give rise to a variety of lesions, such as parenchymal hemorrhage, infarcts, hydrocephalus, and dilation of the deep periventricular veins. Some tumors, such as meningiomas, can compress the deep veins. This information is valuable to the surgeon because complete occlusion of the vein allows it to be sacrificed without danger.[72] Gadolinium can enable better visualization of smaller veins.

Angiography

Conventional catheter cerebral angiography is the gold standard against which other vascular imaging studies are compared. Angiography is the most sensitive test available for the identification of congenital or acquired disorders of the cerebral and extracerebral vasculature. It is superior to MR angiography for evaluation of small vessel disease.

Angiography is absolutely indicated in the evaluation of acute unexplained parenchymal brain hemorrhage. Generally, it should be performed as soon as the patient is stable, and nonvascular causes of the hemorrhage have been ruled out. Identification of an AVM or aneurysm, with early surgical remediation, may reduce the chances of rebleeding and result in a better outcome.[75-77]

Angiography also should be considered in patients with ischemic stroke when the cause of the infarction is unexplained. It can be useful to identify conditions such as moyamoya disease (see Fig. 4-2), fibromuscular dysplasia, atherosclerosis in a young adult, cervicocephalic arterial dissection, and cerebral venous occlusive disease. In these cases, the patient's management would clearly be modified by the results of this procedure (Table 4-2). MR angiography may be just as informative for disorders involving large vessels in the neck and the proximal intracerebral arteries.

Cerebral catheter angiography has greater risk than most of the other diagnostic procedures performed in stroke. General anesthesia or deep sedation is necessary for young children, although the procedure can be done with mild sedation and local anesthetic in older children. Angiography should be undertaken with caution in a patient with impaired renal function. Hyperosmolar contrast medium has been shown to induce in vitro sickling of erythrocytes from patients with sickle cell disorders, so caution must be used with these children as well.[78] The use of low-osmolar contrast medium has reduced the incidence of nephropathy in high-risk patients compared with the use of high-osmolar contrast medium.[79]

In some conditions, there is a risk of additional or worsening brain injury as a result of angiography. In Ehlers-Danlos type IV syndrome, the abnormal collagen in the vascular wall predisposes to aneurysm, which could rupture during angiography.[80] An intra-arterial thrombus in infective endocarditis could be dislodged during angiography causing a further embolic event.[81]

The usual technique in conventional catheter angiography involves catheterization of the femoral artery. When the transfemoral approach is contraindicated, such as in patients without femoral pulses or patients with recent graft surgery, alternative sites, such as the brachial[82] or radial arteries,[83] can be injected for cerebral angiograms.

Patient preparation for conventional angiography requires knowledge of cardiac and renal status. Informed consent must be obtained from the parents or young adult patients. To prevent aspiration, the patient must refrain from solid food for 6 hours before the procedure, but may drink clear liquids up to 2 hours before the procedure. Preprocedure laboratory tests include complete blood count with differential and platelets, prothrombin time (PT) (international normalized ratio), activated partial thromboplastin time (aPTT), and comprehensive metabolic screen, paying attention to serum creatinine and blood urea nitrogen.

TABLE 4-2 **Indications for Catheter Cerebral Angiography**

Absolute Indications

Acute, unexplained parenchymal hemorrhage
Stroke due to suspected small vessel disease that cannot be seen on MR angiography (e.g., vasculitis)

Should Be Considered

In patients with moyamoya disease before surgery
Ischemic stroke of unknown cause
In patients in whom MR angiography is inconclusive

Must Be Used with Caution in Patients with

Impaired renal function
Inconclusive MR angiography or carotid Doppler studies
Ehlers-Danlos syndrome type IV
Pseudoxanthoma elasticum

Carotid Ultrasound

B-mode ultrasonography has been widely used to examine the carotid artery.[84] This method provides real-time information about the lumen and the vessel wall and microscopic characteristics of carotid lesions. Two sonographic methods have been developed for improved understanding of the anatomy and function of the carotid artery. Color Doppler flow imaging has enabled display of the velocity and flow direction of red blood cells and vascular structures. Power Doppler imaging provides homogeneous color signals and generates angiography-like visualization of the vascular lumen surface. Consequently, color Doppler flow imaging and power Doppler imaging have made measurement of the residual lumen of carotid stenosis more reliable than conventional B-mode imaging.

In children, carotid ultrasound imaging requires expert interpretation because values of blood flow and vessel diameter for children differ from those of adults.[85] If pediatric carotid ultrasound interpretation is possible, and MR angiography is unavailable, carotid and transcranial ultrasound imaging should be considered in the evaluation of patients with stroke who are not candidates for standard angiography.[86,87] Carotid ultrasound has the greatest utility in evaluation of atherosclerotic disease of the large vessels, a condition uncommon in children and young adults.[87]

Carotid ultrasound also can be used to follow decimalization of blood vessels, such as after extracorporeal membrane oxygenation (ECMO) or carotid dissection. ECMO is a lifesaving procedure for neonates that involves permanent ligation of the right common carotid artery. Carotid ultrasound is routinely used in many centers to see if the right internal carotid has recanalized.[88,89] Results of a large multicenter study comparing carotid ultrasound with angiography in adults showed that ultrasound was able to differentiate normal from abnormal arteries with a sensitivity of 88% (1077 of 1233 arteries) and accuracy of 79% (1251 of 1578 arteries). Angiographic stenoses equal to or greater than 50% diameter was accurately identified by ultrasound in 72% (1133 of 1578 arteries) of cases.[90] Application of color Doppler imaging and power Doppler imaging includes identification of high-grade stenosis of the internal carotid

artery.[91] Power Doppler imaging has been developed further into three-dimensional visualization, which has been applied to the vertebrobasilar arteries[92] and intracranial vessels (see later).

Transcranial Doppler

Transcranial Doppler (TCD) uses relatively echolucent "windows" of the skull, such as the temporal bone, to image the arteries at the base of the brain. Stenosis is diagnosed on the basis of blood flow velocity. In children and neonates, the Doppler evaluation of the intracranial vessels is complicated further by variation of normal flow velocity according to age, behavioral state, hematocrit, and possibly gender.[86,93] Inability to show forward flow in a vessel and reversed or increased blood flow in related vessels suggests occlusion. TCD predicts the risk of stroke for children with sickle cell disease.[94] Children with abnormal Doppler results who were randomly assigned to receive long-term transfusion therapy had a 92% lower risk of stroke than children randomly assigned to usual care.[95] This finding resulted in early termination of this trial. TCD has been used in many centers to screen children with sickle cell disease. Physicians are employing the results of TCD velocity together with other data such as MRI/MR angiography in determining the need for long-term transfusion treatment in these patients.[96] The successful application of power TCD in the assessment of children with sickle cell disease has afforded superior visualization of intracranial vessels compared with standard Doppler techniques, and is likely to be used more routinely in the future.[97]

Functional Neuroimaging

Proton MR spectroscopy is a neuroimaging method of identifying spectra of brain chemicals. It can be used to identify brain injury secondary to stroke or ischemia. After stroke or asphyxia, tissue injury is seen by an increase in lactate from anaerobic glycolysis and a loss of *N*-acetyl aspartate from neuronal death.[98]

Other types of functional neuroimaging, such as positron emission tomography (PET) and single photon emission computed tomography (SPECT), have been used in research settings with small groups of children who have had stroke. These techniques may have limited clinical application because of the radiation exposure involved in their use. In several cases, functional neuroimaging has identified regions of brain injury not seen by structural neuroimaging. In an outcome study of 11 preterm infants, Tc 99m ECD SPECT perfusion deficits predicted cerebral palsy with 82% sensitivity, 70% specificity, and 74% accuracy.[99] In older children with spastic diplegia, including patients with neonatal strokes, Tc 99m HMPAO SPECT detected hypoperfusion corresponding to CT abnormalities, but this perfusion deficit extended beyond the boundaries of the anatomic deficits.[100]

In a study of 10 children with stroke associated with Sturge-Weber syndrome, HMPAO SPECT and fluorodeoxyglucose (FDG) PET detected bilateral disease in four patients who did not show brain calcification on MRI.[101] In a study of FDG PET in six children with sickle cell disease and stroke, PET showed a corresponding abnormality and identified an area of hypometabolism extending beyond the anatomic lesions detected by MRI for patients with large vessel disease ($n = 4$). PET did not show abnormality in the two patients with small vessel disease.[102]

Laboratory Examination

Cerebral Ischemia

Table 4-3 outlines tests to be considered in the evaluation of ischemic stroke. For any individual patient, clinical judgment determines which diagnostic studies to order.

Because cardiac disorders are common causes of ischemic infarction in children, a noninvasive evaluation of the cardiopulmonary system is indicated for every patient with unexplained stroke. Cardiac disorders associated with stroke are reviewed in detail in Chapter 7. Transthoracic echocardiography (TTE) is an important step in the evaluation of any child or young adult with unexplained cerebral infarction. Contrast echocardiography (echocardiography done

TABLE 4-3 **Laboratory Evaluation of Unexplained Ischemic Stroke**

Complete blood count, including platelets
Prothrombin time (international normalized ratio), activated partial thromboplastin time
Erythrocyte sedimentation rate
Lipid profile
Protein C
Protein S
Elevated plasma level of factor VIII
Homocystinuria
Hyperhomocysteinemia
Serum lactate*
Mitochondrial DNA analysis*
Hemoglobin electrophoresis*
Blood cultures*
Fasting glucose*
Urinalysis
Urine drug screen
Urine and serum amino acids*
Urine for sulfur-containing amino acids (cyanide nitroprusside test)*
Urinary organic acids*
Chest x-ray
Electrocardiogram
Transthoracic echocardiogram
Cervical spine x-ray or CT*
Transesophageal echocardiogram*
Contrast echocardiogram*
Tuberculosis skin testing*
Lumbar puncture*

*Indicates studies that are appropriate only in selected cases.

after intravenous injection of normal saline looking for passage of microbubbles from right to left) has been useful in documenting patent foramen ovale associated with stroke.[103,104] Transesophageal echocardiography (TEE) allows a more accurate evaluation of the interatrial septum, the left atrial body and appendage, cardiac valves, and aortic arch. This study is indicated when there is a high suspicion of a cardiac source of stroke, and the transthoracic study is normal. Numerous studies have shown nearly 100% detection of valvular vegetations with TEE, whereas the sensitivity of TTE may be 25% with very small vegetations.[105-108] TEE is uncomfortable and at this time technically impossible to perform on small children because the transducers are too large. Occasionally, cardiac catheterization is needed to confirm or clarify abnormalities identified by noninvasive techniques.

Prothrombotic Disorders

Prothrombotic disorders are important risk factors for ischemic stroke and sinovenous thrombosis in neonates, children, and young adults. A prothrombotic state is an impairment in the normal hemostatic system in which the balance has shifted toward thrombosis. It is most commonly caused by an abnormality or impairment of the vascular endothelium, the coagulation cascade, the fibrinolytic system, or platelets. Even if the patient has cardiac disease, the hematologic evaluation should still be undertaken because patients with cardiac disease may have a concomitant hypercoagulable state.[109]

Cerebral infarction can occur with deficiency of protein C, protein S, antithrombin (formerly antithrombin III), and plasminogen, or the presence of activated protein C resistance. Protein C, protein S, and antithrombin deficiency may be inherited or acquired. Infections, medications such as asparaginase, and hepatic or renal disease, such as the nephrotic syndrome, are the most common causes of acquired deficiency. Presence of mutations such as factor V Leiden mutation, prothrombin G20210A mutation, homozygous methylene tetrahydrofolate reductase (MTHFR) polymorphism, antiphospholipid antibodies, hyperhomocysteinemia, and elevated lipoprotein (a) are other risk factors.[48] Test results must be compared with age-appropriate reference tables because the hemostatic system is different in infants and children compared with adults.[110]

Neonates

Prothrombotic disorders have been associated with perinatal or neonatal ischemic stroke. Gunther and coworkers[111] evaluated protein C, protein S, antithrombin, factor V Leiden G1691A mutation, prothrombin G20210A gene mutation, lipoprotein (a), and MTHFR c677T in 91 term neonates with ischemic stroke and 182 age-matched and sex-matched controls. They found at least one prothrombotic abnormality in 68% of neonates with ischemic stroke compared with 24% of healthy controls, yielding an odds ratio of 6.7. Other tests of prothrombotic disorders have shown abnormality in neonates with ischemic stroke—plasminogen, activated protein C resistance, IgG and IgM anticardiolipin antibodies, and lupus anticoagulant.[29] Antiphospholipid antibodies should be checked in the mother and the infant in perinatal stroke. Homozygous deficiencies of protein C and protein S usually manifest in the neonatal period, whereas heterozygous deficiencies manifest after puberty.[110]

In the largest study of sinovenous thrombosis in children, deVeber and colleagues[14] reported that neonates accounted for 43% of cases of sinovenous thrombosis in Canadian children, which occurred at a rate of 0.67 cases per 100,000 children per year. Sinovenous thrombosis tends to occur later in the perinatal period than ischemic stroke and can be associated with fetal coagulopathy.[14] Additionally, neonatal sinovenous thrombosis has been associated with protein C deficiency, protein S deficiency, antithrombin deficiency, factor V Leiden mutation, and MTHFR mutation.[28]

Children and Young Adults

The overall incidence of prothrombotic states in children with ischemic strokes is reported to be 10% to 50%.[112-114] Factor V Leiden mutation occurs in 5% to 12% of the general pediatric population. Factor V Leiden gene mutation results in resistance to activated protein C. Heterozygous carriers have a 7-fold increased risk for thrombosis, whereas the risk for homozygous individuals is increased 80-fold.[115]

Children with antiphospholipid antibodies have a significantly increased risk for arterial and venous thrombosis, of which 50% occur in the CNS.[115] Antiphosphatidylethanolamine antibody in particular has been linked to ischemic stroke in young adults (Fig. 4-4).[116] Lipoprotein (a) is a low-density lipoprotein–like lipoprotein that is usually associated with hypercholesterolemia and is an independent risk factor.[117] Lipoprotein (a) levels are increased in children with arterial strokes compared with control subjects.

Pregnancy and the puerperium period are prothrombotic states for healthy young women.[118] As gestation progresses through the second and third trimesters, the levels of vitamin K–dependent factors II, VII, and X increase. The levels of free and total

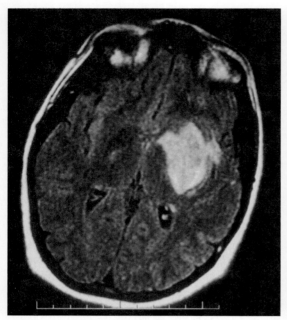

FIGURE 4-4 Axial fluid-attenuated inversion recovery (FLAIR) brain MRI shows infarction involving the left lenticular nucleus, caudate nucleus, and periopercular region in a 16-year-old girl who presented with fever, rash, and left hemiparesis. She was found to have antiphospholipid antibody in her serum and cerebrospinal fluid.

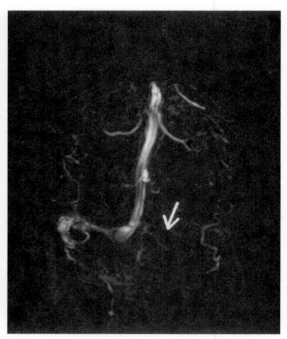

FIGURE 4-5 MR venography showing left transverse sinus and sigmoid sinus thrombosis (*arrow*) in a 22-year-old woman who presented with headaches and vomiting. She was found to have elevated factor VIII activity.

protein S decrease, and a decrease in the activated protein C–sensitivity ratio is noted. There is an increased level of circulating von Willebrand factor. Triglyceride and lipoprotein (a) levels increase, which may contribute to increased thrombin formation and decreased fibrinolysis.[119] These factors contribute to the increased maternal risk of arterial ischemic stroke and sinovenous thrombosis around the time of delivery.[120]

Deficiency of protein C, protein S, and antithrombin; factor V Leiden mutation; and antiphospholipid antibodies have been associated with sinovenous thrombosis in children.[121] Acquired or hereditary prothrombotic conditions, particularly elevation in plasma factor VIII, have been associated with sinovenous thrombosis in adults.[122] Figure 4-5 shows left transverse sinus and sigmoid sinus thrombosis in a 22-year-old woman with elevated factor VIII level.

Cerebral Hemorrhage

Cerebral hemorrhage may occur by two mechanisms: ischemic strokes evolving to hemorrhagic transformation, and hemorrhage caused by a bleeding diathesis. In the first case, thrombus not only causes ischemia, but also can damage large vessel walls, resulting in hemorrhagic stroke. In this circumstance, the prothrombotic evaluation (as described earlier) must be undertaken. Hemorrhagic stroke also can result from primary deficiencies in clotting mechanisms or platelet function. These deficiencies include defects in factors VII, VIII, IX, X, XI, and XIII and von Willebrand factor.[123] Defects in fibrinogen and platelet function also predispose to hemorrhagic stroke. Evaluation for a bleeding diathesis must be undertaken for neonates, children, or young adults presenting with hemorrhagic stroke (Table 4-4).

Bleeding Diathesis

Neonates

The hematologic evaluation includes tests to identify a bleeding diathesis or underlying systemic illness or both leading to hemorrhagic stroke. A common cause of hemorrhagic stroke in the newborn, vitamin K deficiency should be considered in every

TABLE 4-4 **Laboratory Evaluation in Hemorrhagic Stroke***

Complete blood count
Platelet count
PT (international normalized ratio)
aPTT
  If PT elevated—factor VII level
  If aPTT elevated—factor VIII, IX, XI, XII levels and
    von Willebrand activity
  If PT and aPTT elevated—factor II, V, X levels and
    fibrinogen
Serum electrolytes
Blood glucose
Blood urea nitrogen and serum creatine
Liver enzyme levels
Serum calcium
Bleeding time
  If elevated—von Willebrand factor, platelet
    function studies
Drug screen
Erythrocyte sedimentation rate
Luetic and HIV tests
Blood cultures
Sickle cell screen
Hemoglobin electrophoresis
Thick and thin smear of peripheral blood
Fibrinogen, fibrin split products
PAI-1 (plasminogen activity inhibitor-1)

*Consultation with a pediatric hematologist is advised in case of hematologic disorders.

aPTT, activated partial thromboplastin time; PT, prothrombin time.

Adapted from Biller J, Garg B. Stroke in children. In Noseworthy JH, ed. Neurological Therapeutics. London: Martin Dunitz, 2003.

neonate presenting with hemorrhagic stroke. A hematologic consultation is suggested to determine further causes of hypocoagulable states and hemophilia (see later).

Children and Young Adults

Hemophilia must be considered as a possible cause of hemorrhagic stroke. The most common form, factor VIII deficiency, and other forms such as factor IX deficiency are transmitted via X-linked dominant inheritance so that males only are affected. Female carriers may have factor VIII or IX deficiencies, however, and mild bleeding tendencies,[124] which could result in hemorrhagic stroke. In about half of new cases, there is no family history of abnormal bleeding, and the hemophilia is a result of a spontaneous genetic mutation within a recent generation.[125] Other clotting factor deficiencies,

such as factor V or VII and von Willebrand disease, are autosomal and occur equally in men and women.

When a bleeding disorder is suspected, a coagulation workup includes a complete blood cell count, PT, and aPTT. The aPTT may be prolonged if factor VIII or IX levels are less than 20% to 30% and should be prolonged with factor levels less than 15%; the aPTT is a good screening test for all but very mild types of hemophilia.[124] Platelet counts and bleeding times are normal because primary hemostasis is not affected by hemophilia. A prolonged PT indicates factor VII or final common pathway deficiencies (i.e., factors X, V, prothrombin, thrombin, or fibrin). Hematology consultation should be obtained so that specific factor assays can be performed as soon as possible to diagnose the type of hemophilia.

Acquired disorders of coagulation may result from many different conditions, including sepsis, pregnancy, malignancy, or rheumatologic disease.[126] The screening studies outlined (PT [international normalized ratio], aPTT, complete blood count with differential and platelets), erythrocyte sedimentation rate, antinuclear antibodies, and history and physical examination generally detect some abnormality requiring a more aggressive search for one of these underlying conditions.

Metabolic Conditions

Evaluation for metabolic conditions includes a comprehensive metabolic panel, urine screen for organic and amino acids, gene test for homozygous homocystinuria, and methionine loading test for heterozygous homocystinuria. Fasting lipid profile should be performed. Serum or cerebrospinal fluid (or both) lactate may be abnormal in mitochondrial disease.

Pathology

Surgical specimens from children and young adults with strokes are obtained from carotid endarterectomy in patients with accelerated atherosclerosis and from removal of vascular lesions such as AVM or clots from brain parenchyma. Carotid endarterectomy specimens usually show features of complicated atherosclerosis. Fragile, often ulcerated atheroma, strategically located within cervical arteries, may lead to artery-artery emboli of either platelet-fibrin or atheromatous material causing ischemic stroke. Rarely, severe atheroma in the circle of Willis—especially involving the basilar artery—may cause ectasia or fusiform enlargement of the artery. This aneurysmal dilation may result in symptoms caused by compression of nearby structures, such as the brainstem in the case of a basilar artery aneurysm. Surgical pathologic specimens can be used to diagnose other rare arteriopathies affecting large arteries (e.g., fibromuscular dysplasia, moyamoya disease, HIV-associated vasculopathy).[127]

Clots removed surgically must be examined for other diseases that may have caused the bleed, such as primary or metastatic neoplasm or vasculitis. Microangiopathies associated with spontaneous intracerebral hemorrhage can be diagnosed from seemingly trivial surgical material and may influence subsequent patient management. Rarely, a surgically evacuated blood clot may contain evidence of a vascular malformation.

Miscellaneous Evaluations

A chest CT scan is necessary to uncover a pulmonary AVM in Rendu-Osler-Weber/hereditary hemorrhagic telangiectasia.[128] MR venography of the lower extremities and pelvis may be necessary to detect a paradoxical embolism in May-Turner syndrome. In this uncommon condition, there is impaired venous return because of compression of the left common iliac vein by the overlying right common iliac artery, resulting in iliofemoral deep venous thrombosis. Such an obstruction to venous return would be missed if only structures proximal to the heart were investigated.[129] Diagnosis of fibromuscular dysplasia, associated with ischemic stroke, may be confirmed with renal MR angiography to detect beading of the renal arteries.[130]

Conclusion

The approach to a young patient with stroke involves differentiation between ischemic versus hemorrhagic conditions, visualization of the cerebral vasculature, and determination of underlying etiology. This process usually begins with an ultrasound in an infant with an open fontanelle and a CT scan in older patients. The head CT scan is used to rule out hemorrhagic stroke and determine mass effect/midline shift. More sensitive MRI, supplemented with DWI and perfusion-weighted imaging analysis, is used to assess the extent of the stroke. MR angiography detects large and medium artery anatomy; MR venography detects venous anatomy. Catheter angiography is used to identify the cause of cerebral hemorrhage or to visualize small vessel ischemic disease such as vasculitis. The search for a condition that predisposed the patient to stroke begins with a careful history and physical examination combined with a series of screening tests. The results of this initial evaluation may direct additional studies to be done. The nature and extent of the diagnostic testing must be individualized for each patient.

REFERENCES

1. Gabis LV, Yangala R, Lenn NJ. Time lag to diagnosis of stroke in children. Pediatrics 2002;110:924.
2. Volpe JJ. Neurology of the Newborn. Philadelphia: WB Saunders, 2001.
3. Allan WC, Riviello JJ. Perinatal cerebrovascular disease in the neonate. Pediatr Neurol 1992;39:621.
4. Bouza H, Rutherford M, Acolet D, et al. Evolution of early hemiplegic signs in full term infants with unilateral lesions in the neonatal period: a prospective study. Neuropediatrics 1994;25:201.
5. Shevell MI, Silver K, O'Gorman AM, et al. Neonatal dural sinus thrombosis. Pediatr Neurol 1989;5:161.
6. Schoenberg BS, Mellinger JF, Schenberg DG. Cerebrovascular disease in infants and children: a study of incidence, clinical features, and survival. Neurology 1978;28:763.
7. Preter M, Tzourio C, Ameri A, et al. Long-term prognosis in cerebral venous thrombosis: follow-up of 77 patients. Stroke 1996;27:243.
8. Patel H, Smith RR, Garg BP. Spontaneous extracranial artery dissection in children. Pediatr Neurol 1995;13:55.
9. Takeoka M, Takahashi T. Infectious and inflammatory disorders of the circulatory system and stroke in childhood. Curr Opin Neurol 2002;15:159.
10. de Veber G. Cerebrovascular disease in children. In Swaiman KF, ed. Pediatric Neurology: Principles and Practice, 3rd ed. St. Louis, Mosby, 1999.
11. Chabrier S, Rodesch G, Lasjaunias P, et al. Transient cerebral arteriopathy: a disorder recognized by serial angiograms in children with stroke. J Child Neurol 1998;13:27.
12. Askalan R, Laughlin S, Mayank S, et al. Chickenpox and stroke in childhood: a study of frequency and causation. Stroke 2001;32:1257.

13. Joshi VV, Pawel B, Connor E, et al. Arteriopathy in children with acquired immune deficiency syndrome. Pediatr Pathol 1987;7:261.
14. deVeber G, Andrew M, Adams C, et al. For the Canadian Pediatric Ischemic Stroke Study Group. Cerebral sinovenous thrombosis in children. N Engl J Med 2001;345:417.
15. deVeber G, Roach ES, Riela AR, et al. Stroke in children: recognition, treatment and future directions. Semin Pediatr Neurol 2000;7:301.
16. Ohkuma H, Suzuki S, Organe K. Study Group of the Association of Cerebrovascular Disease in Tokeo, Japan. Dissecting aneurysms of intracranial carotid circulation. Stroke 2002;33:941.
17. Higgins JJ, Kammerman LA, Fits CR. Predictors of survival and characteristics of childhood stroke. Neuropediatrics 1991;22:190.
18. Lopez-Yunez AM, Garg BP. Non-infectious cerebral vasculitis in children. Semin Cerebrovasc Dis Stroke 2001;1:249.
19. Chabriat H, Vahedi K, Iba-Zizen MT. Cerebral autosomal dominant arteriopathy and subcortical infarcts with leukoencephalopathy (CADASIL). Lancet 1995;346:934.
20. Sloan MA, Kittner SJ, Feeser BR, et al. Illicit drug-associated ischemic stroke in the Baltimore-Washington Young Stroke Study. Neurol 1998;50:1688.
21. Stadel BV. Oral contraceptives and cardiovascular disease. N Engl J Med 1981;305:612.
22. Kernan WM, Viscoli CM, Brass LM. Phenylpropanolamine and the risk of hemorrhagic stroke. N Engl J Med 2000;343:1826.
23. Saphner T, Tormey DC, Gray R. Venous and arterial thrombosis in patients who received adjuvant tamoxifen therapy for breast cancer. J Clin Oncol 1991;9:286.
24. Dignam JJ, Fisher B. Occurrence of stroke with tamoxifen in NSABP B-24. Lancet 2000;355:848.
25. Shaver DC, Bada HS, Korones SB, et al. Early and late intraventricular hemorrhage: the role of obstetric factors. Obstet Gynecol 1992;80:831.
26. Haskin L, Levit O, Klinger G, et al. Risk factors for intraventricular hemorrhage in very low birth weight premature infants: a retrospective case-control study. Pediatrics 2003;111:590.
27. Shankaran S, Bauer CR, Bain R, et al. Prenatal and perinatal risk and protective factors for neonatal intracranial hemorrhage. National Institute of Child Health and Human Development Neonatal Research Network. Arch Pediatr Adolesc Med 1996;150:491.
28. Golomb MR. Sinovenous thrombosis in neonates. Semin Cerebrovasc Dis Stroke 2001;1:216.
29. deVeber G, Monagle P, Chan A, et al. Prothrombotic disorders in infants and children with cerebral thromboembolism. Arch Neurol 1998;55:1539.
30. Becroft DM, Thompson JM, Mitchell EA. The epidemiology of placental infarction at term. Placenta 2002;23:343.
31. Kanhai HH, Porcelijn L, Zoeren D, et al. Antenatal care in pregnancies at risk of alloimmune thrombocytopenia: a report of 19 cases in 16 families. Eur Obstet Gynecol Reprod Biol 1996;68:67.
32. Redline RW, Wilson-Costello D, Borawshi E, et al. Placental lesions associated with neurologic impairment and cerebral palsy in very low birth-weight infants. Arch Pathol Lab Med 1998;122:1091.
33. Burke CJ, Tanneberg AE. Prenatal brain damage and placental infarction—an autopsy study. Dev Med Child Neurol 1995;37:555.
34. Berg BO. Unusual neurocutaneous syndromes. Neurol Clin 1985;3:165.
35. Barkovich AJ, Hallam D. Neuroimaging in perinatal hypoxic-ischemic injury. MRDD Res Rev 1997;3:28.
36. Inder TE, Anderson NJ, Spencer C, et al. White matter injury in the premature infant: a comparison between serial cranial sonographic and MR findings at term. AJNR Am J Neuroradiol 2003;24:805.
37. Carson SC, Hertzberg BS, Bowie JD, et al. Value of sonography in the diagnosis of intracranial hemorrhage and periventricular leukomalacia: a postmortem study of 35 cases. AJNR Am J Neuroradiol 1990;11:677.
38. Maalouf EF, Duggan PJ, Counsell SJ, et al. Comparison of findings on cranial ultrasound and magnetic resonance imaging in preterm infants. Pediatrics 2001;107:719.
39. Rumack CM, Manco-Johnson ML, Manco-Johnson MJ. Timing and course of neonatal intracranial hemorrhage using real-time ultrasound. Radiology 1985;154:101.
40. Papile LA, Burstein J, Burstein R, et al. Incidence and evolution of subependymal and intraventricular hemorrhage: a study of infants with birth weights less than 1,500 gm. J Pediatr 1978;92:529.
41. Allan WC, Holt PJ, Sawyer LR, et al. Ventricular dilation after neonatal periventricular intraventricular hemorrhage: natural history and therapeutic implications. Am J Dis Child 1982;136:589.
42. Golomb MR, Dick PT, MacGregor DL, et al. Cranial ultrasonography has a low sensitivity for detecting arterial ischemic stroke in term neonates. J Child Neurol 2003;18:98.
43. Kazam E, Rudelli R, Monte W, et al. Sonographic diagnosis of cisternal subarachnoid hemorrhage in the premature infant. AJNR Am J Neuroradiol 1994;15:1009.
44. Grant EG, White EM. Pediatric neurosonography. J Child Neurol 1986;1:319.
45. Urback H, Flacke S, Keller E, et al. Detectability and detection rate of acute cerebral hemisphere infarcts on CT and diffusion weighted MRI. Neuroradiology 2000;42:722.
46. Marks MP, Holmgren HB, Fox AJ, et al. Evaluation of early computed tomographic findings in acute ischemic stroke. Stroke 1999;30:389.
47. Mullins ME, Lev MH, Schellingerhout D, et al. Influence of availability of clinical history on detection of early stroke using unenhanced CT and diffusion-weighted MR imaging. AJR Am J Roentgenol 2002;179:223.

48. Carvalho KS, Garg BP. Cerebral venous thrombosis and venous malformations in children. Neurol Clin North Am 2002;20:1061.
49. Perez-Arjona EA, DelProposto Z, Sehgal V, et al. New techniques in cerebral imaging. Neurol Res 2002;24(suppl 1):S17.
50. Mayer TE, Hamann GF, Garanczyk J, et al. Dynamic CT perfusion imaging of acute stroke. AJNR Am J Neuroradiol 2000;21:1441.
51. Hunter JV. Magnetic resonance imaging in pediatric stroke. Top Magn Reson Imaging 2002;13:23.
52. Barkovich AJ. Destructive brain disorders of childhood. In Barkovich AJ, ed. Pediatric Neuroimaging, 2nd ed. New York: Raven Press, 1995.
53. Blankenberg FG, Norbash AM, Lane B, et al. Neonatal intracranial ischemia and hemorrhage: diagnosis with US, CT, and MR imaging. Radiology 1996;99:253.
54. Hill A, Volpe JJ. Hypoxic-ischemic cerebral injury in the newborn. In Swaiman K, ed. Pediatric Neurology, 3rd ed. St. Louis: Mosby, 1999.
55. Bryan RN, Levy LM, Whitlow WD, et al. Diagnosis of acute cerebral infarction: comparison of CT and MRI imaging. AJNR Am J Neuroradiol 1991;12:611.
56. Fisher M, Sotak CH, Minematsu K, et al. New magnetic resonance techniques for evaluating cerebrovascular disease. Ann Neurol 1992;21:115.
57. Yuh WTC, Grain MR, Loes DJ, et al. MR imaging of cerebral ischemia: findings in the first 24 hours. AJNR Am J Neuroradiol 1991;12:621.
58. Koelfen W, Wentz U, Konig S, et al. Magnetic resonance angiography in 140 neuropediatrics patients. Pediatr Neurol 1995;12:31.
59. Kugler S, Anderson B, Cross D, et al. Abnormal cranial magnetic resonance imaging scans in sickle-cell disease: neurological correlates and clinical implications. Arch Neurol 1993;50:629.
60. Bruno A, Yuh WTC, Biller J, et al. Magnetic resonance imaging in young adults with cerebral infarction due to moyamoya. Arch Neurol 1988;45:303.
61. Ameri A, Bousser MG. Cerebral venous thrombosis. Neurol Clin 1992;10:87.
62. Zimmerman RA, Bogdan AR, Gusnard DA. Pediatric magnetic resonance angiography: assessment of stroke. Cardiovasc Interv Radiol 1992;15:60.
63. Hayman LA, Taber KH, Ford JJ, Bryan RN. Mechanisms of MR signal alteration by acute intracerebral blood: old concepts and new theories. AJNR Am J Neuroradiol 1991;12:899.
64. Mugler JP. Overview of MR pulse sequences. Magn Reson Imaging Clin N Am 1999;7:661.
65. Darby DG, Barber PA, Gerraty RP. Pathophysiology topography of acute ischemia by combined diffusion-weighted and perfusion MRI. Stroke 2000;30:2043.
66. Bydder GM, Rutherford MA, Hajnal JV. How to perform diffusion-weighted imaging. Child Nerv Syst 2001;17:195.
67. Mader I, Schoning M, Klose U, Kuker W. Neonatal cerebral infarction diagnosed by diffusion-weighted

68. Kelly PJ, Hedley-Whyte ET, Primavera J, et al. Diffusion MRI in ischemic stroke compared to pathologically verified infarction. Neurology 2001;56:914.
69. Lansberg MG, Albers GW, Beaulieu C, et al. Comparison of diffusion-weighted MRI and CT in acute stroke. Neurology 2000;4:1557.
70. Schlaug G, Benfield A, Baird AE, et al. The ischemic penumbra: operationally defined by diffusion and perfusion MRI. Neurology 1999;53:1528.
71. Ross JS, Masaryk TJ, Modic MT, et al. Magnetic resonance angiography of the extracranial carotid arteries and intracranial vessels: a review. Neurology 1989;39:1369.
72. Sellar RT. Imaging blood vessels of the head and neck. J Neurol Neurosurg Psychiatry 1995;59:225.
73. Wiznitzer M, Ruggieri PM, Masaryk TJ, et al. Diagnosis of cerebrovascular disease in sickle cell anemia by magnetic resonance angiography. J Pediatr 1990;117:551.
74. Polak JF, Bajakian RL, O'Leary DH, et al. Detection of internal carotid artery stenosis: comparison of MR angiography, color Doppler sonography, and arteriography. Radiology 1992;182:35.
75. Brust JCM, Dickinson PCT, Hughes JEO, et al. The diagnosis and treatment of cerebral mycotic aneurysms. Ann Neurol 1990;27:238.
76. Heros RC, Tu YK. Is surgical therapy needed for unruptured arteriovenous malformations? Neurology 1987;37:279.
77. Miller C, Bissonnette B, Humphreys RP. Cerebral arteriovenous malformations in children. Can J Anaesth 1994;41:321.
78. Rao AK, Thompson R, Dunlacher L, et al. Angiographic contrast-induced acute hemolysis in a patient with hemoglobin SC disease. Arch Intern Med 1985;145:759.
79. Aspelin P, Aubrey P, Fransson SG, et al. Nephrotoxic effects in high-risk patients undergoing angiography. N Engl J Med 2003;348:491.
80. North KN, Whiteman DA, Pepin MG, et al. Cerebrovascular complications in Ehlers-Danlos syndrome type IV. Ann Neurol 1995;38:960.
81. van der Meulen JH, Westrate W, van Gijn J, et al. Is cerebral angiography indicated in infective endocarditis? Stroke 1992;23:1662.
82. Heehan SD, Grubnic S, Buckenham TM. Transbrachial arteriography: indications and complications. Clin Radiol 1996;51:205.
83. Levy EI, Boulos AS, Fessler RD. Transradial cerebral angiography: an alternative route. Neurosurgery 2002;51:335.
84. Umemona A, Kazuo Y. B-mode flow imaging of the carotid artery. Stroke 2001;32:2055.
85. Kojo M, Ogawa T, Yamada K. Normal developmental changes in carotid arterial blood flow measured by Doppler flowmetry in children. Pediatr Neurol 1996;4:313.
86. Adams RJ, Nichols FT, McKie VC, et al. Transcranial Doppler: influence of hematocrit in children with

sickle cell anemia without stroke. J Cardiovasc Tech 1989;8:97.

87. Adams RJ, Aaslid R, El Gammal T, et al. Detection of cerebral vasculopathy in sickle cell disease using transcranial Doppler ultrasonography and magnetic resonance imaging: case report. Stroke 1988;19:518.

88. Gomez CR. Diagnostic evaluation of patients with cerebral ischemic events. In Adams HP Jr, ed. Handbook of Cerebrovascular Diseases. New York: Marcel Dekker, 1993.

89. Crombleholme TM, Adzick NS, deLorimier AA, et al. Carotid artery reconstruction following extracorporeal membrane oxygenation. Am J Disabled Child 1990;144:872.

90. Ricotta JJ, Bryan FA, Bond MG, et al. Multicenter validation study of real-time (B-mode) ultrasound, arteriography, and pathologic examination. J Vasc Surg 1987;6:512.

91. Schmidt P, Sliwka U, Stefan-Georg S, et al. High grade stenosis of the internal artery assessed by color and power Doppler imaging. J Clin Ultrasound 1998;26:85.

92. Koga M, Kimura K, Yasaka M, et al. Three dimensional power Doppler imaging of vertebrobasilar circulation in adults. AJNR Am J Neuroradiol 1999;20:943.

93. Raju TNK. Cerebral Doppler studies in the fetus and newborn infant. J Pediatr 1991;119:165.

94. Adams RJ, McKie V, Nichols F, et al. The use of transcranial ultrasonography to predict stroke in sickle cell disease. N Engl J Med 1992;326:605.

95. Adams RJ, McKie VC, Hsu L, et al. Prevention of first stroke by transfusions in children with sickle cell anemia and abnormal results on transcranial Doppler ultrasonography. N Engl J Med 1998;339:5.

96. Lane PA, Buchanan GR, Ware RE. Variable approaches to therapeutic options for children with sickle cell disease (SCD): a practice survey of the American Society of Pediatric Hematology/Oncology. Blood 2001;98:784.

97. Malouf AJ, Hamrick-Turner JE, Doherty MC, et al. Implementation of the STOP protocol for stroke prevention in sickle cell anemia by using duplex power Doppler imaging. Radiology 2001;219:359.

98. Zimmerman RA. Pediatric cerebrovascular disease. JBR-BTR (Organe de la Societe Royale Belge de Radiologie) 2000;83:245.

99. Valkama AM, Ahonen A, Vainionpaa L, et al. Brain single photon emission computed tomography at term age for predicting cerebral palsy after preterm birth. Biol Neonate 2001;79:27.

100. Sztriha L, al Suhaili AR, Prais V, Nork M. Regional cerebral blood perfusion in children with hemiplegia: a SPECT study. Neuropediatrics 1996;4:178.

101. Maria BL, Neufeld JA, Rosainz LC, et al. High prevalence of bihemispheric structural and functional defects in Sturge-Weber syndrome. J Child Neurol 1998;13:595.

102. Reed W, Jagust W, Al-Mateen M, et al. Role of positron emission tomography in determining the extent of CNS ischemia in patients with sickle cell disease. Am J Hematol 1999;60:268.

103. Bogousslavsky J, Cachin C, Regli F, et al. Cardiac sources of embolism and cerebral infarction—clinical consequences and vascular concomitants. The Lausanne Stroke Registry. Neurology 1991;41:855.

104. Biller J, Adams Jr HP, Johnson MR, et al. Paradoxical cerebral embolism: eight cases. Neurology 1986;36:1356.

105. Gutterman DD, Ayres RW. Use of echocardiography in detecting cardiac sources of embolus. Echocardiography 1993;10:311.

106. Erbel R, Rohmann S, Drexler M, et al. Improved diagnostic value of echocardiography in patients with infective endocarditis by transesophageal approach: a prospective study. Eur Heart J 1988;9:43.

107. Daniel WG, Schroeder E, Mugge A, et al. Transesophageal-echocardiography in infective endocarditis. Am J Cardiol Imaging 1988;2:78.

108. Porembka DT, Hoit BD. Transesophageal echocardiography in the intensive care patient. Crit Care Med 1991;19:826.

109. Roach ES, Garcia JC, McLean WT Jr. Cerebrovascular disease in children. Am Fam Physician 1984;30:215.

110. Andrew M, Monagle PT, Brooker L. Thromboembolic Complications during Infancy and Childhood. Hamilton, Ontario: BC Decker, 2000.

111. Gunther G, Junker R, Strater R, et al. Symptomatic ischemic stroke in full term neonates: role of acquired and genetic prothrombotic risk factors. Stroke 2000;31:2437.

112. Macchi PJ, Grossman RI, Gomori JM, et al. High field MR imaging of cerebral venous thrombosis. J Comput Assist Tomogr 1986;10:10.

113. Bauer WM, Einhaupl K, Heyaring S, et al. MR of venous sinus thrombosis: a case report. AJNR Am J Neuroradiol 1987;8:713.

114. Baram TZ, Butler IJ, Nelson Jr MD, McArdle CB. Transverse sinus thrombosis in newborns: clinical and magnetic resonance imaging findings. Ann Neurol 1988;24:792.

115. Pohl M, Zimmerbackl LB, Heinen F, et al. Bilateral renal vein thrombosis and venous sinus thrombosis in a neonate with factor V mutation (FV Leiden). J Pediatr 1998;132:159.

116. Sokol DK, MacIntyre J, Short RA, et al. Antiphosphatidyl-ethanolamine antibody in CSF and serum. Neurology 2000;14:1245.

117. Scanu AM. Atherothrombogenicity of lipoprotein (a): the debate. Am J Cardiol 1998;82:Q26.

118. Golomb MR. The contributions of prothrombotic disorders to peri- and neonatal ischemic stroke. Semin Thromb Hemost 2003;29:415.

119. Clark P, Greer IA, Walker ID. Interaction of the protein C/proteins anticoagulant system, the endothelium and pregnancy. Blood Rev 1999;13:127.

120. Skidmore FM, Williams LS, Fradkin KD, et al. Presentation, etiology, and outcome of stroke in pregnancy and puerperium. J Stroke Cerebrovasc Dis 2001;10:1.

121. Carvalho KS, Bodensteiner JB, Connolly PJ, et al. Cerebral venous thrombosis in children. J Child Neurol 2001;16:574.

122. Cakmak S, Derex MD, Berruyer M, et al. Cerebral venous thrombosis. Neurology 2003;60:1175.
123. Roach ES. Etiology of stroke in children. Semin Pediatr Neurol 2000;7:244.
124. Hathaway WE, Goodnight SH. Disorders of Hemostasis and Thrombosis. New York: McGraw-Hill, 1994.
125. Bush MT, Roy N. Hemophilia emergencies. J Emerg Nursing 1995;21:531.
126. Schafer AI. The hypercoagulable states. Ann Intern Med 1985;102:814.
127. Vinters HV. Cerebrovascular disease: practical issues in surgical and autopsy pathology. Curr Top Pathol 2001;95:51.
128. Guttmacher AE, Marchuk DA, White RI. Hereditary hemorrhagic telangiectasia. N Engl J Med 1995; 333:918.
129. Way J, Lopez-Yunez A, Beristain X, et al. Paradoxical embolism the basilar apex associated with May-Turner syndrome. Arch Neurol 2000; 57:1761.
130. Leventer RJ, Kornberg AJ, Coleman LT, et al. Stroke and fibromuscular dysplasia confirmation by renal magnetic resonance angiography. Pediatr Neurol 1998;18:112.

CHAPTER 5

Atherosclerotic Cerebral Infarction in Young Adults

José Biller • Rima M. Dafer

KEY TERMS	
CEA	carotid endarterectomy
CNS	central nervous system
CT	computed tomography
DBP	diastolic blood pressure
DM	diabetes mellitus
DWI	diffusion-weighted imaging
HDL	high-density lipoprotein
LDL	low-density lipoprotein
MRI	magnetic resonance imaging
SBP	systolic blood pressure
TIA	transient ischemic attacks

Pathogenesis

Atherosclerosis affects millions of adults. Ischemic heart disease, hypertensive heart disease, cerebrovascular disease, and atherosclerosis in the arteries of the lower limbs constitute major public health problems. Coronary and cerebral atherosclerotic vascular diseases are the major causes of morbidity and mortality in the industrialized world. Atherosclerosis, although uncommon before 40 years of age, has its onset in infancy and childhood.[1-4] Atherosclerosis tends to affect the large and medium-sized arteries, such as the aorta, and iliac, superficial femoral, coronary, and cerebral arteries. Autopsy studies of men in their 20s killed during wartime indicated that more than two thirds had moderately advanced coronary atherosclerosis.

The earliest morphologic arterial change in atherosclerosis is the juvenile (flat) fatty streak, commonly seen in children and adolescents. Raised fatty streaks (fatty plaque) represent the lesion intermediate between the juvenile (flat) fatty streak and the raised lesion of atherosclerosis. Many fatty streaks do not progress to fibrous plaques or complicated (ulcerative, thrombosed, hemorrhagic) atheromatous lesions. Although the progression from fatty streaks through fibrous plaques and complicated atheromatous lesions cannot be documented longitudinally in humans, such progression is presumed to occur.[5,6] Long-range prevention of atherosclerosis should begin in childhood or adolescence.[4]

Risk Factors

Vascular injury and thrombus formation are key events in the pathogenesis of ischemic cerebrovascular disease. Atherosclerotic cerebral infarction in young individuals almost always occurs in individuals who already have significant risk factors for atherosclerosis, such as arterial hypertension, diabetes mellitus (DM), asymptomatic carotid bruits, asymptomatic carotid stenosis, previous transient ischemic attacks (TIAs), and cigarette smoking.[7] Other disorders reported to be associated with an increased risk of accelerated atherosclerosis in early childhood include familial hypercholesterolemia, chronic and end-stage renal disease, congenital heart disease, cardiac transplantation, Kawasaki disease, and chronic inflammatory diseases.

Hypertension affects approximately 1 billion people worldwide, and in the United States, approximately 30% of the population is hypertensive.[8] Although hypertension is infrequent among young stroke patients, childhood blood pressure predicts adult blood pressure; children with elevated blood pressure are more likely to have arterial hypertension as adults. Arterial hypertension is a major factor in the acceleration of atherosclerosis; it also increases cardiovascular morbidity and mortality, especially stroke. Because stroke is one of the major consequences of arterial hypertension, control of hypertension is one of the best strategies for stroke prevention.[9-11]

Reducing the systolic blood pressure (SBP) by a few torrs decreases the rate of ischemic stroke by 38%. More importantly, a key strategy in stroke prevention is the primary prevention of arterial hypertension; evidence comes from dietary and lifestyle studies of stroke risk factors, particularly the relationship between salt intake (sodium chloride) and blood pressure in adults.[12,13] When hypertension occurs in children and young adults, it is often the result of secondary causes. An age-specific blood pressure distribution from birth to 18 years of age is shown in Table 5-1.[14] The JNC7 Report emphasizes that patients at risk, including patients with DM or a history of stroke, should be treated with a reduction in salt intake combined with lifestyle changes and medications.[15]

Approximately 18 million Americans have DM, and at least 10% to 15% have been diagnosed with prediabetes. Cardiovascular disease is the leading cause of morbidity and mortality in diabetics. DM is a prominent risk factor for ischemic stroke and is reported to be second in importance only to arterial hypertension.[16-18] DM increases the risk of arterial hypertension by twofold,

TABLE 5-1   Age-Specific Blood Pressure Distributions from Birth to 18 Years Old: High Normal 90th to 94th Percentile (mm Hg)

Age	SBP	DBP
Infants 0-2 yr	104-111	70-73
Children 3-5 yr	108-115	70-75
Children 6-9 yr	114-121	74-77
Children 10-12 yr	122-125	78-81
Children 13-15 yr	130-135	80-85
Adolescents 16-18 yr	136-141	84-91

DBP, diastolic blood pressure; SBP, systolic blood pressure.

Adapted from The Fifth Report of the Joint National Committee on Detection, Evaluation, and Treatment of High Blood Pressure (JNC V). Bethesda, MD: National Heart, Lung, and Blood Institute, National Institutes of Health, 1992.

cardiac disease by twofold, and ischemic cerebrovascular disease by twofold to fourfold compared with nondiabetics. Patients with DM are at least two times more likely to have an atherothrombotic stroke than nondiabetics. In the Honolulu Heart Program, men with DM had an increased risk for stroke; men with glucosuria without a diabetic history also were at increased risk for stroke.[16] Atherosclerotic vascular disease occurs more commonly, advances more rapidly, and strikes at a younger age in diabetic patients than in nondiabetic individuals.[19] Although tight glycemic control reduces microvascular complications (i.e., retinopathy, nephropathy, and peripheral neuropathy), as yet, there is no compelling evidence that it significantly reduces stroke risk.[20]

Asymptomatic carotid bruits are found in 3% to 4% of the general population older than 45 years of age. The prevalence increases with age, hypertension, and DM. The risk of stroke in patients with asymptomatic bruits is 2% per year; subsequent strokes are not always ipsilateral to the involved vessel.[21] Asymptomatic carotid artery stenosis is identified in 10% to 20% of patients with symptomatic carotid atherosclerosis in other vascular territories, and in 25% to 40% of patients undergoing contralateral carotid endarterectomy (CEA). The rate of ipsilateral TIA or stroke is 3% to 5% per year. Progression to high-grade carotid artery stenosis correlates with ischemic cerebrovascular symptoms. When carotid artery stenosis is 75% or less, the stroke rate is 1.3% per year. When carotid stenosis is greater than 75%, however, the rate of TIA and stroke is 10.5% per year.[22]

Independently of other risk factors, the risk of a subsequent stroke is at least three times greater for individuals with a history of TIA than for individuals without such a history.[23] The risk of stroke after a TIA is less in individuals younger than age 50 years than in older individuals.[24]

China and India now account for 40% of the world's cigarette smokers. Prospective data accumulated over the last decades show a strong relationship between cigarette smoking and all types of stroke.[25-33] Individuals who smoke cigarettes have a twofold to threefold greater risk of having an ischemic stroke compared with nonsmokers.[26-28] The increased stroke risk among cigarette smokers is dose related and independent of arterial hypertension.[29] Smoking may be a particularly important risk factor for premature atherosclerosis and is an important risk factor for cerebral infarction in young adults.[33] Second-hand smoke also increases the risk of cardiovascular disease, whereas smoking cessation lessens the risks of cardiovascular complications and death in older and younger individuals.[34,35]

High total cholesterol, especially high low-density lipoprotein (LDL) cholesterol concentration, correlates with atherosclerosis. The association between dyslipidemia and coronary artery and peripheral vascular atherosclerotic disease is well established. Patients with coronary or peripheral vascular atherosclerotic disease often have one of the following alterations of serum lipids: increased LDL cholesterol concentration, decreased high-density lipoprotein (HDL) cholesterol concentration, increased triglyceride values, or increased lipoprotein (a) concentration.[1,2]

In the United States, the National Cholesterol Education Program has defined dyslipidemia in children as total cholesterol greater than 200 mg/dL and LDL cholesterol greater than 130 mg/dL.[36,37] Caution is needed not to overinterpret serum lipoprotein abnormalities during the acute phase of stroke.[38] According to some epidemiologic data, serum cholesterol levels have an inverse relationship to intracranial hemorrhage.[39] High serum triglyceride levels may be associated with an increased risk of ischemic stroke in young patients.[40] Some studies suggest that increased serum lipoprotein (a), a lipid-containing particle similar to LDL, and decreased HDL are major risk factors for ischemic cerebrovascular disease, even in patients with normal serum cholesterol and triglycerides.[41-46] Others failed to show such an association, however, particularly among young women with ischemic stroke.[47] The American Heart Association recommends lipid screening for overweight or obese children, children with a history of dyslipidemia and early-onset cardiovascular disease, and children with disorders potentially associated with premature atherosclerotic cardiovascular disease.[48,49]

Other inherited conditions, such as Tangier disease and Fabry disease, also carry a risk of stroke.[50] Patients with Tangier disease develop premature atherosclerosis. Tangier disease is an autosomal recessive disorder characterized by deficiency or absence of plasma HDL cholesterol. Serum cholesterol is low, and triglycerides are normal or elevated. Cardiovascular involvement (angina, myocardial infarction, stroke) is thought to be related to the deposition of cholesterol esters.[51]

Fabry disease (Anderson-Fabry disease, angiokeratoma corporis diffusum, ceramide trihexosidosis), a disorder of glycolipid metabolism, involves the skin, eyes, kidneys, heart, gastrointestinal tract, peripheral nervous system, and central nervous system (CNS). The prevalence of Fabry disease has been estimated to be 1 in 40,000, although more recent studies suggest a higher prevalence. Fabry disease is inherited as a sex-linked recessive trait and leads to an accumulation of glycosphingolipids. Fabry disease is caused by α-galactosidase A (ceramide trihexosidase) deficiency (Fig. 5-1). Cardiovascular and cerebrovascular complications include arterial hypertension, myocardial infarction, congestive heart failure, cerebral infarction, a dilated/ectatic arteriopathy with preferential involvement for the vertebrobasilar circulation, and cerebral hemorrhage.[52-57] Diagnosis is made by measuring the amount of α-galactosidase activity in the blood. Enzyme replacement therapy with agalsidase α and agalsidase β is now available.[58-61] Whether therapy with these enzymes changes the natural history of a stroke attributable to Fabry disease is unclear.

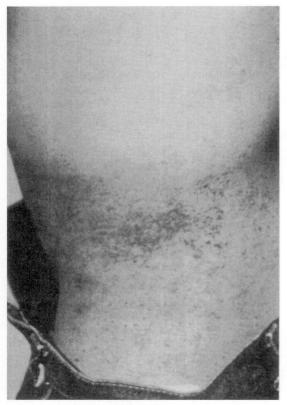

FIGURE 5-1   Punctate, nonblanching, dark red cutaneous vascular lesions consistent with angiokeratoma corporis diffusum in a patient with Fabry disease.

Obesity is a risk factor for stroke. Children and adolescents who are overweight (body mass index >85th percentile) or obese (body mass index >95th percentile) are at greater risk to be hypertensive, to have dyslipidemia and insulin resistance, and to develop type 2 DM. Examination of university medical records of former medical students identified four precursors of fatal and nonfatal stroke in later life: arterial hypertension, cigarette smoking, short body stature, and increased weight for height.[62-65] Because higher salt intake increases soft drink consumption, reducing salt intake and reducing obesity may prevent the development of hypertension and cardiovascular disease.[65,66]

The relationship between alcohol intake and stroke is conflicting.[67-69] Probable explanations of alcohol intake as a stroke risk factor may relate to several mechanisms, including arterial hypertension, hemostatic alterations, cardiac arrhythmias, and worsening of underlying cardiomyopathy.[67-72]

The conflicting epidemiologic information about alcohol intake and the risk of cerebral infarction may stem from the confounding effects of cigarette smoking. Restriction of alcohol consumption to less than two drinks daily is recommended for light to moderate drinkers and nonpregnant women.

Increasing evidence indicates that genetic factors are associated with stroke. Numerous genetic polymorphisms have been identified. A fivefold increase in stroke prevalence among monozygotic compared with dizygotic male twin pairs suggests a genetic etiology in stroke. The proband concordance rates between the proband and presence of stroke for monozygotic and dizygotic pairs have been reported to be 17.7% and 3.6%.[73] The Siblings With Ischemic Stroke Study (SWISS) is currently investigating the genetic component of stroke among probands, concordant siblings, and discordant siblings.[74]

Rarely, the development of a presumed atherosclerotic cerebral infarction in a very young patient may warrant investigations for rare premature aging syndromes.[75] The association of homocystinuria, Hutchinson-Gilford syndrome (progeria), and Tangier disease with premature atherosclerosis and cardiovascular and cerebrovascular events is well documented.

Homocystinuria is a rare autosomal recessive inborn error of metabolism caused by a deficiency of cystathionine synthase. Children and young adults with homocystinuria have a marfanoid appearance; mental retardation; ectopia lentis; and a propensity to intracranial, retinal, arterial, and venous thrombosis.[76-81] Management of homocystinuria includes a methionine-restricted cysteine-supplemented diet, high-dose pyridoxine, folic acid, betaine, cyanocobalamin, and symptomatic measures. Elevated plasma homocysteine levels have been associated with increased risk for cardiovascular and cerebrovascular disease. Homozygosity for methylene tetrahydrofolate reductase (MTHFR) C677T is associated with hyperhomocysteinemia.[81] Hyperhomocysteinemia can be reduced by alteration of diet or by supplementation with folic acid along with pyridoxine and vitamin B_{12}. Whether this approach decreases cardiovascular events or death is not yet proven.

An unusual group of disorders featuring premature aging have been associated with abnormal mitochondrial function. Among them, progeria and Werner syndrome are known as segmental aging disorders.[82] Patients with progeria have short stature, alopecia, craniofacial disproportion, beaked nose, micrognathia, prominent eyes, high-pitched voice, progressive loss of subcutaneous fat, and overt signs of premature aging.[75] Progeria is thought to represent an inherited disorder with autosomal recessive or dominant trait. Patients appear normal until 18 months of age (range 12 to 24 months), and most have a mutation on the gene that encodes the protein lamin A (LMNA). DeBusk[83] estimated the incidence of progeria as 1 in 8 million births. Most patients die in the second decade of life, usually as a consequence of coronary or cerebrovascular disease. A DNA-based diagnostic test for children suspected to have progeria is available. Presently, there is no available treatment for this condition. Werner syndrome, a rare autosomal recessive condition due to a mutation in a DNA helicase belonging to the RecQ family, is characterized by premature aging, bilateral cataracts, scleroderma-like changes of the skin, dwarfism, hypogonadism, severe atheroma, hyperlipidemia, an increased risk of thrombosis, and a propensity for malignant tumors.[75]

Clinical Features

Cerebrovascular atherosclerosis falls into two categories: atherosclerosis of the large extracranial and intracranial vessels and penetrating intracranial small vessel cerebrovascular disease. A lower prevalence of carotid bifurcation atherosclerosis has been reported among blacks. Likewise, intracranial stenosis is more common than extracranial stenosis among Asians. Most atherothrombotic ischemic strokes result from large artery thrombotic or embolic occlusions or occlusion of small penetrating branches of the anterior, middle, and posterior cerebral arteries and the basilar artery. The most common locations for these small deep infarcts are the internal capsule, pons, caudate nucleus, putamen, thalamus, and adjacent white matter. Most atherosclerotic cerebral infarctions involve the territory of the internal carotid artery and its branches. There has been an increased recognition, however, of vertebrobasilar distribution strokes in young patients (Fig. 5-2).[84-88] A few of these children have had vertebral artery dissections, Klippel-Feil syndrome, or subluxation of the upper cervical spine. Other risk factors included hypertension and thrombophilic predisposition.

Most young subjects with atherosclerotic cerebral infarction tend to be men in their 30s or 40s, obese, with a background history of DM or glucose intolerance, hyperuricemia, or coronary or peripheral vascular disease. Because atherothrombosis is multifactorial, comorbidities frequently overlap, and risk factors are often additive. Many have warning TIAs before cerebral infarction. They often have a family history of premature cardiovascular disease or genetic abnormalities of lipid metabolism. Some of these patients may have xanthomas, xanthelasmas, and corneal arcus. There is often radiographic evidence of aortic calcification and associated electrocardiographic abnormalities.

A presumed or definite atherosclerotic etiology of cerebral infarction is often established if the patient has two or more risk factors for atherosclerosis, or when typical atherosclerotic lesions are found by arteriography, surgery, or autopsy. In 245 necropsied cases of cerebrovascular lesions, Aring and Merritt[89] found that 1% of cerebral thrombosis cases occurred in patients younger than 40 years of age. Irish,[90] reviewing 361 thrombotic cerebrovascular lesions in a series of 12,000 autopsies, found 37 (10.2%) thrombotic strokes in patients younger than 40 years old. Wells and Timberger[91] reported 77 patients younger than 50 years with clinically diagnosed cerebral thrombosis; 22 of them were younger than 40 years. It is unclear, however, whether these patients had atherosclerotic cerebral infarction, or the arterial thrombosis had a nonatherosclerotic mechanism.

Berlin and associates[92] described 13 patients with cerebral infarction, most of whom were 20 to 30 years old. None was hypertensive, diabetic, or hyperlipidemic. Arteriography performed in seven patients showed evidence of either stenosis or occlusion of the internal carotid artery or its branches in four cases.

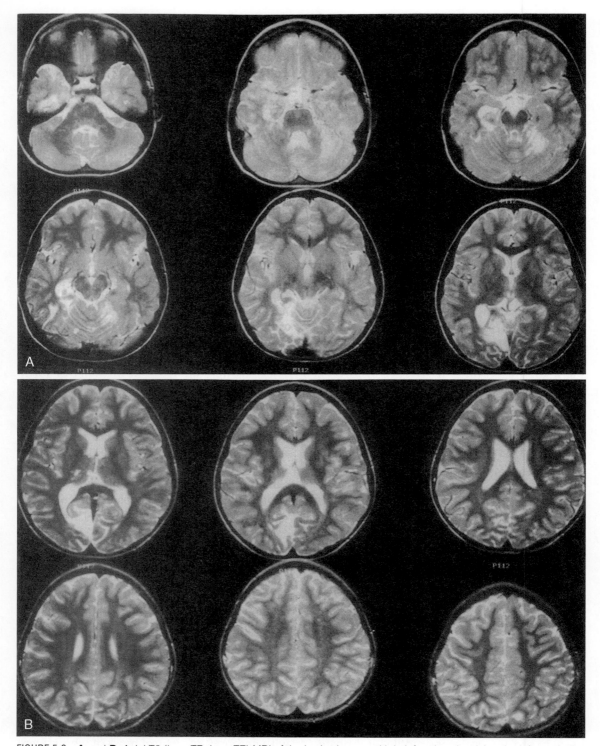

FIGURE 5-2 **A** and **B,** Axial T2 (long TR, long TE) MRI of the brain shows multiple infarctions involving the left cerebellar hemisphere, right occipital lobe, and right thalamus in a 4-year-old boy.

Haerer and Smith[93] evaluated 207 consecutive stroke patients 15 to 50 years of age. Although patients with TIAs and cerebral thrombosis had the best prognosis, one sixth of the patients with TIAs and 30% of the patients with cerebral thrombosis died during the follow-up period. Seneviratne and Ameratunga[94] studied 44 rural Ceylonese patients, 12 to 45 years old, with ischemic stroke, including 19 men with atherothrombotic internal carotid artery occlusion. None was hypertensive, diabetic, or hypercholesterolemic. All consumed a calorically marginal diet that did not include coconut fat, and this possibly led to carbohydrate-induced hyperlipidemia. Carolei and colleagues[95] studied 333 patients, 15 to 44 years old, presenting with their first episode of TIA or stroke. Cerebral ischemia was attributed to atherothrombosis in one third of cases, and in this group men outnumbered women. The authors suspected an atherothrombotic etiology when typical atherosclerotic lesions were shown by angiography, or when patients had two or more atherogenic risk factors and no other identifiable etiology. A definite or presumed atherosclerotic etiology of cerebral infarction is often found in 20% to 25% of young adults with ischemic stroke.[96-116]

Paraclinical Evaluation

Detailed cardiovascular and neurologic assessments including the NIH Stroke Scale are obtained in all patients before proceeding with neuroimaging techniques. Cardiovascular risks are evaluated in each patient. Many approaches to the noninvasive neuroimaging evaluation of young patients with presumed atherosclerotic cerebrovascular lesions have been recommended.[117] B-mode real-time ultrasound offers valuable measurements of the degree of carotid atherosclerosis. Pulsed Doppler with spectral analysis provides accurate quantification of the hemodynamic significance of carotid artery disease. Transcranial Doppler ultrasonography assesses the hemodynamic characteristics of the basal cerebral vessels. Neuroimaging evaluation should include unenhanced cranial computed tomography (CT). Magnetic resonance imaging (MRI) is

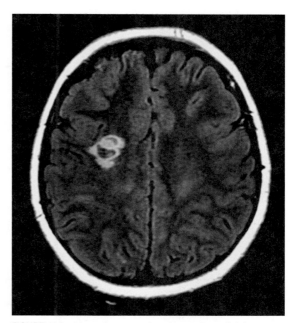

FIGURE 5-3 Hyperintense signal noted on fluid attenuated inversion recovery in the right centrum semiovale consistent with remote infarction in an 11-year-old child with hyperlipidemia.

superior to CT in the detection of early infarctions, small infarctions, and posterior fossa infarctions (Fig. 5-3). Diffusion, perfusion, and gradient echo MRI sequences can rapidly detect early ischemic and hemorrhagic lesions and describe the amount of "at-risk" tissue ("ischemic penumbra") (Fig. 5-4). MR angiography or multidetector CT angiography offers

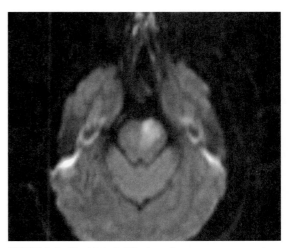

FIGURE 5-4 Restricted diffusion changes are present on diffusion-weighted imaging in the left paramedian pons consistent with an acute ischemic lesion in a young patient with diabetes mellitus and hyperlipidemia.

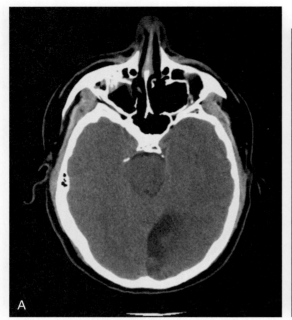
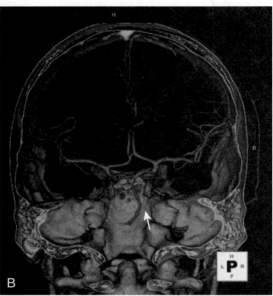

FIGURE 5-5   **A,** Remote left occipital infarction in a 35-year-old patient with an occluded left vertebral artery. **B,** CT angiogram shows absent left vertebral artery (*arrow*).

valuable visualization of large and medium-sized vessels. Cervicocerebral catheter angiography is associated with complications, and its use is being challenged by the increasing quality of MR angiography and multidetector CT angiography (Fig. 5-5). The main disadvantage of MR angiography is that it overestimates the degree of arterial stenosis. A disadvantage of multidetector CT angiography is the amount of radiation, volume of contrast dye used, and bony artifacts in the petrous and cavernous sections of the skull. Cerebral angiography is indicated to determine the location and extent of arterial stenosis and the underlying cause of stroke (Figs. 5-6 and 5-7). Suggested paraclinical evaluation of a patient with presumed atherosclerotic cerebral infarction is detailed in Tables 5-2 and 5-3.

Management

Preventing Stroke Recurrence

Medical Therapy

Dietary and lifestyle changes, platelet anti-aggregants, antihypertensive agents, and statin therapy remain the mainstays of

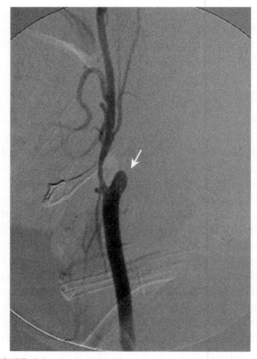

FIGURE 5-6   Occlusion of the postbulbar right internal carotid artery (*arrow*) seen on catheter cerebral angiogram after right common carotid artery injection in a young man with a history of hypertension.

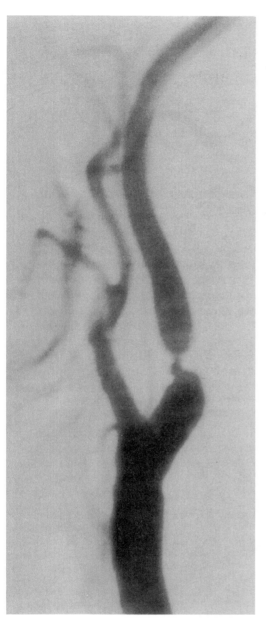

FIGURE 5-7   Catheter cerebral angiography shows irregular narrowing of the internal carotid artery distal to the common carotid artery bifurcation consistent with atherosclerosis.

TABLE 5-2   **Initial Tests for Potential Atherosclerotic Cerebral Infarction in Young Adults**

Complete blood count with differential and platelet count
Prothrombin time, activated partial thromboplastin time
Blood glucose, hemoglobin A_{1C}, serum electrolytes, blood chemistries, plasma homocysteine
Total cholesterol, triglycerides, lipoprotein fractionation
Erythrocyte sedimentation rate
Urinalysis
Chest radiograph
Electrocardiogram
Two-dimensional echocardiogram
Transesophageal echocardiogram (in some instances)
Duplex ultrasound of the carotid arteries
Transcranial Doppler ultrasonography
Cranial CT
MRI of brain
MR angiography
Multidetector CT angiography
Catheter cerebral angiography (in some instances)

TABLE 5-3   **More Selective Tests for Potential Atherosclerotic Cerebral Infarction Depending on Clinical Findings**

Urine for lipid-laden epithelial cells (Fabry disease)
Apolipoprotein quantification
Plasma homocysteine after oral loading with methionine
Measurement of cystathionine β-synthase activity in biopsied tissue (skin biopsy with fibroblast culture or liver biopsy with an enzyme assay)
Leukocyte α-galactosidase activity

medical therapy for stroke prevention. Lifestyle interventions include smoking cessation, limitation of alcohol intake to no more than two drinks daily for men and no more than one drink daily for nonpregnant women, limitation of saturated fats and salt, and physical activity aiming for an ideal body mass index.

Optimal level of lipid and lipoprotein is LDL cholesterol less than 100 mg/dL or HDL cholesterol greater than 50 mg/dL. For high-risk patients, LDL cholesterol less than 70 mg/dL is recommended.

Data from meta-analysis in patients with prior stroke or TIA show a 28% relative risk reduction in nonfatal stroke, and a 16% reduction in fatal stroke with use of platelet antiaggregant therapy. Of these agents, three are currently viable options to prevent stroke: aspirin, clopidogrel, and aspirin plus extended-release dipyridamole.[117]

Surgical Therapy

Carotid Endarterectomy

Stroke remains the third leading cause of death in the United States, and approximately 15% of strokes are the result of extracranial carotid artery atherosclerotic disease. CEA is the standard procedure for the invasive management of carotid artery atherosclerotic occlusive disease. Results from major prospective studies provide compelling evidence of the benefit of CEA performed by experienced surgeons in improving the chance of stroke-free survival in high-risk symptomatic patients. Compared with symptomatic carotid artery stenosis, asymptomatic carotid artery stenosis is associated with relatively low risk for ipsilateral cerebral infarction. Based on current guidelines, and ongoing controversies, some experts recommend CEA only when the degree of stenosis is greater than 80%, provided that surgery is performed by an experienced surgeon with a complication rate (combined arteriographic and surgical) of 3% or less.[118-122]

Stenting of the Carotid Artery

Carotid artery angioplasty and stenting may offer an alternative treatment to CEA. Although the more recent development of embolic protection techniques has improved the results of carotid artery stenting, carotid artery angioplasty and stenting should still be regarded as experimental (Fig. 5-8).

Management of Acute Ischemic Stroke

Modern therapy for acute ischemic stroke is currently approached in two different ways. First and most important are general measures aimed at prevention and treatment of complications. Second are reperfusion strategies directed at arterial recanalization. In June 1996, the U.S. Food and Drug Administration (FDA) approved the use of intravenous tissue plasminogen activator for ischemic stroke within 3 hours of symptom

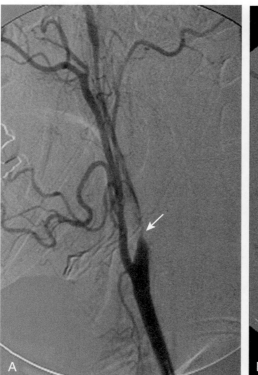
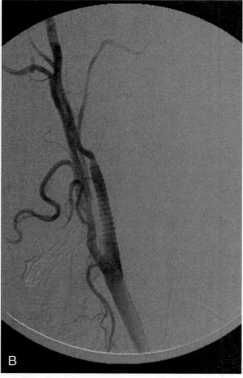

FIGURE 5-8   **A,** Near-complete occlusion of the proximal postbulbar left internal carotid artery along a 2-cm segment (*arrow*), with diffusely small caliber of the cervical segment internal carotid artery. **B,** Successful transarterial stent-assisted reconstruction of severe left carotid stenosis.

onset. Intravenous tissue plasminogen activator improved clinical outcomes in treated patients compared with placebo with no increase in mortality, despite an increased risk of symptomatic intracerebral hemorrhage. Hemorrhagic complications are the major adverse event associated with thrombolytic therapy. Intravenous tissue plasminogen activator administration requires strict dose adherence to protocol guidelines.[123]

REFERENCES

1. Kannel WB, Dawber TR. Atherosclerosis as a pediatric problem. Pediatrics 1972;80:544.
2. Strong WB. Is atherosclerosis a pediatric problem? An overview. In Strong WB, ed. Atherosclerosis: Its Pediatric Aspects. Clinical Cardiology Monographs. New York: Grune & Stratton, 1978.
3. Berenson GS, Srinivasan SR, Bao W, et al. Association between multiple cardiovascular risk factors and atherosclerosis in children and young adults. The Bogalusa Heart Study. N Engl J Med 1998;338:1650.
4. McGill HC Jr, McMahan CA, Zieske AW, et al. Associations of coronary heart disease risk factors with the intermediate lesion of atherosclerosis in youth. The Pathobiological Determinants of Atherosclerosis in Youth (PDAY) Research Group. Arterioscler Thromb Vasc Biol 2000;20:1998.
5. Ross R. The pathogenesis of atherosclerosis—an update. N Engl J Med 1986;314:488.
6. Newman WP, Strong JP. Natural history, geographic pathologic, and pediatric aspects of atherosclerosis. In Strong WB, ed. Atherosclerosis: Its Pediatric Aspects. Clinical Cardiology Monographs. New York: Grune & Stratton, 1978.
7. Wolf PA, Kannel WB, Verter J. Current status of risk factors for stroke. Neurol Clin 1983;1:317.
8. Kearney PM, Whelton M, Reynolds K, et al. Global burden of hypertension: analysis of worldwide data. Lancet 2005;365:217.
9. Garraway WM, Whisnant JP. The changing pattern of hypertension and the declining incidence of stroke. JAMA 1987;258:214.
10. SHEP Cooperative Research Group. Prevention of stroke by antihypertensive drug treatment in older persons with isolated systolic hypertension: final results of the Systolic Hypertension in the Elderly Program (SHEP). JAMA 1991;265:3255.
11. Sacco R, Adams R, Albers G, et al. Guidelines for prevention of stroke in patients with ischemic stroke or transient ischemic attack: a statement of healthcare professionals from the American Heart Association/American Stroke Association Council on Stroke: co-sponsored by the Council on Cardiovascular Radiology and Intervention: the American Academy of Neurology affirms the value of the guideline. Stroke 2006;37:516.
12. Law MR, Frost CD, Wald NJ. By how much does dietary salt reduction lower blood pressure? I:

analysis of observational data among population. BMJ 1991;302:811.
13. He SJ, MacGregor GA. Importance of salt in determining blood pressure in children: meta-analysis of controlled trials. Hypertension 2006;48:861.
14. The Fifth Report of the Joint National Committee on Detection, Evaluation, and Treatment of High Blood Pressure (JNC V). Bethesda, MD: National Heart, Lung, and Blood Institute, National Institutes of Health, 1992.
15. Chobanian AV, Bakris GL, Glack HR, et al. The Seventh Report of the Joint National Committee on Prevention, Detection, Evaluation, and Treatment of High Blood Pressure: the JNC 7 report. JAMA 2003;289:2560.
16. Abbott RD, Donahue RP, MacMahon SW, et al. Diabetes and the risk of stroke. The Honolulu Heart Program. JAMA 1987;257:949.
17. Barrett-Connor E, Khaw KT. Diabetes mellitus: an independent risk factor for stroke. Am J Epidemiol 1988;128:116.
18. Brand FN, Abbott RD, Kannel WB. Diabetes, intermittent claudication, and risk of cardiovascular events: the Framingham study. Diabetes 1989;38:504.
19. Biller J, Love BB. Diabetes and stroke. Med Clin North Am 1993;77:95.
20. UK Prospective Diabetes Study Group. Intensive blood-glucose with sulphonylureas or insulin compared with conventional treatment and risk of complications in patients with type 2 diabetes (UKPDS 33). Lancet 1999;352:837.
21. Chambers RC, Norris JW. Outcome in patients with asymptomatic neck bruits. N Engl J Med 1986;315:860.
22. Norris JW, Zhu CZ, Bornstein NM, Chambers BR. Vascular risks of asymptomatic carotid stenosis. Stroke 1991;22:1485.
23. Davis PH, Dambrosia JM, Schoenberg BS, et al. Risk factors for ischemic stroke: a prospective study in Rochester, Minnesota. Ann Neurol 1987;22:319.
24. Marshall J. The cause and prognosis of strokes in people under 50 years. J Neurol Sci 1982;53:473.
25. Molgaard CA, Bartock A, Peddecord KM, Rothrock J. The association between cerebrovascular disease and smoking: a case-control study. Neuroepidemiology 1986;5:88.
26. Abbott RD, Yin TY, Reed DM, Yano K. Risk of stroke in male cigarette smokers. N Engl J Med 1986;315:717.
27. Bonita R, Scragg R, Stewart A, et al. Cigarette smoking and risk of premature stroke in men and women. BMJ 1986;293:6.
28. Colditz GA, Bonita RA, Stampfer MJ, et al. Cigarette smoking and risk of stroke in middle-aged women. N Engl J Med 1988;318:937.
29. Wolf PA, D'Agostino RB, Kannel WB, et al. Cigarette smoking as a risk factor for stroke: the Framingham study. JAMA 1988;259:1025.
30. Donnan GA, McNeil JJ, Adena MA, et al. Smoking as a risk factor for cerebral ischemia. Lancet 1989;1:643.
31. Shinton R, Beevers G. Meta-analysis of relation between cigarette smoking and stroke. BMJ 1989;298:789.
32. Whisnant JP, Homer D, Ingall TJ, et al. Duration of cigarette smoking is the strongest predictor of

severe extracranial carotid atherosclerosis. Stroke 1990;21:707.

33. Love BB, Biller J, Jones MP, et al. Cigarette smoking as a risk factor for cerebral infarction in young adults. Arch Neurol 1990;47:693.

34. Wells AJ. Heart disease from passive smoking in the workplace. J Am Coll Cardiol 1998;31:1.

35. Hermanson B, Omenn GS, Kronmal RA, Gersh BJ. Beneficial six-year outcome of smoking cessation in older men and women with coronary artery disease: results from the CASS registry. N Engl J Med 1988;319:1365.

36. National Cholesterol Education Program (NCEP). Highlights of the Report of the Expert Panel on Blood Cholesterol Levels in Children and Adolescents. Pediatrics 1992;89:495.

37. McCrindle BW, Urbina EM, Dennison BA, et al. Drug therapy of high-risk lipid abnormalities in children and adolescents: a scientific statement from the American Heart Association Atherosclerosis, Hypertension, and Obesity in Youth Committee, Council of Cardiovascular Disease in the Young, with the Council on Cardiovascular Nursing. Circulation 2007;115:1948.

38. Woo J, Lam CKW, Kay R, et al. Acute and long-term changes in serum lipids after acute stroke. Stroke 1990;21:1407.

39. Iso H, Jacobs DR Jr, Wentworth D, et al. Serum cholesterol levels and six year mortality from stroke in 350,977 men screened for the multiple risk factor intervention trial. N Engl J Med 1989;320:904.

40. Fogelholm R, Aho K. Ischaemic cerebrovascular disease in young adults, 2: serum cholesterol and triglyceride values. Acta Neurol Scand 1973;49:428.

41. Mathew NT, Davis D, Meyer JS, Chandar K. Hyperlipoproteinemia in occlusive cerebrovascular disease. JAMA 1975;232:262.

42. Sirtori CR, Gianfranceschi G, Gritti I, et al. Decreased high-density lipoprotein cholesterol levels in male patients with transient ischemic attacks. Atherosclerosis 1979;32:205.

43. Glueck CJ, Daniels SR, Bates S, et al. Pediatric victims of unexplained stroke and their families: familial lipid and lipoprotein abnormalities. Pediatrics 1982;69:308.

44. Zenker G, Koltringer P, Bone G, et al. Lipoprotein (a) as a strong indicator for cerebrovascular disease. Stroke 1986;17:942.

45. Jurgens G, Koltringer P. Lipoprotein (a) in ischemic cerebrovascular disease: a new approach to the assessment of risk for stroke. Neurology 1987;37:513.

46. Woo J, Lau E, Lam CWK, et al. Hypertension, lipoprotein (a), and apolipoprotein A-I as risk factors for stroke in the Chinese. Stroke 1991;22:203.

47. Wityk RJ, Kittner SJ, Jenner JL, et al. Lipoprotein (a) and the risk of ischemic stroke in young women. Atherosclerosis 2000;150:389.

48. American Academy of Pediatrics Committee on Nutrition. Cholesterol in childhood. Pediatrics 1998;101(1 Pt 1):141.

49. Kavey RE, Allada V, Daniels SR, et al. Cardiovascular risk reduction in high-risk pediatric patients: a scientific statement from the American Heart Association Expert Panel on Population and Prevention Science; the Councils on Cardiovascular Disease in the Young, Epidemiology and Prevention, Nutrition, Physical Activity and Metabolism, High Blood Pressure Research, Cardiovascular Nursing, and the Kidney in Heart Disease; and the Interdisciplinary Working Group on Quality of Care and Outcomes Research: endorsed by the American Academy of Pediatrics. Circulation 2006;114:2710.

50. Natowicz M, Kelley RI. Mendelian etiologies of stroke. Ann Neurol 1987;22:175.

51. Schaefer EJ, Zech LA, Schwartz DE, Brewer HB Jr. Coronary heart disease prevalence and other clinical features in familial high-density lipo protein deficiency (Tangier disease). Ann Intern Med 1980;93:261.

52. Serfaty-Lacrosniere C, Civeira F, Lanzberg A, et al. Homozygous Tangier disease and cardiovascular disease. Atherosclerosis 1994;107:85.

53. Maisey DN, Cosh JA. Basilar artery aneurysm and Anderson-Fabry disease. J Neurol Neurosurg Psychiatry 1980;43:85.

54. Mitsias P, Levine SR. Cerebrovascular complications of Fabry's disease. Ann Neurol 1996;40:8.

55. Moore DF, Scott LT, Gladwin MT, et al. Regional cerebral hyperperfusion and nitric oxide pathway dysregulation on Fabry disease: reversal by enzyme replacement therapy. Circulation 2001;104:1506.

56. Garzuly F, Marodi L, Erdos M, et al. Megadolichobasilar anomaly with thrombosis in a family with Fabry's disease and a novel mutation in the alpha-galactosidase A gene. Brain 2005;128(Pt 9):2078.

57. Rofts A, Bottcher T, Zschiesche M, et al. Prevalence of Fabry disease in patients with cryptogenic stroke: a prospective study. Lancet 2005;366:1794.

58. Schiffmann R, Murray GJ, Treco D, et al. Infusion of alpha-galactosidase A reduces tissue globotriaosylceramide storage in patients with Fabry disease. Proc Natl Acad Sci U S A 2000;97:365.

59. Eng CM, Guffon N, Wilcox WR, et al. Safety and efficacy of recombinant human alpha-galactosidase A—replacement therapy in Fabry's disease. N Engl J Med 2001;345:9.

60. Schiffmann R, Kopp JB, Austin HA 3rd, et al. Enzyme replacement therapy in Fabry disease: a randomized controlled trial. JAMA 2001;285:2743.

61. Eng CM, Banikazemi M, Gordon RE, et al. A phase 1/2 clinical trial of enzyme replacement in Fabry disease: pharmacokinetic, substrate clearance, and safety studies. Am J Hum Genet 2001;68:711.

62. van Dam RM, Willett WC, Manson JE, Hu FB. The relationship between overweight in adolescence and premature death in women. Ann Intern Med 2006;145:91.

63. Folsom AR, Prineas RJ, Kaye SA, Munger RG. Incidence of hypertension and stroke in relation to body fat distribution and other risk factors in older women. Stroke 1990;21:701.

64. Paffenbarger RS Jr, Wing AL. Chronic disease in former college students, XI: early precursors of nonfatal stroke. Am J Epidemiol 1971;94:524.

65. He SJ, Markandu MD, Sagnella GA, MacGregor GA. Effect of salt intake on renal excretion of water in humans. Hypertension 2001;38:317.
66. He SJ, Marrero NM, MacGregor GA. Salt and blood pressure in children and adolescence. J Hum Hypertens 2008;22:4.
67. Gorelick PB. Alcohol and stroke. Stroke 1987;18:267.
68. Gorelick PB, Rodin MB, Langenberg P, et al. Is acute alcohol ingestion a risk factor for ischemic stroke? Results of a controlled study in middle-aged and elderly stroke patients at three urban medical centers. Stroke 1987;18:359.
69. Gorelick PB, Rodin MB, Langenberg P, et al. Weekly alcohol consumption, cigarette smoking, and the risk of ischemic stroke: results of a case control study at three urban medical centers in Chicago, Illinois. Neurology 1989;39:339.
70. Hilbom ME, Kaste M. Ethanol intoxication: a risk factor for ischemic brain infarction. Stroke 1983;14:694.
71. Gill JS, Zezulka AV, Shipley MJ, et al. Stroke and alcohol consumption. N Engl J Med 1986;315:1041.
72. Benshlomo Y, Markowe H, Shipley M, Parot G. Stroke risk for alcohol consumption using different control groups. Stroke 1992;23:1093.
73. Brass LM, Isaacsohn JL, Merikangas KR, Robinette CD. A study of twins and stroke. Stroke 1992;23:221.
74. Meschia JF, Kissela BM, Brott TG, et al. The Siblings With Ischemic Stroke Study (SWISS): a progress report. Clin Med Res 2006;4:12.
75. Neufeld HN, Blieden LC. Pediatric atherosclerosis: genetic aspects. In Strong WB, ed. Atherosclerosis: Its Pediatric Aspects. Clinical Cardiology Monographs. New York: Grune & Stratton, 1978.
76. Carson NAJ, Dent CE, Field CMB, Gaull GE. Homocystinuria. J Pediatr 1965;3:565.
77. Harker LA, Ross R, Slichter SJ, Scott CR. Homocysteine-induced arteriosclerosis: the role of endothelial cell injury and platelet response in its genesis. J Clin Invest 1976;58:731.
78. De Groot PG, Willems C, Boers GHJ, et al. Endothelial cell dysfunction in homocystinuria. Eur J Clin Invest 1983;13:405.
79. Newman G, Mitchell JRA. Homocystinuria presenting as multiple arterial occlusions. QJM 1984;210:251.
80. Mudd SH, Skovby F, Levy HL, et al. The natural history of homocystinuria due to cystathionine β-synthase deficiency. Am J Hum Genet 1985;37:1.
81. Boers GHJ, Smals AGH, Trijbels FJM, et al. Heterozygosity for homocystinuria in premature peripheral and cerebral occlusive arterial disease. N Engl J Med 1985;313:709.
82. Navarro CL, Cau P, Levy N. Molecular bases of progeroid syndromes. Hum Mol Genet 2006;15(Spec No 2): R151.
83. DeBusk FI. The Hutchinson-Gilford progeria syndrome. J Pediatr 1972;80:697.
84. DeVivo DC, Farrell FW Jr. Vertebrobasilar occlusive disease in children: a recognizable clinical entity. Arch Neurol 1972;26:278.
85. Ganesan V, Chong WK, Cox TC, et al. Posterior circulation stroke in childhood: risk factors and recurrence. Neurology 2002;59:1552.

86. Rosman NP, Adhami S, Mannheim GB, et al. Basilar Artery occlusion in children: misleading presentations, "locked-in" state, and diagnostic importance of accompanying vertebral artery occlusion. J Child Neurol 2003;18:L450.
87. Karimi M, Razavi M, Fattal D. Rubral lateropulsion due to vertebral artery dissection in a patient with Klippel-Feil syndrome. Arch Neurol 2004;61:583.
88. Vohra S, Johnston BC, Cramer K, Humphreys K. Adverse events associated with pediatric spinal manipulation: a systematic review. Pediatrics 2007;119:e275.
89. Aring C, Merritt HH. Differential diagnosis between cerebral hemorrhage and cerebral thrombosis. Arch Intern Med 1935;56:435.
90. Irish CW. Cerebral vascular lesions in newborn infants and young children: with report of 40 among 1,000 necropsied cases with spontaneous vascular encephalopathy. J Pediatr 1939;15:64.
91. Wells CE, Timberger RJ. Cerebral thrombosis in patients under fifty years of age. Arch Neurol 1961;4:268.
92. Berlin L, Tumarkin B, Martin HL. Cerebral thrombosis in young adults. N Engl J Med 1955;252:162.
93. Haerer AF, Smith RR. Cerebrovascular disease of young adults in a Mississippi teaching hospital. Stroke 1970;1:466.
94. Seneviratne BIB, Ameratunga B. Strokes in young adults. BMJ 1972;3:791.
95. Carolei A, Marini C, Ferranti E, et al. A prospective study of cerebral ischemia in the young: analysis of pathogenic determinants. Stroke 1993;24:362.
96. Louis S, McDowell F. Stroke in young adults. Ann Intern Med 1967;66:932.
97. Abraham J, Shetty G, Jose CJ. Strokes in the young. Stroke 1971;2:259.
98. Jolly SS, Rai B, Singh N, et al. Cerebrovascular accidents in young adults (15-40 years): a study of 253 cases. Indian J Med Sci 1971;25:518.
99. Hindfelt B, Nilsson O. Brain infarction in young adults. Acta Neurol Scand 1977;55:145.
100. Grindal AB, Cohen RJ, Saul RF, Taylor JR. Cerebral infarction in young adults. Stroke 1978;9:39.
101. Schoenberg BS, Mellinger JF, Schoenberg DG. Cerebrovascular disease in infants and children: a study of incidence, clinical features, and survival. Neurology 1978;28:763.
102. Chopra JS, Prabhakar S. Clinical features and risk factors in stroke in young. Acta Neurol Scand 1979;60:289.
103. Snyder BD, Ramirez-Lassepas M. Cerebral infarction in young adults. Stroke 1980;11:149.
104. Hart LU, Miller VT. Cerebral infarction in young adults: a practical approach. Stroke 1983;14:110.
105. Franck G, Doyen F, Grisar T, Moonen G. Les accidents ischémiques cérébraux du sujet jeune, âgé de moins de quarante-cinq ans. Semin Hop Paris 1983;59:2642.
106. Klein GM, Seland TP. Occlusive cerebrovascular disease in young adults. Can J Neurol Sci 1984;11:302.
107. Hilton-Jones D, Warlow CP. The causes of stroke in the young. J Neurol 1985;232:137.

108. Hachinski V, Norris JW. The young stroke. In Idem, eds. The Acute Stroke. Philadelphia: FA Davis, 1985.
109. Adams HP, Butler MJ, Biller J, et al. Nonhemorrhagic cerebral infarction in young adults. Arch Neurol 1986;43:793.
110. Radhakrishnan K, Ashok PP, Sridharan R, Mousa ME. Stroke in the young: incidence and pattern in Benghazi, Libya. Acta Neurol Scand 1986;73:434.
111. Bogousslavsky J, Regli F. Ischemic stroke in adults younger than 30 years of age. Arch Neurol 1987;44:479.
112. Alvarez J, Matias-Guiu J, Sumalla J, et al. Ischemic stroke in young adults, I: analysis of the etiological subgroups. Acta Neurol Scand 1989;80:28.
113. Gautier JC, Pradat-Diehl P, Loron PH, et al. Accidents vasculaires cérébraux des sujets jeunes: une étude de 133 patients âgés de 9 a 45 ans. Rev Neurol 1989;6-7:437.
114. Bevan H, Sharma K, Bradley W. Stroke in young adults. Stroke 1990;21:382.
115. Lisovoski F, Rousseaux P. Cerebral infarction in young people: a study of 148 patients with early cerebral angiography. J Neurol Neurosurg Psychiatry 1991;54:576.
116. Lanzino G, Andreoli A, Di Pasquale G, et al. Etiopathogenesis and prognosis of cerebral ischemia in young adults: a survey of 155 treated patients. Acta Neurol Scand 1991;84:321.
117. Biller J, Love BB, Schneck MJ. Vascular diseases of the nervous system: ischemic cerebrovascular disease. In Bradley WJ, Daroff RB, Fenichel GM, Jankovic J, eds. Neurology of Clinical Practice, 5th ed. Butterworth Heinemann, 2008. The efficacy and safety of intravenous thrombolysis administered between 3 and 4.5 hours is currently under active investigation.
118. North American Symptomatic Carotid Endarterectomy Trial Collaborators. Beneficial effect of carotid endarterectomy in symptomatic patients with high-grade carotid stenosis. N Engl J Med 1991;325:445.
119. Mayberg MR, Wilson SE, Yatsu F, et al. Carotid endarterectomy and prevention of cerebral ischemia in symptomatic carotid stenosis. JAMA 1991;266:3289.
120. European Carotid Surgery Trialists Collaborative Group. Risk of stroke in the distribution of an asymptomatic carotid artery. Lancet 1995;345:209.
121. European Carotid Surgery Trialists Collaborative Group. Endarterectomy for moderate symptomatic carotid stenosis: interim results from the MRC European Carotid Surgery Trial. Lancet 1996;347:1591.
122. Biller J, Feinberg WM, Castaldo JE, et al. Guidelines for carotid endarterectomy. A Statement for Healthcare Professionals from a Special Writing Group of the Stroke Council. American Heart Association. Stroke 1998;29:554.
123. National Institute of Neurological Disorders and Stroke rt-PA Stroke Study Group. Tissue plasminogen activator for acute ischemic stroke. N Engl J Med 1995;333:1581.

CHAPTER 6

Nonatherosclerotic Cerebral Vasculopathies

Rima M. Dafer • José Biller

Causes of ischemic stroke are multiple, especially in children and young adults. Although atherosclerosis of the cerebral vasculature and cardioembolic arterial occlusions are the most common causes of stroke, approximately 5% of strokes are due to other conditions, such as nonatherosclerotic vasculopathies and thrombophilic states, and approximately 30% remain cryptogenic. Although uncommon, nonatherosclerotic vasculopathies are well-recognized causes of stroke mainly in children and young adults, accounting for 14% to 25% of stroke in subjects 14 to 47 years of age.[1,2] A large variety of nonatherosclerotic causes can lead to ischemic stroke through diverse mechanisms. Exploring these etiologies particularly in children and young adults is in order. These nonatherosclerotic causes include cervicocephalic arterial dissections (CCADs), fibromuscular dysplasia (FMD), infectious vasculitides, moyamoya disease, nonamyloid vasculopathy, and many others.

Hypoplasia and Agenesis of the Internal Carotid Artery

Embryologically, the internal carotid artery (ICA) originates from the third aortic arch and the dorsal aorta. Agenesis of the ICA (unilateral or bilateral) is a rare developmental malformation, which results from failure of the embryonic primordium of the ICA to develop before 3 to 5 weeks of embryonic life. The incidence of unilateral agenesis of ICA is estimated at 0.36%. This abnormality is usually asymptomatic, and a rare cause of cerebral ischemia from arterial compression or dilated vascular channels. Associated intracranial aneurysms

115

occur in 25% to 35% of patients and are often responsible for intracranial hemorrhage. Rupture of these malformations may account for intracerebral hemorrhage or subarachnoid hemorrhage (SAH).[3-5] Cerebral infarctions are uncommon.[6-9]

Arterial Fenestrations

Fenestrations of the intracranial arteries are extremely rare congenital anomalies associated with pediatric stroke (Fig. 6-1).[10-12] Vertebrobasilar junction fenestrations are the most frequently observed fenestrations of the cerebral arteries, often associated with saccular aneurysm formation and arteriovenous malformations, with an increased risk of SAH.[13-16]

Coils and Kinks

Redundant length of the cervical carotid artery causes coils and kinks and other forms of tortuosity. The incidence of coiling and kinking of the ICA in the general population is estimated at 10% to 16%.[17] By definition, coiling is elongation and redundancy of an ICA resulting in an exaggerated S-shaped curvature or a circular configuration. A kink is an angulation of one or more segments of the ICA associated with stenosis of the affected segment (Fig. 6-2). Unilateral or bilateral aberrant tortuosity of the ICAs may become more pronounced with aging, especially among hypertensive individuals, and can present unsuspected surgical risks for the

otolaryngologist and head and neck surgeon.[18-20] The clinical importance of these abnormalities is controversial. Kinks and coils are exceedingly rare causes of cerebral ischemia secondary to combined obstruction, neck rotation and head position, and microembolization. Careful judgment should be employed when considering surgical intervention procedures to correct a coiled or kinked ICA in asymptomatic subjects. Surgical correction of isolated carotid elongations with coiling or kinking may be considered in selected patients with recurrent symptoms when all other risk factors for stroke have been excluded or controlled.[17,20-23]

Moyamoya Disease

Moyamoya disease is a chronic progressive noninflammatory occlusive intracranial vasculopathy of unknown etiology.[24-29] Moyamoya disease has been associated with neonatal anoxia; head trauma; basilar meningitis; postinfectious or postradiation vasculopathies; phakomatoses including tuberous sclerosis, neurofibromatosis 1, Sturge-Weber syndrome, phakomatosis pigmentovascularis type IIIB, pseudoxanthoma elasticum, and hypomelanosis of Ito; and hematologic disorders including sickle cell anemia, β-thalassemia, Fanconi anemia, and hereditary spherocytosis. Other conditions associated with moyamoya disease include brain tumors, polyarteritis nodosa, Marfan syndrome, Turner syndrome, Williams syndrome, arteriosclerosis, use of oral contraceptives, FMD, cerebral dissecting and saccular aneurysms, Sneddon syndrome, homocystinuria, type I glycogenosis, Alpert syndrome, primary oxalosis, sarcoidosis, Hirschsprung disease, Alagille syndrome, hyperphosphatasia, Graves disease, coarctation of the aorta, factor XII deficiency, renal artery stenosis, and Down syndrome.[23-40]

Moyamoya disease is more frequent in Japanese, but has been reported in all ethnic groups.[30-36] The disease is seen in children and adults, especially women, often in the first or third decades of life. Familial cases have been reported with autosomal dominant inheritance, with the locations on the gene encoding tissue inhibitor of metalloproteinase (TIMP) 4 and TIMP2 spanning chromosomes 3p24.2-p26 and 17q25.[37-43]

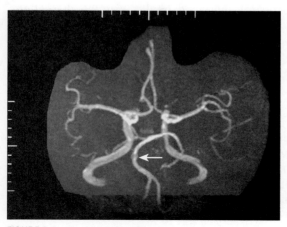

FIGURE 6-1   Fenestration in the mid–basilar artery (*arrow*).

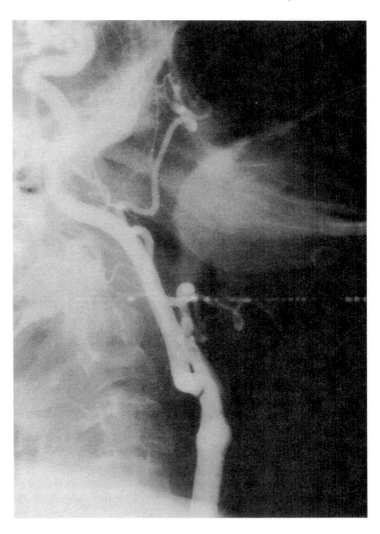

FIGURE 6-2 Common carotid angiography (lateral projection) shows a kink of the proximal left internal carotid artery. (Courtesy of Eric Russell, M.D.)

The distal segments of the ICAs at the bifurcation are most commonly involved, resulting in the formation of a fine network of collateral neovasculature. Pathologically, there is intimal thickening of the cerebral arterial trunks, endothelial hyperplasia and fibrosis, tortuosity and duplication of the internal elastic lamina, thinning of the media, normal adventitia, and lack of inflammatory reaction. The endothelial thickening starts at the terminal segment of the ICA and spreads to the proximal portions of the anterior cerebral artery (ACA) and middle cerebral artery (MCA) (occasionally to the posterior cerebral arteries), causing a progressive stenosis of the major cerebral vessels and abundant angiogenesis for collateral blood supplies.[44-49]

Clinical manifestations of moyamoya disease include transient ischemic attacks (TIAs), headaches, seizures, mental retardation, involuntary movements, cerebral infarction, and intracranial hemorrhage or SAH. In children, the disease most often causes TIAs or ischemic strokes. Recurrent strokes are common. Seizures can be the presenting symptom.[50-52] SAH is the most common presentation in adults secondary to ruptured intracerebral aneurysms, with subependymal or intraventricular hemorrhages.[53-56] Cerebral infarctions are common.[57,58]

Hematologic, biochemical, and serologic findings are nonspecific. Diagnosis is based on a distinct angiographic appearance of a telangiectatic pattern of "puff of smoke" in the basal ganglia region—hence the

Japanese name of moyamoya. There is bilateral stenosis or occlusion of the supraclinoid segment of the ICAs and the proximal parts of the ACA and MCA. An extensive parenchymal, transdural, and leptomeningeal collateral network may be seen. The vertebrobasilar circulation is rarely involved. Intracranial aneurysms occur in one fourth of patients.[59-67]

Common neuroimaging findings on computed tomography (CT) and magnetic resonance imaging (MRI) of brain include infarctions, often bilateral, in the watershed territories between the anterior, middle, and posterior cerebral arteries and basal ganglia, thalami, and centrum semiovale in distal beds of supply of the penetrating branches of the ACA and MCA. Other findings include diffuse cerebral atrophy and hemosiderin deposition as a result of silent hemorrhages. Diffusion-weighted MRI allows early detection of cerebral infarctions and may be beneficial in monitoring the progression of ischemia. Transcranial Doppler ultrasonography may be useful in detecting microembolic signals at the distal portion of stenotic arteries. 3-Tesla system time of flight MR angiography, CT angiography, and cerebral angiography may show narrowing or occlusion of the proximal segments of the ACA and MCA (Fig. 6-3). Susceptibility-weighted imaging is useful for detection of hemorrhagic lesions.[70-82]

The optimal treatment of moyamoya disease is unclear. Medical management includes platelet antiaggregants, corticosteroids, and antiepileptic drugs for patients with seizures. Anticoagulants are not useful. Patients with recurrent and progressive focal cerebral ischemic symptoms may benefit from surgical intervention aimed at improving cerebral blood flow through direct and indirect revascularization procedures, such as superficial temporal artery to MCA bypass, encephalomyosynangiosis, omental pedicle transposition, encephaloduroarteriosynangiosis, and dural inversion procures or burr holes without vessel synangiosis.[2,25,68-88]

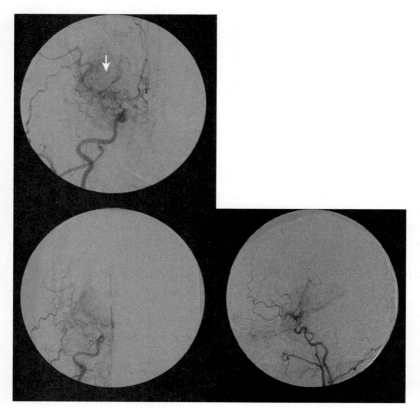

FIGURE 6-3 Angiographic pattern consistent with moyamoya disease, with puff of smoke appearance (*arrowhead*), and stenosis of the distal internal carotid artery and proximal middle cerebral artery.

Fibromuscular Dysplasia

FMD is a nonatheromatous segmental noninflammatory angiopathy of unknown etiology. The disease usually affects the medium-sized and small arteries, predominantly the renal and extracranial segment of the ICAs, with medial fibrodysplasia or, less commonly, intimal fibrodysplasia. Other arterial beds may be involved, including hepatic, celiac, mesenteric, axillary, and external iliac arteries. The vertebrobasilar system and the intracranial segments of the ICAs are rarely involved. Bilateral involvement is common. FMD is more common in young women, especially in individuals with a history of migraines. Familial cases have been reported. Childhood FMD is rare. The natural history of FMD is unknown, and most cases are asymptomatic.

Clinical symptoms are broad: Patients may present with headaches, dizziness, pulsatile tinnitus, vertigo, or TIAs. Focal neurologic symptoms may include Horner syndrome secondary to cervicocephalic arterial dissection (CCAD), cranial nerve palsies, and other focal neurologic deficits (Table 6-1) when cerebral infarction occurs secondary to stenosis, dissection, or embolization from a major involved artery. Associated intracranial aneurysms are common and may lead to SAH.

Three characteristic angiographic patterns are recognized; the most common is multifocal short stenoses with multiple mural dilations predominantly involving the

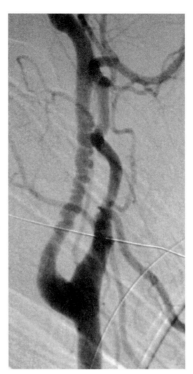

FIGURE 6-4 "String of beads" of the extracranial internal carotid artery on carotid angiography in a patient with cervicocephalic fibromuscular dysplasia.

middle portion of the ICA, 2 to 3 cm distal to its origin, producing the typical "string of beads" appearance owing to medial fibroplasias, seen in at least 80% of type I cases (Fig. 6-4). Less common angiographic patterns are unifocal or multifocal tubular or concentric stenoses with cerebral aneurysms (type II) and atypical FMD (type III). Involvement of the ICA is often adjacent to the level of the second cervical vertebra, and frequently spares the proximal segment of the vessel.[89-92]

Patients with hypertension and a history of cigarette smoking are predisposed to FMD. Polymorphisms of the renin-angiotensin system may play a role in the development of FMD.[93] FMD has been reported in association with various syndromes, including Ehlers-Danlos syndrome type IV, Alport syndrome, pheochromocytoma, Marfan syndrome, and Takayasu arteritis.[94-98] The differential diagnosis encompasses a variety of conditions causing irregularities and variation in the caliber of the ICAs, including atherosclerosis, cerebral vasospasm, giant cell arteritides,

TABLE 6-1 **Extracranial Cervicocephalic Arterial Dissection—Clinical Picture**

Ipsilateral headache
Lightheadedness and syncope
Tinnitus
Horner syndrome
Scintillations
Carotidynia
Ocular/orbital pain
Amaurosis fugax
Anterior and posterior ischemic optic neuropathy
Central retinal artery occlusion
Ophthalmic artery occlusion
Cranial nerves III, IV, VI palsies
Cranial nerves IX to XII palsies (Vernet and Collet-
  Sicard syndromes)
Cerebral infarction

stationary arterial waves, circular spastic contractions, arterial hypoplasia,[99] and decreased distal arterial flow.[91,100]

The optimal treatment of symptomatic cervicocephalic FMD is unclear; antiaggregants or anticoagulants are often used in symptomatic patients. Surgical intervention is seldom warranted. Percutaneous interventions for symptomatic stenosis with balloon angioplasty and stenting or surgical graduated endoluminal dilation combined with carotid endarterectomy may be considered in patients with recurrent symptoms. Other surgical options include coiling of associated cerebral aneurysms, excision of fibromuscular tissue with primary anastomosis or patch grafting, and rarely extracranial-intracranial bypass.[101-104]

Cervicocephalic Arterial Dissections

CCADs are a common cause of ischemic stroke, particularly in young and middle-aged patients in the absence of known vascular risk factors. CCADs account for 10% to 20% of ischemic strokes in young adults and for 2.5% of all ischemic strokes.[105-109] Incidence rates for CCADs have been reported to be 2.6 to 5 per 100,000 with higher prevalence in the fall and winter, with a long-term recurrence rate estimated at approximately 1% per year.[110-113]

Pathologically, a tear in the intimal layer of the carotid or vertebral arteries may occur, with subsequent subintimal penetration of blood and longitudinal extension of the intramural hematoma, leading to tapering, focal stenosis, or occlusion of the affected vessel. If it proceeds between the media and adventitia, a pseudoaneurysm results.[114,115] Impaired endothelium-dependent vasodilation abnormalities may be a predisposing factor for CCADs.[116] The extracranial segments of the carotid and vertebral arteries are more commonly involved. Less commonly, CCADs may extend intracranially toward the petrous canal, often involving the horizontal segment of the MCA or the supraclinoid ICA.[117] Vertebrobasilar circulation dissections most often affect the extracranial vertebral artery in its third segment. Bilateral involvement is frequent. Involvement of the intracranial vertebral artery, basilar artery, or posterior cerebral artery is rare.

In most cases of spontaneous intracranial ICA dissections, the lesions are subintimal, whereas in intracranial vertebrobasilar circulation dissections they tend to occur between the media and adventitia.[114,118-120]

CCADs may occur spontaneously or secondary to antecedent trauma (Table 6-2). Blunt trauma accounts for only 3% to 10% of all carotid injuries, predominantly secondary to motor vehicle collisions. CCADs also have been reported after minor trauma or neck maneuvering with rapid head tilt during chiropractic manipulation, head banging, childbirth, boxing, and many other mechanisms of rapid neck flexion or extension.[121-128] Most carotid artery trauma is due to penetrating injuries, primarily the results of projectile injuries. The pathogenesis of spontaneous dissections is unknown, although a history of trivial trauma or other precipitating event is frequently elicited. Recent respiratory tract infections have been thought to trigger CCADs, a finding supported by the seasonal variation in the incidence of spontaneous CCADs.[113,129]

Various risk factors for CCADs have been reported, including tobacco use, oral contraceptives, migraine, α_1-antitrypsin deficiency, hyperhomocysteinemia, methylene tetrahydrofolate reductase (MTHFR) genotype, arterial hypertension, and large aortic root diameter.[130-137] CCADs also are common among patients with collagen vascular disease

TABLE 6-2 **Traumatic Causes of Extracranial Arterial Dissections**

Carotid Artery Dissection	Vertebral Artery Dissection
Direct blow	Atlantoaxial
Damage to artery	subluxation
Mandibular fracture	Cervical spine
Stretching of lateral	fracture
processes of C2-3	Cervical
Basal skull fracture	osteoarthritis
Peritonsillar trauma	Cervical spine
Strangulation	hyperextension
Craniocerebral trauma	or hyper-rotation
	Chiropractic
	manipulation
	Foramen magnum
	tumor
	Head banging
	(heavy metal
	rockers)

or other arteriopathies, including cervico-cephalic arterial FMD, autosomal dominant polycystic kidney disease, osteogenesis imperfecta, Ehlers-Danlos syndrome type IV, cystic medial degeneration, luetic arteritis, moya-moya disease, pharyngeal infections, and Marfan syndrome.[97,138-140]

The clinical picture varies, and some CCADs remain asymptomatic (see Table 6-1). Symptoms may result from direct compression by dissecting aneurysm, stenosis, or occlusion of the affected vessel. Ipsilateral headache is common, occurring in 83% of patients. The headache is usually retro-orbital when the ICA is affected, associated with oculosympathetic palsy (Horner syndrome), and occipital in location with vertebral dissection. Multiple cranial nerve palsies are common, with lower cranial nerves most commonly involved. Dysgeusia may occur as a result of involvement of the chorda tympani.[141] Amaurosis fugax and other transient neurologic deficits may result. Although ischemic stroke remains the most common serious complication of CCAD, intracranial extension may cause SAH in 25% of patients.[142] The pathogenesis of the clinical deficits is often due to intimal disruption with distal embolism, luminal narrowing leading to flow-related symptoms, disruption of sympathetic nerve fibers causing an oculosympathetic palsy, compression or stretching of the nerve by the expanded artery in the upper cervical parapharyngeal space, and rarely extension of the dissection intracranially or interruption of the nutrient vessels supplying the nerve.[141,143-146]

Clinical suspicion should be high in young patients presenting with ischemic stroke in the absence of other cerebrovascular risk factors. MRI may show signal void abnormalities in the lumen of the affected artery representing the intramural hematoma. Although conventional angiography remains the gold standard in the diagnosis of arterial disease, helical CT angiography and MR angiography are alternative noninvasive studies, which may show tapering or occlusion of the affected artery, and may help in determining intracranial extension (Figs. 6-5, 6-6, and 6-7). Characteristic angiographic features of CCAD include the presence of pseudoaneurysm or a double lumen, seen in less than 10% of cases.[147]

The appropriate management of CCAD is still unknown. Intravenous thrombolysis with tissue plasminogen activator should be considered in patients presenting with acute ischemic strokes within 3 hours of the onset of symptoms only after intradural extension is ruled out.[148] The appropriate secondary prevention measure after the diagnosis of CCAD is confirmed remains unknown in

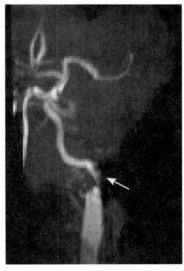

FIGURE 6-5   MR angiography showing focal stenosis of the left internal carotid artery suggestive of cervicocephalic arterial dissection (*arrow*).

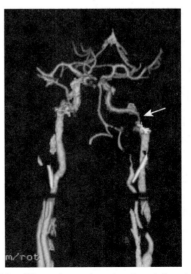

FIGURE 6-6   CT angiography showing left extracranial internal carotid artery dissection (*arrow*).

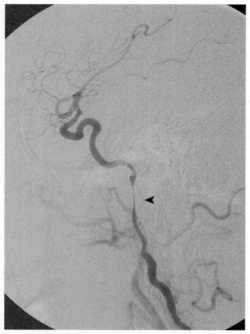

FIGURE 6-7   Left internal carotid artery dissection extending to the petrous segment shown on lateral view of catheter carotid angiogram (*arrowhead*).

the absence of randomized clinical studies to determine the best medical management. The use of antithrombotic or anticoagulation therapy in CCADs is empirical, rather than evidence based. The collaborating members of the Canadian Stroke Consortium reported the results of prospectively collected data on patients with angiographically proven acute vertebral or carotid arterial dissection followed for 1 year. Fifteen percent of patients had recurrent ischemic events (TIA, stroke, or death) mainly in the weeks immediately after the dissection. The event rate in patients treated with anticoagulants was not significantly different than that in patients treated with aspirin (8.3% versus 12.4%).[149] Data from a Cochrane analysis of the literature from nonrandomized trials did not show a significant difference between the two treatment modalities.[150]

Medical management is first line in most patients. Treatment decisions should be customized based on clinical characteristics, recurrent event rate, pathophysiologic mechanisms, and imaging findings of CCAD. The presence of intracranial or intradural extension should warrant caution against the use of anticoagulation because of the high risk of SAH. In contrast, pseudo-occlusion or pseudoaneurysm, high-intensity transient signals on transcranial Doppler studies, and the presence of thrombus in the dissected artery favor the use of anticoagulation.[151] Given the greatest risk of symptom recurrence and cerebral ischemia in the first few weeks after dissection, and the risk of thrombus formation and early embolization or occlusion, it is reasonable to recommend anticoagulation with intravenous heparin or low-molecular-weight heparin followed by dose-adjusted warfarin for 3 to 6 months in patients with extracranial CCADs who present acutely. In patients presenting late after the index event, antiplatelet therapy should be considered. Endovascular or surgical interventions should be reserved for a few patients with recurrent events despite appropriate medical therapy, or when the use of anticoagulation is contraindicated.[152-155] The natural history and incidence of carotid and vertebral arterial dissections is unknown. CCADs seem to recur within the first 2 months after the initial event.[156] CCADs have a favorable outcome with good recovery rate, with a better prognosis in vertebral dissection compared with carotid dissection.[157]

Radiation-induced Vasculopathies

Radiation-induced vasculopathy and arteritis are two of the complications of whole-brain radiation therapy, which may occur many years after radiation therapy. Although the incidence of radiation-induced vasculopathy is correlated with the patient's age and radiation dose, the mechanism by which vasculopathy occurs after cranial irradiation remains unclear. Progressive cerebral arteriopathy with transdural anastomoses may lead to moyamoya disease. Patients may present with encephalopathy, seizures, and focal neurological deficits. MRI usually shows thickening and prominent ring enhancement of the wall of the affected large cerebral arteries, and angiography reveals multiple medium-sized arterial wall irregularities and focal arterial stenoses.[158-163]

Central Nervous System Vasculitides

Central nervous system (CNS) vasculitides are a serious uncommon cause of ischemic and hemorrhagic stroke in children and young adults, which present a diagnostic challenge for physicians. CNS vasculitides account for 19% of ischemic stroke in children and young adults. This heterogeneous group of disorders may be a manifestation of a systemic disorder, or may primarily involve the CNS (primary or isolated CNS angiitis [PACNS]) where the vascular inflammation is limited to the brain and spinal cord. Secondary CNS vasculitides occur in various conditions, including infections and noninfectious inflammatory disorders (Table 6-3), collagen vascular diseases, systemic vasculitides, and malignancies. Patients may present with constitutional symptoms, such as fever, malaise, and weight loss; unexplained skin lesions; glomerulopathy; arthropathy; or cardiac or pulmonary manifestations. Common neurologic symptoms include headaches usually with nonspecific characteristics, recurrent TIAs or stroke (ischemic or hemorrhagic), cognitive disorders, encephalopathies, and multifocal neurologic deficits. Myelopathy, myopathy, and peripheral neuropathy may occur.

PACNS is a rare disease, the pathogenesis of which remains unknown. Various pathogens have been documented in association with PACNS, including viral, bacterial, spirochetal, fungal, and protozoal organisms.[164-167] The disorder involves the small and medium-sized leptomeningeal and cortical arteries. PACNS is characterized by headache and cognitive impairment, seizures, chronic meningitis, multifocal neurologic deficits, and recurrent strokelike presentations. Pathologic findings include classic granulomatous angiitis with Langhans cells and lymphocytic and necrotizing vasculitis.

Laboratory tests and cerebrospinal fluid (CSF) analysis are nondiagnostic. Findings on MRI of the brain are nonspecific and usually show multiple cortical and subcortical infarctions. Angiographic yield is low, with a specificity of less than 25%; however, when present, the findings of vessel stenosis or occlusion in the setting of the suspected clinical picture are vital for the diagnosis (Fig. 6-8). Definitive diagnosis is histologic, and a brain

TABLE 6-3 **Classification of Cerebral Vasculitis**

Infectious vasculitis
  Spirochetal (syphilis)
  Mycobacterial
  Fungal
  Rickettsial
  Bacterial (purulent) meningitis
  Viral
  Other organisms
Necrotizing vasculitides
  Classic polyarteritis nodosa
  Wegener granulomatosis
  Allergic angiitis and granulomatosis
    (Churg-Strauss)
  Necrotizing systemic vasculitis—overlap
    syndrome
  Lymphomatoid granulomatosis
Vasculitis associated with collagen vascular diseases
  Systemic lupus erythematosus
  Rheumatoid arthritis
  Scleroderma
  Sjögren syndrome
Primary central nervous system vasculitis
Giant cell arteritis
  Takayasu arteritis
  Temporal (cranial) arteritis
Hypersensitivity vasculitides
  Henoch-Schönlein purpura
  Drug-induced vasculitides
  Chemical vasculitides
  Essential mixed cryoglobulinemia
Miscellaneous
  Vasculitis associated with neoplasia
  Vasculitis associated with radiation
  Cogan syndrome
  Dermatomyositis-polymyositis
  X-linked lymphoproliferative syndrome
  Thromboangiitis obliterans
  Kawasaki syndrome
Vasculitis associated with other systemic diseases
  Behçet disease
  Ulcerative colitis
  Sarcoidosis
  Relapsing polychondritis
Kohlmeier-Degos disease

Adapted from Biller J, Sparks LH. Diagnosis and Management of Cerebral Vasculitis. In: Handbook of Cerebrovascular Diseases. Maral Dekker, Inc, pp 549–568, 1993. H.P. Adams, Jr (editor).

(corticomeningeal) biopsy with a sampling of the leptomeninges is necessary. The yield of a biopsy is low, however, and a negative biopsy result does not preclude the diagnosis of PACNS. If untreated, the disease carries a poor prognosis. Treatment includes intravenous cyclophosphamide in association with oral prednisone.[165,166]

Infections are well-known causes of cerebral infarcts or hemorrhages in children

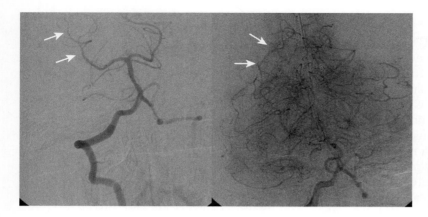

FIGURE 6-8 Irregularity in the right posterior cerebral artery (*arrows*) in a patient diagnosed with primary CNS vasculitis or angiitis.

and young adults. Prompt diagnosis and therapy are needed to reduce the severity of brain damage and to avoid recurrent strokes. This chapter highlights the most common infections associated with CNS vasculitis.

Acute purulent bacterial meningitis may result in intracranial arteritis and thrombophlebitis, with impaired consciousness, elevated intracranial pressure, hydrocephalus, and seizures.[168] Activation of coagulation and attenuation of fibrinolysis in the CSF are important features of bacterial meningitis that may contribute to the development of cerebral infarctions predominantly in children.[169] Early aggressive treatment with antibiotic therapy is lifesaving. Varicella-zoster virus usually spreads to the CNS via hematogenous or direct extension, or through invasion of the cerebral vessels, most commonly the MCA.[170,171] The diagnosis is made by angiographic findings of multiple focal arterial stenosis and the presence of oligoclonal varicella IgG antibodies in the CSF. Antiviral therapy may be beneficial in halting the progression of the disease and reversal of symptoms and is associated with a favorable outcome.

Stroke is a common neurologic complication of human immunodeficiency virus (HIV) infection and acquired immunodeficiency syndrome (AIDS). Mechanisms of stroke in HIV-infected patients vary, with HIV vasculopathy reported in 20% of cases, followed by coagulopathies, hyperviscosity, endocarditis, and ruptured mycotic aneurysms. Cerebral infarctions are more common than intraparenchymal hemorrhage.[172-181]

Tuberculosis remains a major health problem in the developing countries around the world and is a growing concern in HIV-infected individuals in the United States. The most severe form of the disease is tuberculous meningitis, often affecting children and young adults, followed by tuberculoma, tuberculous abscess, tuberculous encephalopathy/encephalitis, and rarely cerebral arteritis of the supraclinoid carotid arteries and proximal segments of the ACA and MCA. Diagnosis is usually based on clinical features, and the CSF findings of moderate pleocytosis, with mononuclear predominance of neutrophils, elevated protein, and hypoglycorrhachia. Acid-fast bacilli cultures are positive in only 10% to 20% of proven cases. Radiologic imaging discloses cerebral infarctions, usually with bilateral involvement in the territory of the lenticulostriate and thalamoperforating territories. Tuberculomas may be present, predominantly infratentorially. Angiographic studies may show intracranial occlusion or narrowing of the ICA or its branches. Early diagnosis and prompt institution of antituberculous treatments and dexamethasone may prevent permanent deficit and fatal outcome.[176,182-190]

Syphilitic arteritis is an obliterative endarteritis most commonly affecting the large and medium-sized vessels (Heubner arteritis) or less frequently the small vessels (Nissl arteritis) of the brain, meninges, and spinal cord.[191] Although meningovascular syphilis occurs 5 to 10 years after the onset of untreated syphilis, early symptomatic manifestations of the disease are often identified in patients with HIV coinfection.[192] Patients often have a subacute encephalopathic presentation, rather than sudden-onset strokelike symptoms. Manifestations range from progressive personality changes to seizures and focal neurologic deficit. The most frequently involved vessel is the MCA. CSF shows pleocytosis and increased protein content, and reactive serology is suggestive. Cerebral angiography often shows a diffuse angiopathy with concentric narrowing of the large vessels and focal narrowing and dilation of the small vessels. Aortic dissection may occur secondary to aortitis.[170,171,191-196] Penicillin remains the drug of choice for neurosyphilis.

Common neurologic manifestations of Lyme disease (neuroborreliosis) include lymphocytic meningitis, cranial mononeuropathies or mononeuritis multiplex, radiculoneuritis, peripheral neuropathy, encephalopathy, and myelitis. Stroke is an uncommon presentation of neuroborreliosis and may occur in the late persistent stage of the disease. The diagnosis of neuroborreliosis is established with serologic testing. Treatment with antibiotics should be initiated immediately when the diagnosis is confirmed.[197-199]

Aspergillosis and mucormycosis are common fungal infections. They usually involve the CNS in approximately 1.2% to 3% of immunocompromised and transplant patients. Ischemic and hemorrhagic strokes may occur owing to fungal invasion of the leptomeningeal vessels. Other infections associated with CNS vasculitis include tuberculosis, cryptococcosis, coccidioidomycosis, cat-scratch disease, Rocky Mountain spotted fever, candidiasis, mycoplasmosis, toxoplasmosis, and amebiasis.[170,188,200-207]

Drug abuse is a major medical, legal, and social problem in the world today. Ischemic and hemorrhagic stroke is a complication of illicit drug use. Most commonly, the implicated substances are amphetamines, cocaine, heroin, phenylpropanolamine hydrochloride, and pentazocine lactate injection in combination with tripelennamine. Symptoms frequently develop immediately or within hours of administration of the offending drug, but may be delayed for 2 to 3 weeks after exposure. Complications of stroke caused by illicit drug use have been attributed to drug-induced sympathomimetic pressor effects, hypersensitivity-mediated arterial hypotension, enhanced platelet aggregation, decreased fibrinolytic activity, infective endocarditis, cardiac arrhythmias, foreign particle embolization, vasospasm, direct arterial injection, AIDS, and drug-induced vasculitis. Beading of the intracranial vessels has been described in young individuals with a diagnosis of stroke who were suspected of being users of amphetamines (dextroamphetamines and methamphetamine hydrochloride) alone or in combination with other drugs. A necrotizing vasculitis, pathologically similar to periarteritis nodosa, was shown. Fatal intracranial hemorrhage has been reported after the use of intravenous, oral, or intranasal amphetamines. The findings suggest that intracranial hemorrhage is due to an immunologically mediated vasculitis or amphetamine-related hypertensive crisis or both.

There has been a significant increase in the number of case reports describing stroke associated with cocaine use, especially among HIV-infected patients. Ischemic and hemorrhagic strokes occur equally with alkaloidal "crack" cocaine, whereas cocaine hydrochloride is more likely to cause intraparenchymal hemorrhage (80% compared with ischemic stroke). The exact mechanism of cocaine-induced stroke remains unclear: Mechanisms include enhanced platelet aggregation, cardioembolism, and hypertensive surges owing to its sympathomimetic properties, resulting in altered cerebral autoregulation and ruptured cerebral saccular aneurysms or vascular malformations. Less commonly, cerebral vasospasm and vasculitis may occur.[208-210]

Heroin use has been associated with spongiform leukoencephalopathy and ischemic and hemorrhagic strokes, mainly watershed infarctions. Strokes in heroin abusers may be due to infective endocarditis, foreign particle embolization, mycoses, cerebral arteritis, hypersensitivity reaction with arterial hypotension, or positional vascular compression.[211-213]

Phenylpropanolamine is a synthetic sympathomimetic drug structurally and functionally similar to amphetamine and ephedrine. It is an ingredient in numerous over-the-counter preparations, including cough and cold remedies and diet pills. Cases of intracerebral hemorrhage with angiographic features of vasculitis have been described after phenylpropanolamine exposure, particularly in women.[214-216] Some patients who intravenously inject pentazocine lactate and tripelennamine develop brain infarcts. Stroke also can result from the intravenous or the inadvertent intra-arterial administration of methylphenidate hydrochloride. Vascular spasm has been implicated in the etiology of stroke after the oral ingestion of lysergic acid diethylamide (LSD), after intoxication with phencyclidine (PCP), and after glue sniffing.[217-220]

Secondary noninfectious inflammatory vasculitides may be divided into necrotizing autoimmune vasculitis, hypersensitivity vasculitis, giant cell arteritis, and vasculitis associated with collagen vascular disorders. In this chapter, we review only multisystem selective vasculitides that may manifest as stroke in this particular group of patients.

Polyarteritis nodosa is an uncommon systemic necrotizing panarteritis of small and medium-sized arteries. Cerebral vessels are rarely involved, occurring late in the course of the disease, with intraparenchymal hemorrhage or SAH more common than ischemic stroke.[170,193,196]

Vasculitis occurs in at least 20% of patients with systemic lupus erythematosus. True immune complex–mediated CNS vasculitis is uncommon, however. Strokes may result from local vasculopathy, vascular irritation, and leakage caused by circulating immune complexes. Strokes also may occur from thrombotic arterial occlusions associated with the presence of circulating antiphospholipid antibodies, premature atherosclerosis, arterial hypertension, thrombophilia associated with nephrotic syndrome (lupus nephritis), or cardiac embolism associated with Libman-Sacks endocarditis.[204,221-225]

Behçet disease is a multisystem inflammatory disease characterized by relapsing oral and genital ulcerations, iritis, uveitis, synovitis, and cutaneous vasculitis. Neuropathologic features with lymphocytic vasculitis of the small vessels have been reported, although vessels of all sizes may be affected. Cerebral vein thrombosis may occur. Cerebral vasculitis is rare.[193,226]

Sarcoid angiitis is rare; it primarily affects the eyes, meninges, cerebral arteries, and veins. Cerebral infarctions and TIA rarely may be the presenting manifestations of the disease.[165,170,171]

Kohlmeier-Degos disease or malignant atrophic papulosis is a rare systemic vaso-occlusive disease of the medium-sized and small vessels of unknown etiology. The disease is characterized by gastrointestinal and neurologic involvement and, almost invariably, a fatal outcome. Necrotizing arteritic skin lesions often precede the neurologic manifestations. Intracranial hemorrhage occurs secondary to intracranial vessel rupture.[195,227-229]

Takayasu arteritis or pulseless disease is a chronic panarteritis localized in the large arteries, predominantly the aortic arch or its branches, the ascending thoracic aorta, the abdominal aorta, or the entire aorta. Most cases occur in young women (Fig. 6-9). Laboratory abnormalities include

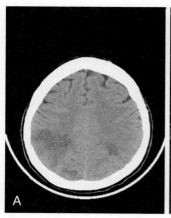
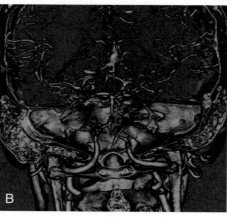

FIGURE 6-9 **A** and **B,** CT of brain showing bilateral wedge-shaped hypodensities in the cortical and subcortical white matter of the posterior frontal and parietal areas in a cardiac recipient after cyclosporine therapy (**A**); diffuse "vasospasm" of the basilar, posterior cerebral, middle cerebral, and anterior cerebral arteries (**B**).

normochromic or hypochromic anemia, leukocytosis, increased erythrocyte sedimentation rate, and elevated C-reactive protein. Angiography usually reveals irregular dilation of the aortic arch and its major branches, with focal narrowing at the origin of the major arteries.[196,226,230]

Henoch-Schönlein purpura is a nonthrombocytopenic, small vessel hypersensitivity vasculitis, most frequently seen in children. The disease represents a variety of leukocytoclastic hypersensitivity conditions, characterized by IgA, C3, and immune complex deposition in arterioles, capillaries, and venules. Neurologic involvement is rare. Cases of cerebral infarction and intracranial hemorrhage have been described. Some studies suggest a widespread arteritis and arteriolitis.[231,232]

Kawasaki syndrome may rarely be associated with stroke. This vasculitic syndrome in infants and young children is characterized by fever, lymphadenitis, mucosal and cutaneous inflammation, and widespread aneurysmal formation.[233-237]

Strokelike syndromes have been reported after treatment with various immunosuppressants in organ recipients and cancer patients, mainly asparaginase, methotrexate, BCNU, cisplatin, cyclophosphamide, cyclosporine, and tacrolimus.[157,238-241]

The diagnosis of cerebral vasculitis is often inferential, based on clinical presentation, presence of multisystem organ involvement, and abnormal serologic tests. Neurologic symptoms and laboratory tests are nonspecific. Serologic findings may support the presence of a systemic inflammatory state, but are often nonspecific. CSF can be normal or show nonspecific changes of increased protein and pleocytosis, indicating inflammatory CNS activity. Electroencephalography may be normal, show focal or diffuse slow-wave abnormality, or show epileptiform activity.[165,193] Cranial CT/CT angiography and MRI/MR angiography help delineate the anatomic extent of CNS involvement and arteriopathic changes in the vessels of the circle of Willis. Digital angiography is useful to detect changes in the arterial calibers, although sensitivity and specificity are limited. Such angiographic findings may be seen with various mimics, including vasospasm secondary to migraine or after aneurysmal SAH, brain tumors, intracerebral hematomas, pyogenic meningitides, intracranial atherosclerosis, head trauma, vascular anomalies associated with neurocutaneous syndromes, moyamoya disease, or sickle cell disease.

Histopathologic diagnosis with brain tissue and leptomeningeal biopsy specimens is the gold standard for the diagnosis of isolated angiitis of the CNS. Leptomeningeal biopsy is often for the definitive diagnosis of cerebral vasculitis.[165,166,170,171,193] Differential diagnosis includes metabolic, demyelinating, vascular, infectious, and other causes of stroke in children and young adults. Tables 6-4 and 6-5 present the suggested laboratory evaluation of patients with suspected noninfectious vasculitides. Treatment of the infectious cerebral vasculitides is beyond the scope of this chapter and is not discussed.

Management of CNS vasculitis includes treatment of the primary disorders. Treatment with corticosteroids and immunosuppressant agents has been shown to produce favorable clinical responses in patients with systemic vasculitides and may prove beneficial in patients with PACNS. Immunoglobulin therapy and plasma exchange have shown modest benefit in recurrent stroke refractory

TABLE 6-4 **Evaluation of Patients with Suspected Noninfectious Vasculitis: Basic Evaluation**

Complete blood count with differential and platelet count
Prothrombin time and activated partial thromboplastin time
Serum creatinine and blood urea nitrogen levels
Drug screen
Plasma glucose levels
Serum calcium
Erythrocyte sedimentation rate
High sensitivity C-reactive protein
Liver function tests
Serum bilirubin
Aspartate aminotransferase
γ-Glutamyl transpeptidase
Alanine aminotransferase
Lactate dehydrogenase
Alkaline phosphatase
Creatine kinase
Serum immunoelectrophoresis
Urinalysis with microscopic evaluation

Adapted from Biller J, Sparks LH. Diagnosis and Management of Cerebral Vasculitis. In: Handbook of Cerebrovascular Diseases. Maral Dekker, Inc, pp 549–568, 1993. H.P. Adams, Jr (editor).

TABLE 6-5 **Additional Evaluation of Patients with Suspected Cerebral Vasculitis**

Drug screen
Fluorescent treponemal antibody absorption
Venereal Disease Research Laboratory
Serum *Borrelia* antibodies
Human immunodeficiency virus serology
Antinuclear antibodies, extractable nuclear antigens
  (Sm, nRNP, antibody to double-stranded DNA,
  only if antinuclear antibody positive)
Rheumatoid factor
Anticardiolipin antibodies (IgG, IgM, IgA) and
  anti-β_2 glycoprotein 1 antibodies
Lupus inhibitor screening
C_3, C_4, CH_{50}
Antineutrophilic cytoplasmic antibody
Hepatitis B surface antigen
Sd 70 antibody (anti-isomerase antibody)
Anticentromere antibodies
Serum angiotensin-converting enzyme
Serum immunoglobulin levels
Cryoglobulins Coombs test
Schirmer test
Cerebrospinal fluid examination
Skin test for allergy
Pulmonary function tests (spirometry, lung volumes,
  diffusing capacity)
Paranasal sinus x-rays
Gallium 647 scanning
Visceral angiography (renal, hepatic, mesenteric
  circulation)
Tissue biopsy

Adapted from Biller J, Sparks LH. Diagnosis and Management of Cerebral Vasculitis. In: Handbook of Cerebrovascular Diseases. Maral Dekker, Inc, pp 549–568, 1993. H.P. Adams, Jr (editor).

to aggressive immunosuppressive therapy. Platelet antiaggregants should be considered in patients with ischemic strokes.

Conclusion

Nonatherosclerotic cerebral vasculopathies (inflammatory and noninflammatory) are frequent causes of cerebral infarction in young adults, accounting for 16% of all strokes in patients younger than age 45. Spontaneous or traumatic CCADs are among the most commonly encountered nonatherosclerotic vasculopathies. Accurate diagnosis and appropriate management reduce the morbidity and mortality and improve outcome. Although newer neuroimaging technologies such as MR angiography or CT angiography are becoming widely used noninvasive diagnostic tools, cerebral angiography remains the gold standard and is often required for definitive diagnosis.

REFERENCES

1. Rasura M, Spalloni A, Ferrari M, et al. A case series of young stroke in Rome. Eur J Neurol 2006;13:146.
2. Biller J, Adams HP Jr, Bruno A, et al. Mortality in acute cerebral infarction in young adults—a ten-year experience. Angiology 1991;42:224.
3. Dinc H, Gumele HR, Kuzeyli K, Baykal S. Unilateral agenesis of internal carotid artery with subarachnoid hemorrhage: report of two cases. Int J Angiol 1999;8:157.
4. Fukui S, Katoh H, Nawashiro H, et al. Anomalous internal carotid artery associated with ipsilateral cerebral arteriovenous malformation—case report. Neurol Med Chir (Tokyo) 2001;41:607.
5. Tangchai P, Khaoborisut V. Agenesis of internal carotid artery associated with aneurysm of contralateral middle cerebral artery. Neurology 1970;20:809.
6. Cali RL, Berg R, Rama K. Bilateral internal carotid artery agenesis: a case study and review of the literature. Surgery 1993;113:227.
7. Lee JH, Oh CW, Lee SH, Han DH. Aplasia of the internal carotid artery. Acta Neurochir (Wien) 2003;145:117.
8. Savastano S, Feltrin GP, Chiesura-Corona M, Miotta D. Cerebral ischemia due to congenital malformations of brachiocephalic arteries—case reports. Angiology 1992;43:76.
9. Wang PJ, Liu HM, Young C, et al. Agenesis of internal carotid artery associated with symptomatic partial epilepsy. Epilepsia 1994;35:1337.
10. Erro Aguirre ME, Gallego J, Aymerich N, et al. Paramedian pontine infarct secondary to basilar artery dissection. Cerebrovasc Dis 2003;16:178.
11. Gailloud P, Carpenter J, Heck DV, Murphy KJ. Pseudofenestration of the cervical internal carotid artery: a pathologic process that simulates an anatomic variant. AJNR Am J Neuroradiol 2004;25:421.
12. Kloska SP, Schlegel PM, Strater R, Niederstadt TU. Causality of pediatric brainstem infarction and basilar artery fenestration? Pediatr Neurol 2006;35:436.
13. Yoon SM, Chun YI, Kwon Y, Kwun BD. Vertebrobasilar junction aneurysms associated with fenestration: experience of five cases treated with Guglielmi detachable coils. Surg Neurol 2004;61:248.
14. Uchino A, Kato A, Takase Y, Kudo S. Basilar artery fenestrations detected by MR angiography. Radiat Med 2001;19:71.
15. Uchino A, Kato A, Abe M, Kudo S. Association of cerebral arteriovenous malformation with cerebral arterial fenestration. Eur Radiol 2001; 11:493.
16. Tasker AD, Byrne JV. Basilar artery fenestration in association with aneurysms of the posterior cerebral circulation. Neuroradiology 1997;39:185.
17. Poulias GE, Skoutas B, Doundoulakis N, et al. Kinking and coiling of internal carotid artery with and without associated stenosis: surgical considerations and long-term follow-up. Panmin Med 1996;38:22.
18. Derrick JR, Kirksey TD, Estess M, Williams D. Kinking of the carotid arteries: clinical considerations. Am Surg 1966;32:503.

19. Sarkari NB, Holmes JM, Bickerstaff ER. Neurological manifestations associated with internal carotid loops and kinks in children. J Neurol Neurosurg Psychiatry 1970;33:194.
20. Oliviero U, Scherillo G, Casaburi C, et al. Prospective evaluation of hypertensive patients with carotid kinking and coiling: an ultrasonographic 7-year study. Angiology 2003;54:169.
21. Ballotta E, Thiene G, Baracchini C, et al. Surgical vs medical treatment for isolated internal carotid artery elongation with coiling or kinking in symptomatic patients: a prospective randomized clinical study. J Vasc Surg 2005;42:838.
22. Cioffi FA, Meduri M, Tomasello F, et al. Kinking and coiling of the internal carotid artery: clinical-statistical observations and surgical perspectives. J Neurosurg Sci 1975;19(1-2):15.
23. Koskas F, Bahnini A, Walden R, Kieffer E. Stenotic coiling and kinking of the internal carotid artery. Ann Vasc Surg 1993;7:530.
24. Asumal KB, Akhtar N, Syed NA, et al. Moyamoya disease: an elusive diagnosis. J Pak Med Assoc 2003;53:160.
25. Han DH, Nam DH, Oh CW. Moyamoya disease in adults: characteristics of clinical presentation and outcome after encephalo-duro-arterio-synangiosis. Clin Neurol Neurosurg 1997;99(suppl 2): S151.
26. Khan N, Schuknecht B, Boltshauser E, et al. Moyamoya disease and moyamoya syndrome: experience in Europe; choice of revascularisation procedures. Acta Neurochir (Wien) 2003;145:1061.
27. Suzuki J, Kodama N. Moyamoya disease—a review. Stroke 1983;14:104.
28. Yamashiro Y, Takahashi H, Takahashi K. Cerebrovascular Moyamoya disease. Eur J Pediatr 1984;142:44-50.
29. Yilmaz EY, Pritz MB, Bruno A, et al. Moyamoya: Indiana University Medical Center experience. Arch Neurol 2001;58:1274.
30. Klasen H, Britton J, Newman M. Moyamoya disease in a 12-year-old Caucasian boy presenting with acute transient psychosis. Eur Child Adolesc Psychiatry 1999;8:149.
31. Linfante I, Ciarmiello A, Fusco C, et al. Similar TIAs and corresponding alterations in regional cerebral perfusion in Caucasian monozygotic twins with moyamoya disease. Clin Imaging 2002;26:378.
32. Spengos K, Kosmaidou-Aravidou Z, Tsivgoulis G, et al. Moyamoya syndrome in a Caucasian woman with Turner's syndrome. Eur J Neurol 2006;13:e7.
33. Fuchs FD, Francesconi CR, Caramori PR, et al. Moyamoya disease associated with renovascular disease in a young African-Brazilian patient. J Hum Hypertens 2001;15:499.
34. Oppenheim JS, Gennuso R, Sacher M, Hollis P. Acute atraumatic subdural hematoma associated with moyamoya disease in an African-American. Neurosurgery 1991;28:616.
35. Andreone V, Ciarmiello A, Fusco C, et al. Moyamoya disease in Italian monozygotic twins. Neurology 1999;53:1332.
36. Dhopesh VP, Dunn DP, Schick P. Moyamoya and Hageman factor (factor XII) deficiency in a black adult. Arch Neurol 1978;35:396.
37. Kaneko Y, Imamoto N, Mannoji H, Fukui M. Familial occurrence of moyamoya disease in the mother and four daughters including identical twins. Neurol Med Chir (Tokyo) 1998;38:3494.
38. Kang HS, Kim SK, Cho BK, et al. Single nucleotide polymorphisms of tissue inhibitor of metalloproteinase genes in familial moyamoya disease. Neurosurgery 2006;58:1074.
39. Mineharu Y, Takenaka K, Yamakawa H, et al. Inheritance pattern of familial moyamoya disease: autosomal dominant mode and genomic imprinting. J Neurol Neurosurg Psychiatry 2006;77:1025.
40. Nanba R, Kuroda S, Tada M, et al. Clinical features of familial moyamoya disease. Childs Nerv Syst 2006;22:258.
41. Paez MT, Yamamoto T. Single nucleotide polymorphisms of tissue inhibitor of metalloproteinase genes in familial moyamoya disease. Neurosurgery 2007;60:E582, author reply E582.
42. Shetty-Alva N, Alva S. Familial moyamoya disease in Caucasians. Pediatr Neurol 2000;23:445.
43. Zafeiriou DI, Ikeda H, Anastasiou A, et al. Familial moyamoya disease in a Greek family. Brain Dev 2003;25:288.
44. Rao M, Zhang H, Liu Q, et al. Clinical and experimental pathology of Moyamoya disease. Chin Med J (Engl) 2003;116:1845.
45. Serdaru M, Gray F, Merland JJ, et al. Moyamoya disease and intracerebral hematoma: clinical pathological report. Neuroradiology 1979;18:47.
46. Takekawa Y, Umezawa T, Ueno Y, et al. Pathological and immunohistochemical findings of an autopsy case of adult moyamoya disease. Neuropathology 2004;24:236.
47. Coakham HM, Duchen LW, Scaravilli F. Moyamoya disease: clinical and pathological report of a case with associated myopathy. J Neurol Neurosurg Psychiatry 1979;42:289.
48. Lamas E, Diez Lobato R, Cabello A, Abad JM. Multiple intracranial arterial occlusions (moyamoya disease) in patients with neurofibromatosis: one case report with autopsy. Acta Neurochir (Wien) 1978;45(1-2):133.
49. Oka K, Yamashita M, Sadoshima S, Tanaka K. Cerebral haemorrhage in Moyamoya disease at autopsy. Virchows Arch A Pathol Anat Histol 1981;392:247.
50. Robertson NP, Compston DA, Kirkpatrick P. Moyamoya disease presenting as Valsalva related partial seizures. J Neurol Neurosurg Psychiatry 1999;66:111.
51. Schoenberg BS, Mellinger JF, Schoenberg DG, Barringer FS. Moyamoya disease presenting as a seizure disorder: a case report. Arch Neurol 1977;34:511.
52. Yasukawa M, Yasukawa K, Akagawa S, et al. Convulsions and temporary hemiparesis following spinal anesthesia in a child with moyamoya disease. Anesthesiology 1988;69:1023.
53. Aoki N. Moyamoya disease and subarachnoid hemorrhage. Surg Neurol 1985;23:202.

54. Cholankeril JV, Cenizal JS, Huda R, et al. Moya-moya disease: a cause of intracerebral and sub-arachnoid hemorrhage. J Med Soc N J 1982;79:559.

55. Marushima A, Yanaka K, Matsuki T, et al. Sub-arachnoid hemorrhage not due to ruptured aneu-rysm in moyamoya disease. J Clin Neurosci 2006;13:146.

56. Somasundaram S, Thamburaj K, Burathoki S, Gupta AK. Moyamoya disease with cerebral arte-riovenous malformation presenting as primary subarachnoid hemorrhage. J Neuroimaging 2007; 17:251.

57. Bruno A, Yuh WT, Biller J, et al. Magnetic resonance imaging in young adults with cerebral infarction due to moyamoya. Arch Neurol 1988;45:303.

58. Kim SK, Seol HJ, Cho BK, et al. Moyamoya disease among young patients: its aggressive clinical course and the role of active surgical treatment. Neurosurgery 2004;54:840.

59. Halpern EJ, Nack TL. Prospective diagnosis of moyamoya disease with Doppler ultrasonography. J Ultrasound Med 1995;14:157.

60. Houkin K, Aoki T, Takahashi A, Abe H. Diagnosis of moyamoya disease with magnetic resonance angi-ography. Stroke 1994;25:2159.

61. Tsuchiya K, Makita K, Furui S. Moyamoya disease: diagnosis with three-dimensional CT angiography. Neuroradiology 1994;36:432.

62. Weiller C, Mullges W, Leibold M, et al. Infarctions and non-invasive diagnosis in moyamoya disease: two case reports. Neurosurg Rev 1991;14:75.

63. Yamada I, Matsushima Y, Suzuki S. Moyamoya dis-ease: Diagnosis with three-dimensional time-of-flight MR angiography. Radiology 1992;184:773.

64. Yamada I, Nakagawa T, Matsushima Y, Shibuya H. High-resolution turbo magnetic resonance angiog-raphy for diagnosis of Moyamoya disease. Stroke 2001;32:1825.

65. Jayakumar PN, Vasudev MK, Srikanth SG. Radio-logical findings in moyamoya disease. Indian Pediatr 1995;32:461.

66. Jayakumar PN, Vasudev MK, Srikanth SG. Posterior circulation abnormalities in moyamoya disease: a radiological study. Neurol India 1999;47:112.

67. Kuroda S, Hashimoto N, Yoshimoto T, Iwasaki Y. Radiological findings, clinical course, and outcome in asymptomatic moyamoya disease: results of multicenter survey in Japan. Stroke 2007;38:1430.

68. Sencer S, Poyanli A, Kiris T, et al. Recent experience with Moyamoya disease in Turkey. Eur Radiol 2000;10:569.

69. Scott RM. Moyamoya syndrome: a surgically treat-able cause of stroke in the pediatric patient. Clin Neurosurg 2000;47:378.

70. Yamada I, Matsushima Y, Suzuki S. Childhood moyamoya disease before and after encephalo-duro-arterio-synangiosis: an angiographic study. Neuroradiology 1992;34:318.

71. Matsushima Y, Aoyagi M, Koumo Y, et al. Effects of encephalo-duro-arterio-synangiosis on childhood moyamoya patients—swift disappearance of ische-mic attacks and maintenance of mental capacity. Neurol Med Chir (Tokyo) 1991;31:708.

72. Matsushima T, Inoue TK, Suzuki SO, et al. Surgical techniques and the results of a fronto-temporo-parietal combined indirect bypass procedure for children with moyamoya disease: a comparison with the results of encephalo-duro-arterio-synangiosis alone. Clin Neurol Neurosurg 1997;99 (suppl 2):S123.

73. Matsushima T, Fukui M, Kitamura K, et al. Ence-phalo-duro-arterio-synangiosis in children with moyamoya disease. Acta Neurochir (Wien) 1990;104 (3-4):96.

74. Isono M, Ishii K, Kamida T, et al. Long-term out-comes of pediatric moyamoya disease treated by encephalo-duro-arterio-synangiosis. Pediatr Neurosurg 2002;36:14.

75. Touho H. A simple surgical technique of direct anastomosis for treatment of moyamoya disease: technical note. Surg Neurol 2004;62:366.

76. Takahashi A, Kamiyama H, Houkin K, Abe H. Surgi-cal treatment of childhood moyamoya disease—comparison of reconstructive surgery centered on the frontal region and the parietal region. Neurol Med Chir (Tokyo) 1995;35:231.

77. Smith ER, Scott RM. Surgical management of moyamoya syndrome. Skull Base 2005;15:15.

78. Scott RM. Surgical treatment of moyamoya syndrome in children. Pediatr Neurosurg 1995; 22:39.

79. Matsushima Y, Inaba Y. The specificity of the collaterals to the brain through the study and surgical treatment of moyamoya disease. Stroke 1986;17:117.

80. Matsushima Y, Fukai N, Tanaka K, et al. A new sur-gical treatment of moyamoya disease in children: a preliminary report. Surg Neurol 1981;15:313.

81. Kuroda S, Houkin K, Kamiyama H, Abe H. Effects of surgical revascularization on peripheral artery aneurysms in moyamoya disease: report of three cases. Neurosurgery 2001;49:463.

82. Kim DS, Kang SG, Yoo DS, et al. Surgical results in pediatric moyamoya disease: angiographic revas-cularization and the clinical results. Clin Neurol Neurosurg 2007;109:125.

83. Kim CY, Wang KC, Kim SK, et al. Encephaloduroar-teriosynangiosis with bifrontal encephalogaleo (periosteal)synangiosis in the pediatric moyamoya disease: the surgical technique and its outcomes. Childs Nerv Syst 2003;19(5-6):316.

84. Karasawa J, Kikuchi H, Furuse S, et al. A surgical treatment of "moyamoya" disease "encephalo-myo synangiosis." Neurol Med Chir (Tokyo) 1977;17(1 Pt 1):29.

85. Houkin K, Kamiyama H, Abe H, et al. Surgical ther-apy for adult moyamoya disease: can surgical revascularization prevent the recurrence of intra-cerebral hemorrhage? Stroke 1996;27:1342.

86. Fujita K, Tamaki N, Matsumoto S. Surgical treat-ment of moyamoya disease in children: which is more effective procedure, EDAS or EMS? Childs Nerv Syst 1986;2:134.

87. Houkin K, Kuroda S, Nakayama N. Cerebral revas-cularization for moyamoya disease in children. Neurosurg Clin N Am 2001;12:575.

88. Dauser RC, Tuite GF, McCluggage CW. Dural inversion procedure for moyamoya disease: technical note. J Neurosurg 1997;86:719.
89. Furie DM, Tien RD. Fibromuscular dysplasia of arteries of the head and neck: imaging findings. AJR Am J Roentgenol 1994;162:1205.
90. de Monye C, Dippel DW, Dijkshoorn ML, et al. MDCT detection of fibromuscular dysplasia of the internal carotid artery. AJR Am J Roentgenol 2007;188:W367.
91. Slovut DP, Olin JW. Fibromuscular dysplasia. N Engl J Med 2004;350:1862.
92. Sandok BA. Fibromuscular dysplasia of the internal carotid artery. Neurol Clin 1983;10:39.
93. Bofinger A, Hawley C, Fisher P, et al. Polymorphisms of the renin-angiotensin system in patients with multifocal renal arterial fibromuscular dysplasia. J Hum Hypertens 2001;15:185.
94. Schievink WI, Limburg M. Angiographic abnormalities mimicking fibromuscular dysplasia in a patient with Ehlers-Danlos syndrome, type IV. Neurosurgery 1989;25:482.
95. Hudgins LB, Limbacher JP. Fibromuscular dysplasia in Alport's syndrome. J Tenn Med Assoc 1982;75:733.
96. de Mendonca WC, Espat PA. Pheochromocytoma associated with arterial fibromuscular dysplasia. Am J Clin Pathol 1981;75:749.
97. Schievink WI, Bjornsson J, Piepgras DG. Coexistence of fibromuscular dysplasia and cystic medial necrosis in a patient with Marfan's syndrome and bilateral carotid artery dissections. Stroke 1994;25:2492.
98. Janzen J, Vuong PN, Rothenberger-Janzen K. Takayasu's arteritis and fibromuscular dysplasia as causes of acquired atypical coarctation of the aorta: retrospective analysis of seven cases. Heart Vessels 1999;14:277.
99. Lamis PA, Carson WP, Wilson JP, Letton AH. Recognition and treatment of fibromuscular hyperplasia of the internal carotid artery. Surgery 1971;69:498.
100. Kishore PR, Lin JP, Kricheff II. Fibromuscular hyperplasia and stationary waves of the internal carotid artery. Acta Radiol Diagn (Stockh) 1971;11:619.
101. Van Damme H, Sakalihasan N, Limet R. Fibromuscular dysplasia of the internal carotid artery: personal experience with 13 cases and literature review. Acta Chir Belg 1999;99:163.
102. Rosset E, Albertini JN, Magnan PE, et al. Surgical treatment of extracranial internal carotid artery aneurysms. J Vasc Surg 2000;31:713.
103. Assadian A, Senekowitsch C, Assadian O, et al. Combined open and endovascular stent grafting of internal carotid artery fibromuscular dysplasia: long term results. Eur J Vasc Endovasc Surg 2005;29:345.
104. Slovut DP, Olin JW. Fibromuscular dysplasia. Curr Treat Options Cardiovasc Med 2005;7:159.
105. Schievink WI. Spontaneous dissection of the carotid and vertebral arteries. N Engl J Med 2001;344:898.
106. Fisher CM, Ojemann RG, Roberson GH. Spontaneous dissection of cervico-cerebral arteries. Can J Neurol Sci 1978;5:9.
107. Mokri B, Sundt TM Jr, Houser OW. Spontaneous internal carotid dissection, hemicrania, and Horner's syndrome. Arch Neurol 1979;36:677.
108. Schievink WI, Mokri B, Piepgras DG. Spontaneous dissections of cervicocephalic arteries in childhood and adolescence. Neurology 1994;44:1607.
109. Ducrocq X, Lacour JC, Debouverie M, et al. [Cerebral ischemic accidents in young subjects: a prospective study of 296 patients aged 16 to 45 years]. Rev Neurol (Paris) 1999;155:575.
110. Giroud M, Fayolle H, Andre N, et al. Incidence of internal carotid artery dissection in the community of Dijon. J Neurol Neurosurg Psychiatry 1994;57:1443.
111. Schievink WI, Mokri B, Whisnant JP. Internal carotid artery dissection in a community: Rochester, Minnesota, 1987-1992. Stroke 1993;24:1678.
112. Schievink WI, Roiter V. Epidemiology of cervical artery dissection. Front Neurol Neurosci 2005;20:12.
113. Caso V, Paciaroni M, Bogousslavsky J. Environmental factors and cervical artery dissection. Front Neurol Neurosci 2005;20:44.
114. Saver JL, Easton JDH, Hart RG. Dissection and trauma of cervicocerebral arteries. In Barnett HJM, Mohr JP, Stein BM, Yatsu FM, eds. Stroke: Pathophysiology, Diagnosis and Management, 2nd ed. New York: Churchill Livingstone, 1992.
115. Bostrom K, Liliequist B. Primary dissecting aneurysm of the extracranial part of the internal carotid and vertebral arteries: a report of three cases. Neurology 1967;17:179.
116. Baumgartner RW, Lienhardt B, Mosso M, et al. Spontaneous and endothelial-independent vasodilation are impaired in patients with spontaneous carotid dissection: a case-control study. Stroke 2007;38:405.
117. Mokri B, Sundt TM Jr, Houser OW, Piepgras DG. Spontaneous dissection of the cervical internal carotid artery. Ann Neurol 1986;19:126.
118. Biller J, Hingtgen WL, Adams HP Jr, et al. Cervicocephalic arterial dissections: a ten-year experience. Arch Neurol 1986;43:1234.
119. Hart RG. Vertebral artery dissection. Neurology 1988;38:987.
120. Deck JH. Pathology of spontaneous dissection of intracranial arteries. Can J Neurol Sci 1987;14:88-91.
121. Benedict WJ, Prabhu V, Viola M, Biller J. Carotid artery pseudoaneurysm resulting from an injury to the neck by a fouled baseball. J Neurol Sci 2007;256(1-2):94.
122. Schievink WI, Atkinson JL, Bartleson JD, Whisnant JP. Traumatic internal carotid artery dissections caused by blunt softball injuries. Am J Emerg Med 1998;16:179.
123. Davis JM, Zimmerman RA. Injury of the carotid and vertebral arteries. Neuroradiology 1983;25:55.
124. Jackson MA, Hughes RC, Ward SP, McInnes EG. "Headbanging" and carotid dissection. BMJ (Clin Res Ed) 1983;287:1262.

125. Mourad JJ, Girerd X, Safar M. Carotid-artery dissection after a prolonged telephone call. N Engl J Med 1997;336:516.

126. Schellhas KP, Latchaw RE, Wendling LR, Gold LH. Vertebrobasilar injuries following cervical manipulation. JAMA 1980;244:1450.

127. Weintraub MI. Beauty parlor stroke syndrome: report of five cases. JAMA 1993;269:2085.

128. Wiebers DO, Mokri B. Internal carotid artery dissection after childbirth. Stroke 1985;16:956.

129. Grau AJ, Brandt T, Buggle F, et al. Association of cervical artery dissection with recent infection. Arch Neurol 1999;56:851.

130. Paciaroni M, Georgiadis D, Arnold M, et al. Seasonal variability in spontaneous cervical artery dissection. J Neurol Neurosurg Psychiatry 2006;77:677.

131. Guillon B, Berthet K, Benslamia L, et al. Infection and the risk of spontaneous cervical artery dissection: a case-control study. Stroke 2003;34:e79.

132. Vila N, Millan M, Ferrer X, et al. Levels of alpha1-antitrypsin in plasma and risk of spontaneous cervical artery dissections: a case-control study. Stroke 2003;34:E168.

133. Pezzini A, Del Zotto E, Archetti S, et al. Plasma homocysteine concentration, C677T MTHFR genotype, and 844ins68bp CBS genotype in young adults with spontaneous cervical artery dissection and atherothrombotic stroke. Stroke 2002;33:664.

134. Pezzini A, Caso V, Zanferrari C, et al. Arterial hypertension as risk factor for spontaneous cervical artery dissection: a case-control study. J Neurol Neurosurg Psychiatry 2006;77:95-97.

135. Rubinstein SM, Peerdeman SM, van Tulder MW, et al. A systematic review of the risk factors for cervical artery dissection. Stroke 2005;36:1575.

136. Pezzini A, Granella F, Grassi M, et al. History of migraine and the risk of spontaneous cervical artery dissection. Cephalalgia 2005;25:575.

137. Tzourio C, Benslamia L, Guillon B, et al. Migraine and the risk of cervical artery dissection: a case-control study. Neurology 2002;59:435.

138. Schievink WI, Michels VV, Piepgras DG. Neurovascular manifestations of heritable connective tissue disorders: a review. Stroke 1994;25:889.

139. Finsterer J, Strassegger J, Haymerle A, Hagmuller G. Bilateral stenting of symptomatic and asymptomatic internal carotid artery stenosis due to fibromuscular dysplasia. J Neurol Neurosurg Psychiatry 2000;69:683.

140. Schievink WI, Wijdicks EF, Michels VV, et al. Heritable connective tissue disorders in cervical artery dissections: a prospective study. Neurology 1998;50:1166.

141. Mokri B, Silbert PL, Schievink WI, Piepgras DG. Cranial nerve palsy in spontaneous dissection of the extracranial internal carotid artery. Neurology 1996;46:356.

142. Pelkonen O, Tikkakoski T, Pyhtinen J, Sotaniemi K. Cerebral CT and MRI findings in cervicocephalic artery dissection. Acta Radiol 2004;45:259.

143. Mateen F, Boes C, Kumar N. Unilateral headache and hypoglossal nerve palsy: a report of three cases. Cephalalgia 2007;27:840.

144. Olzowy B, Lorenzl S, Guerkov R. Bilateral and unilateral internal carotid artery dissection causing isolated hypoglossal nerve palsy: a case report and review of the literature. Eur Arch Otorhinolaryngol 2006;263:390.

145. Mattioni A, Paciaroni M, Sarchielli P, et al. Multiple cranial nerve palsies in a patient with internal carotid artery dissection. Eur Neurol 2007;58:125.

146. Mokri B, Schievink WI, Olsen KD, Piepgras DG. Spontaneous dissection of the cervical internal carotid artery: presentation with lower cranial nerve palsies. Arch Otolaryngol Head Neck Surg 1992;118:431.

147. Houser OW, Mokri B, Sundt TM Jr, et al. Spontaneous cervical cephalic arterial dissection and its residuum: angiographic spectrum. AJNR Am J Neuroradiol 1984;5:27.

148. Derex L, Nighoghossian N, Turjman F, et al. Intravenous tPA in acute ischemic stroke related to internal carotid artery dissection. Neurology 2000;54:2159.

149. Beletsky V, Nadareishvili Z, Lynch J, et al. Cervical arterial dissection: time for a therapeutic trial? Stroke 2003;34:2856.

150. Lyrer P, Engelter S. Antithrombotic drugs for carotid artery dissection. Cochrane Database Syst Rev 2003;3:CD000255.

151. Engelter ST, Brandt T, Debette S, et al. Antiplatelets versus anticoagulation in cervical artery dissection. Stroke 2007;38:2605.

152. Kadkhodayan Y, Jeck DT, Moran CJ, et al. Angioplasty and stenting in carotid dissection with or without associated pseudoaneurysm. AJNR Am J Neuroradiol 2005;26:2328.

153. Zhao WY, Krings T, Alvarez H, et al. Management of spontaneous haemorrhagic intracranial vertebrobasilar dissection: review of 21 consecutive cases. Acta Neurochir (Wien) 2007;149:585.

154. Liu AY, Paulsen RD, Marcellus ML, et al. Long-term outcomes after carotid stent placement treatment of carotid artery dissection. Neurosurgery 1999;45:1368.

155. Malek AM, Higashida RT, Phatouros CC, et al. Endovascular management of extracranial carotid artery dissection achieved using stent angioplasty. AJNR Am J Neuroradiol 2000;21:1280.

156. Dittrich R, Nassenstein I, Bachmann R, et al. Polyarterial clustered recurrence of cervical artery dissection seems to be the rule. Neurology 2007;69:180.

157. Chandra A, Suliman A, Angle N. Spontaneous dissection of the carotid and vertebral arteries: the 10-year UCSD experience. Ann Vasc Surg 2007;21:178.

158. Grenier Y, Tomita T, Marymont MH, et al. Late postirradiation occlusive vasculopathy in childhood medulloblastoma: report of two cases. J Neurosurg 1998;89:460.

159. Ferroir JP, Marro B, Belkacemi Y, et al. [Cerebral infarction related to intracranial radiation arteritis twenty-four years after encephalic radiation therapy]. Rev Neurol (Paris) 2007;163:96.

160. Bitzer M, Topka H. Progressive cerebral occlusive disease after radiation therapy. Stroke 1995;26:131.

161. Ishikawa N, Tajima G, Yofune N, et al. Moyamoya syndrome after cranial irradiation for bone marrow transplantation in a patient with acute leukemia. Neuropediatrics 2006;37:364.
162. Aoki S, Hayashi N, Abe O, et al. Radiation-induced arteritis: thickened wall with prominent enhancement on cranial MR images report of five cases and comparison with 18 cases of Moyamoya disease. Radiology 2002;223:683.
163. Omura M, Aida N, Sekido K, et al. Large intracranial vessel occlusive vasculopathy after radiation therapy in children: clinical features and usefulness of magnetic resonance imaging. Int J Radiat Oncol Biol Phys 1997;38:241.
164. Ceccarelli A, De Blasi R, Pavone I, et al. Primary angiitis of the central nervous system: a misinterpreted clinical onset of CNS vasculitis. Eur Neurol 2005;53:40.
165. Calabrese LH. Diagnostic strategies in vasculitis affecting the central nervous system. Cleve Clin J Med 2002;69(suppl 2):SII-105.
166. Calabrese L. Primary angiitis of the central nervous system: the penumbra of vasculitis. J Rheumatol 2001;28:465.
167. Calabrese LH, Duna GF, Lie JT. Vasculitis in the central nervous system. Arthritis Rheum 1997;40:1189.
168. Igarashi M, Gilmartin RC, Gerald B, et al. Cerebral arteritis and bacterial meningitis. Arch Neurol 1984;41:531.
169. Weisfelt M, Determann RM, de Gans J, et al. Procoagulant and fibrinolytic activity in cerebrospinal fluid from adults with bacterial meningitis. J Infect 2007;54:545.
170. Carolei A, Sacco S. Central nervous system vasculitis. Neurol Sci 2003;24(suppl 1):S8.
171. West SG. Central nervous system vasculitis. Curr Rheumatol Rep 2003;5:116.
172. Atalaia A, Ferro J, Antunes F. Stroke in an HIV-infected patient. J Neurol 1992;239:356.
173. Keeling DM, Birley H, Machin SJ. Multiple transient ischaemic attacks and a mild thrombotic stroke in a HIV-positive patient with anticardiolipin antibodies. Blood Coagul Fibrinolysis 1990;1:333.
174. Legido A, Lischner HW, de Chadarevian JP, Katsetos CD. Stroke in pediatric HIV infection. Pediatr Neurol 1999;21:588.
175. Menge T, Neumann-Haefelin T, von Giesen HJ, Arendt G. Progressive stroke in an HIV-1-positive patient under protease inhibitors. Eur Neurol 2000;44:252.
176. Mochan A, Modi M, Modi G. Protein S deficiency in HIV associated ischaemic stroke: an epiphenomenon of HIV infection. J Neurol Neurosurg Psychiatry 2005;76:1455.
177. Modi G, Modi M, Mochan A. Stroke and HIV—causal or coincidental co-occurrence? S Afr Med J 2006;96:1247.
178. Ortiz G, Koch S, Romano JG, et al. Mechanisms of ischemic stroke in HIV-infected patients. Neurology 2007;68:1257.
179. Patel VB, Sacoor Z, Francis P, et al. Ischemic stroke in young HIV-positive patients in Kwazulu-Natal, South Africa. Neurology 2005;65:759.
180. Qureshi AI. HIV infection and stroke: if not protein S deficiency then what explains the relationship? J Neurol Neurosurg Psychiatry 2005;76:1331.
181. Restrepo L, McArthur J. Stroke and HIV infection. Stroke 2003;34:e176, author reply e176.
182. Katti MK. Pathogenesis, diagnosis, treatment, and outcome aspects of cerebral tuberculosis. Med Sci Monit 2004;10:RA215.
183. Rohr-Le Floch J, Myers P, Gauthier G. [Cerebral ischemic accidents and tuberculous meningitis]. Rev Neurol (Paris) 1992;148:779.
184. Kumar N, Singh W. Thalamic haemorrhage due to tuberculous arteritis. J Assoc Physicians India 1991;39:573.
185. Poltera AA. Thrombogenic intracranial vasculitis in tuberculous meningitis: a 20 year "post mortem" survey. Acta Neurol Belg 1977;77:12.
186. Renard D, Morales R, Heroum C. Tuberculous meningovasculitis. Neurology 2007;68:1745.
187. Uesugi T, Takizawa S, Morita Y, et al. Hemorrhagic infarction in tuberculous meningitis. Intern Med 2006;45:1193.
188. Kouame-Assouan AE, Cowppli-Bony P, Aka-Anghui Diarra E, et al. [Two cases of cryptococcal meningitis revealed by an ischemic stroke]. Bull Soc Pathol Exot 2007;100:15.
189. Leiguarda R, Berthier M, Starkstein S, et al. Ischemic infarction in 25 children with tuberculous meningitis. Stroke 1988;19:200.
190. Hsieh FY, Chia LG, Shen WC. Locations of cerebral infarctions in tuberculous meningitis. Neuroradiology 1992;34:197.
191. Simon RP. Neurosyphilis. Arch Neurol 1985;42:606.
192. Flood JM, Weinstock HS, Guroy ME, et al. Neurosyphilis during the AIDS epidemic, San Francisco, 1985-1992. J Infect Dis 1998;177:931.
193. Borhani Haghighi A, Pourmand R, Nikseresht AR. Neuro-Behcet disease: a review. Neurologist 2005;11:80.
194. Bousser MG, Biousse V. Small vessel vasculopathies affecting the central nervous system. J Neuro-ophthalmol 2004;24:56.
195. Benseler S, Schneider R. Central nervous system vasculitis in children. Curr Opin Rheumatol 2004;16:43.
196. Frankel SK, Sullivan EJ, Brown KK. Vasculitis: Wegener granulomatosis, Churg-Strauss syndrome, microscopic polyangiitis, polyarteritis nodosa, and Takayasu arteritis. Crit Care Clin 2002;18:855.
197. Defer G, Levy R, Brugieres P, et al. Lyme disease presenting as a stroke in the vertebrobasilar territory: MRI. Neuroradiology 1993;35:529.
198. Reik L Jr. Stroke due to Lyme disease. Neurology 1993;43:2705.
199. Zhang Y, Lafontant G, Bonner FJ Jr. Lyme neuroborreliosis mimics stroke: a case report. Arch Phys Med Rehabil 2000;81:519.
200. de Carvalho CA, Allen JN, Zafranis A, Yates AJ. Coccidioidal meningitis complicated by cerebral arteritis and infarction. Hum Pathol 1980;11:293.
201. Pruitt AA. Nervous system infections in patients with cancer. Neurol Clin 2003;21:193.
202. Saul RF, Gallagher JG, Mateer JE. Sudden hemiparesis as the presenting sign in cryptococcal meningoencephalitis. Stroke 1986;17:753.

203. Bonawitz C, Castillo M, Mukherji SK. Comparison of CT and MR features with clinical outcome in patients with Rocky Mountain spotted fever. AJNR Am J Neuroradiol 1997;18:459.

204. Fox JW, Studley JK, Cohen DM. Recurrent expressive aphasia as a presentation of cat-scratch encephalopathy. Pediatrics 2007;119:e760.

205. Alarcon F, Vanormelingen K, Moncayo J, Vinan I. Cerebral cysticercosis as a risk factor for stroke in young and middle-aged people. Stroke 1992;23:1563.

206. del Brutto OH. [Central nervous system mycotic infections]. Rev Neurol 2000;30:447.

207. Griesemer DA, Barton LL, Reese CM, et al. Amebic meningoencephalitis caused by Balamuthia mandrillaris. Pediatr Neurol 1994;10:249.

208. Treadwell SD, Robinson TG. Cocaine use and stroke. Postgrad Med J 2007;83:389.

209. Levine SR, Brust JC, Futrell N, et al. A comparative study of the cerebrovascular complications of cocaine: alkaloidal versus hydrochloride—a review. Neurology 1991;41:1173.

210. Levine SR, Brust JC, Futrell N, et al. Cerebrovascular complications of the use of the "crack" form of alkaloidal cocaine. N Engl J Med 1990;323:699.

211. Neiman J, Haapaniemi HM, Hillbom M. Neurological complications of drug abuse: pathophysiological mechanisms. Eur J Neurol 2000;7:595.

212. Buttner A, Mall G, Penning R, Weis S. The neuropathology of heroin abuse. Forensic Sci Int 2000;113(1-3):435.

213. Niehaus L, Meyer BU. Bilateral borderzone brain infarctions in association with heroin abuse. J Neurol Sci 1998;160:180.

214. Yoon BW, Bae HJ, Hong KS, et al. Phenylpropanolamine contained in cold remedies and risk of hemorrhagic stroke. Neurology 2007;68:146.

215. Delorio NM. Cerebral infarcts in a pediatric patient secondary to phenylpropanolamine, a recalled medication. J Emerg Med 2004;26:305.

216. Kernan WN, Viscoli CM, Brass LM, et al. Phenylpropanolamine and the risk of hemorrhagic stroke. N Engl J Med 2000;343:1826.

217. Caplan LR, Hier DB, Banks G. Current concepts of cerebrovascular disease—stroke: stroke and drug abuse. Stroke 1982;13:869.

218. Lawson TM, Rees A. Stroke and transient ischaemic attacks in association with substance abuse in a young man. Postgrad Med J 1996;72:692.

219. Altura BT, Quirion R, Pert CB, Altura BM. Phencyclidine ("angel dust") analogs and sigma opiate benzomorphans cause cerebral arterial spasm. Proc Natl Acad Sci U S A 1983;80:865.

220. Altura BT, Altura BM. Phencyclidine, lysergic acid diethylamide, and mescaline: cerebral artery spasms and hallucinogenic activity. Science 1981;212:1051.

221. Freire BF, da Silva RC, Fabro AT, dos Santos DC. Is systemic lupus erythematosus a new risk factor for atherosclerosis? Arq Bras Cardiol 2006;87:300.

222. Chartash EK, Lans DM, Paget SA, et al. Aortic insufficiency and mitral regurgitation in patients with systemic lupus erythematosus and the antiphospholipid syndrome. Am J Med 1989;86:407.

223. Fluture A, Chaudhari S, Frishman WH. Valvular heart disease and systemic lupus erythematosus: therapeutic implications. Heart Dis 2003;5:349.

224. Fung CW, Kwong KL, Tsui EY, Wong SN. Moyamoya syndrome in a child with Down syndrome. Hong Kong Med J 2003;9:63.

225. Laversuch CJ, Brown MM, Clifton A, Bourke BE. Cerebral venous thrombosis and acquired protein S deficiency: an uncommon cause of headache in systemic lupus erythematosus. Br J Rheumatol 1995;34:572.

226. Moore PM, Cupps TR. Neurological complications of vasculitis. Ann Neurol 1983;14:155.

227. Burrow JN, Blumbergs PC, Iyer PV, Hallpike JF. Kohlmeier-Degos disease: a multisystem vasculopathy with progressive cerebral infarction. Aust N Z J Med 1991;21:49.

228. Dastur DK, Singhal BS, Shroff HJ. CNS involvement in malignant atrophic papulosis (Kohlmeier-Degos disease): vasculopathy and coagulopathy. J Neurol Neurosurg Psychiatry 1981;44:156.

229. Fernandez-Perez ER, Grabscheid E, Scheinfeld NS. A case of systemic malignant atrophic papulosis (Kohlmeier-Degos' disease). J Natl Med Assoc 2005;97:421.

230. Kohrman MH, Huttenlocher PR. Takayasu arteritis: a treatable cause of stroke in infancy. Pediatr Neurol 1986;2:154.

231. Sokol DK, McIntyre JA, Short RA, et al. Henoch-Schonlein purpura and stroke: antiphosphatidylethanolamine antibody in CSF and serum. Neurology 2000;55:1379.

232. Ruiter M. Purpura rheumatica: a type of allergic cutaneous arteriolitis. Br J Dermatol 1956;68:16.

233. Fujiwara S, Yamano T, Hattori M, et al. Asymptomatic cerebral infarction in Kawasaki disease. Pediatr Neurol 1992;8:235.

234. Lapointe JS, Nugent RA, Graeb DA, Robertson WD. Cerebral infarction and regression of widespread aneurysms in Kawasaki's disease: case report. Pediatr Radiol 1984;14:1-5.

235. Suda K, Matsumura M, Ohta S. Kawasaki disease complicated by cerebral infarction. Cardiol Young 2003;13:103.

236. Templeton PA, Dunne MG. Kawasaki syndrome: cerebral and cardiovascular complications. J Clin Ultrasound 1987;15:483.

237. Wada Y, Kamei A, Fujii Y, et al. Cerebral infarction after high-dose intravenous immunoglobulin therapy for Kawasaki disease. J Pediatr 2006;148:399.

238. Reddy AT, Witek K. Neurologic complications of chemotherapy for children with cancer. Curr Neurol Neurosci Rep 2003;3:137.

239. Macdonald DR. Neurologic complications of chemotherapy. Neurol Clin 1991;9:955.

240. Armstrong T, Gilbert MR. Central nervous system toxicity from cancer treatment. Curr Oncol Rep 2004;6:11.

241. Schiff D, Wen P. Central nervous system toxicity from cancer therapies. Hematol Oncol Clin North Am 2006;20:1377.

CHAPTER 7

Cardiac Disorders and Stroke in Children and Young Adults

José Biller • Michael J. Schneck • Betsy B. Love

Of the 700,000 to 750,000 annual strokes in the United States, approximately 5% affect young adults between 15 and 45 years of age.[1,2] The incidence of stroke in children is estimated to be 2.5 to 3.1 events per 100,000 children annually.[3-6] The impact of cardiovascular disease is substantial in this age group. Heart disease is the underlying cause in 15% to 30% of strokes.[7] For children and young adults, atherosclerotic cerebrovascular disease is much less common compared with cardiac causes of stroke. A definite or presumed cardiac etiology of cerebral infarction is found in 4.7% to 35.4% of young adults.[2-28]

These figures may be too conservative, however, because some cardioembolic events may be clinically unrecognized by routine imaging studies, and misclassified as strokes of "undetermined" mechanism. With advanced cardiac imaging, such as transesophageal echocardiography (TEE), Doppler color flow studies, ultrafast cardiac computed tomography (CT), and magnetic resonance imaging (MRI) of the heart, identification of cardiac sources of cerebral embolism should increase.[29]

Cardiac disease in children accounts for approximately 25% of ischemic strokes. Although nonvalvular atrial fibrillation, ischemic cardiomyopathy, coronary heart disease, and prosthetic valvular heart disease are the most common causes of cardioembolic stroke in older individuals, the causes in young adults are more diverse, and unusual disorders need to be considered more seriously, including congenital cardiac anomalies and genetic disorders. Additionally, in young adults, a right-to-left shunt from an underlying patent foramen ovale (PFO) is probably a common cause of cardiac (transcardiac) stroke, and congenital heart disease is probably the most common cause of ischemic stroke in children.[3-6]

Clinical Features

Diagnosis of cardioembolic stroke remains inferential; the clinical pattern is nonspecific. The classic presentation involves an abrupt onset of focal neurologic impairment occurring while the patient is awake, often during activity. Abrupt onset of neurologic deficit after a Valsalva maneuver or in conjunction with acute pulmonary hypertension suggests the possibility of a transcardiac source and paradoxical embolism. The neurologic deficit is characteristically maximal at onset. Stuttering or progressive neurologic impairment may occur in a few patients, however, as a result of dissolution and migration of emboli.

Emboli frequently lodge in the middle cerebral artery, posterior cerebral artery, or top of the basilar artery, and often cause a severe neurologic deficit (Fig. 7-1). Cardioembolic strokes are seldom preceded by transient ischemic attacks in the same vascular territory. Previous cortical strokes in other vascular territories or multiple acute strokes in separate vascular territories, and, foremost, the presence of systemic embolism are additional supportive clinical evidence for a cardioembolic source (Fig. 7-2). Sites of systemic embolization in the upper or lower extremities or viscera should be sought by a detailed history, careful palpation of peripheral pulses, and selective paraclinical investigations. Identification of a potential embolic cardiac source and the exclusion of an arterial source of embolism is helpful. Historical clues, such as paroxysms of atrial fibrillation or sick sinus syndrome in a patient with episodic palpitations, lightheadedness, or dizziness, may suggest occult cardiac disease.[29] Table 7-1 lists clinical and diagnostic features suggestive of cardioembolic stroke. Table 7-2 presents the evaluation for a cardiac embolic source of cerebral infarction in young adults.

Causes

Although all types of heart disease may predispose to cerebral embolism, certain cardiac disorders are more commonly associated with cerebral embolism in children and young adults (Table 7-3). Valvular heart disease and congenital cardiac disease is probably the second most common cause of cardioembolic stroke, after atrial fibrillation, in children and adults.

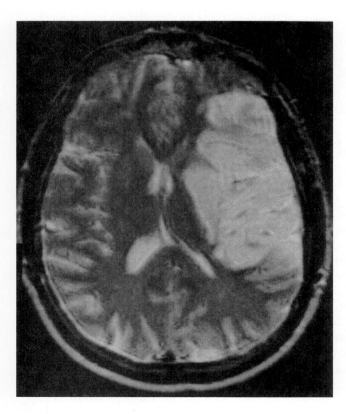

FIGURE 7-1   MRI shows a large left middle cerebral artery territory infarction with associated mass effect in a 44-year-old man with a left atrial appendage thrombus on transesophageal echocardiography.

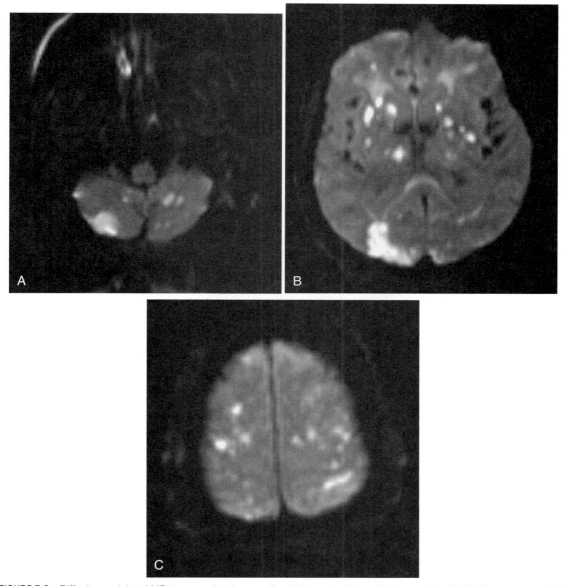

FIGURE 7-2   Diffusion-weighted MR images showing small multiple emboli in multiple vascular distributions as a result of cardiac embolism. **A,** Image of brainstem and cerebellum. **B,** Image showing multiple small subcortical and cortical ischemic infarcts and a larger right occipital lobe infarct at the level of the third ventricle. **C,** Image showing multiple small high cortical infarcts in the carotid distributions bilaterally.

Valvular Heart Disease

Valvular heart disease may result from rheumatic, prosthetic, myxomatous, inflammatory, infective, marantic, traumatic, degenerative, or congenital etiologies.[30] Stroke risk after heart valve surgery is determined by numerous factors, including valve location (aortic versus mitral), presence of atrial fibrillation, adequacy of anticoagulation, and patient comorbid factors. The main causes of aortic and mitral stenosis are congenital, calcific, and rheumatic. Congenital disorders of the aortic valve are much more common compared with mitral valve disorders. In contrast, infectious and degenerative disorders more commonly affect the mitral valve.

TABLE 7-1   **Clinical and Paraclinical Criteria Suggesting Cardioembolic Stroke**

Clinical Criteria

Sudden onset in an awake patient; fluctuating or progressive deficit may occur

Absence of prior TIAs in the same vascular territory

Previous cortical strokes in other vascular territories

Evidence of systemic embolism

Abnormal cardiac examination

Absence of an arterial source of emboli

Paraclinical Criteria

Bland or hemorrhagic infarction in a cortical arterial distribution on CT or MRI

Branch artery occlusion, but no proximal extracranial arterial source on MR angiography, CT angiography, carotid ultrasound, or catheter cervicocerebral angiography, if performed

Likely source of embolism on cardiac imaging studies

Absence of a hemodynamically consequential extracranial or intracranial arterial source on carotid ultrasound, TCD, CT angiography, MR angiography, or catheter angiography, if performed

CT, computed tomography; MRI, magnetic resonance imaging; TCD, transcranial Doppler; TIA, transient ischemic attack.

TABLE 7-2   **Suggested Evaluation for Potential Cardiac Causes of Stroke in Young Adults**

Routine*	Selected Patients
Cardiac enzymes and troponins	Contrast CT scan of the chest
Chest x-ray	Cardiac MRI
12-lead ECG	MR venography of pelvic and proximal lower extremity veins (rule out May-Thurner syndrome in cases of suspected paradoxical embolism)
TTE	24-hour ambulatory ECG (Holter) monitoring
TEE (in most instances)	Blood cultures (e.g., infective endocarditis)
CT head (noncontrast)	Genetic studies (e.g., mitochondrial disorders)
MRI of the brain and MR angiography of the cervicocerebral vessels and aorta *or* CT angiography of the cervicocerebral vessels	Hypercoagulable profile (e.g., APAS)
	Autoimmune studies (e.g., SLE)

*All patients with suspected ischemic stroke should have the following ancillary investigations: complete blood count, platelet count, electrolytes, blood urea nitrogen, creatinine, serum glucose, prothrombin time and international normalized ratio, and activated partial thromboplastin time.

APAS, antiphospholipid antibody syndrome; CT, computed tomography; ECG, electrocardiogram; MRI, magnetic resonance imaging; SLE, systemic lupus erythematosus; TEE, transesophageal echocardiography; TTE, transthoracic echocardiography.

Rheumatic Valvular Heart Disease

Although the incidence of rheumatic heart disease is declining in the industrialized nations, it continues to be a prevalent cause of acquired cardiac morbidity and mortality in children and young adults worldwide. More recent reports note a resurgence of acute rheumatic fever (RF) in the United States. RF begins with a group A streptococcal tonsillopharyngeal infection in a susceptible host. After a latency period, the untreated host, usually a young child, develops signs and symptoms of acute RF, often manifested as migratory arthritis usually involving the large joints (knees, ankles, elbows, wrists), pericarditis, chorea (Sydenham chorea), painless subcutaneous nodules, erythema marginatum, or some combination of the above.[31,32] Acute RF with pericarditis often causes marked valvular deformities characterized by mitral or aortic regurgitation or by early development of mitral stenosis. The mitral valve is the most commonly affected valve, followed by the aortic valve. The other less commonly involved valves, in decreasing order, are the tricuspid and pulmonic valves.

Mitral stenosis is usually a sequela of RF. Other etiologies are very rare and include congenital disease, collagen vascular–induced stenosis (related to systemic lupus erythematosus or rheumatoid arthritis), malignant carcinoid, mucopolysaccharidoses, Fabry disease, Whipple disease, and methysergide therapy.[30,33-36]

Patients with symptomatic mitral stenosis have a 5-year mortality rate of 45% to 60%. The murmur of mitral stenosis is usually apparent a decade after onset of RF. Then, in another decade, symptoms of

TABLE 7-3 **Cerebral Infarction of Cardiac Origin**

Valvular heart disease
  Rheumatic
  Prosthetic
  Mitral valve prolapse
  Infective endocarditis
  Nonbacterial thrombotic marantic endocarditis
  Libman-Sacks endocarditis
  Calcific heart valves
  Congenital valvular heart disease
  Mitral valve strands
  Aneurysm of the sinus of Valsalva
Other congenital heart disease
  Transposition of the great vessels
  Ventricular septal defect
  Atrial septal defect
  Pulmonary stenosis
  Tetralogy of Fallot
  Eisenmenger complex
  Truncus arteriosus with decreased flow
  Patent ductus arteriosus
  Endocardial cushion defect
  Hypoplastic left ventricle
  Ebstein anomaly
  Pulmonary atresia
  Coarctation of the aorta
Cardiac arrhythmias
  Atrial fibrillation
  Sick sinus syndrome
Other myocardial causes
  Cardiomyopathies—dilated, hypertrophic, restric-
    tive, arrhythmogenic right ventricle, unclassified
  Myocardial infarction
  Left ventricular aneurysm
  Kawasaki disease
Intracardiac tumors
  Atrial myxomas
  Rhabdomyomas
  Cardiac papillary fibroelastoma
Paradoxical embolism
  Patent foramen ovale
  Atrial septal defect
  Atrial septal aneurysm
Cardiac procedures (including ECMO) and heart
  transplantation

ECMO, extracorporeal membrane oxygenation.

pulmonary congestion develop. Systemic embolism may be the first manifestation of mitral stenosis, particularly if it is associated with atrial fibrillation. The lifetime risk of a clinically detectable embolic episode with rheumatic mitral stenosis is 20%. It has been estimated that embolism in rheumatic heart disease is cerebral in 60%, peripheral in 30%, and visceral in 10% of cases.[30-32,37-38] The risk is increased if concomitant atrial fibrillation, left atrial enlargement, low cardiac output, or severe mitral stenosis is present. In mitral stenosis, thrombi are found most frequently in the atria and are often restricted to the left atrial appendage. Extensive evaluation for the presence of a left atrial body or appendage thrombus is indicated. TEE has special advantages when investigating this possible source.

Long-term anticoagulation decreases the rate of recurrent embolization. It also has been suggested that percutaneous balloon mitral valve commissurotomy may reduce the incidence of ischemic stroke. In one series, patients with symptomatic rheumatic mitral valve disease who underwent commissurotomy had significantly fewer strokes than patients treated with medical therapy alone (2% versus 13%; $P = .043$).[39]

Prosthetic Heart Valves

Each year, thousands of operations are performed worldwide to replace malfunctioning or diseased cardiac valves with mechanical or biologic prosthetic heart valves. In the United States, approximately 99,000 patients receive cardiac valve replacements each year.[1] The choice of a biologic versus a mechanical prosthetic heart valve is based on considerations of durability, thrombogenicity, and the hemodynamic profile of the artificial heart valve. Mechanical heart valves are highly durable but thrombogenic, whereas biologic prosthetic heart valves are less thrombogenic, but also less durable. Approximately 30% of biologic heterografts and 10% to 20% of homografts require replacement within 10 to 15 years.[30]

Most clinically detected thromboembolic events arising from cardiac valvular prostheses involve the central nervous system (CNS). The overall rate of systemic embolism ranges from 0.87% to 3% after cardiac valve surgery. The rate of cerebral thromboembolism in patients with mechanical heart valves receiving anticoagulation is 4% per year in the mitral position and 2% per year in the aortic position.[2,3,30,40] The frequency is higher in cases with mitral valve prostheses and inadequate anticoagulation.[30,40-44] The incidence of thromboembolism is greater if there is associated atrial fibrillation, seriously impaired left ventricular function, or a history of prior thromboembolism.[30,45,46]

Two-dimensional echocardiography combined with Doppler or color blood flow mapping or both can supply useful information on the presence of a thrombus or vegetation and on the structural features and flow characteristics of prosthetic heart valves.

Reverberations and other artifacts produced by metallic valves can make a thrombus or vegetation difficult to distinguish from the prosthetic apparatus. TEE with Doppler color flow studies is particularly useful in assessing prosthetic heart valve malfunction under those circumstances.

The risk of embolization is less in patients with biologic prosthetic heart valves, with most events occurring in the perioperative period. Patients with mechanical prosthetic heart valves require long-term anticoagulant therapy. Patients with biologic prosthetic heart valves require long-term anticoagulant therapy if they have a history of atrial fibrillation, left atrial enlargement, prior thromboembolism, or left atrial thrombus. Although converting patients with atrial fibrillation to normal sinus rhythm may reduce the stroke incidence in these patients, it does not decrease the need for continued anticoagulation because these patients are at very high risk for spontaneous reversion to atrial fibrillation.[35,40,45-48]

Although anticoagulation decreases the stroke risk after cardiac valve surgeries, anticoagulation depends not only on the specific valve type, but also on its location. Most experts recommend a 3 months course of anticoagulant therapy after placement of a biologic prosthetic heart valve in the mitral position, but not in the aortic position. Although mechanical prosthetic heart valves are much more thrombogenic compared with biologic prosthetic heart valves, thromboembolic events actually occur with equal frequency in patients with either valve with adequate anticoagulation.[30,48-50]

Currently, patients with mechanical prosthetic heart valves receive long-term anticoagulants, and patients with biologic prosthetic heart valves may be anticoagulated only for the first 3 months after surgery, with aspirin prescribed thereafter because these valves are thought to be less thrombogenic.[30,51] Goal international normalized ratio values for anticoagulation with aortic mechanical prosthetic heart valves range from 2.0 to 3.0, and

2.5 to 3.5 for mechanical prosthetic heart values in the mitral position.[30,50-56] All patients with prosthetic heart valves also require endocarditis prophylaxis for even minor procedures such as dental care. Guidelines exist for antithrombotic therapies following prosthetic heart valves, and the current American College of Chest Physicians and the American College of Cardiology/American Heart Association recommendations are briefly summarized in Table 7-4.[30,55,56]

Mitral Valve Prolapse

Mitral valve prolapse (MVP) affects 2% to 6% of the general population and, when uncomplicated, does not have an increased risk for stroke.[30,57,85] There is evidence favoring an autosomal dominant inheritance pattern, with many affected individuals having a tall, slender body habitus, with prominent skeletal abnormalities.[59-61] Associated complications are rare, and in the absence of mitral regurgitation, MVP does not seem to increase the risk of arrhythmias, stroke, or sudden death.[57] Stroke in patients with MVP, regardless of age, is probably due to other causes.[57] MVP is an uncommon cause of stroke in young adults; the risk is 1 per 6000 per year.[61-63] MVP is a common cause of mitral regurgitation.

Classic auscultatory findings of MVP, not always audible, include a midsystolic click and a late-systolic murmur, but this examination finding has a low sensitivity for diagnosis of MVP.[57] Transthoracic echocardiography with parasternal and apical long axis imaging is sensitive and possibly more specific than apical imaging in the evaluation of MVP (Fig. 7-3). Thickened and elongated chordae, chamber enlargement, mitral valve leaflets with marked myxomatous changes, and associated mitral regurgitation by echocardiography may increase the risk for the development of cerebral emboli.[64]

The source of CNS embolization in patients with MVP may be from fibrin-platelet emboli formed in the myxomatous valve leaflets or chordal tissue, infective endocarditis, or associated arrhythmias. Many young adults with MVP and cerebral infarction seem to have another cause for the cerebral infarction. Before diagnosing MVP as the cause of a cerebral infarction, other causes need to be

TABLE 7-4 **Current Recommendations for Antithrombotic Therapy in Patients with Prosthetic Heart Valves**

Mechanical Valves*	Therapy	Evidence Class
St. Jude Medical bileaflet AV	W (INR 2.0-3.0)	I
CarboMedics bileaflet AV or Medtronic Hall tilting disk AV[†]	W (INR 2.0-3.0)	I
Tilting disk and bileaflet MV	W (INR 2.5-3.5)	I
Caged ball or caged disc valves	W (INR 2.5-3.5) + ASA (75-100 mg/day)	I
Mechanical AV or MV with additional risk factors[‡]	W (INR 2.5-3.5) + ASA (75-100 mg/day)	I
Mechanical AV or MV with systemic embolism despite therapeutic INR on W alone	W (INR 2.5-3.5) + ASA (75-100 mg/day)	I
Biologic MV without additional risk factors[‡]	W (INR 2.0-3.0) for 3 mo followed by ASA (75-100 mg/day)	I
Biologic AV without additional risk factors[‡]	W (INR 2.0-3.0) for 3 mo followed by ASA 75-100 mg/day	IIa

Note: For patients who cannot take W, ASA at a dose of 75-325 mg daily is recommended (class I evidence). In high-risk patients for whom ASA cannot be used, W monotherapy to a goal INR of 3.5-4.5 or the addition of clopidogrel 75 mg/day may be considered (class IIb evidence).

*For all of these patients, low-molecular-weight heparin should be considered if W must be discontinued.

[†]With normal left atrium size and normal sinus rhythm.

[‡]Additional risk factors include atrial fibrillation, myocardial infarction, endocardial damage, or low left ventricular ejection fraction.

ASA, aspirins; AV, aortic valve; INR, international normalized ratio; MV, mitral valve; W, warfarin.

From Bonow RO, Carabello BA, Chatterjee K, et al. ACC/AHA 2006 guidelines for the management of patients with valvular heart disease. A report of the American College of Cardiology/American Heart Association. J Am Coll Cardiol 2006;48(3):598.

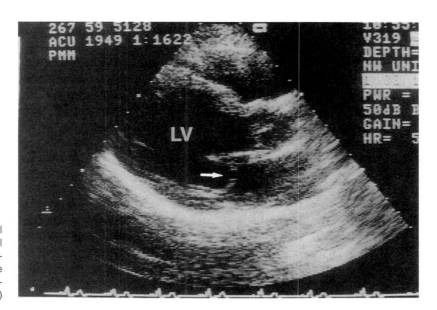

FIGURE 7-3 Two-dimensional echocardiogram, parasternal long-axis view, showing posterior leaflet mitral valve prolapse (*arrow*). LV, left ventricle. (Courtesy of David McPherson, M.D.)

excluded. Antiplatelet therapy is indicated as the initial measure to prevent recurrent CNS embolization. Patients with MVP and recurrent cerebral embolization despite platelet antiaggregants, or recurrent or persistent atrial fibrillation, must be considered for anticoagulant therapy.[65]

Infective Endocarditis

Infective endocarditis is a rare cause of stroke in young individuals except for cases associated with intravenous drug abuse. Neurologic complications are common with infective endocarditis; cerebrovascular events account for about half of neurologic complications. Cerebrovascular complications include transient ischemic attacks, cerebral infarction, intracerebral hemorrhage, subarachnoid hemorrhage, and subdural hemorrhages.[66-72] Associated systemic symptoms suggestive of infective endocarditis include fever, fatigue, malaise, weight loss, tachycardia, or tachypnea. The pathophysiologic mechanisms include septic embolization, infective (mycotic) aneurysm formation, and vasculitis. Symptomatic emboli commonly involve the middle cerebral artery territory. The diagnosis should be suspected when a stroke occurs in the setting of a febrile illness or new or changing murmurs, or when there is evidence of systemic embolization. The classic signs of native valve endocarditis (petechiae, Roth spots, Janeway lesions, and Osler nodes) are often absent. Splenomegaly is present in 25% of patients in the early stages and 40% in the later stages.

Infective endocarditis has been described in patients with almost every type of congenital or acquired cardiac abnormality and in patients with previously normal heart valves. The mitral and aortic valves are most commonly involved. Cerebrovascular events account for more than half of the complications associated with infective endocarditis, with meningitis, encephalitis, and cerebral abscesses constituting most of the remaining complications.[72] Neurologic complications are more common in patients with native valve or prosthetic valve endocarditis compared with patients with drug addiction or

pacemaker-related endocarditis.[72] The risk of prosthetic valve endocarditis is greater in the first 3 months after valve replacement, with a cumulative risk of 3% to 6%.

Virtually any species of bacteria or fungi can cause infective endocarditis. Viridans streptococci, *Staphylococcus aureus,* and *Enterococcus* species account for most native valve endocarditis cases. Culture-negative endocarditis is most commonly the result of prior use of antibiotics and less commonly bacterial strains, including *Haemophilus* subspecies, *Actinobacillus actinomycetemcomitans, Cardiobacterium hominis, Eikenella* subspecies, and *Kingella kingae.*[72]

Echocardiography, in particular TEE, is useful in detecting vegetations and local suppurative complications.[71-75] A negative echocardiogram (transthoracic echocardiography or TEE) does not completely exclude prosthetic valve endocarditis, however. Large, bulky, and mobile vegetations (i.e., fungal endocarditis) are easier to visualize by echocardiography and are associated with a higher incidence of embolic events (Fig. 7-4).

Long-term parenteral, bactericidal antibiotics are the appropriate treatment, and initiation of antibiotic therapy is associated with a decrease in the incidence of stroke, with the risk of stroke declining substantially over the course of treatment.[76] Anticoagulants are contraindicated in patients with native valve endocarditis complicated with cerebral embolism.[30,66,77,78] Anticoagulant therapy is controversial in cases of prosthetic valve endocarditis.[79-81] Patients requiring

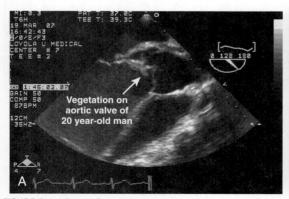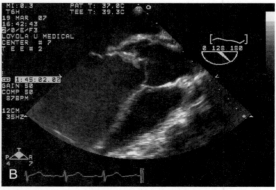

FIGURE 7-4   **A** and **B,** A 20-year-old man with infective endocarditis and multiple central nervous system infarcts. Transesophageal echocardiography shows aortic vegetation. (Courtesy of William Jacobs, M.D.)

cardiac valve replacement with stroke complicated by meningitis, hemorrhage, or brain abscess had a higher perioperative mortality rate compared with patients with uncomplicated ischemic stroke and endocarditis, but the neurologic complication rate was similar in both groups.[77] Mechanical prosthetic valve endocarditis is an indication for surgical removal of the prosthesis with implantation of a homograft, if possible.[30,72]

Nonbacterial Thrombotic Marantic Endocarditis

Nonbacterial thrombotic marantic endocarditis is characterized by the presence of multiple, small, sterile, fibrin-platelet valvular thrombi, most frequently involving the mitral and aortic valves in patients with mucin-producing malignancies leading to fibrin deposition (e.g., pancreas, colon, lung) and disseminated intravascular coagulation. This condition is an uncommon cause of stroke in young adults.[82] Premortem diagnosis is often difficult because the valvular lesions are often small and below the resolution of two-dimensional echocardiography. TEE is more sensitive in the evaluation of patients with marantic vegetations. Treatment consists of treating the underlying malignancy. It is unknown whether antiplatelet therapy or anticoagulants alter the course of this disorder or are effective in preventing recurrent embolization.[66]

Libman-Sacks Endocarditis

Libman-Sacks endocarditis is a rare type of noninfectious endocarditis that occurs in association with systemic lupus erythematosus and is characterized by verrucous, fibrinous valvular lesions, involving the mitral or aortic valves. The predominant abnormality is regurgitation; stenosis is rare. Arterial embolization is rare.[66] Embolic stroke resulting from noninfectious endocarditis also has been reported in Wegener disease and antiphospholipid syndrome.[83,84]

Calcific Heart Valves

Mitral annular calcification and isolated degenerative or calcific aortic stenosis are rare potential sources of cerebral embolism in young adults.[30,85,86] Mitral annulus calcification may double the risk of stroke.[87] Two-dimensional echocardiography is the procedure of choice to evaluate mitral annulus calcification and to assess aortic valve calcification. Optimal treatment of calcareous embolization is currently unknown. Likewise, a congenital bicuspid aortic valve, one of the most common causes of aortic stenosis in young patients, estimated to exist in 1% to 2% of the population, is rarely the cause of embolic phenomena.[88]

Congenital Heart Disease

The incidence of congenital heart disease is estimated at 1 in 125 live births. More than 1 million Americans may be affected with these disorders.[5] In the past, owing to progressive cardiac failure or hypoxemia, only 50% of these individuals survived to adolescence. Survival for children with congenital heart disease has markedly improved, however, and 85% of newborns may be expected to survive to adulthood. These patients are at significant increased risk for stroke, cerebral abscess, and developmental delay. It is estimated that strokes may occur in one quarter of children with congenital heart disease. In one study, 86% of adults with congenital heart disease had at least one major complication, including thromboembolic strokes, endocarditis, or arrhythmias.[89]

Of infants and children with cerebral ischemic arterial strokes, 70% of infants younger than 6 months old and 30% of children have an underlying cardiac disorder.[89] Ischemic strokes in these patients may be due to structural anomalies of the heart chambers or valves with thrombus formation on the abnormal structures. Alternatively, strokes may occur as a result of accompanying right-to-left cardiac shunts. Hyperviscosity syndromes caused by polycythemia or microcytic anemia and associated hypercoagulable states may be associated with ischemic stroke in patients with congenital heart disease. Finally, strokes may occur as a result of complications from endovascular diagnostic and therapeutic cardiac procedures in these children.

Cardiac embryogenesis begins at around 6 to 7 weeks of gestation, and it is during this time that many of the major cardiac structural disorders arise, although anomalies continue to arise throughout the middle and late trimesters as well.[90] The disorders include conotruncal lesions (i.e., tetralogy of Fallot), other transpositions of the great arteries, coarctation of the aorta and other vascular stenoses, and ventricular disorders.

Some of the most common cardiac malformations may not produce symptoms until early adulthood. In a series of 1875 patients with congenital heart disease, 72 patients (3.8%) had strokes, mostly occurring during the first 20 months of life.[91] The highest incidence of strokes occurred in patients who had the most severe hypoxemia or polycythemia. In selected series of stroke in young adults, congenital heart disease accounts for 1% to 7% of thrombotic or embolic cerebral infarctions.[91-93]

The mechanisms by which congenital heart defects may produce cerebral infarction include polycythemia, elevated hematocrit levels, high whole-blood viscosity, hypochromic microcytic anemia, hypoxemia, cardiac arrhythmias, cardiomyopathy, infective endocarditis, intracardiac shunt, or fragmentation of intracardiac thrombus at time of cardiac catheterization.[94-96] Coarctation of the aorta may cause strokes as a result of associated intracranial aneurysms of the circle of Willis, and less commonly as a result of thrombosis or embolization of cerebral vessels (Fig. 7-5).[97,98] A cerebral infarction also may occur in association with corrective cardiac surgery.[99] In some conditions, more than one mechanism is present.

Tetralogy of Fallot is the most common cyanotic heart defect, although transposition of the great vessels is the most common cause of cyanotic congenital heart disease discovered at birth.[2,93,100,101] Both of these disorders are being primarily repaired much earlier with a resultant decrease in ischemic stroke during childhood related to these lesions. With advances in surgical techniques

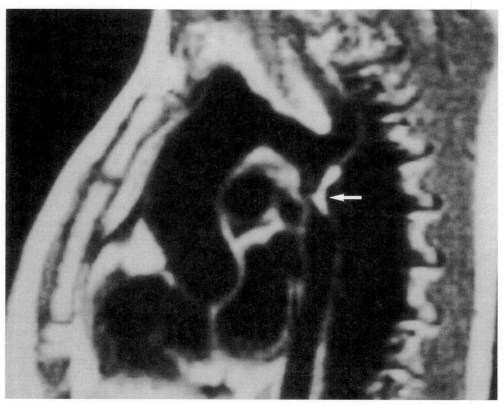

FIGURE 7-5   MRI of aortic coarctation (*arrow*), distal to the left subclavian artery. Note dilation of ascending aorta proximal to coarctation. (Courtesy of Maria Mendelson, M.D.)

for repair of transposition, mortality is less than 5%, and currently the greatest risk of stroke in patients with cyanotic congenital heart disease is for children with single ventricles who previously would have died shortly after birth. Among these latter congenital heart disease disorders are hypoplastic left heart syndrome, pulmonary atresia, tricuspid atresia, and an unbalanced atrioventricular canal. Typically, these patients have severe right-to-left cardiac shunts with cyanosis and associated high risk of embolic events. The treatment involves the Fontan procedure whereby systemic blood is routed from the venous system directly to the pulmonary arteries and then to the remaining functional single ventricle with resulting involvement in cardiac output and oxygenation. These patients remain at high risk for cardiac embolism, although there are no data for the use of warfarin as opposed to aspirin in these children.[3,100-102]

Coarctation of the aorta may occur proximal to the left subclavian artery, or may occur in the abdominal aorta, but is usually a focal stenosis of the thoracic aorta just distal to the left subclavian artery.[3,6,103] Coarctation of the aorta is more common in males and is frequently associated with a bicuspid aortic valve. Likewise, coarctation of the aorta is the most common cardiovascular anomaly in patients with Turner syndrome (45 X/O). Coarctation of the aorta represents approximately 6% to 8% of all congenital heart disease cases and is usually sporadic, although it can be associated with cerebrovascular malformations because the aortic arch and cervicocerebral blood vessels arise from neural crest tissues. Cerebral arterial aneurysms may occur in half of patients with coarctation of the aorta, and these patients are at higher risk of intracranial hemorrhage during adolescence and young adult years. Patients also may have perioperative strokes as a result of posterior circulation embolism or focal vertebral artery injury during repair or angioplasties around the left subclavian artery. Even with successful repair of coarcted aortas, there is an increased risk of systemic hypertension, and small vessel ischemic strokes may occur at a younger age.

Coarctation of the aorta associated with a bicuspid aortic valve may lead to aortic root dilation, aortic dissection, and ascending aortic aneurysm with the potential of spinal cord ischemia as a result of these lesions.[103,104] Isolated bicuspid aortic valves are the most common form of isolated aortic valvular stenoses in young adults with a familiar clustering of bicuspid aortic valves; 35% of these patients have an additional family member with a similar valvular abnormality.[6,30,105] Other, less common forms of aortic valve anomalies include unicuspid aortic valves and aortic annular hypoplasia. Other left ventricular outflow tract lesions include subvalvular aortic stenosis (with or without hypertrophic obstructive cardiomyopathy) and supravalvular stenosis.[6,105] Supravalvular aortic stenosis may occur sporadically. It also may be present in Williams syndrome, which is associated with several abnormalities in addition to supravalvular aortic stenosis, including defects in visuospatial cognition, mental retardation, hypercalcemia, renovascular hypertension, facial abnormalities (upturned nose, long philtrum, wide mouth, and small chin), and short stature.[106] Other genetic disorders associated with supravalvular stenosis include an autosomal dominant familial form without features of Williams syndrome, and patients with homozygous and less frequently heterozygous familial hypercholesterolemia.[105] The prognosis of untreated supravalvular aortic stenosis is poor.

Data regarding stroke prophylaxis in patients with structural congenital heart disease are limited, and guidelines for antithrombotic therapies are derived from adult cardiac and stroke patients.[6] Based on the bleeding complication rates for children with prosthetic valves of 12.2% on anticoagulation therapy, the tendency is to use aspirin, as opposed to warfarin, in children with cardioembolic strokes secondary to congenital heart disease. Whether other antiplatelet agents are superior to aspirin in children with congenital heart disease is unknown at this time.

Cardiac Arrhythmias

Focal cerebral ischemia is uncommon in patients with cardiac arrhythmias except in patients with atrial fibrillation or sick sinus syndrome. Heart block is common in patients with Kearns-Sayre syndrome. Polymorphic ventricular arrhythmias (torsades de pointes) may occur in patients with Jervell and Lange-Nielsen syndrome, characterized by congenital deafness and cardiac arrhythmias (long Q-T interval).

Atrial Fibrillation

Overall, almost half of all cases of cardioembolic stroke are related to atrial fibrillation, although the incidence of atrial fibrillation increases with age.[7] Atrial fibrillation is found in 0.4% of adults younger than 60 years. The prevalence of atrial fibrillation in residents of Rochester, Minnesota, was zero in the 35- to 44-year age group.[107] Although atrial fibrillation is a common cause of stroke in the elderly, it is an uncommon cause in young adult series.[108] Atrial fibrillation may be encountered in children, however, with rheumatic heart disease, hyperthyroidism, cardiomyopathies,

atrial tumors, Marfan syndrome with mitral regurgitation, endocardial fibroelastosis, congenital heart malformations, or after surgical repair of congenital heart disease.[109]

Patients with nonvalvular atrial fibrillation have a risk of stroke that is at least five times greater than that of patients with normal sinus rhythm. When atrial fibrillation complicates rheumatic valvular heart disease, the risk of ischemic stroke is increased by approximately 17-fold.[110] Reports of familial occurrence of atrial fibrillation are uncommon.[111]

Two-dimensional echocardiography is often obtained in patients with atrial fibrillation to determine left atrial size, to assess the presence of left atrial thrombus, to evaluate the cardiac valves, and to estimate left ventricular function (Fig. 7-6). Left atrial thrombi often reside in the left atrial appendage, however, which are poorly visualized by this technique. TEE should be used in these circumstances.[112]

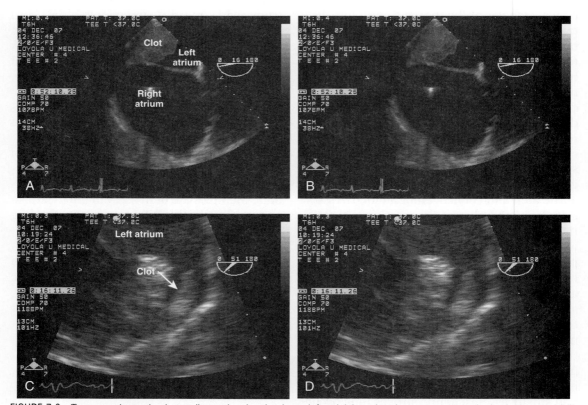

FIGURE 7-6   Transesophageal echocardiography showing large left atrial thrombus in a young man who had a large middle cerebral artery territory ischemic stroke secondary to the acute onset of atrial fibrillation. **A** and **B,** Transesophageal echocardiography image with views of the left and right atria showing left atrial thrombus. **C** and **D,** Transesophageal echocardiography showing view of the left atrial appendage with echodense material consistent with clot. (Courtesy of William Jacobs, M.D.)

TABLE 7-5 **CHADS2 Stroke Risk Score for Atrial Fibrillation**

Congestive heart failure	1
Hypertension	1
Age >75 yr	1
Diabetes Mellitus	1
Prior Stroke or TIA	2
Low risk	0-1
Moderate risk	2-3
High risk	4-6

TIA, transient ischemic attack.

From Gage BF, Waterman AD, Shannon W, et al. Validation of clinical classification schemes for predicting stroke: results from the National Registry of Atrial Fibrillation. JAMA 2001;285:2864.

The role of oral anticoagulation with warfarin in nonvalvular atrial fibrillation has been addressed by five major studies. All of the studies showed a reduced risk of stroke with oral anticoagulation with warfarin.[113-119] Long-term anticoagulation is indicated after a cerebral embolic event attributed to atrial fibrillation.[119-121] The risk of stroke in the context of atrial fibrillation has been quantified via the CHADS2 score (Table 7-5).[122] Patients with "lone" atrial fibrillation and otherwise low-risk patients may be treated with aspirin, 325 mg daily. Although younger patients, especially with lone atrial fibrillation, are at lower risk of stroke, the presence of prior stroke or transient ischemic attack alone puts patients into a moderate-risk category, and the presence of cardiovascular risk factors increases the risk of stroke further. These moderate-risk or high-risk patients should be treated with full-dose warfarin (goal international normalized ratio 2.0 to 3.0).

Sick Sinus Syndrome

The sick sinus syndrome encompasses a variety of rhythm disorders caused by extrinsic or intrinsic dysfunction of the sinus node. Sick sinus syndrome is most often caused by idiopathic disease of the sinoatrial node. This condition occurs rarely in young adults. Causes include various congenital and acquired heart disorders. Sick sinus syndrome in a young adult may be associated with cardiomyopathies, pericardial disease, surgical injury to the sinoatrial node, hemochromatosis, amyloidosis,

Friedreich ataxia, myotonic dystrophy, fascioscapulohumeral dystrophy, scapuloperoneal dystrophy, the surdocardiac syndrome, and degenerative myopia. The "tachy-brady" syndrome has the greatest risk of embolization.[123-128]

A similar approach to that outlined in the evaluation for patients with atrial fibrillation, supplemented with 24-hour ambulatory electrocardiogram monitoring, may be used in patients with sick sinus syndrome. Implantation of a permanent demand pacemaker is the preferred therapy for symptomatic sick sinus syndrome. A variety of conduction disturbances, including complete heart block, have been reported with the Kearns-Sayre syndrome, a mitochondrial disorder characterized by chronic progressive external ophthalmoplegia, pigmentary retinal degeneration with onset by age 20, which may be a rare source of cerebral embolization.

Cardiomyopathies

Primary cardiomyopathies are broadly classified into dilated cardiomyopathy, hypertrophic cardiomyopathy, restrictive cardiomyopathy, arrhythmogenic right ventricular cardiomyopathy, and unclassified types.[128,129,132] Dilated cardiomyopathy is the most prevalent.[129-132] Approximately one third of dilated cardiomyopathies are familial, and some are associated with sensorineural hearing loss. Stroke also has been associated with the rare syndrome of Takotsubo (named for the Japanese octopus trap—*tako-tsubo*) cardiomyopathy, a stress-induced reversible form of left ventricular dysfunction.[133] Systemic emboli occur at an annual rate of approximately 4%. Cardiomyopathy also may be a component of various neuromuscular disorders, particularly Fabry disease, Refsum disease, glycogenoses, mucopolysaccharidoses, certain lipid storage diseases, carnitine deficiency, Friedreich ataxia, mitochondrial myopathy, and most muscular dystrophies.

Affected patients may present with symptoms of congestive heart failure, cardiac arrhythmias, or symptoms secondary to pulmonary or systemic embolism.[9] The mechanism of embolization is likely multifactorial; left ventricular mural thrombus is probably the most important. Mural thrombi occur in approximately two thirds of patients.[128–132] Cerebral embolism is an uncommon complication of peripartum cardiomyopathy and infectious myocarditis.[134,135] Peripartum cardiomyopathy found in the last month of pregnancy or in the first 5 months postpartum is discussed in more detail in Chapter 10. Cardiac amyloidosis rarely causes cerebral embolism.[136] Cardiomyopathy also is a frequent manifestation of Chagas disease (caused by *Trypanosoma cruzi*), a disorder prevalent in some regions of Central and South America.[137]

Two-dimensional echocardiography is currently the procedure of choice to identify left ventricular thrombi in patients with dilated cardiomyopathy (Fig. 7-7). The presence of left ventricular thrombus by echocardiography is a significant and independent marker for stroke with an odds ratio of 3.4 for increased stroke risk.[138]

In a retrospective study, systemic embolism occurred in 18% of patients with dilated cardiomyopathy not receiving anticoagulants and in none of the patients who were receiving anticoagulants.[139] Some authors believe all patients with dilated cardiomyopathy should receive anticoagulants; others suggest anticoagulant therapy only for patients with atrial fibrillation. To date, there has not been a prospective, double-blind, randomized clinical trial to define the role of anticoagulant therapy in this group.[140]

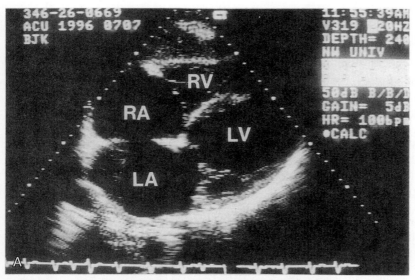

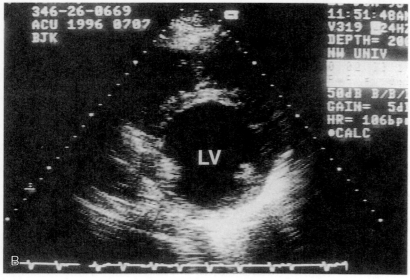

FIGURE 7-7 **A,** Two-dimensional echocardiogram showing subcostal–four chamber view of a young patient with dilated cardiomyopathy. **B,** Two-dimensional echocardiogram showing parasternal short-axis view of same patient. LA, left atrium; LV, left ventricle; RA, right atrium; RV, right ventricle. (Courtesy of David McPherson, M.D.)

Optimal antithrombotic therapy remains unclear, and pooled data from the more recently completed inconclusive Warfarin and Antiplatelet Therapy in Chronic Heart Failure (WATCH) study and the Warfarin versus Aspirin in Reduced Cardiac Ejection Fraction (WARCEF) may shed light on whether warfarin is beneficial compared with antiplatelet therapy in patients with heart failure with reduced ejection fractions without concomitant atrial fibrillation.[140,141]

Myocardial Infarction

Cerebrovascular disease and coronary heart disease are complications of a common generalized atherosclerotic process and represent major causes of death in most industrialized nations. Pathologic studies have shown a high correlation between the degree of coronary atherosclerosis and the degree of atherosclerosis of the extracranial and intracranial vessels. Patients with acute stroke sometimes develop an acute myocardial infarction (MI), and patients with acute MI also develop acute strokes. In the United States, approximately 1.5 million individuals per year have an acute MI.

Acute MI is complicated by cerebral embolism in approximately 2% to 6% of patients. Cerebral embolism accompanying MI is very rare in children. The major underlying causes are anomalous origin of the left coronary artery from the pulmonary artery, ostial coronary artery, stenosis after surgical correction of transposition of the great arteries, inflammatory disease of coronary arteries, medial calcification with fibroblastic proliferation of the intima, Kawasaki syndrome (mucocutaneous lymph node syndrome), and Fabry disease.[155-157] Kawasaki syndrome is an acute febrile illness of young children characterized by the development of coronary arteritis or coronary artery aneurysms (Fig. 7-8). Fabry disease, an X-linked recessive lysosomal storage disease with a resultant α-galactosidase A deficiency, can be associated with multifocal cerebral infarctions (see Chapter 11).

Cerebral infarction after MI may result from the dislodgment of fragments from a left ventricular thrombus (Fig. 7-9) or, less frequently, may be due to complicating hemodynamic disturbances. Cerebral embolism after MI usually develops within 1 month and is most common within the first 2 weeks after MI. The risk of cerebral embolism is greatest with transmural or anterior MIs, extensive infarctions with markedly elevated cardiac enzymes, presence of congestive heart failure, atrial fibrillation, and major septal compromise.[9,142-147]

A meta-analysis of patients with non–ST segment elevation acute coronary syndrome noted a low event rate for this type of MI, with a rate of 0.7% all-cause strokes (0.5% ischemic and 0.06% hemorrhagic). The only significant predictors were age, prior stroke

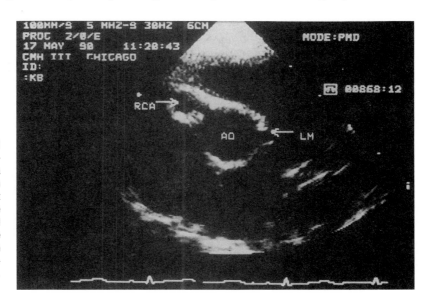

FIGURE 7-8 Two-dimensional echocardiogram shows cross-sectional view of the aorta (AO), and take-off of left main coronary artery (LM) and right coronary artery (RCA). Note large size of RCA compared with LM, which is compatible with aneurysmal dilation as seen in patients with Kawasaki syndrome. (Courtesy of Farooq A. Chaudry, M.D.)

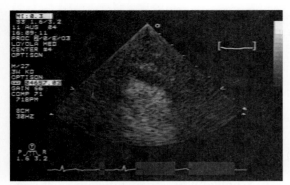

FIGURE 7-9 Two-dimensional echocardiogram in a young man with left hemispheric ischemic stroke secondary to "occult" left ventricular thrombus.

history, and elevated heart rate.[148] In the Valsartan in Acute Myocardial Infarction (VALIANT) registry of post-MI patients, without initial neurologic symptoms, the risk of stroke 6 weeks after MI was 0.94% (95% confidence interval 0.78 to 1.09). Elevated baseline estimated glomerular filtration rate and heart rate in sinus rhythm were the most powerful risk predictors for early stroke (within 45 days after MI), whereas elevated diastolic blood pressure greater than 90 mm Hg, a history of stroke before qualifying MI, and atrial fibrillation were the most powerful overall predictors of stroke after MI. Age also was a significant predictor of stroke risk.[149]

Thrombi usually are located in the left ventricular apex in an area of wall motion abnormality. Although echocardiography is typically diagnostic, it may be missed sometimes in young adults for whom left ventricular thrombus might otherwise be unexpected (see Fig. 7-7).[150] Embolization is greatest with protruding and mobile thrombi.[151,152] Because thrombi tend to develop between days 3 and 5 after MI, it has been suggested that the optimal times to perform echocardiography are by day 3 and again at days 10 to 14. If a protruding, mobile thrombus is identified, a 3- to 6-month course of anticoagulant therapy is indicated. Prophylactic treatment with anticoagulants is controversial. Several more recent studies have helped define the role of anticoagulants after MI. Heparin at a dosage of 12,500 U subcutaneously every 12 hours has been shown to be more effective than

5000 U every 12 hours in preventing left ventricular thrombus in patients with anterior transmural MI. Another study has shown a 55% reduction in cerebral infarction after MI with long-term warfarin therapy.[153,154]

Left Ventricular Aneurysm

Left ventricular aneurysms occur in about 7% to 10% of patients after MI (Fig. 7-10). After an anterior left ventricular aneurysm develops, mural thrombus formation may be found by two-dimensional echocardiography in 35% to 50% of patients. Left ventricular thrombus formation occurs infrequently in an inferior left ventricular aneurysm. Although left ventricular aneurysms commonly have associated thrombi, the risk of cerebral embolization is low. Most experts do not recommend anticoagulation of left ventricular thrombi associated with apical aneurysms. Limited data are inconclusive about the emboligenic risk of later forming left ventricular thrombus.[158-160]

Intracardiac Tumors

Atrial myxomas are a potentially curable form of serious heart disease.[161-174] They are the most common primary cardiac tumors, found

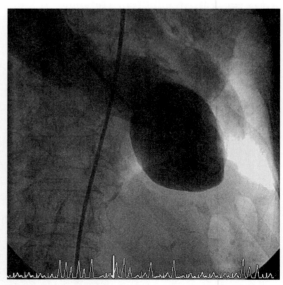

FIGURE 7-10 Cardiac catheterization showing a left ventricular aneurysm in a patient who had a myocardial infarction and subsequent ischemic stroke. (Courtesy of Robert Dieter, M.D.)

in approximately 1 per 100,000 autopsies. Most atrial myxomas are sporadic, but there is evidence favoring a dominant mode of inheritance, with frequent cases reported in families, as is the case with the Carney complex, localized to chromosome 17q2.[175] Myxomas tend to be solitary tumors originating in the left atrium near the fossa ovalis. Atrial myxomas can cause embolic cerebral infarction or intracranial hemorrhage, which may be the initial manifestation of the disease. Half of patients with atrial myxomas experience clinically detectable embolism, and most of these involve the cerebral circulation.

Affected patients present with constitutional, obstructive, or embolic symptoms. Cerebral embolism may occur before onset of other symptoms and may lead to the formation of multiple intracranial aneurysms that may be found before or after the excision of the myxoma. The incidence of atrial myxomas in several series of young adults is 0% to 2%. In most instances, diagnosis can be easily, reliably, and accurately made with two-dimensional echocardiography (Fig. 7-11). Prompt surgical excision is curative.

Rhabdomyomas are benign primary cardiac tumors often found in association with tuberous sclerosis complex. Patients seldom present with cerebral embolism.[176] Numerous other rare tumors involving the heart are associated with cardioembolic stroke. Primary cardiac lymphoma, cardiac hemangioma, cardiac paraganglioma, and cardiac papillary fibroelastoma all have been associated with cardioembolic cerebral ischemic events.[177-183]

Intracardiac Defects with Paradoxical Embolism

Patients with tetralogy of Fallot or Eisenmenger syndrome have right-to-left shunts; most have the defects corrected during childhood. Other potential right-to-left intracardiac communications are common, although they are usually clinically insignificant. The patent foramen ovale (PFO) is probably the most common "congenital heart disease." A PFO results when the primum and secundum atrial septa fail to seal together in the postpartum period with a flap, which then persists over the fossa ovalis that can function as a one-way valve. The PFO is a part of normal perinatal development, however, and probably should not be considered a true congenital disorder. A PFO, atrial septal defects (ostium secundum, sinus venosus, and ostium primum), or atrial septal aneurysms may be a transcardiac source for paradoxical embolism.[184-192]

The significance of a PFO as a cause of stroke is controversial. Physiologic shunting may be present in 10% to 18% of normal individuals, but the prevalence of PFO shown by contrast echocardiography has been found to be higher in young adults with otherwise unexplained strokes.[193] PFO may be present in 25% to 40% of all adults. Using contrast echocardiography, Lechat and coworkers[194] showed a PFO in 40% of patients with no other source for an embolic stroke, whereas only 10% of controls had a PFO. There have been multiple images of in

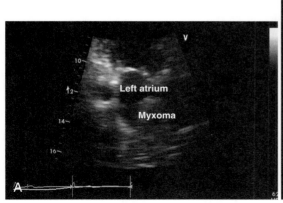 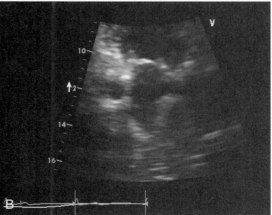

FIGURE 7-11   **A** and **B,** Echocardiography showing left atrial myxoma. (Courtesy of William Jacobs, M.D.)

situ thrombus, and echocardiography often shows a clear right-to-left shunt. Although PFO is frequently identified in the context of an ischemic stroke, a causal embolic source, such as venous thromboembolism, associated with the discovered PFO is rarely identified.

A PFO is probably the most frequent potential source of cardiac embolism in young (Fig. 7-12) and middle-aged adults, although the relationship in older adults is less clear.[195,196] The relationship of PFO and ischemic stroke is mainly based on associations from multiple case series and case-control studies. In one meta-analysis, the odds ratio was 5.01 among patients younger than 56 years old with no statistically significant association among older individuals (odds ratio 1.20).[195-197] A more recent study of 503 consecutive patients suggested that the prevalence of a PFO was significantly greater in patients younger (odds ratio 4.70) and older than age 55 (odds ratio 2.92) with cryptogenic stroke. The association of cryptogenic stroke and PFO was even stronger if an atrial septal aneurysm was present. For patients younger than 55 years old with cryptogenic stroke and atrial septal aneurysm, the odds ratio was 7.36; the odds ratio was 3.88 for patients older than 55.[198] Overall, the annual risk of first-ever cryptogenic stroke in patients with a PFO is less than 0.1%, and other factors, such as occult arrhythmias or hypercoagulable states, must be considered in patients with PFO and ischemic stroke. Because of the very low incidence of first-ever stroke, prophylactic therapeutic interventions for primary prevention of stroke in patients with PFO are not recommended.[197]

Recurrent stroke rates in patients with PFO-related stroke are low. In only one other study was there a significantly increased risk of recurrent stroke, and that occurred in the context of PFO with an associated atrial septal aneurysm.[199] This finding has not been replicated in many other studies. Antiplatelet therapy, anticoagulants, and surgical or transcatheter closure of PFO all have been used in secondary stroke prevention for these patients. Randomized trials are under way of medical versus transcatheter closure of PFO, but there is no current evidence to support interventional procedures preferentially.

The Patent Foramen Ovale in Cryptogenic Stroke Study (PICSS) remains the largest observation study of medical interventions with blinded randomization of patients to warfarin or aspirin, as part of the larger Warfarin-Aspirin Recurrent Stroke Study (WARSS).[200,201] In that study, there was a trend toward benefit of warfarin, compared with aspirin, in a cohort of older patients with cryptogenic stroke and PFO. Of the 630 patients in the PICSS study who had a TEE, however, only 98 patients were found to have a cryptogenic stroke. Two smaller observational studies of approximately 50 patients each with PFO-related stroke also found a beneficial trend with warfarin, but both of these studies were not randomized studies.[202-203] As such, there is insufficient evidence for warfarin compared with aspirin at this time.[199]

Transcatheter closure may seem to be a logical alternative to medical therapy for patients with PFO at risk for recurrent strokes because the 1-year rates for recurrent events

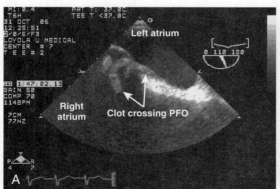
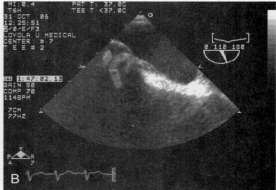

FIGURE 7-12   **A** and **B,** Transesophageal echocardiography showing thrombus crossing a patent foramen ovale (*arrows*) in a young woman with a presumptive embolic stroke. (Courtesy of William Jacobs, M.D.)

are reported as 0 to 4.9% with device closure and 3.8% to 12% with medical therapy.[195-197,204,205] Complications of device deployment generally are reported as low, but the actual rate is unclear, and current evidence does not support device closure versus medical therapies. Clinical trials are under way to define whether transcatheter closure of PFO is superior to medical therapy. Outside of those clinical trials, the American Academy of Neurology and the American Stroke Association guidelines do not support routine transcatheter device closure of PFO for cryptogenic stroke.[197,204,205]

In contrast to PFO, atrial septal defects represent a true form of congenital heart disease. Atrial septal defects are one of the most common congenital heart lesions found in adults. Left-to-right and right-to-left shunting may occur. Shunting increases during pregnancy. Atrial septal aneurysms are localized malformations of the interatrial septum. Defects of the septum secundum occur in 70% of atrial septal defects. There is a wide range in the size of discovered secundum atrial septal defects, and these tend to be isolated defects.[6,206,207] In contrast, primum septum atrial septal defects are usually associated with ventricular septal defects and atrioventricular canal defects. The defect may be congenital or acquired. The mechanism of cerebral embolism may be due to thrombus formation or interatrial shunting. In children, as opposed to young adults, paradoxical embolism through a right-to-left shunt from a PFO or atrial septal defect is considered to be rare.

Pulmonary arteriovenous malformations occur in 15% to 20% of patients with hereditary hemorrhagic telangiectasia (Rendu-Osler-Weber syndrome) and may be the source of paradoxical emboli causing cerebral ischemia. The Rendu-Osler-Weber syndrome is an autosomal dominant disorder characterized by fibrovascular dysplasia of mucus membranes, skin, and viscera. Contrast echocardiography and ultrafast chest CT scans are used to localize single and multiple pulmonary arteriovenous malformations before selective pulmonary angiography.[207-211]

Paradoxical embolism is believed to be an underdiagnosed source of embolic stroke.[212-214] TEE with contrast enhancement is the procedure of choice to evaluate for possible paradoxical embolism (see Fig. 7-11). Transcranial Doppler ultrasonography may help identify patients with right-to-left cardiac or pulmonary shunts.[215] Paradoxical embolism should be suspected in young adults with cryptogenic strokes; in cases of strokes associated with the Valsalva maneuver; in cases of strokes in young women taking oral contraceptives; and in cases of strokes associated with recent immobilization, venous thrombosis excluding thrombosis of the pulmonary veins, or acute increase in right atrial pressure with pulmonary hypertension.

Miscellaneous Causes

Patients undergoing cardiac catheterization, coronary artery bypass surgery, percutaneous transluminal coronary angioplasty, percutaneous transluminal valvuloplasty, intra-aortic balloon pump insertion, ventricular assist device placement, or cardiac transplantation are at risk for cerebral embolization.[216-219] Embolism is a particular concern with intra-aortic balloon pumps and ventricular assist devices, and vigilant monitoring for thromboembolism, including spinal cord ischemia, is essential in patients with these devices. Fat embolism to the brain can complicate cardiopulmonary bypass and, more rarely, myelodysplasia, juvenile rheumatoid arthritis, collagen vascular disease, and osteoporotic conditions.[220,221] The mechanisms of cerebral infarction include release of microaggregates into the circulation during coronary artery bypass surgery; catheter-induced endothelial trauma or shearing of a plaque; systemic hypotension with cerebral hypoperfusion; or embolization of calcific, fat, or fibrin-platelet material.

Conclusion

Numerous cardiac conditions can lead to cerebral infarction in young adults. Detection of these abnormalities requires a detailed history, cardiac examination, and often extensive cardiologic diagnostic studies. TEE is superior to transthoracic echocardiography in showing potential cardiac sources of emboli, especially in patients younger than 45 years of age.

REFERENCES

1. American Heart Association. Heart Disease and Stroke Statistics, 2007 Update. Dallas, TX: American Heart Association, 2007.
2. Hachinski V, Norris JW. The young stroke. In Idem, eds. The Acute Stroke. Philadelphia: FA Davis, 1985.
3. Caldwell RL. Strokes and congenital heart disease in infants and children. Semin Cerebrovasc Dis 2003;3:200.
4. Broderick J, Talbot GT, Prenger E, et al. Stroke in children within a major metropolitan area: the surprising importance of intracerebral hemorrhage. J Child Neurol 1993;8:250.
5. Green A. Outcomes of congenital heart disease: a review. Pediatr Nurs 2004;30:280.
6. Brickner ME, Hillis LD, Lange RA. Congenital heart disease in adults. First of two parts. N Engl J Med 2000;342:256.
7. Sila CA. Heart diseases and stroke. Curr Neurol Neurosci Rep 2006;6:23.
8. Levine J, Swanson PD. Non-atherosclerotic causes of stroke. Ann Intern Med 1969;70:807.
9. Abraham J, Shetty G, Jose CJ. Strokes in the young. Stroke 1971;2:259.
10. Hindfelt B, Nilsson O. Brain infarction in young adults. Acta Neurol Scand 1977;55:145.
11. Grindal AB, Cohen RJ, Saul RF, Taylor JR. Cerebral infarction in young adults. Stroke 1978;9:39.
12. Schoenberg BS, Mellinger JF, Schoenberg DG. Cerebrovascular disease in infants and children: a study of incidence, clinical features, and survival. Neurology 1978;28:763.
13. Chopra JS, Prabhakar S. Clinical features and risk factors in stroke in young. Acta Neurol Scand 1979;60:289.
14. Snyder BD, Ramirez-Lassepas M. Cerebral infarction in young adults. Stroke 1980;11:149.
15. Hart RJ, Miller VT. Cerebral infarction in young adults: a practical approach. Stroke 1983;14:110.
16. Franck G, Doyen P, Grisar T, Moonen G. Les accidents ischemiques cerebraux du sujet jeune, age de moins de quarante-cinq ans. Sem Hop Paris 1983;59:2642.
17. Klein GM, Seland TP. Occlusive cerebrovascular disease in young adults. Can J Neurol Sci 1984;11:302.
18. Hilton-Jones D, Warlow CP. The causes of stroke in the young. J Neurol 1985;232:137.
19. Adams HP, Butler MJ, Biller J, et al. Nonhemorrhagic cerebral infarction in young adults. Arch Neurol 1986;43:793.
20. Radhakrishnan K, Ashok PP, Sridharan R, Mousa ME. Stroke in the young: incidence and pattern in Benghazi, Libya. Acta Neurol Scand 1986;73:434.
21. Bogousslavsky J, Regli F. Ischemic stroke in adults younger than 30 years of age. Arch Neurol 1987;44:479.
22. Alvarez J, Matias-Guiu J, Sumalla J, et al. Ischemic stroke in young adults, I: analysis of the etiological subgroups. Acta Neurol Scand 1989;80:28.
23. Gautier JC, Pradat-Diehl P, Loron PH, et al. Accidents vasculaires cerebraux des sujets jeunes: une étude de 133 patients agés de 9 a 45 ans. Rev Neurol 1989;6-7:437.
24. Bevan H, Sharma K, Bradley W. Stroke in young adults. Stroke 1990;21:382.
25. Lisovoski F, Rousseaux P. Cerebral infarction in young people: a study of 148 patients with early cerebral angiography. J Neurol Neurosurg Psychiatry 1991;54:576.
26. Lanzino G, Andreoli A, Di Pasquale G, et al. Etiopathogenesis and prognosis of cerebral ischemia in young adults: a survey of 155 treated patients. Acta Neurol Scand 1991;84:321.
27. Carolei A, Marmni C, Ferranti E, et al. A prospective study of cerebral ischemia in the young: analysis of pathogenic determinants. Stroke 1993;24:362.
28. Vandenberg B, Biller J. Cardiac investigations after acute stroke. Cerebrovasc Dis 1991;1(suppl 1):73.
29. Cohen BA, Hildebrand F, Biller J. Cardioembolic stroke, part I: clinical patterns and associated cardiac conditions. ACC Current J Rev 1993;Jan/Feb:51.
30. Bonow RO, Carabello BA, Chatterjee K, et al. ACC/AHA 2006 guidelines for the management of patients with valvular heart disease. A report of the American College of Cardiology/American Heart Association. J Am Coll Cardiol 2006;e1.
31. Jones TD. Diagnosis of rheumatic fever. JAMA 1944;126:481.
32. Special Writing Group of the Committee on Rheumatic Fever, Endocarditis, and Kawasaki Cardiac Disorders and Stroke Disease of the Council on Cardiovascular Disease in the Young of the American Heart Association. Guidelines for the diagnosis of rheumatic fever. Jones Criteria, 1992 Update. JAMA 1992;268:2069.
33. Liu YT, Sinert R. Mitral stenosis. 2006. Available at: http://www.emedicine.com /EMERG/topics315.htm.
34. Zalzstein E, Hamilton R, Zucker N, et al. Presentation, natural history, and outcome in children and adolescents with double orifice mitral valve. Am Cardiol 2004;93:1067.
35. Amital H, Langevitz P, Levy Y, et al. Valvular deposition of antiphospholipid antibodies in the antiphospholipid syndrome: a clue to the origin of the disease. Clin Exp Rheumatol 1999;17:99.
36. Gibson SC, Pathi VL. Mitral valve replacement for mitral stenosis secondary to Hunter's syndrome. Ann Thorac Surg 2005;80:1911.
37. Jordan RA, Scheifley CH, Edwards JE. Mural thrombosis and arterial embolism in mitral stenosis: a clinicopathologic study of fifty-one cases. Circulation 1951;111:363.
38. Wood P. An appreciation of mitral stenosis, part I: clinical features. BMJ 1954;1:1051.
39. Lai HC, Lee WL, Wang KY, et al: Percutaneous balloon commissurotomy reduces incidence of ischemic cerebral stroke in patients with symptomatic rheumatic mitral stenosis. Int J Cardiol 2008;23:189.
40. Vongpatanasin W, Hillis LD, Lange RA. Prosthetic heart valves. N Engl J Med 1996;335:407.
41. Barebetseas J, Pitsavos C, Aggeli C, et al. Comparison of frequency of left atrial thrombus in patients with mechanical prosthetic cardiac valves and stroke versus transient ischemic attacks. Am J Cardiol 1997;80:526.

42. Puvimanasinghe JP, Steyerberg EW, Takkenberg JJ, et al. Prognosis after aortic valve replacement with a bioprosthesis: predictions based on meta-analysis and microsimulation. Circulation 2001;103:1535.

43. Remadi JP, Baron O, Roussel C, et al. Isolated mitral valve replacement with St Jude medical prosthesis: long-term results: a follow-up of 19 years. Circulation 2001;103:1542.

44. Deviri E, Sareli P, Wisenbaugh T, et al. Obstruction of mechanical heart prosthesis: clinical aspects of surgical management. J Am Coll Cardiol 1991;17:646.

45. Edmiston A, Harrison CC, Duick G, et al. Thromboembolism in mitral porcine valve recipients. Am J Cardiol 1978;41:508.

46. Hart RG, Sherman DG, Miller VT, Easton JD. Diagnosis and management of ischemic stroke, part II: selected controversies. Curr Probl Cardiol 1983;7:25.

47. Bando K, Kobayashi J, Hirata M, et al. Early and late stroke after mitral valve replacement with a mechanical prosthesis: risk factor analysis of a 24-year experience. J Thorac Cardiovasc Surg 2003;126:358.

48. Wyse DG, Waldo AL, DiMarco JP, et al; for the Atrial Fibrillation Follow-up Investigation of Rhythm Management (AFFIRM) Investigators. A comparison of rate control and rhythm control in patients with atrial fibrillation. N Engl J Med 2002;347:1825.

49. Hammermeister KE, Sethi GK, Henderson WG, et al. A comparison of outcomes in men 11 years after heart valve replacement with a mechanical valve or bioprosthesis. Veterans Affairs Cooperative Study on Valvular Heart Disease. N Engl J Med 1993;328:1289.

50. Roudaut R, Lafitte S, Roudaut MF, et al. Fibrinolysis of mechanical prosthetic valve thrombosis: a single-center study of 127 cases. J Am Coll Cardiol 2003;41:653.

51. Bloomfield P, Wheatley DJ, Prescott RJ, et al. Twelve-year comparison of Bjork-Shiley mechanical heart valve with porcine bioprostheses. N Engl J Med 1991;324:573.

52. Cannegieter SC, Rosendaal FR, Wintzen AR, et al. Optimal oral anticoagulation therapy in patients with mechanical heart valves. N Engl J Med 1995;333:11.

53. Horstkotte D, Schulte JD, Bircks W, et al. Lower intensity anticoagulation therapy results in lower complication rates with the St Jude Medical Prosthesis. J Thorac Cardiovas Surg 1994;107:1136.

54. Acar J, Iung B, Boissel JP, et al. AREVA: Multi-center randomized comparison of low-dose versus standard dose anticoagulation in patients with mechanical prosthetic heart valves. Circulation 1996;94:2107.

55. Salem DN, Stein PD, Al-Ahmad A, et al. Antithrombotic therapy in valvular heart disease—native and prosthetic. The Seventh ACCP Conference on Antithrombotic and Thrombolytic Therapy. Chest 2004;126:457S.

56. Butchart EG, Gohlke-Barwolf C, Antunes MJ, et al. Recommendations for the management of patients after heart valve surgery. Eur Heart J 2005;26:2463.

57. Savage DD, Garrison RJ, Devereux RB, et al. Mitral valve prolapse in the general population, I: epidemiologic features. The Framingham Study. Am Heart J 1983;3:571.

58. Hayek E, Griffin B. Mitral valve prolapse: old beliefs yield to new knowledge. Cleve Clin J Med 2002;69:889.

59. Pickering NJ, Brody JI, Barrett MJ. Von Willebrand syndromes and mitral-valve prolapse: linked mesenchymal dysplasias. N Engl J Med 1981;305:131.

60. Devereux RB, Brown WT, Kramer-Fox R, Sachs I. Inheritance of mitral valve prolapse: effect of age and sex on gene expression. Ann Intern Med 1982;97:826.

61. Loehr JP, Synhorst DP, Wolfe RR, Hagerman RJ. Aortic root dilatation and mitral valve prolapse in the fragile X syndrome. Am J Med Genet 1986;23:189.

62. Barnett HJM, Boughner DR, Taylor DW, et al. Further evidence relating mitral-valve prolapse to cerebral ischemic events. N Engl J Med 1980;302:139.

63. Rice GPA, Ebers GC, Bondar RL, Boughner DR. Mitral valve prolapse: a cause of stroke in children? Dev Med Child Neurol 1981;23:352.

64. Kouvaras G, Bacoulas G. Association of mitral valve leaflet prolapse with cerebral ischaemic events in the young and middle-aged patient. QJM New Series 1985;55:387.

65. Chesler E, King RA, Edwards JE. The myxomatous mitral valve and sudden death. Circulation 1983; 67:632.

66. Levine HJ, Pauker SG, Salzman EW, Eckman MH. Antithrombotic therapy in valvular heart disease. Chest 1992;102(suppl):434S.

67. Greenlee JE, Mandell GL. Neurological manifestations of infective endocarditis. Stroke 1973;4:958.

68. Brandenburg RO, Giuliani ER, Wilson WR, Geraci JE. Infective endocarditis: a 25 year overview of diagnosis and therapy. J Am Coll Cardiol 1983;1:280.

69. Silverman NA, Levitsky R, Mammana R. Acute endocarditis in drug addicts: surgical treatment for multiple valve infection. J Am Coll Cardiol 1984;4:680.

70. Keys TF. Infective endocarditis: a continuing challenge: update on causes, presentation, treatment, and prophylaxis. J Crit Illness 1987;2:18.

71. Lerner P. Neurologic complications of infective endocarditis. Med Clin North Am 1985;69:385.

72. Hacek DT, Lukes AS, Bright DK; Duke Endocarditis Service. New criteria for diagnosis of infective endocarditis: utilization of specific echocardiographic findings. Am J Med 1994;96:200.

73. Corral I, Martin-Davila P, Fortun J, et al. Trends in neurological complications of endocarditis. J Neurol 2007;254:1253.

74. O'Brien JT, Geiser EA. Infective endocarditis and echocardiography. Am Heart J 1984;108:386.

75. Mugge A, Daniel WG, Frank G, Lichtlen PR. Echocardiography in infective endocarditis: reassessment of prognostic implications of vegetation size determined by the transthoracic and the transesophageal approach. J Am Coll Cardiol 1989;14:631.

76. Dickerman SA, Abrutyn E, Barsic B, et al. The relationship between the initiation of antimicrobial therapy and the incidence of stroke in infective endocarditis: an analysis from the ICE Prospective Cohort Study (ICE-PCS). Am Heart J 2007;154:1086.

77. Ruttmann E, Weilleit J, Ulmer H, et al. Neurological outcome of septic cardioembolic stroke after infective endocarditis. Stroke 2006;37:2094.

78. Robbins MJ, Eisenberg ES, Frishman WH. Infective endocarditis: a pathophysiologic approach to therapy. Cardiol Clin 1987;5:545.

79. Wilson WR, Geraci JE, Danielson GK, et al. Anticoagulant therapy and central nervous system complications in patients with prosthetic valve endocarditis. Circulation 1978;57:1004.

80. Carpenter JL, McAllister CK; and the US Army Collaborative Group. Anticoagulation in prosthetic valve endocarditis. South Med J 1983;76:1372.

81. Dalen JE. Valvular heart disease, infected valves and prosthetic heart valves. Am J Cardiol 1990;65:29C.

82. Biller J, Challa VR, Toole JF, Howard VJ. Non-bacterial thrombotic endocarditis: a neurologic perspective of clinicopathologic correlations of 99 patients. Arch Neurol 1982;39:95.

83. Jimenez Caballero PE, Segura MT. Cardioembolic stroke secondary to non-bacterial endocarditis in Wegener disease. Eur J Neurol 2007;14:683.

84. Letsas KP, Filippatos GS, Kounas SP, et al. Primary antiphospholipid syndrome and factor V Leiden mutation in a young patient with non-bacterial thrombotic endocarditis and transient ischemic stroke. Thromb Haemost 2005;94:1331.

85. Jespersen CM, Egeblad H. Mitral annulus calcification and embolism. Acta Med Scand 1987;222:37.

86. Lin CS, Schwartz IS, Chapman I. Calcification of the mitral annulus fibrosus with systemic embolization. Arch Pathol Lab Med 1987;111:411.

87. Benjamin EJ, Plehn JF, D'Agostino RB, et al. Mitral annular calcification and the risk of stroke in an elderly cohort: the Framingham study. N Engl J Med 1992;327:374.

88. Braverman AC, Guven H, Beardslee MA, et al. The bicuspid aortic valve. Curr Probl Cardiol 2005;30:470.

89. Monagle P. Anticoagulation in the young. Heart 2004;90:808.

90. Trines J, Hornberger LK. Evolution of heart disease in utero. Pediatr Cardiol 2004;25:287.

91. Tyler HR, Clark DB. Cerebrovascular accidents in patients with congenital heart disease. AMA Arch Neurol Psychology 1957;77:483.

92. Cohen MM. The central nervous system in congenital heart disease. Neurology 1960;10:452.

93. Martelle RR, Linde LM. Cerebrovascular accidents with tetralogy of Fallot. Am J Dis Child 1961;101:206.

94. Terpian KL. Patterns of brain damage in infants and children with congenital heart disease. Am J Dis Child 1973;125:175.

95. Phornphutkul C, Rosenthal A, Nadas AS, Berenberg W. Cerebrovascular accidents in infants and children with cyanotic congenital heart disease. Am J Cardiol 1973;32:329.

96. Kurlan R, Griggs RC. Cyanotic congenital heart disease with suspected stroke: should all patients receive antibiotics? Arch Neurol 1983;40:209.

97. Reifenstein GH, Levine SA, Gross RE. Coarctation of the aorta: a review of 104 autopsied cases of the "adult type," 2 years of age or older. Am Heart J 1947;33:146.

98. Shearer WT, Rutman JY, Weinberg WA, Goldring D. Coarctation of the aorta and cerebrovascular accident: a proposal for early corrective surgery. Pediatrics 1970;77:1004.

99. Folger GM, Shah KD. Subclavian steal in patients with Blalock-Taussig anastomosis. Circulation 1965;31:241.

100. Wu JC, Child JS. Common congenital heart disorders in adults. Curr Probl Cardiol 2004;29:641.

101. Brickner ME, Hillis LD, Lange RA. Congenital heart disease in adults. Second of two parts. N Engl J Med 2000;342:334.

102. Barker PC, Nowak C, King K, et al. Risk factors for cerebrovascular events following Fontan palliation in patients with a functional single ventricle. Am J Cardiol 2005;96:587.

103. Jenkins NP, Ward C. Coarctation of the aorta: natural history and outcome after surgical treatment. QJM 1997;92:365.

104. Braverman AC, Guven H, Beardslee MA, et al. The bicuspid aortic valve. Curr Probl Cardiol 2005;30:470.

105. Latson LA. Aortic stenosis: valvar, supravalvar, and fibromuscular subvalvar. In Garson A, Bricker JT, Fisher DJ, Neish SR, eds. The Science and Practice of Pediatric Cardiology. Baltimore: Williams & Wilkins, 1998.

106. Pagon RA, Bennett FC, LaVeck B, et al. Williams syndrome: features in late childhood and adolescence. Pediatrics 1987;80:85.

107. Phillips SJ, Whisnant JP, O'Fallon WM, Frye RL. Prevalence of cardiovascular disease and diabetes mellitus in residents of Rochester, Minnesota. Mayo Clin Proc 1990;65:344.

108. Sherman DG, Goldman L, Whiting RB, et al. Thromboembolism in patients with atrial fibrillation. Arch Neurol 1984;41:708.

109. Radford DJ, Izukawa T. Atrial fibrillation in children. Pediatrics 1977;59:250.

110. Wolf PA, Dawber TR, Thamer Jr HE, Kannel WB. Epidemiologic assessment of chronic atrial fibrillation and risk of stroke. The Framingham study. Neurology 1978;28:973.

111. Hinton RC, Kistler JP, Fallon JT, et al. Influence of etiology of atrial fibrillation on incidence of systemic embolism. Am J Cardiol 1977;40:509.

112. Stroke Prevention in Atrial Fibrillation (SPAF) Investigators (B). Predictors of thromboembolism in atrial fibrillation, II: echocardiographic features of patients at risk. Ann Intern Med 1992;116:6.

113. Petersen P, Boysen G, Godtfredsen J, et al. Placebo-controlled, randomized trial of warfarin and aspirin for prevention of thromboembolic complications in chronic atrial fibrillation. The Copenhagen AFASAK Study. Lancet 1989;1:176.

114. Stroke Prevention in Atrial Fibrillation (SPAF) Investigators. Preliminary report of the Stroke Prevention in Atrial Fibrillation Study. N Engl J Med 1990;322:863.

115. Boston Area Anticoagulation Trial for Atrial Fibrillation (BAATAF) Investigators. The effect of low dose warfarin on the risk of stroke in patients with nonrheumatic atrial fibrillation. N Engl J Med 1990;323:1505.

116. Connolly SI, Laupacis A, Gent M, et al; for the CAFA Study coinvestigators. Canadian Atrial Fibrillation Anticoagulation (CAFA) Study. J Am Coll Cardiol 1991;18:340.
117. Ezekowitz MD, Bridgers SL, James KE, et al; for the Veterans Affairs Stroke Prevention in Non-rheumatic Atrial Fibrillation Investigators. Warfarin in the prevention of stroke associated with non-rheumatic atrial fibrillation. N Engl J Med 1992;11:1406.
118. Laupacis A, Albers G, Dunn M, Feinberg W. Antithrombotic therapy in atrial fibrillation. Chest 1992;102(suppl):426S.
119. Albers GW, Sherman DC, Gress DR, et al. Stroke prevention in non-valvular atrial fibrillation: a review of prospective randomized trials. Ann Neurol 1991;30:511.
120. Sherman DG, Dyken ML, Fisher M, et al. Antithrombotic therapy for cerebrovascular disorders. Chest 1992;102(suppl):529S.
121. Singer DE, Albers GW, Dalen JE, et al. Antithrombotic therapy in atrial fibrillation: The seventh ACCP conference on antithrombotic and thrombolytic therapy. Chest 2004;3(suppl):429S.
122. Gage BF, Waterman AD, Shannon W, et al. Validation of clinical classification schemes for predicting stroke. Results from the National Registry of Atrial Fibrillation. JAMA 2001;285:2864.
123. Rubenstein JL, Schulman CL, Yurchak PM, DeSanctis RW. Clinical spectrum of the sick sinus syndrome. Circulation 1972;46:5.
124. Fairfax AJ, Lambert CD, Leatham A. Systemic embolism in chronic sinoatrial disorder. N Engl J Med 1976;295:190.
125. Fairfax AJ, Lambert CD. Neurological aspects of sinoatrial heart block. J Neurol Neurosurg Psychiatry 1976;39:576.
126. Greenspan AJ, Hart RG, Dawson D, et al. Predictors of stroke in patients paced for sick sinus syndrome. J Am Coll Cardiol 2004;43:1617.
127. Ferrer MI. Sick sinus syndrome. J Cardiovasc Med 1981;6:743.
128. Ghali JK, Shanes JG. A review of dilated cardiomyopathy. Compr Ther 1987;13:46.
129. Varon J, Fromm RE. Cardiomyopathies in the ICU. Hosp Physician 1992;March:23.
130. Johnson RA, Palacios I. Dilated cardiomyopathies of the adult. First of two parts. N Engl J Med 1982;307:1051.
131. Johnson RA, Palacios I. Dilated cardiomyopathies of the adult. Second of two parts. N Engl J Med 1982;307:1119.
132. Maron BJ, Towbin JA, Thiene G, et al. Contemporary definitions and classification of the cardiomyopathies. An American Heart Association Scientific Statement. Circulation 2006;113:1807.
133. Grabowski A, Kilian J, Strank C, et al. Takotsubo cardiomyopathy—a rare cause of cardioembolic stroke. Cerebrovasc Dis 2007;24:146.
134. Hodgman MT, Pessin MS, Homans DC, et al. Cerebral embolism as the initial manifestation of peripartum cardiomyopathy. Neurology 1982;32:668.
135. Ashkenazi A, Frydman M, Weitz R, et al. Myocarditis and acute infantile hemiparesis. Helv Paediat Acta 1984;39:491.
136. Rice GPA, Ebers GC, Newland F, Wysocki GP. Recurrent cerebral embolism in cardiac amyloidosis. Neurology 1981;31:904.
137. Bern C, Montgomery SP, Herwaldt BL, et al. Evaluation and treatment of Chagas disease in the United States: a systematic review. JAMA 2007;298:2171.
138. Crawford TC, Smith WT 4th, Velazquez EJ, et al. Prognostic usefulness of left ventricular thrombus by echocardiography in dilated cardiomyopathy in predicting stroke, transient ischemic attack, and death. Am J Cardiol 2004;93:500.
139. Fuster V, Gersh BJ, Giuliani ER, et al. The natural history of idiopathic dilated cardiomyopathy. Am J Cardiol 1981;47:525.
140. Pullicino PM, Halperin JL, Thompson JL. Stroke in patients with heart failure and reduced left ventricular ejection fraction. Neurology 2000;54:288.
141. Thatai D, Ahooja V, Pullicino PM. Pharmacological prevention of thromboembolism in patients with left ventricular dysfunction. Am J Cardiovasc Drugs 2006;6:41.
142. McAllen PM, Marshall J. Cerebrovascular incidents after myocardial infarction. J Neurol Neurosurg Psychiatry 1977;40:951.
143. Thompson PL, Robinson JS. Stroke after acute myocardial infarction: relation to infarct size. BMJ 1978;2:457.
144. Komrad MS, Coffey E, Coffey KS, et al. Myocardial infarction and stroke. Neurology 1984;34:1403.
145. Puletti M, Morocutti C, Tronca M, et al. Cerebrovascular accidents in acute myocardial infarction. Ital J Neurol Sci 1987;8:245.
146. O'Connor CM, Califf RM, Massey EW, et al. Stroke and acute myocardial infarction in the thrombolytic era: clinical correlates and long-term prognosis. J Am Coll Cardiol 1990;16:533.
147. Behar S, Tanne D, Abinader E, et al. Cerebrovascular accident complicating acute myocardial infarction: incidence, clinical significance, and short-and-long-term mortality rates. Am J Med 1991;91:45.
148. Westerhout CM, Hernandez AV, Steyerberg EW, et al. Predictors of stroke within 30 days in patients with non-ST-segment elevation acute coronary syndromes. Eur Heart J 2006;27:2956.
149. Sampson UK, Pfeffer MA, McMurray JJ, et al. Predictors of stroke in high-risk patients after acute myocardial infarction: insights from the VALIANT Trial. Eur Heart J 2007;28:685.
150. Marriott E, Schneck MJ, Barron L, et al. Left ventricular thrombus discovered on chest computed tomography for presumed cryptogenic stroke. J Stroke Cerebrovasc Dis 2006;15:41.
151. Asinger RW, Mikeli FL, Elsperger J, Hodges M. Incidence of left ventricular thrombosis after acute transmural myocardial infarction. N Engl J Med 1981;305:297.

152. Stratton JR, Resnick AD. Increased embolic risk in patients with left ventricular thrombi. Circulation 1987;75:1004.

153. Ezekowitz MD. Acute infarction, left ventricular thrombus and systemic embolization: an approach to management. J Am Coll Cardiol 1985;5:1281.

154. Cairns JA, Hirsh J, Lewis HD, et al. Antithrombotic agents in coronary artery disease. Chest 1992;102 (suppl):456S.

155. Kawasaki T. Acute febrile mucocutaneous syndrome with lymphoid involvement with specific desquamation of the fingers and toes in children (Japanese). Jpn J Allergy 1967;16:178.

156. Nakashima M, Takashima S, Hashimoto K, Shiraishi M. Association of stroke and myocardial infarction in children. Neuropediatrics 1982;13:47.

157. Zeluff GW, Caskey CT, Jackson D. Heart attack or stroke in a young man? Think Fabry's disease. Heart Lung 1978;7:1056.

158. Davis RW, Ebert PA. Ventricular aneurysm—a clinical-pathologic correlation. Am J Cardiol 1972;29:1.

159. Simpson MT, Oberman A, Kouchoukos NT, Rogers WJ. Prevalence of mural thrombi and systemic embolization with left ventricular aneurysm: effect of anticoagulation therapy. Chest 1980;77:463.

160. Lapeyre AC III, Steele PM, Kazmier FJ, et al. Systemic embolism in chronic left ventricular aneurysm: incidence and the role of anticoagulation. J Am Coll Cardiol 1985;6:534.

161. Kleid JJ, Klugman J, Haas J, Battock D. Familial atrial myxoma. Am J Cardiol 1973;32:361.

162. Siltanen P, Tuuteri L, Norio R, et al. Atrial myxoma in a family. Am J Cardiol 1976;38:252.

163. Farah MG. Familial atrial myxoma. Ann Intern Med 1975;83:358.

164. Powers JC, Falkoff M, Heinle RA, et al. Familial cardiac myxoma: emphasis on unusual clinical manifestations. J Thorac Cardiovasc Surg 1979;5:782.

165. Ekinci EI, Donnan GA. Neurological manifestations of cardiac myxoma: a review of the literature and report of cases. Intern Med J 2004;34:243.

166. Steinmetz EF, Calanchini PR, Aguilar MJ. Left atrial myxoma as a neurological problem: a case report and review. Stroke 1973;4:451.

167. Damasio H, Seabra-Gomes R, da Silva JP, et al. Multiple cerebral aneurysms and cardiac myxoma. Arch Neurol 1975;32:269.

168. Desousa AL, Muller J, Campbell RL, et al. Atrial myxoma: a review of the neurological complications, metastases, and recurrences. J Neurol Neurosurg Psychiatry 1978;41:1119.

169. Sandok BA, von Estorff I, Giuliani ER. CNS embolism due to atrial myxoma. Arch Neurol 1980;37:485.

170. Sutton MGSJ, Mercier LA, Giuliani ER, Lie JT. Atrial myxomas: a review of clinical experience in 40 patients. Mayo Clin Proc 1980;55:371.

171. Sandok BA, von Estorff I, Giuliani ER. Subsequent neurological events in patients with atrial myxoma. Ann Neurol 1980;3:305.

172. Knepper LE, Biller J, Adams HP Jr, Bruno A. Neurologic manifestations of atrial myxoma: a 12-year experience and review. Stroke 1988;11:1435.

173. Pinede L, Duhaut P, Loire R. Clinical presentation of left atrial cardiac myxoma: a series of 112 consecutive cases. Medicine 2001;80:159.

174. Herbst M, Wattjes MP, Urbach H, et al. Cerebral embolism from left atrial myxoma leading to cerebral and retinal aneurysms: a case report. AJNR Am J Neuroradiol 2005;26:666.

175. Casey M, Mah C, Merliss AD, et al. Identification of a novel genetic locus for familial cardiac myxomas and Carney complex. Circulation 1998;98:2560.

176. Kandt RS, Gebarski SS, Goetting MG. Tuberous sclerosis with cardiogenic cerebral embolism: magnetic resonance imaging. Neurology 1985;35:1223.

177. Quigley MM, Schwartzman E, Boswell PD, et al. A unique atrial primary cardiac lymphoma mimicking myxoma presenting with embolic stroke—a case report. Blood 2003;101:4708.

178. Burri H, Vuille C, Sierra J. Papillary fibroelastoma as a cause of cardioembolic stroke. Heart 2002;88:216.

179. Kanarek SE, Wright P, Liu J, et al. Multiple fibroelastomas: a case report and review of the literature. J Am Soc Echocardiogr 2003;16:373.

180. Dehnee AE, Brizendine S, Herrera CJ. Recurrent strokes in a young patient with papillary fibroelastoma: a case report and literature review. Echocardiography 2006;23:592.

181. Pasquino S, Balucani C, di Bella I, et al. Cardiac hemangioma of the right atrium: a possible cause of cerebellar stroke. Cerebrovasc Dis 2007;24:154.

182. Hayek ER, Hughes MM, Speakman ED, et al. Cardiac paraganglioma presenting with acute myocardial infarction and stroke. Ann Thorac Surg 2007;83:1882.

183. Binder J, Pfleger S, Schwarz S. Images in cardiovascular medicine: right atrial primary cardiac lymphoma presenting with stroke. Circulation 2004;110:e451.

184. Royden Jones H, Caplan LR, Come PC, et al. Cerebral emboli of paradoxical origin. Ann Neurol 1983;13:314.

185. Biller J, Adams HP Jr, Johnson MR, et al. Paradoxical cerebral embolism: eight cases. Neurology 1986;36:1356.

186. Biller J, Johnson MR, Adams HP Jr, et al. Further observations on cerebral or retinal ischemia in patients with right-left intracardiac shunts. Arch Neurol 1987;44:740.

187. Lynch JJ, Schuchard GH, Gross CM, Wann LS. Prevalence of right-to-left atrial shunting in a healthy population: detection by Valsalva maneuver contrast echocardiography. Am J Cardiol 1984;53:1478.

188. Movsowitz C, Podolsky LA, Meyerowitz CB, et al. Patent foramen ovale: a nonfunctional embryological remnant or a potential cause of significant pathology? J Am Soc Echocardiogr 1992;5:259.

189. Feldman T, Borow KM. Atrial septal defect in adults: symptoms, signs, and natural history. Cardiovasc Med 1985;7:31.

190. Harvey JR, Teague SM, Anderson JL, et al. Clinically silent atrial septal defects with evidence for cerebral embolization. Ann Intern Med 1986;105:695.

191. Belkin RN, Hurwitz BJ, Kisslo J. Atrial septal aneurysm: association with cerebrovascular and peripheral embolic events. Stroke 1987;18:856.

192. Di Pasquale G, Andreoli A, Grazi P, et al. Cardioembolic stroke from atrial septal aneurysm. Stroke 1988;19:640.

193. Webster MWI, Chancellor AM, Smith HJ, et al. Patent foramen ovale in young stroke patients. Lancet 1988;2:11.

194. Lechat PH, Mas JL, Lascault G, et al. Prevalence of patent foramen ovale in patients with stroke. N Engl J Med 1988;318:1148.

195. Kizer JR, Deveruex RB. Patent foramen ovale in young adults with unexplained stroke. N Engl J Med 2005;353:2361.

196. Horton SC, Bunch TJ. Patent foramen ovale and stroke. Mayo Clin Proc 2004;79:79.

197. Messe SR, Silverman IE, Kizer JR, et al: Practice parameter: recurrent stroke with patient foramen ovale and atrial septal aneurysm: report of the Quality Standards Subcommittee of the American Academy of Neurology. Neurology 2004;62:1042.

198. Handke M, Harloff A, Olschewski M, et al. Patent foramen ovale and cryptogenic stroke in older patients. N Engl J Med 2007;357:2262.

199. Mas J-L, Arquizan C, Lamy C, et al. Recurrent cerebrovascular events associated with patent foramen ovale, atrial septal aneurysm or both. N Engl J Med 2001;345:1740.

200. Homma S, Sacco RL, Di Tullio MR, et al. Effect of medical treatment in stroke patients with PFO. PFO in Cryptogenic Stroke Study. Circulation 2002;105:2625.

201. Mohr JP, Thompson JLP, Lazar RM, et al. Warfarin-Aspirin Recurrent Stroke Study. N Engl J Med 2001;345:1444.

202. Cujec B, Mainra R, Johnson DH. Prevention of recurrent cerebral ischemic events in patients with patent foramen ovale and cryptogenic strokes or transient ischemic attacks. Can J Cardiol 1999;15:57.

203. Schneck MJ, DiSavino EM, Moore CG, et al. Recurrence rates in patients with patent foramen ovale (PFO) and cryptogenic stroke or transient ischemia (TIA). American Heart Association Scientific Sessions, 2002.

204. Maisel WH, Laskey WK. Patent foramen ovale closure devices: moving beyond equipoise. JAMA 2005;294:366.

205. Flachskampf FA, Daniel WG. Closure of patent foramen ovale: is the case really closed as well. Heart 2005;91:449.

206. McDaniel NL. Ventricular and atrial septal defects. Pediatr Rev 2001;22:265.

207. Wu JC, Child JS. Common congenital heart disorders in adults. Curr Probl Cardiol 2004;29:641.

208. Adams HP Jr, Bosch EP. Neurologic aspects of hereditary hemorrhagic telangiectasia: report of two cases. Arch Neurol 1977;34:101.

209. Roman G, Fisher M, Perl DP, et al. Neurological manifestations of hereditary hemorrhagic telangiectasia (Rendu-Osler-Weber disease): report of two cases and review of the literature. Ann Neurol 1978;4:130.

210. Shub C, Tajik AJ, Seward JB, Dines DE. Detecting intrapulmonary right-to-left shunt with contrast echocardiography: observations in a patient with diffuse pulmonary arteriovenous fistulas. Mayo Clin Proc 1976;51:81.

211. Love BB, Biller JB, Landas SK, Hoover WH. Diagnosis of pulmonary arteriovenous malformation by ultrafast chest computed tomography in Rendu-Osler-Weber syndrome with cerebral ischemia: a case report. Angiology 1992;6:522.

212. Biller J, Johnson MR, Adams HPJr, et al. Echocardiographic evaluation of young adults with nonhemorrhagic cerebral infarction. Stroke 1986;17:608.

213. Sirna S, Biller J, Skorton D, Seabold JE. Cardiac evaluation of the patient with stroke. Stroke 1990;21:14.

214. Barinagarrementeria F, Diaz F, Vargas J, Samayoa E. Prevalence of patent foramen ovale in young patients with stroke: role of color-flow echocardiography. J Stroke Cerebrovasc Dis 1992;2:7.

215. Chimowitz MI, Nemec JJ, Marwick TH, et al. Transcranial Doppler ultrasound identifies patients with right-to-left cardiac or pulmonary shunts. Neurology 1991;41:1902.

216. Breuer AC, Furlan AJ, Hanson MR, et al. Central nervous system complications of coronary artery bypass surgery: prospective analysis of 421 patients. Stroke 1983;14:682.

217. Sila CA, Furlan AJ. Neurological complications in patients with cardiovascular procedures. In Adams HP Jr, ed. Handbook of Cerebrovascular Diseases. New York: Marcel Dekker, 1993.

218. Jarquin-Valdivia AA, Wijdicks EF, McGregor C. Neurologic complications following heart transplantation in the modern era: decreased incidence, but postoperative stroke remains prevalent. Transplant Proc 1999;31:2161.

219. Inoue K, Luth JU, Pottkamper D, et al. Incidence and risk factors of perioperative cerebral complications: heart transplantation compared to coronary artery bypass grafting and valve surgery. J Cardiovasc Surg 1998;39:201.

220. Drummond DS, Salter RB, Boone J. Fat embolism in children: its frequency and relationships to collagen disease. Can Med Assoc J 1969;101:200.

221. Limbird TI, Ruderman RJ. Fat embolism in children. Clin Orthop 1978;136:267.

CHAPTER 8

Cerebral Infarction and Migraine

Rima M. Dafer • José Biller

KEY TERMS

CADASIL	cerebral autosomal dominant arteriopathy with subcortical infarcts and leukoencephalopathy
CADASILM	cerebral autosomal dominant arteriopathy with subcortical infarcts, leukoencephalopathy, and migraine
CSD	cortical spreading depression
CT	computed tomography
ICHD-II	*International Classification of Headache Disorders, second edition*
MELAS	mitochondrial encephalopathy, lactic acidosis, and strokelike episodes
MERRF	mitochondrial encephalopathy and ragged red fibers
MRI	magnetic resonance imaging
MTHFR	methylene tetrahydrofolate reductase
PFO	patent foramen ovale

Migraine is a common paroxysmal headache disorder of uncertain pathogenesis, which has been linked to cerebral ischemia. The occurrence of cerebral infarction during the course of a typical migraine attack has been well described based on clinical, radiologic, and pathologic evidence. It remains unclear whether migraine is a risk factor for ischemic stroke, or whether migraine may occur as a consequence of conditions that are known to cause stroke. It is unclear whether ischemia results in migraine, or whether migraine results in ischemia. Data from observational studies identified migraine as an independent risk factor for ischemic stroke. Young patients with migraine, particularly with aura, are at increased risk for ischemic stroke, particularly in the subgroup of patients of childbearing age and on oral contraceptives. More recent data have shown that migraineurs, in particular those who report auras, are at higher risk of showing white matter abnormalities on magnetic resonance imaging (MRI) than subjects without migraine.

The new *International Classification of Headache Disorders* (ICHD-II) has permitted a more homogeneous separation of cases on which more accurate epidemiologic, clinical, and therapeutic data are being obtained (Table 8-1).[1] Migrainous stroke is diagnosed when a patient develops persistent irreversible aura, with neuroimaging findings consistent with infarction in the appropriate brain territory, and when all other possible causes and mechanisms of stroke have been eliminated.

TABLE 8-1 **Classification of Migraine as Proposed by the International Headache Society**

1.1	Migraine without aura
1.2	Migraine with aura
1.2.1	Typical aura with migraine headache
1.2.2	Typical aura with nonmigraine headache
1.2.3	Typical aura without headache
1.2.4	Familial hemiplegic migraine
1.2.5	Sporadic hemiplegic migraine
1.2.6	Basilar-type migraine
1.3	Childhood periodic syndromes that are commonly precursors of migraine
1.3.1	Cyclic vomiting
1.3.2	Abdominal migraine
1.3.3	Benign paroxysmal vertigo of childhood
1.4	Retinal migraine
1.5	Complications of migraine
1.5.1	Chronic migraine
1.5.2	Status migrainosus
1.5.3	Persistent aura without infarction
1.5.4	Migraine-triggered seizure
1.6	Probable migraine
1.6.1	Probable migraine without aura
1.6.2	Probable migraine with aura
1.6.3	Probable chronic migraine

Note that in the ICHD-II ophthalmoplegic migraine is classified under cranial neuralgias and central causes of facial pain (13.17).

From The International Classification of Headache Disorders, 2nd ed. Cephalalgia 2004;24(suppl 1):9.

The causal relationship between migraine and stroke is likely complex, and the precise pathophysiologic mechanisms leading to cerebral infarction remain obscure. This chapter summarizes the epidemiologic, clinical, and therapeutic aspects of migrainous infarction. We specifically discuss the link of migraine to ischemic stroke because the occurrence of other types of stroke, such as intracerebral hemorrhage or subarachnoid hemorrhage, during an attack of migraine is very rare and remains controversial.[2] Well-documented cases of intracerebral hemorrhage in association with a migrainous attack have been reported to occur, which, given the prevalence of migraine in the population at large, hardly constitute enough evidence to implicate an association between them.[3-8]

Diagnostic Criteria for Migrainous Infarction

The current diagnostic criteria for migrainous infarction are those set forth by the

TABLE 8-2 **Diagnostic Criteria for Migrainous Infarction**

Previously established diagnosis of migraine with aura
Infarction must occur during the course of a typical migraine aura attack
One or more aura symptoms persist for >60 min
Neuroimaging confirmation of ischemic infarction in relevant location
Other causes of infarction must be excluded

From The International Classification of Headache Disorders, 2nd ed. Cephalalgia 2004;24(suppl 1):9.

ICHD-II classification[1] and depicted in Table 8-2. Charcot has been given credit for making the observation that any of the transient neural dysfunctions of migraine, such as hemianopsia, aphasia, sensory disorders, and paralyses, could become permanent, setting the stage for establishing migraine as a potential cause of cerebral infarction.[9] As our concepts of this phenomenon have evolved, it has become evident that a cerebral infarction may occur during the course of a typical migraine attack, constituting a true migrainous infarction. Other circumstances may prevail, however, such as the coexistence of other risk factors for ischemic infarction, including hypertension, diabetes, heart disease, tobacco use, oral contraceptive use, presence of antiphospholipid antibodies, and presence of a patent foramen ovale (PFO), in a patient who also has migraine.

In such cases, it is difficult to establish what role, if any, migraine has in the causation of the infarction, or whether it acts together with the other risk factors to promote cerebral ischemia. In other instances, new or established structural nervous system disease (i.e., arteriovenous malformation, cerebral contusion, meningoencephalitis, metabolic encephalopathies, cerebral ischemia from atherosclerotic and nonatherosclerotic vasculopathies) may mimic the symptoms of migraine and lead to a cerebral infarction as well. In such cases, the morbid structural disturbance triggers a migrainous attack as part of its clinical presentation, which may culminate in a fixed neurologic ischemic deficit. These situations constitute the basis of the current classification of migrainous infarction initially postulated by Welch and Levine (Table 8-3).[10]

TABLE 8-3 **Classification of Migrainous Infarction**

Coexisting infarction and migraine (e.g., patent foramen ovale)
Infarction with clinical features of migraine
Established (symptomatic migraine) (e.g., CADASIL, MELAS)
New onset (migraine mimic) (e.g., cervicocephalic arterial dissection, vasculitis)
Migraine-induced infarction
    Without risk factors
    With risk factors
    Uncertain/complex

From Welch KM, Levine SR. Migraine-related stroke in the context of the International Headache Society classification of head pain. Arch Neurol 1990;47:458.

Epidemiology of Migrainous Infarction

Migraine and stroke are common neurologic conditions, with 1-year prevalence for migraine of 121 per 1000 in the general population, and a stroke incidence of 750,000 a year in the United States. The real lifetime risk of stroke among migraineurs is unknown. It is estimated that 1% to 17% of strokes in patients younger than age 50 years can be attributed to migraine. Previous series have included cases that do not fulfill the strict criteria of the International Headache Society classification and are likely to be misleading probably by having overdiagnosed the condition. Without specific criteria, one is likely to diagnose a migrainous infarction in every migraineur who has a stroke, rather than labeling it as cryptogenic. True migrainous infarction is a rare event, however, and an idea of its true incidence can be gleaned from the following available data: The annual incidence of ischemic cerebral infarctions in young adults (i.e., <45 years old) is roughly 24 cases per year per 100,000.[11-14] In the United States, the average annual incidence rates of all strokes in individuals younger than age 55 years was 113.8 per 100 000, whereas that for cerebral infarction was 73.1 per 100, 000.[15-21] A report of the World Health Organization (WHO) MONICA Project documented that stroke incidence varied from 48 to 240 per 100,000 individuals 45 to 54 years old in 10 countries involved.[22]

The point prevalence of migraine in the United States is about 11%, which translates to about 33 million people,[23] with migraine with aura accounting for one third of cases, which is the type of migraine that most likely would lead to cerebral infarction; about 8 million people are at risk of having a migrainous infarction.[24,25] The incidence of migrainous infarction is 1.44 cases per year per 100,000 population, increasing to 3.36 cases per year per 100,000 in the presence of other stroke risk factors. The average annual incidence rate was 11.4 per 100,000 among individuals 15 to 49 years old, whereas the average annual incidence rate among individuals 15 to 44 years old was 6.9 per 100,000. In the Women's Health Study, migraine with aura was associated with increased risk of major cardiovascular disease, myocardial infarction, ischemic stroke, and death due to ischemic cardiovascular disease, and with coronary revascularization and angina. Such association was not present in migraine without aura.[26] Such risk is more common in women, in patients 45 years old or younger,[13,20,21,27-30] and in women on oral contraceptives,[31-36] and is less well recognized in children[37] and elderly individuals.[38]

Clinical Picture

The spectrum of neurologic symptoms that may be seen as part of migraine is varied and is a subject that has been pondered to the point of exhaustion.[39,40] When migraine is associated with neurologic symptoms, other than the headache, it is referred to as migraine with aura. When only premonitory symptoms occur in association with the headache, it is referred to as migraine without aura. As depicted in Table 8-1, the migraine aura may occur without a headache.

Based on the 2004 ICHD-II, migrainous infarctions occur in the setting of typical prolonged and persistent aura. The most common migrainous auras involve the visual and somatosensory systems, occurring in 40% and 30% of patients with migraine with aura. A full range of strokelike symptoms in migraine encompasses visual and sensory hallucinations, symptoms of brainstem dysfunction, motor symptoms, and abnormalities in higher integrative functions (perception, ideation, memory, and speech).[39,40]

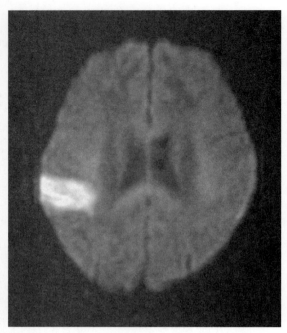

FIGURE 8-1 MRI showing an area of restricted diffusion in the territory of the right middle cerebral artery consistent with acute infarction in a migraine patient with patent foramen ovale.

Permanent visual field deficits from infarcts in the territory of the posterior cerebral arteries and sensorimotor deficits with or without language disturbances from infarcts in the territory of the middle cerebral arteries constitute greater than 80% of the cases (Fig. 8-1). Most of the remaining cases predominantly involve the vertebrobasilar arterial territory. Another salient feature of migrainous infarcts is that they have only rarely been associated with a fatal outcome,[41,42] and generally have a good functional outcome.

Pathophysiology

The mechanism of stroke in migraine is complex and remains unclear. As previously alluded to, the main problem yet to be resolved regarding the role of migraine in cerebral infarction is whether it is directly responsible for inducing ischemia, or whether it merely acts as a risk factor, which when associated with other risk factors or abnormalities may act in concert with them to produce the infarct. Data obtained from the clinical profile of patients having a neurologic deficit during a migraine attack together with paraclinical information obtained from cerebral blood flow measurements, cerebral angiograms, computed tomography (CT) and MRI, and hematologic studies, all point to migraine as being responsible for the infarct. The problem is how?

The prevalent theories surrounding migraine pathogenesis are the vascular, the neurochemical, and the neural theories.[43-49] None of these is sufficiently persuasive to account for the clinical behavior of the complex and varied symptoms. The most appealing explanation is to combine all three theories because the attack of migraine is a complex cascade of events (premonitory symptoms, prodrome, aura, headache, post-ictal state, and recovery), each one possibly triggered by different mechanisms. A primary "spontaneous" neuronal depolarization (initiated by the many known triggering factors) could lead to a secondary release of myriad neurotransmitters, each responsible for modifying a certain physiologic parameter at the neuronal, vascular, or endocrine levels. Although the occurrence of cerebral infarcts supports the vascular hypothesis, the point to be made is that the vascular phenomena are probably secondary to neural activity with the intermediary action of neurotransmitters. Exactly why this sequence of events may lead to infarction in only a small percentage of migraineurs has not been deciphered.

There is preliminary clinical evidence to suggest that cerebral ischemia induced by atherosclerotic or nonatherosclerotic vasculopathies may be responsible for triggering a migraine attack with aura (symptomatic migraine) more commonly than migraine-induced ischemic insults.[50] These observations make it all the more important to investigate patients who develop permanent neurologic symptoms during a migraine attack to exclude disease that may be triggering it.

More recent data suggest that brain ischemia in migraine patients may be induced by cortical spreading depression (CSD).[51,52] Magnetoencephalography and blood oxygen level–dependent MRI data strongly suggest that an electrophysiologic event such as CSD generates the aura in the human visual cortex.[53] This neuroelectric event may arise spontaneously, or may be visually triggered in widespread regions of hyperexcitable occipital cortex[54] during a migraine attack, with spreading suppression of initial neuronal activation and increased occipital cortex oxygenation.[55] This phenomenon suggests that oligemia plays a role in the mechanism of infarction in migraine and potentially may explain the predilection of strokes among migraineurs to the posterior circulation.[56] Other potential mechanisms include disruption of the blood-brain barrier via a matrix metalloproteinase-2, 9 (MMP-9)–dependent mechanism[57] after an intense neuronal and glial depolarization during migraine.[58]

The relationship of changes in platelet activity to the pathophysiology of migraine-induced infarcts seems to have weakened over the years. Despite the weak evidence that a causal relationship exists between platelet physiology and migraine,[59] recent literature suggests that platelet activation and pro-inflammatory platelet adhesion to leukocytes[58,60-63] and elevated von Willebrand factor occurs during the interictal phase of migraine.[64,65]

In association with the concept of focal ischemia triggering migraine with aura is the relationship between migraine and cervicocephalic arterial dissections. It has been postulated that repeated episodes of migraine with aura with its attendant vascular phenomena may, with time, predispose to "spontaneous" dissection by weakening of the intimal–elastic lamina portion of the vessel.[66-69] In most of these cases, however, the migraine attack has not occurred at the same time as the dissection, or, if it did, the neurologic deficit was reversible. Arterial dissections occasionally may trigger or mimic a migraine attack, rather the latter causing the dissection.

Another type of disorder in migraine-like headaches in association with strokelike episodes is the mitochondrial encephalomyopathies, in particular MELAS (mitochondrial encephalopathy, lactic acidosis, and strokelike episodes), which has led to speculation that migraine might be the result of an incomplete defect in mitochondrial DNA.[70] In contrast to this observation is the vascular territorial location of infarcts in migraine versus the nonterritorial

location and the progressive or recurrent nature of the infarcts in the mitochondrial encephalomyopathies.[71-74] This may be another example of a migraine "mimic," rather than a migrainous infarction.

Similarly, migraine with aura is one of the clinical hallmarks of CADASIL (cerebral autosomal dominant arteriopathy with subcortical infarcts and leukoencephalopathy), an adult-onset autosomal dominant disorder, which, in addition to migraine with aura, is characterized by recurrent transient ischemic attacks and subcortical ischemic strokes, cognitive decline, dementia, and prominent white matter signal abnormalities and subcortical infarctions on brain MRI (Fig. 8-2). CADASIL is due to mutations in the *NOTCH3* gene on chromosome 19q12.[75-78] A new acronym, CADASILM (cerebral autosomal dominant arteriopathy with subcortical infarcts, leukoencephalopathy, and migraine), refers to a subvariety of CADASIL characterized by high frequency of migraine, frequency of psychotic disorders, and early neurologic manifestations.[79] The mechanism of this nonarteriosclerotic, nonamyloid microangiopathy is unknown.

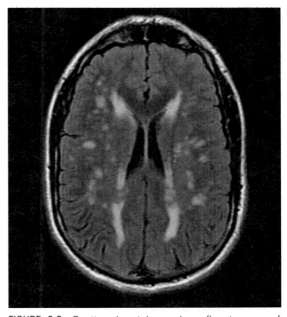

FIGURE 8-2 Scattered patchy and confluent areas of hyperintense signal in the subcortical and periventricular white matter on T2/fluid attenuated inversion recovery MRI in a patient with CADASIL.

Pathologically, there is a characteristic deposition of granular osmiophilic material in arterial walls, including dermal arteries.[80] No treatment is currently available. A clinical trial of cholesterase inhibitor for the treatment of dementia associated with CADASIL has been completed.

Vasospasm has been a frequent angiographic finding during the investigation of patients with a history of migraine-related neurologic symptoms.[81-86] It may be the ultimate derangement in the cascade of events that lead to transient or permanent cerebral ischemia, depending on its duration or compensation from collateral flow or both. The clinician should be cognizant, however, of other pathologic conditions associated with this same angiographic pattern (Table 8-4).

Pari passu, cerebral arteriography has been incriminated as a probable triggering factor for migraine, migrainous infarction, or simply cerebral arterial vasospasm mainly in reports from the 1950s through the 1970s.[87-89] The newer radiologic techniques and safer contrast material later developed have decreased the side effects of angiography for all patients, however. A review of the risks of arteriography in 142 migraine patients during and in between attacks compared with the rate of complications in a prospective series of 1002 patients without migraine revealed no increased risk from arteriography in the patients with migraine.[90] It was suggested in this article that the probable cause of the increased number of complications that was documented in the earlier reports may have been related to the technique of direct carotid arterial puncture used at the time.

Additional risk factors for stroke in migraineurs include history of cigarette smoking,[29,36,91] use of combined oral contraceptives, anticardiolipin antibody immunoreactivity,[92-99] acquired antiphospholipid antibodies and Sneddon syndrome,[100] and hereditary hemorrhagic telangiectasia (Table 8-5).[101] Strokelike migraine attacks also have been described after radiation therapy (SMART syndrome),[102] and migrainous neurologic dysfunction has been described in patients with prosthetic cardiac valves.[103]

The relationship between migraine, estrogen, and stroke in premenopausal women is complex. The risk of ischemic stroke in migraine, in particular migraine with aura, is increased by tobacco smoking and oral contraceptive use. Based on the current evidence, the use of oral contraceptives in young migraineurs is not contraindicated; however, young women with migraine with aura should be warned of the increased risk of stroke while taking oral contraceptives, especially if they are cigarette smokers, and

TABLE 8-4 **Differential Diagnosis of Vasospasm on Angiography**

Subarachnoid hemorrhage
Infectious and noninfectious central nervous system vasculitis
Migraine
Drugs (migraine medications such as ergots, triptans; immunosuppressants such as cyclosporine, cyclophosphamide, tacrolimus; intravenous immunoglobulins, pseudoephedrine, nicotine, phenylpropanolamine, cocaine, amphetamines, lysergic acid derivatives, marijuana)
Severe hypertension (hypertensive encephalopathy, preeclampsia or eclampsia, pheochromocytoma, cocaine)
Cervicocephalic arterial dissection
Central nervous system trauma
Cervicocephalic fibromuscular dysplasia
Cerebral embolization
Postradiation angiitis
Postpartum angiitis
Posterior reversible ischemic encephalopathy
Pregnancy, puerperium, eclampsia, and preeclamptic toxemia of pregnancy

TABLE 8-5 **Migraine and Stroke: Coexisting Disorders and Risk Factors**

Cervicocephalic arterial dissection
Patent foramen ovale
Triptans and ergotamine*
Oral contraceptives and estrogen use
Cigarette smoking
MTHFR deficiency
Hypercoagulability
Mitochondrial disorders (MELAS, MERFF)
CADASIL
Hereditary hemorrhagic telangiectasia
Elevated C-reactive protein
Estrogen receptors
Antiphospholipid antibodies and Sneddon syndrome
Angiotensin-converting enzyme—D allele

*These medications seem to carry low risk of stroke,[104] but should be avoided in individuals with hemiplegic migraine, basilar migraine, vascular risk factors, and prior history of stroke.

should be advised to quit smoking and to switch to low-estrogen formulations or progestagen-only pills.[105]

Several studies have shown that the prevalence of a PFO with a right-to-left shunt in patients with migraine with aura is significantly higher than in patients without migraine.[34,106-108] The prevalence of PFO in patients with migraine with aura is 41% to 48% compared with 16% to 23% in patients with migraine without aura and patients without migraine. Such prevalence is increased in patients younger than age 45 years with a prior history of stroke (52%).

It has been hypothesized that a PFO with right-to-left shunt permits paradoxical microemboli and vasoactive chemicals in the venous circulation to bypass lung filtration, causing excitability of neuronal depolarization and triggering a migraine aura. More recent data from case reports suggested that PFO closure may prevent further attacks of migraine with aura.[34,106-110] A more recently completed randomized, controlled trial failed to reach its primary outcome of resolution of migraine after the intervention, however. Other randomized clinical trials to assess prospectively the benefit of shunt closure in migraine patients are currently ongoing. Nevertheless, the role of PFO closure in stroke prevention per se, regardless of the presence or absence of a history of migraine, remains controversial and is being investigated in randomized clinical trials.

Migraine and White Matter Disease

More recently, data from a population-based, cross-sectional MRI study showed that migraine is an independent risk factor for white matter lesions (adjusted odds ratio 2.1, 95% confidence interval 1.0-4.1) (Fig. 8-3) and subclinical posterior circulation territory infarctions (adjusted odds ratio 13.7, 95% confidence interval 1.7-112), with an increased lesion load with more frequent attacks.[56,111,112]

Investigation of a Patient with a Migraine-Associated Cerebral Infarction

In the clinical setting, "possible" cases of migrainous infarction should undergo an

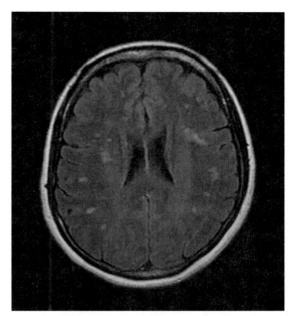

FIGURE 8-3 Subcortical hyperintense signal abnormalities on T2/fluid attenuated inversion recovery in a patient with migraine with aura.

extended diagnostic workup. Because migraine-induced infarction is so rare, and given the other more common eventualities of coexisting stroke and migraine and of stroke with clinical features of migraine, a young migrainous patient who presents with a stroke should be investigated with the assumption in mind that patients with migraine may have strokes caused by many other etiologies, even if it occurred in the throes of a migraine attack, to rule out symptomatic migraine owing to extracranial or intracranial vascular pathology, and to exclude a causal role for other conditions. A complete, yet rational investigation should be performed before attributing the infarct to migraine. In most instances, this investigation requires sophisticated neuroimaging and laboratory testing (Table 8-6).

Management of Migraine-Induced Infarctions

There are insufficient data in the literature to address the acute or long-term management of patients with migraine-induced cerebral infarctions. The reason may be the low incidence of these types of strokes and the difficulty in establishing a firm diagnosis. An empirical approach has been taken in most

TABLE 8-6 **Investigation of a Patient with Suspected Migrainous Infarction**

Laboratory (Update)

Routine: complete blood count, platelet count, serum electrolytes, biochemical profile, erythrocyte sedimentation rate, C-reactive protein, Venereal Disease Research Laboratory, prothrombin time, activated partial thromboplastin time, urinalysis

Special: drug screen, lipid profile, blood cultures, cerebrospinal fluid analysis

Special hematologic studies: hemoglobin electrophoresis, bleeding time, thrombin time

Hypercoagulable state studies: antiphospholipid antibodies (anticardiolipin antibodies IgG, IgA, and IgM) β_2 glycoprotein I antibodies (IgG, IgA, IgM), lupus anticoagulant (or dilute Russell viper venom time), free protein S antigen, protein C activity, antithrombin, prothrombin gene mutation, factor V Leiden, MTHFR, homocysteine, factor VIII, lipoprotein (a), plasminogen activator inhibitor, serum fibrinogen, circulating platelet aggregates, von Willebrand factor antigen and activity

Vasculitis panel: erythrocyte sedimentation rate, antinuclear antibody, antineutrophilic cytoplasmic antibody, anti-SSa and anti-SSb, rheumatoid factor, serum complement level)

Special circumstances: genetic testing for CADASIL, mutation for familial hemiplegic migraine

Imaging Studies

Routine: chest radiograph, carotid duplex ultrasonography, MRI and MR angiography of brain

Special: Transcranial Doppler, cerebral angiography, transesophageal echocardiography, cerebral blood flow metabolism studies (SPECT, PET)

MRI, magnetic resonance imaging; PET, positron emission tomography; SPECT, single photon emission computed tomography.

instances following the general guidelines of preventive migraine therapy. In an acute setting, the management of migraine-induced infarction does not differ from the management of non–migraine-related infarction. Other potential causes for stroke should be excluded. Treatment consists of adequate control of migraine attacks with the reduction of frequency, intensity, and duration. Prophylactic migraine therapy should be initiated.

Because the pathophysiology of migraine-induced infarctions is still marred with the concept that vasospasm is responsible for inducing ischemia, the initial attempt has been to reverse it. Calcium channel antagonists, such as nimodipine, nifedipine, verapamil hydrochloride, and diltiazem hydrochloride, seem promising in the prevention of recurrent migraine attacks, but a definite conclusion regarding their effectiveness cannot yet be made.[113] Flunarizine, a nonselective calcium antagonist that has been extensively studied in numerous controlled clinical studies outside the United States, has been shown to be efficacious in migraine prophylaxis,[114] especially in patients with alternating hemiplegia of childhood. Isolated reports of the reversal of neurologic deficits in hemiplegic migraine using flunarizine are encouraging.[114,115]

β-blockers are commonly used as preventive therapy for recurrent migraine attacks; however, they also have been reported to precipitate strokes.[116-119] Presumably, by blocking central β-receptors, unopposed α-receptor function may lead to further vasoconstriction in individuals with a predisposition to prolonged vasospasm, as may occur in the peripheral circulation in patients with Raynaud phenomenon.[120,121] Further support for this mechanism is the report by Kupersmith and colleagues[122] on the use of the β-antagonist drug isoproterenol hydrochloride to reverse visual auras quickly.

Other migraine preventive therapies, such as topiramate, valproic acid, and amitriptyline, may be useful.[113,123] Lamotrigine was shown to reduce significantly the frequency of aura attacks,[124] and topiramate showed benefit in reducing attacks of alternating hemiplegia of childhood.[125] NR2B-containing N-methyl-D-aspartate receptors, key mediators of CSD, such as memantine and NR2B-selective antagonists, may be useful new therapeutic agents for the treatment of migraine and other CSD-related disorders, such as stroke; however, their efficacy in migraine and migrainous stroke is yet to be determined.[126] Acetazolamide may reduce further attacks of migraine in patients with sporadic and familial hemiplegic migraine[127] and CADASIL.[128,129]

Migraine-specific drugs used to treat acute migraine attacks with marked vasoconstrictive action, such as triptans and ergots, should be avoided. Risk factors should be strictly controlled or, if possible, eliminated, in particular cigarette smoking, and oral contraceptives should be discontinued. Antiplatelet therapies should be administered for secondary stroke prevention. PFO closure in patients with right-to-left shunt is being investigated.

With our current knowledge of the subject, it seems reasonable to state that there is no therapy that has been proved effective in the acute setting of a migraine-induced infarction. Isolated reports of reversal of neurologic deficits with flunarizine warrant further support for its use. None of the other calcium channel antagonists seems encouraging from trials for preventive treatment. Propranolol, topiramate, valproic acid, amitriptyline, and flunarizine are considered to be the most effective compounds for the prophylaxis of migraine in adults. In children, β-blockers, cyproheptadine, amitriptyline, divalproex sodium, topiramate, and levetiracetam lack proof of effectiveness, whereas flunarizine has given positive results in controlled studies. It is probably best to discontinue and avoid further β-blockers in patients in whom the infarct occurs during their administration for prophylaxis. The most crucial point is to exclude other diagnoses associated with vasospasm angiographically in the setting of a migraine attack before instituting any empirical therapy (see Table 8-4).

Conclusion

There is good evidence that migraine with aura is associated with an increased risk of ischemic stroke, mainly among younger individuals. Despite this relationship, migraine remains a benign disorder, and the absolute risk of ischemic stroke is very low. Judicious exclusion of other causes of stroke associated with migraine-like headaches is required. Patients with migraine with aura should be warned of the potential increased risk of stroke while on oral contraceptives. Stroke risk factors should be controlled, and behavioral risk factor modifications, such as smoking cessation, should be encouraged. Although triptans seem to be safe, these medications should be avoided in patients with hemiplegic and basilar migraine and in patients with stroke or cardiac ischemia.[101] Whether patients with migraine with aura should be started on antiplatelets prophylactically, especially

patients with abnormal white matter changes or silent infarctions on MRI, is undetermined.

REFERENCES

1. The International Classification of Headache Disorders, 2nd ed. Cephalalgia 2004;24(suppl 1):9.
2. Carter KN, Anderson N, Jamrozik K, et al. Migraine and risk of subarachnoid haemorrhage: a population-based case-control study. J Clin Neurosci 2005;12:534.
3. Gautier JC, Majdalani A, Juillard JB, Carmi AR. Cerebral hemorrhage in migraine. Rev Neurol (Paris) 1993;149:407.
4. Shuaib A, Metz L, Hing T. Migraine and intracerebral hemorrhage. Cephalalgia 1989;9:59.
5. Furui T, Iwata K. Intracerebral hemorrhage associated with migrainous headache—a case report. Angiology 1993;44:164.
6. Cole AJ, Aube M. Migraine with vasospasm and delayed intracerebral hemorrhage. Arch Neurol 1990;47:53.
7. Nakamura K, Saku Y, Ibayashi S, Fujishima M. Simultaneous multiple brain hemorrhage associated with migraine—a case report. Angiology 1997;48:551.
8. Aldrey JM, Castillo J, Leira R, et al. Cerebral hemorrhage and migraine. Rev Neurol 1996;24:183.
9. Fere C. Contribution a l'étude de la migraine opthalmique. Rev Med Paris 1881;1:40.
10. Welch KM, Levine SR. Migraine-related stroke in the context of the International Headache Society classification of head pain. Arch Neurol 1990;47:458.
11. Levine J, Swanson PD. Non-atherosclerotic causes of stroke. Ann Intern Med 1969;70:807.
12. Hindfelt B, Nilsson O. Brain infarction in young adults (with particular reference to pathogenesis). Acta Neurol Scand 1977;55:145.
13. Snyder B, Ramirez-Lassepas M. Cerebral infarction in young adults. Stroke 1980;11:149.
14. Hart RG, Miller VT. Cerebral infarction in young adults: a practical approach. Stroke 1983;14:110.
15. Weiss W, Weinfeld F. The National Survey of Stroke: introduction. Stroke 1981;12:13.
16. Foulkes MA, Wolf PA, Price TR, et al. The Stroke Data Bank: design, methods, and baseline characteristics. Stroke 1988;19:547.
17. Bogousslavsky J, Pierre P. Ischemic stroke in patients under age 45. Neurol Clin 1992;10:113.
18. Naess H, Nyland HI, Thomassen L, et al. Incidence and short-term outcome of cerebral infarction in young adults in western Norway. Stroke 2002;33:2105.
19. Franck G, Doyen P, Grisar T, Moonen G. Les accidents ischémiques cérébraux du sujet jeune, âgé de moins de quarante-cinq ans. Sem Hop Paris 1983;59:2642.
20. Carolei A, Marini C, De Matteis G. History of migraine and risk of cerebral ischaemia in young adults. The Italian National Research Council

Study Group on Stroke in the Young. Lancet 1996;347:1503.

21. Kurth T, Slomke MA, Kase CS, et al. Migraine, headache, and the risk of stroke in women: a prospective study. Neurology 2005;64:1020.

22. Thorvaldsen P, Asplund K, Kuulasmaa K, et al. Stroke incidence, case fatality, and mortality in the WHO MONICA project. World Health Organization Monitoring Trends and Determinants in Cardiovascular Disease. Stroke 1995;26:361.

23. Kurtzke JF. The current neurologic burden of illness and injury in the United States. Neurology 1982;32:1207.

24. Tentschert S, Wimmer R, Greisenegger S, et al. Headache at stroke onset in 2196 patients with ischemic stroke or transient ischemic attack. Stroke 2005;36:e1.

25. Sochurkova D, Moreau T, Lemesle M, et al. Migraine history and migraine-induced stroke in the Dijon stroke registry. Neuroepidemiology 1999;18:85.

26. Kurth T, Gaziano JM, Cook NR, et al. Migraine and risk of cardiovascular disease in women. JAMA 2006;296:283.

27. Schwaag S, Nabavi DG, Frese A, et al. The association between migraine and juvenile stroke: a case-control study. Headache 2003;43:90.

28. Arboix A, Massons J, Garcia-Eroles L, et al. Migrainous cerebral infarction in the Sagrat Cor Hospital of Barcelona Stroke Registry. Cephalalgia 2003;23:389.

29. Henrich JB, Horwitz RI. A controlled study of ischemic stroke risk in migraine patients. J Clin Epidemiol 1989;42:773.

30. Buring JE, Hebert P, Romero J, et al. Migraine and subsequent risk of stroke in the Physicians' Health Study. Arch Neurol 1995;52:129.

31. Etminan M, Takkouche B, Isorna FC, Samii A. Risk of ischaemic stroke in people with migraine: systematic review and meta-analysis of observational studies. BMJ 2005;330:63.

32. Chang CL, Donaghy M, Poulter N. Migraine and stroke in young women: case-control study. The World Health Organisation Collaborative Study of Cardiovascular Disease and Steroid Hormone Contraception. BMJ 1999;318:13.

33. Donaghy M, Chang CL, Poulter N. Duration, frequency, recency, and type of migraine and the risk of ischaemic stroke in women of childbearing age. J Neurol Neurosurg Psychiatry 2002;73:747.

34. Milhaud D, Bogousslavsky J, van Melle G, Liot P. Ischemic stroke and active migraine. Neurology 2001;57:1805.

35. Tzourio C, Iglesias S, Hubert JB, et al. Migraine and risk of ischaemic stroke: a case-control study. BMJ 1993;307:289.

36. Tzourio C, Tehindrazanarivelo A, Iglesias S, et al. Case-control study of migraine and risk of ischaemic stroke in young women. BMJ 1995;310:830.

37. Ebinger F, Boor R, Gawehn J, Reitter B. Ischemic stroke and migraine in childhood: coincidence or causal relation? J Child Neurol 1999;14:451.

38. Mosek A, Marom R, Korczyn AD, Bornstein N. A history of migraine is not a risk factor to develop an ischemic stroke in the elderly. Headache 2001;41:399.

39. Wilkinson M. Clinical features of migraine. In Vinken PJ, Klawans HL, eds, and Clifford Rose F, co-ed. Handbook of Clinical Neurology. Headache. Amsterdam: Elsevier Science Publishers, 1986.

40. Fernández-Beer E, Saver J, Biller J. Stroke symptoms associated with migraine headaches. Heart Dis Stroke 1993;2:69.

41. Jayamaha JE, Street MK. Fatal cerebellar infarction in a migraine sufferer whilst receiving sumatriptan. Intensive Care Med 1995;21:82.

42. Guest IA, Woolf AL. Fatal infarction of the brain in migraine. BMJ 1964;1:225.

43. Schoenen J. Pathogenesis of migraine: the biobehavioural and hypoxia theories reconciled. Acta Neurol Belg 1994;94:79.

44. Blau JN. Migraine: theories of pathogenesis. Lancet 1992;339:1202.

45. Levine S, Ramadan NM. The relationship of stroke and migraine. In Adams HP, ed. Handbook of Cerebrovascular Diseases. New York: Marcel Dekker, 1993.

46. Welch KM. Pathogenesis of migraine. Semin Neurol 1997;17:335.

47. Welch KM. Concepts of migraine headache pathogenesis: insights into mechanisms of chronicity and new drug targets. Neurol Sci 2003;24(suppl 2):S149.

48. Spierings EL. Pathogenesis of the migraine attack. Clin J Pain 2003;19:255.

49. Longoni M, Ferrarese C. Inflammation and excitotoxicity: role in migraine pathogenesis. Neurol Sci 2006;27(suppl 2):S107.

50. Olesen J, Friberg L, Olsen TS, et al. Ischaemia-induced (symptomatic) migraine attacks may be more frequent than migraine-induced ischaemic insults. Brain 1993;116:187.

51. Olsen TS. Pathophysiology of the migraine aura: the spreading depression theory. Brain 1995;118 (Pt 1):307.

52. Agostoni E, Aliprandi A. The complications of migraine with aura. Neurol Sci 2006;27(suppl 2):S91.

53. Hadjikhani N, Sanchez Del Rio M, Wu O, et al. Mechanisms of migraine aura revealed by functional MRI in human visual cortex. Proc Natl Acad Sci U S A 2001;98:4687.

54. Bowyer SM, Aurora KS, Moran JE, et al. Magnetoencephalographic fields from patients with spontaneous and induced migraine aura. Ann Neurol 2001;50:582.

55. Cao Y, Welch KM, Aurora S, Vikingstad EM. Functional MRI-BOLD of visually triggered headache in patients with migraine. Arch Neurol 1999;56:548.

56. Kruit MC, Launer LJ, Ferrari MD, van Buchem MA. Infarcts in the posterior circulation territory in migraine: the population-based MRI CAMERA study. Brain 2005;128:2068.

57. Gursoy-Ozdemir Y, Qiu J, Matsuoka N, et al. Cortical spreading depression activates and upregulates MMP-9. J Clin Invest 2004;113:1447.

58. Zeller JA, Frahm K, Baron R, et al. Platelet-leuko-cyte interaction and platelet activation in migraine: a link to ischemic stroke? J Neurol Neurosurg Psychiatry 2004;75:984.

59. Joseph R, Welch KM. The platelet and migraine: a nonspecific association. Headache 1987;27:375.

60. Hering-Hanit R, Friedman Z, Schlesinger I, Ellis M. Evidence for activation of the coagulation system in migraine with aura. Cephalalgia 2001; 21:137.

61. Zeller JA, Lindner V, Frahm K, et al. Platelet activation and platelet-leucocyte interaction in patients with migraine: subtype differences and influence of triptans. Cephalalgia 2005;25:536.

62. Sarchielli P, Alberti A, Coppola F, et al. Platelet-activating factor (PAF) in internal jugular venous blood of migraine without aura patients assessed during migraine attacks. Cephalalgia 2004;24:623.

63. Allais G, Facco G, Ciochetto D, et al. Patterns of platelet aggregation in menstrual migraine. Cephalalgia 1997;17(suppl 20):39-41.

64. Tietjen GE, Al-Qasmi MM, Athanas K, et al. Increased von Willebrand factor in migraine. Neurology 2001;57:334.

65. Cesar JM, Garcia-Avello A, Vecino AM, et al. Increased levels of plasma von Willebrand factor in migraine crisis. Acta Neurol Scand 1995;91:412.

66. Mirza Z, Hayward P, Hulbert D. Spontaneous carotid artery dissection presenting as migraine—a diagnosis not to be missed. J Accid Emerg Med 1998;15:187.

67. Duyff RF, Snijders CJ, Vanneste JA. Spontaneous bilateral internal carotid artery dissection and migraine: a potential diagnostic delay. Headache 1997;37:109.

68. D'Anglejan-Chatillon J, Ribeiro V, Mas JL, et al. Migraine—a risk factor for dissection of cervical arteries. Headache 1989;29:560.

69. Ramadan NM, Tietjen GE, Levine SR, Welch KM. Scintillating scotomata associated with internal carotid artery dissection: report of three cases. Neurology 1991;41:1084.

70. Dvorkin G, Andermann F, Carpenter S. Classic migraine, intractable epilepsy, and multiple stroke: a syndrome related to mitochondrial encephalomyopathy. In Andermann F, Lugaresi E, eds. Migraine and Epilepsy. Stoneham, MA: Butterworth, 1987.

71. Barak Y, Arnon S, Wolach B, et al. MELAS syndrome: peripheral neuropathy and cytochrome C-oxidase deficiency: a case report and review of the literature. Isr J Med Sci 1995;31:224.

72. Crimmins D, Morris JG, Walker GL, et al. Mitochondrial encephalomyopathy: variable clinical expression within a single kindred. J Neurol Neurosurg Psychiatry 1993;56:900.

73. Catarci T, Clifford Rose F. Migraine and heredity. Pathol Biol (Paris) 1992;40:284.

74. Montagna P, Gallassi R, Medori R, et al. MELAS syndrome: characteristic migrainous and epileptic features and maternal transmission. Neurology 1988;38:751.

75. Vahedi K, Chabriat H, Levy C, et al. Migraine with aura and brain magnetic resonance imaging abnormalities in patients with CADASIL. Arch Neurol 2004;61:1237.

76. Hutchinson M, O'Riordan J, Javed M, et al. Familial hemiplegic migraine and autosomal dominant arteriopathy with leukoencephalopathy (CADASIL). Ann Neurol 1995;38:817.

77. Gladstone JP, Dodick DW. Migraine and cerebral white matter lesions: when to suspect cerebral autosomal dominant arteriopathy with subcortical infarcts and leukoencephalopathy (CADASIL). Neurologist 2005;11:19.

78. Chabriat H, Tournier-Lasserve E, Vahedi K, et al. Autosomal dominant migraine with MRI white-matter abnormalities mapping to the CADASIL locus. Neurology 1995;45:1086.

79. Verin M, Rolland Y, Landgraf F, et al. New phenotype of the cerebral autosomal dominant arteriopathy mapped to chromosome 19: migraine as the prominent clinical feature. J Neurol Neurosurg Psychiatry 1995;59:579.

80. Kalimo H, Ruchoux MM, Viitanen M, Kalaria RN. CADASIL: a common form of hereditary arteriopathy causing brain infarcts and dementia. Brain Pathol 2002;12:371.

81. Boasso LE, Fischer AQ. Cerebral vasospasm in childhood migraine during the intermigrainous period. J Neuroimaging 2004;14:158.

82. Gonzalez-Alegre P, Tippin J. Prolonged cortical electrical depression and diffuse vasospasm without ischemia in a case of severe hemiplegic migraine during pregnancy. Headache 2003;43:72.

83. Prodan CI, Holland NR, Lenaerts ME, Parke JT. Magnetic resonance angiogram evidence of vasospasm in familial hemiplegic migraine. J Child Neurol 2002;17:470.

84. Spierings EL. Angiographic changes suggestive of vasospasm in migraine complicated by stroke. Headache 1990;30:727.

85. Solomon S, Lipton RB, Harris PY. Arterial stenosis in migraine: spasm or arteriopathy? Headache 1990;30:52.

86. Jensen IW. Unusual angiographic appearance during attack of hemiplegic migraine. Headache 1986;26:295.

87. Rowbotham GF, Hay RK, Kirby AR, et al. Technique and the dangers of cerebral angiography. J Neurosurg 1953;10:602.

88. Prendes JL. Transient cortical blindness following vertebral angiography. Headache 1978;18:222.

89. Patterson R, Goodell H, Dunning H. Complications of cerebral angiography. Arch Neurol 1964;10:513.

90. Shuaib A, Hachinski VC. Migraine and the risks from angiography. Arch Neurol 1988;45:911.

91. Frigerio R, Santoro P, Ferrarese C, Agostoni E. Migrainous cerebral infarction: case reports. Neurol Sci 2004;25(suppl 3):S300.

92. Gupta VK. Migrainous stroke: are antiphospholipid antibodies pathogenetic, a biological epiphenomenon, or an incidental laboratory aberration? Eur Neurol 1996;36:110.

93. Perju-Dumbrava L, Zeiler K, Kapiotis S, Deecke L. Anticardiolipin-antibodies in stroke and in other neurological disorders. Rom J Neurol Psychiatry 1995;33:137.

94. Silvestrini M, Cupini LM, Matteis M, et al. Migraine in patients with stroke and antiphospholipid antibodies. Headache 1993;33:421.

95. Tietjen GE, Levine SR, Brown E, et al. Factors that predict antiphospholipid immunoreactivity in young people with transient focal neurological events. Arch Neurol 1993;50:833.

96. Levine SR, Deegan MJ, Futrell N, Welch KM. Cerebrovascular and neurologic disease associated with antiphospholipid antibodies: 48 cases. Neurology 1990;40:1181.

97. Tietjen GE. The relationship of migraine and stroke. Neuroepidemiology 2000;19:13.

98. Pilarska E, Lemka M, Bakowska A. Prothrombotic risk factors in ischemic stroke and migraine in children. Acta Neurol Scand 2006;114:13.

99. Crassard I, Conard J, Bousser MG. Migraine and haemostasis. Cephalalgia 2001;21:630.

100. Tietjen GE, Al-Qasmi MM, Gunda P, Herial NA. Sneddon's syndrome: another migraine-stroke association? Cephalalgia 2006;26:225.

101. Tietjen GE. The risk of stroke in patients with migraine and implications for migraine management. CNS Drugs 2005;19:683.

102. Black DF, Bartleson JD, Bell ML, Lachance DH. SMART: stroke-like migraine attacks after radiation therapy. Cephalalgia 2006;26:1137.

103. Caplan LR, Weiner H, Weintraub RM, Austen WG. "Migrainous" neurologic dysfunction in patients with prosthetic cardiac valves. Headache 1976;16:218.

104. Hall GC, Brown MM, Mo J, MacRae KD. Triptans in migraine: the risks of stroke, cardiovascular disease, and death in practice. Neurology 2004;62:563.

105. Bousser MG. Estrogens, migraine, and stroke. Stroke 2004;35:2652.

106. Anzola GP, Magoni M, Guindani M, et al. Potential source of cerebral embolism in migraine with aura: a transcranial Doppler study. Neurology 1999;52:1622.

107. Sztajzel R, Genoud D, Roth S, et al. Patent foramen ovale, a possible cause of symptomatic migraine: a study of 74 patients with acute ischemic stroke. Cerebrovasc Dis 2002;13:102.

108. Wilmshurst P, Nightingale S, Pearson M, et al. Relation of atrial shunts to migraine in patients with ischemic stroke and peripheral emboli. Am J Cardiol 2006;98:831.

109. Del Sette M, Angeli S, Leandri M, et al. Migraine with aura and right-to-left shunt on transcranial Doppler: a case-control study. Cerebrovasc Dis 1998;8:327.

110. Wammes-van der Heijden EA, Tijssen CC, Egberts AC. Right-to-left shunt and migraine: the strength of the relationship. Cephalalgia 2006;26:208.

111. Kruit MC, van Buchem MA, Hofman PA, et al. Migraine as a risk factor for subclinical brain lesions. JAMA 2004;291:427.

112. Kruit MC, Launer LJ, Ferrari MD, van Buchem MA. Brain stem and cerebellar hyperintense lesions in migraine. Stroke 2006;37:1109.

113. Silberstein SD, Dodick D, Freitag F, et al. Pharmacological approaches to managing migraine and associated comorbidities—clinical considerations for monotherapy versus polytherapy. Headache 2007;47:585.

114. Alvarez Gomez MJ, Narbona Garcia J, Barona Zamora P. Alternating hemiplegia: partial effectiveness of treatment with flunarizine. Neurologia 1992;7:116.

115. Tobita M, Hino M, Ichikawa N, et al. A case of hemiplegic migraine treated with flunarizine. Headache 1987;27:487.

116. Mendizabal JE, Greiner F, Hamilton WJ, Rothrock JF. Migrainous stroke causing thalamic infarction and amnesia during treatment with propranolol. Headache 1997;37:594.

117. Alvarez Sabin J, Molins A, Turon A, et al. Migraine-infarct in patients treated with beta-blockers. Rev Clin Esp 1993;192:228.

118. Bardwell A, Trott JA. Stroke in migraine as a consequence of propranolol. Headache 1987;27:381.

119. Gilbert GJ. An occurrence of complicated migraine during propranolol therapy. Headache 1982;22:81.

120. Brand FN, Larson MG, Kannel WB, McGuirk JM. The occurrence of Raynaud's phenomenon in a general population: the Framingham study. Vasc Med 1997;2:296.

121. Vale JA, Jefferys DB. Peripheral gangrene complicating beta-blockade. Lancet 1978;1:1216.

122. Kupersmith MJ, Hass WK, Chase NE. Isoproterenol treatment of visual symptoms in migraine. Stroke 1979;10:299.

123. Loder E, Biondi D. General principles of migraine management: the changing role of prevention. Headache 2005;45(suppl 1):S33.

124. D'Andrea G, Nordera GP, Allais G. Treatment of aura: solving the puzzle. Neurol Sci 2006;27(suppl 2):S96.

125. Di Rosa G, Spano M, Pustorino G, et al. Alternating hemiplegia of childhood successfully treated with topiramate: 18 months of follow-up. Neurology 2006;66:146.

126. Peeters M, Gunthorpe MJ, Strijbos PJ, et al Effects of pan- and subtype-selective NMDA receptor antagonists on cortical spreading depression in the rat: therapeutic potential for migraine. J Pharmacol Exp Ther 2007;312:1195.

127. Black DF. Sporadic and familial hemiplegic migraine: diagnosis and treatment. Semin Neurol 2006;26:208.

128. Forteza AM, Brozman B, Rabinstein AA, et al. Acetazolamide for the treatment of migraine with aura in CADASIL. Neurology 2001;57:2144.

129. Weller M, Dichgans J, Klockgether T. Acetazolamide-responsive migraine in CADASIL. Neurology 1998;50:1505.

CHAPTER 9

Hemostatic Disorders Presenting as Cerebral Infarction

Rima M. Dafer • José Biller

Although thrombosis is uncommon in children and young adults, alterations in hemostasis are associated with an increased risk of stroke, particularly venous and less commonly arterial.[1] These disorders have been implicated in 2% to 10% of all strokes, with a higher proportion in young patients, and the discovery of new coagulation disorders has increased the rate of strokes attributable to hypercoagulable states to 19%.[1-6] Numerous primary and secondary hypercoagulable conditions, which may be inherited or acquired (Tables 9-1 and 9-2), may predispose to recurrent episodes of deep venous thromboembolism (VTE), pulmonary embolism, cerebral arterial or venous infarction, and other life-threatening thrombotic events.[1-8] This chapter discusses conditions associated with hypercoagulability, with emphasis on the most commonly encountered conditions in younger patients.

Primary Hypercoagulable States

Inherited disorders predisposing to thrombosis, especially affecting the venous circulation, include antithrombin (AT) deficiency, protein C and protein S deficiencies, methylene tetrahydrofolate reductase (MTHFR) gene mutation, activated protein C (APC) resistance with or without factor V Leiden (FVL) mutation, prothrombin G20210A mutation, heparin cofactor II (HCII) deficiency, and abnormalities of fibrinogen

TABLE 9-1 **Primary Hypercoagulable States**

Antithrombin deficiency
Protein C deficiency
Protein S deficiency
Activated protein C resistance
Factor V Leiden mutation
Prothrombin G20210A mutation
Heparin cofactor II deficiency
Disorders of fibrinogen
   Afibrinogenemia
   Hypofibrinogenemia
   Dysfibrinogenemia
Elevated thrombin-activatable fibrinolysis inhibitor
Elevated factor VIII
Elevated factor IX
Elevated factor XI
Disorders of the fibrinolytic system
   Hypoplasminogenemia
   Plasminogen activators deficiency
   Tissue plasminogen activator defects
MTHFR gene mutation

TABLE 9-2 **Secondary Hypercoagulable States**

Antiphospholipid syndrome
Myeloproliferative disorders
Paraproteinemia
Cancer
Pregnancy
Oral contraceptives
Polycythemia rubra vera
Iron deficiency anemia
Hemoglobinopathies
Sickle cell disease
   Sickle cell anemia (hemoglobin SS)
   Sickle cell disease (hemoglobin SC)
   Sickle cell trait
   Sickle β-thalassemia
Thalassemias
   β-thalassemia major, intermediate and trait
   α-thalassemia major or trait
Platelet disorders
Essential thrombocythemia
Heparin-induced thrombocytopenia
Thrombotic thrombocytopenic purpura
Essential thrombocythemia
Homocystinuria and hyperhomocysteinemia
Paroxysmal nocturnal hemoglobinuria
Diabetes mellitus
Ovarian hyperstimulation syndrome
Nephrotic syndrome
Disseminated intravascular coagulation
Plasma glutathione peroxidase deficiency

and plasminogen.[9-13] These disorders should be suspected in patients with recurrent neonatal purpura fulminans; episodes of deep venous thrombosis; recurrent pulmonary embolism; family history of thrombotic events; neonatal purpura fulminans; unusual sites of venous or arterial thromboses; or thrombotic events occurring during childhood, adolescence, or early adulthood.

Activated Protein C Resistance

Inherited resistance to APC is the most common genetic risk factor for thrombophilia.[14] APC resistance is linked to a single point mutation in the factor V gene, which predicts replacement of Arg (R) at position 506 with a Gln (Q).[15,16] APC resistance is believed to be responsible for 64% of cases of veno-occlusive disorders annually.[17] Approximately 80% of individuals with APC resistance carry a mutation of the FV gene referred to as FVL mutation. Heterozygous FVL is found in 3% to 8% of whites.[18-21] Heterozygous and homozygous carriers of this mutation are at greater risk for VTE (Fig. 9-1). Thrombophilic risk is increased 5 to 10 times in heterozygotes and 50 to 100 times in homozygotes compared with controls.[18,22,23] Less commonly, acquired forms of APC resistance may be associated with elevated levels of factor VIII and fibrinogen, in the absence of FVL, especially in patients with multiple myeloma and cancer.[24,25]

The risk of VTE is higher when APC resistance coexists with another thrombophilic defect, such as protein C or S deficiency, AT deficiency, prothrombin gene mutation, hyperhomocystinemia, or antiphospholipid syndrome (APS).[26-31] Other predisposing factors for VTE in patients with APC resistance include the use of oral contraceptives (OCs), hormonal replacement therapy, cigarette smoking, and pregnancy.[32-36]

The most common veno-occlusive manifestation of APC is deep venous thrombosis, although pulmonary embolism and superficial thrombophlebitis may occur. APC resistance with or without FVL mutation has been associated with ischemic stroke, mainly deep venous thrombosis and cerebral vein thrombosis in young patients.[37-46]

Diagnostic tests include activated partial thromboplastin time, the APC resistance test,

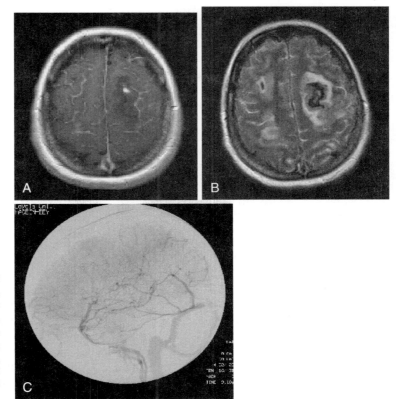

FIGURE 9-1 **A** and **B,** Multiple foci of intraparenchymal hemorrhage in the frontal and parietal lobes bilaterally (**A**) with gyriform cortical enhancement (**B**) consistent with hemorrhagic venous infarctions in a young woman with FVL mutation taking OCs. **C,** Cerebral angiogram shows total occlusion of the superior sagittal sinus.

and the FVL mutation. Carriers for APC resistance who are asymptomatic should receive counseling on the importance of avoiding factors that increase the risk for VTE. Women should stop the use of OCs or hormonal replacement therapy. Smoking cessation is advocated. In subjects at high risk for VTE, such as in cases of pregnant women or after surgery or trauma, prophylaxis with heparin is beneficial. Following VTE, patients receive anticoagulation treatment for 3 to 6 months. Patients with recurrent events may require lifetime anticoagulation therapy with warfarin. Because warfarin-induced skin necrosis has been associated with APC resistance, patients should receive heparin before initiation of warfarin therapy.[47]

Antithrombin Deficiency

AT or AT III is a non–vitamin K–dependent plasma glycoprotein with a molecular weight of 58,000 D. AT inhibits coagulation by inhibiting serine proteases and lysing thrombin

and factor Xa. AT also is believed to exert an anti-inflammatory effect on the vascular endothelium. AT is a hereditary autosomal dominant disorder, affecting individuals of all ethnicities.[48,49] The true prevalence of AT is approximately 1:2000 to 1:5000, whereas it is present in about 4% of patients with a venous thromboembolic event.[50,51] Homozygous AT deficiency is not seen probably because it is lethal to the fetus. Many AT gene mutations have been reported in association with AT deficiency, the most frequent being the A384S mutation among whites.[50,52] Two categories of inherited AT deficiency have been recognized: classic or type I, characterized by decreased immunologic and biologic activity of AT, and type II, characterized by low biologic activity of AT, but essentially normal immunologic activity.

Acquired AT deficiency occurs primarily as a result of consumption and may follow acute thrombosis and disseminated intravascular coagulation (DIC). AT deficiency also has been associated with nephrotic syndrome; liver cirrhosis; microangiopathic hemolytic anemias; use of OCs; and administration of asparaginase, tamoxifen, and heparin therapy. AT deficiency should be suspected in patients with cerebral venous infarction, and rarely in young patients with arterial stroke, especially with coexisting right-to-left cardiac shunt.[1,11,49,53-55]

Acute thrombotic episodes usually are treated with unfractionated or low-molecular-weight heparins, with or without adjunctive human pooled plasma-derived AT concentrate particularly in high-risk circumstances, such as pregnant women, premature infants, and patients in intensive care.[56] Human recombinant AT is currently approved in Europe and may provide a useful alternative treatment option. Prophylactic therapy depends on the individual patient's risk of recurrent thromboembolic disease and usually consists of long-term warfarin administration for 3 to 6 months.

Protein C Deficiency

Protein C is a vitamin K–dependent serine protease with a molecular weight of 62,000 D. Protein C deficiency is inherited as an autosomal dominant disorder and is present in approximately 0.2% of the general population.[57-59] Homozygous protein C deficiency manifests in infancy as neonatal purpura fulminans.[60] Heterozygotes are predisposed to recurrent thrombosis. Thrombotic manifestations are predominantly venous, occur at a young age, and have a tendency to recur. Acquired protein C deficiency has been associated with the administration of asparaginase, liver disease, DIC, postoperative state, and adult respiratory distress syndrome. Skin necrosis is a serious potential complication in patients with protein C deficiency at the initiation of warfarin therapy.[47,61-66] The acute management of thrombosis associated with protein C deficiency consists of prompt administration of heparin followed by incremental doses of warfarin. Long-term therapy requires the administration of warfarin.[67-74]

Protein S Deficiency

Protein S is a vitamin K–dependent protein with a molecular weight of approximately

69,000 D. Protein S deficiency has an autosomal dominant mode of inheritance. Homozygous protein S deficiency occurs with venous thromboembolic disease. Heterozygotes are prone to recurrent thrombosis (venous and possibly arterial), including cerebral venous thrombosis (Fig. 9-2). Childhood strokes rarely are associated with familial protein S deficiency.[74-78] Acquired protein S deficiency occurs in association with pregnancy, acute thromboembolic episodes, DIC, nephrotic syndrome, systemic lupus erythematosus, the use of OCs, and administration of asparaginase. Acquired free protein S deficiency also is common among hospitalized patients in the absence of a recognized predisposing condition, and rarely is associated with thrombotic complications.[78]

Levels should be rechecked within a few months of the acute thrombotic event before committing patients for long-term anticoagulation therapy. Heparin therapy is effective in the management of acute thrombotic events followed by long-term anticoagulation with warfarin for preventing recurrent thromboembolism. Warfarin therapy should be initiated with caution because it may reduce free protein S to critically low levels, predisposing to recurrent thrombosis, and rarely may cause warfarin-induced skin necrosis.[62,63,66,79]

Prothrombin G20210A Mutation

Factor II is a vitamin K–dependent coagulation factor and the precursor of thrombin. A variant in prothrombin factor II, a G-to-A transition at nucleotide position 20210, is a common congenital abnormality associated with a twofold to fivefold increase in the risk for VTE, including cerebral venous sinus thrombosis.[80-83] Its role in arterial thrombosis is still undefined; cases of arterial strokes or myocardial infarctions have been reported especially in children and young women.[68,84-88] Mutations in the prothrombin gene mutation are present in approximately 2% of the northern European population. The prevalence for the heterozygote prothrombin G20210A mutation is 1%

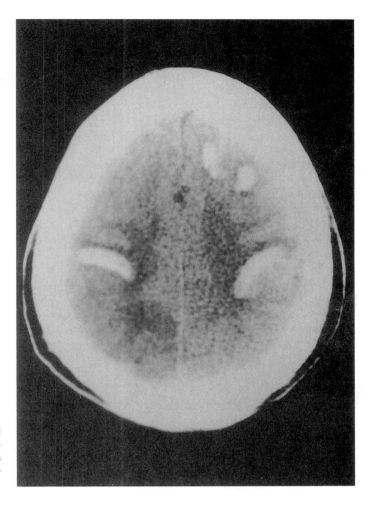

FIGURE 9-2 Non–contrast-enhanced axial CT scan shows bilateral hemorrhagic infarctions suggesting superior sagittal sinus thrombosis, confirmed by MRI and angiography, in a patient with protein S deficiency.

to 6% among whites, and it is very rare or absent in other ethnic groups.[83,89] A new prothrombin gene variant C20209T was not found to be an important risk factor for thromboembolism.[90]

Heparin Cofactor II Deficiency

HCII is a hepatic serpin plasma glycoprotein with a molecular weight of approximately 65,600 D. HCII has a significant AT activity through inhibition of binding of an acidic domain in HCII to thrombin exosite I.[7,91] HCII deficiency has been implicated in DIC, inflammatory reaction, atherosclerosis, liver disease, and wound repair.[4,91-94] Inherited deficiencies of HCII (probably in autosomal dominant fashion) and thrombophilia have been described in several families.[95-97]

Homocystinuria, Hyperhomocysteinemia, and Methylene Tetrahydrofolate Reductase Deficiency

Homocystinuria is an autosomal recessive inborn error of metabolism caused by a deficiency of cystathionine synthase, an enzyme essential in the methionine-to-cysteine pathway. Platelet functional abnormalities have been noted in patients with this condition. Patients with homocystinuria have a marfanoid appearance, fair complexion with brittle hair, malar flush, mental retardation, dislocation of the crystalline lens, and a propensity for intracranial arterial and venous thrombosis. Thromboembolic episodes may occur at any age. Death may result from pulmonary embolism, myocardial infarction, or stroke.[98-101] Approximately half of patients respond to large doses of pyridoxine (vitamin B_6). Patients who do not respond are treated with trimethylglycine (betaine) and a low-methionine diet supplemented with cysteine.

Hyperhomocysteinemia is determined by genetic or dietary factors and is an independent risk factor for arterial and venous thrombosis.[102-104] Two polymorphic genetic mutations in the gene coding MTHFR predominantly homozygous C677T, an autosomal recessive disorder, play a crucial role in modulating the levels of plasma homocysteine, and have been associated with increased risk of hemorrhagic and ischemic stroke (Fig. 9-3).[105] The prevalence of the mutated homozygous C677T MTHFR and heterozygous C677T/A1298C genotypes in patients with arterial stroke is 1.4% and 31.88%, with a higher frequency of 16.6% and 33.3% in venous infarctions.[106-117] The benefit of reduction of total homocysteine with high doses of folic acid, pyridoxine, and cobalamin (vitamin B_{12}) on vascular outcomes in patients with arterial thrombosis remains controversial.[118,119] Patients with homozygous C677T mutation with recurrent thrombotic events may require long-term anticoagulation therapy.

Acquired hyperhomocysteinemia in the absence of any mutation or polymorphism may be associated with cigarette smoking, renal failure, diabetes mellitus, hypothyroidism, carcinoma, pernicious anemia, folate and vitamins B_6 and B_{12} deficiencies, or inflammatory bowel disease. It also may occur as the result of methotrexate, theophylline, or phenytoin therapy. This topic is not discussed further in this chapter.

Disorders of Fibrinogen

Abnormalities in the fibrinolytic system have been associated with an increased risk for stroke. Fibrinogen is composed of a three-pair polypeptide chain with a molecular weight of approximately 340,000 D. High and low concentrations of fibrinogen increase the risk for stroke and myocardial infarction. Afibrinogenemia is probably transmitted as an autosomal recessive trait; complications include umbilical cord bleeding, gastrointestinal hemorrhage, and cerebral hemorrhage. Hypofibrinogenemia represents the heterozygous form of afibrinogenemia; bleeding is rare. Dysfibrinogenemia reflects a qualitative disorder in the fibrinogen molecule and may be associated with hemorrhagic and thrombotic events. Hereditary dysfibrinogenemia is inherited in an autosomal dominant fashion. Decreased concentrations of fibrinogen are found in association with DIC; liver failure; snake bite; and treatment with asparaginase, ancrod, fibrinolytic drugs, and valproic acid. Treatment consists of infusion of cryoprecipitate.[120-123]

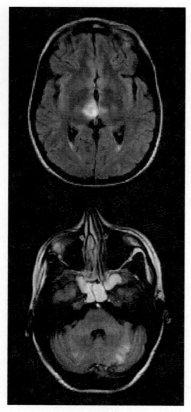

FIGURE 9-3 Fluid attenuated inversion recovery MRI shows right thalamic and bilateral cerebellar high signal intensity lesions consistent with infarctions in a young woman with heterozygous mutation for MTHFR C677T and patent foramen ovale taking OCs.

Plasminogen Abnormalities

Plasminogen is a plasma glycoprotein with a molecular weight of 90,000 D. Decreased levels of plasminogen, qualitative abnormalities in the plasminogen molecule, and defective release of plasminogen activators have been described in families with recurrent thrombotic events.[1,8,124-126] Impaired fibrinolytic function secondary to elevated levels of the plasminogen activator inhibitor type gene 1 polymorphism 4G/5G is associated with an increased risk for thrombotic diseases, predominantly ischemic stroke.[127-131] The underlying mechanism of stroke remains undetermined. Deficiency of tissue plasminogen activator also may exacerbate ischemia-induced cerebrovascular thrombosis, especially after thrombolytic therapy with intravenous tissue plasminogen activator for acute ischemic stroke.[132]

A novel pro-carboxypeptidase B–like proenzyme thrombin-activatable fibrinolysis inhibitor has been described more recently as a potent inhibitor of tissue plasminogen activator–induced fibrinolysis. It is thought to play an important role in coagulation/fibrinolysis balance. Its relevance in thromboembolic disease remains unclear.[133-138]

Other rare hypercoagulable causes of stroke include elevated factors VIII, IX, and XI.[139-147] Table 9-3 presents a suggested paraclinical evaluation of a patient with presumed hypercoagulable cause of cerebral infarction.

Secondary Hypercoagulable States

The acquired or secondary hypercoagulable states consist of a heterogeneous group of disorders with an increased risk for developing thrombosis.

Antiphospholipid Syndrome

APS, or Hughes syndrome, is an acquired prothrombotic syndrome characterized by recurrent arterial thromboembolism or VTE, unexplained fetal loss usually within the first 10 weeks of gestation, and thrombocytopenia. APS is associated with the presence of circulating antiphospholipid antibodies against protein antigens that bind to membrane anionic phospholipid anticardiolipins.[148] APS is encountered in association with common autoimmune rheumatologic disorders; after exposure to certain drugs, including procainamide, propranolol, hydralazine, quinine,

TABLE 9-3 **Evaluation for Potential Hypercoagulable Cause of Cerebral Infarction in Young Adults**

Complete blood count with differential and peripheral smear
Hemoglobin electrophoresis
Prothrombin time and international normalized ratio, activated partial thromboplastin time
Thrombin time
Plasma antithrombin activity
Protein C activity and total and free protein S antigen levels
Homocysteine level
Methylene tetrahydrofolate reductase C677T and A1298
Activated protein C resistance and factor V Leiden
Prothrombin G20210A mutation
Antiphospholipid antibodies (lupus anticoagulant, anticardiolipin antibodies, β_2-glycoprotein antibodies)
Heparin cofactor II levels
Heparin antibodies
Plasma fibrinogen
Euglobulin clot lysis time
Plasminogen levels
Plasmin functional activity
Inhibitors of plasminogen activation
Factors V, VII, VIII, IX, X, XI, and XIII assay
Circulating platelet aggregates and spontaneous platelet aggregation
Functional fibrinogen assay
Fibrin monomers
Fibrin degradation products
Fibrinolytic activity
Sucrose hemolysis test (if positive, acidified serum lysis test)
Plasma homocysteine
Measurement of cystathionine β-synthase activity in biopsy tissue obtained

phenytoin, chlorpromazine, interferon alfa, amoxicillin, and quinidine; and in systemic illnesses, such as infections and malignancy.

Primary APS is an immune-mediated coagulopathy associated with cerebral ischemia in young adults. Several antiphospholipid antibodies have been described, mainly lupus anticoagulant; anticardiolipin IgG, IgA, and IgM isotypes; and β_2 glycoprotein 1 antibodies (β2GP1).[149] The antiphospholipid antibodies are important independent risk factors for cerebral ischemia in children and young adults.[150-160] Arterial and venous infarctions may occur. Magnetic resonance imaging (MRI) of the brain may show

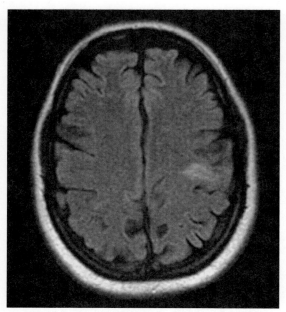

FIGURE 9-4 Fluid attenuated inversion recovery MRI shows abnormal high signal intensity lesion in the cortical and subcortical white matter of the left frontoparietal region consistent with acute infarction in a young woman with APS.

diffuse subcortical white matter ischemic changes, cerebral infarctions, or sinovenous occlusive disease (Fig. 9-4).[161,162] Catastrophic APS or Asherson syndrome is a rare life-threatening fulminant thrombotic condition seen in less than 1% of patients. Patients with catastrophic APS have cerebral infarctions and multiorgan failure. A lethal outcome has been reported in more than 40% of cases.[163]

The best therapeutic strategy for preventing stroke in patients with APS is unclear. Treatment of APS should focus on the management of the underlying disorder. Aspirin is effective for preventing recurrent cerebral arterial events in patients with first stroke.[164] Anticoagulants are indicated in patients with venous thrombosis and recurrent arterial thrombosis who failed antiplatelet therapy.[165,166] Plasmapheresis and intravenous immunoglobulin therapy combined with corticosteroids and anticoagulation may improve outcome in patients with recurrent VTE or with catastrophic APS.[167-170] Other options include the use of immunosuppressants, such as cyclophosphamide and rituximab.[171-173]

Systemic Conditions That May Induce Changes in the Coagulation System

Malignancies

Cancer in children is uncommon. The types of malignant diseases in children differ from those encountered in adults. The most frequently seen tumors in children include leukemias, central nervous system (CNS) tumors, lymphomas, soft tissue sarcomas, neuroblastomas, Wilms tumor, bone tumors, and retinoblastomas. Hypercoagulability is a common finding in patients with malignancy, especially with mucin-secreting adenocarcinomas, myeloproliferative disorders, acute promyelocytic leukemia, and brain tumors.[174-181] Cerebral infarction in patients with malignancy may be due to thrombosis associated with the hypercoagulable state.

The cause of the hypercoagulable state is often multifactorial. The pathophysiology is believed to be due to a state of low-grade intravascular coagulation induced by the cancer and secondary fibrinolysis, but with the balance shifted toward "clotting." Other potential mechanisms of stroke include cancer-enhanced atherothrombosis, direct tumor effects through invasion of the arterial and venous sinuses by tumor cells, and leptomeningeal infiltrates. There also is the possibility of embolism arising from septic (fungal or bacterial) or tumoral emboli, bone marrow embolization, emboli originating from mural thrombi, or emboli arising from marantic vegetations associated with nonbacterial thrombotic endocarditis (Fig. 9-5). This condition is characterized by the presence of multiple, small, sterile thrombotic vegetations varying in size from 3 mm to 1.5 cm or larger, most frequently involving the mitral and aortic valves. Ischemic and hemorrhagic strokes also may occur secondary to vascular injury induced by chemotherapy or radiation therapy. Anticoagulants and platelet antiaggregants have been used with variable success.[1,7,8,175,182-184]

Paroxysmal Nocturnal Hemoglobinuria

Paroxysmal nocturnal hemoglobinuria (Marchiafava-Micheli syndrome) is an acquired clonal stem cell disorder characterized

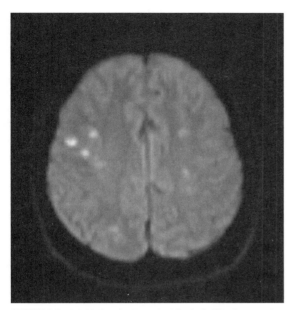

FIGURE 9-5   Multiple small cortical foci of diffusion restriction on MRI involving the frontal and parietal lobes consistent with acute infarction in a young man with marantic endocarditis associated with non–small cell carcinoma of the lung.

by hemolytic anemia occurring only occasionally during the night and hemosiderinuria. A rare feared complication is cerebral arterial or venous thrombosis. Cerebral venous thrombosis and portal vein thrombosis are the most frequent causes of death. The cause of thrombophilia is not firmly established. If hemolytic anemia is significant, treatment consists of corticosteroids. There is no effective antithrombotic treatment for paroxysmal nocturnal hemoglobinuria. Heparin should be used with caution in the presence of thrombocytopenia. Danaparoid, a low-molecular-weight heparinoid, is an alternative option.[181,185-189]

Disorders of Platelets

Heparin-induced Thrombocytopenia

Thrombocytopenia may be secondary to immune or nonimmune disorders associated with increased platelet destruction or consumption, or congenital or acquired disorders associated with impaired platelet production. Heparin is a sulfated glycosaminoglycan with a mean molecular weight of 10,000 to 15,000 D (range 4000 to 40,000 D) isolated from either bovine lung or porcine intestinal mucosa. Heparin is commonly used in the intensive care unit for preventing and treating thromboembolic disease. A significant complication of heparin use is heparin-induced thrombocytopenia (HIT).

There are two types of HIT. Type I HIT, a non–immune-mediated transient benign condition associated with platelet counts around $100,000/mm^3$, tends to resolve spontaneously. Type II HIT, an immune-mediated disorder, is a potentially devastating complication of unfractionated or low-molecular-weight heparins and is associated with increased risk of venous and arterial thrombosis. Despite HIT being rare (affecting <1% of intensive care unit patients), it is a serious condition associated with increased risk for venous and arterial thrombosis with high fatality rates.[190] Stroke is a rare complication of HIT type II; it is encountered more commonly among women and in patients with more severe thrombocytopenia occurring within the first 2 weeks of initiation of heparin therapy.[191-199]

When HIT type II is clinically suspected, heparin should be stopped immediately, and a direct thrombin inhibitor therapy with lepirudin, argatroban, or danaparoid should be initiated alone or in combination with warfarin, even before laboratory confirmation.[200] Thrombocytopenia is no longer an essential criterion for the diagnosis of HIT because the condition has been reported with a normal platelet count.[201] A 50% decrease in the platelet count may be a more specific indicator for HIT. The risk of major hemorrhage with direct thrombin inhibitors is directly related to the activated partial thromboplastin time ratio, which should be monitored closely.[202] Warfarin should not be used until the platelet count has recovered. Severe anaphylactic shock and anaphylactoid reactions have been reported with various direct thrombin inhibitors.[203-205] Guidelines for the management of HIT have been published in the United Kingdom.[202]

Thrombotic Thrombocytopenic Purpura

Thrombotic thrombocytopenic purpura (TTP), or Moschcowitz disease, is a life-threatening condition of undetermined etiology. TTP is characterized by the systemic deposition of platelet microthrombi in the arterioles, with abundance of von Willebrand factor in the arterioles and capillaries in numerous organs, especially the heart, kidneys, and brain. The main neuropathologic changes include variable degrees of CNS ischemic changes and parenchymal and subarachnoid hemorrhages. More recently, von Willebrand factor protease (ADAMTS13) activity was found to be severely deficient in hereditary and acquired idiopathic TTP.[206,207] TTP has been reported as a complication of treatment with ticlopidine and rarely with clopidogrel.[208-210] Patients with TTP may present with pyrexia, thrombocytopenic purpura, microangiopathic hemolytic anemia, renal dysfunction, strokelike symptoms, and fluctuating neurologic manifestations. Neurologic symptoms include headache, seizures, mental changes, hemiparesis, hemisensory deficits, aphasia, visual changes, and cranial nerve deficits.[3,211-218] Therapy is with fresh frozen plasma, therapeutic plasma exchange, corticosteroids, and platelet antiaggregants. Rituximab may improve outcome in patients with CNS involvement or with refractory relapsing TTP.[216,219,220]

Disorders of Red Blood Cells and Hemoglobinopathies

Sickle Cell Disease

Sickle cell disease (SCD) is a chronic hemolytic anemia associated with a hyperviscosity state and sludging within the small vessels resulting in microinfarctions of the affected organs. At low oxygen tensions, erythrocytes containing hemoglobin S (HbS) assume a sickle-like appearance. HbS forms as a result of a potent mutation in codon 6 of the β globin gene, causing a change in the amino acid encoded from glutamine to valine. Children with SCD present with a wide variety of neurologic syndromes, including arterial and venous strokes, transient ischemic attacks, seizures, headache, and altered mental status. Primary hemorrhagic stroke is an uncommon complication of SCD. Intracranial hemorrhage is more common in patients receiving corticosteroids, patients with systemic hypertension, or patients with

recent transfusion.[221-223] Although there is pathologic evidence that small vessel occlusion and sludging as a result of sickling does occur in the brain, the clinical and neurodiagnostic findings are more consistent with a large vessel arterial occlusive disease affecting the major intracranial arteries, often bilaterally, and frequently involving the distal internal carotid and anterior cerebral–middle cerebral arterial border zones. Fat embolism and spinal cord infarction also may occur.

A complicated pathogenesis of cerebral infarction is postulated and involves intra-arterial embolization, perfusion failure, and intravascular sickling, in particular, in individuals with low hemoglobin value, hypertension, and high white blood cell count. The evaluation of a stroke patient with sickle cell anemia includes blood cell count, peripheral blood smear, hemoglobin electrophoresis, and sickling test. Transcranial Doppler (TCD) is a sensitive and specific noninvasive technique for the detection of arterial vasculopathy and a key test in identifying high risk and in determining the need for prophylactic blood transfusion. High arterial blood flow velocity rates of 200 cm/sec or greater on TCD are associated with high stroke rates of more than 10% per year. Computed tomography (CT) and MRI may show subclinical lesions or cerebral infarctions, and angiographic studies may show extent of intracranial arterial involvement. Although there is a theoretical risk that the hypertonic contrast media can cause sickling, cerebral angiography can be performed safely when indicated. SCD commonly causes an angiographic pattern resembling moyamoya disease. Cerebral infarction is an infrequent complication of sickle trait; when it occurs, it is often associated with dehydration, severe hypoxia, or heat stress.

There have been no acute stroke treatment studies in SCD. Meticulous hydration, adequate oxygenation, and analgesia are necessary. TCD screening of all children with SCD is routine continuing care to detect intracranial stenosis. Periodic blood transfusion has proven beneficial in primary stroke prevention in patients with abnormal blood flow velocities on TCD with a target HbS less than 30%. Blood transfusion also may prevent the

Hemostatic Disorders Presenting as Cerebral Infarction **183**

progression of silent cerebral infarcts. Transfusion should be continued for 5 years or at least until the child is 18 years old. Indefinite blood transfusion to maintain a level of HbS less than 30% in the high-risk group is the only proven secondary stroke prevention strategy so far in SCD patients, with stroke risk reduction of less than 1% per year. Measures to prevent iron overload should be taken. Secondary stroke prevention with hydroxyurea and phlebotomy is currently being tested as an alternative approach to long-term transfusion in a multicenter trial. The use of antiplatelet agents or anticoagulants in secondary ischemic stroke prevention has not proved beneficial. Data to support bone marrow transplantation in SCD are limited.[222-233]

Iron Deficiency Anemia

Iron deficiency anemia in children may develop because of inadequate iron intake, malabsorption, or blood loss. Iron deficiency anemia may be associated with neurologic complications, including developmental delay, breath-holding episodes, pseudotumor cerebri, and cranial nerve palsies. Stroke is a serious complication of iron deficiency anemia in healthy children and young adults, affecting the arterial and venous systems.[6,234-239]

Myeloproliferative Disorders

Chronic myeloproliferative disorders are typically disorders of middle-aged or elderly patients, although many cases are seen in younger individuals. They are rare causes of ischemic stroke.

Essential Thrombocythemia

Essential thrombocythemia is a chronic clonal myeloproliferative disorder characterized by thrombocytosis and abnormal megakaryocyte proliferation. Essential thrombocythemia is associated with increased risk of thrombosis, hemorrhage, and vasomotor symptoms. Ischemic arterial and venous strokes are common complications of essential thrombocythemia. Patients may have splenomegaly, persistently elevated platelet count (usually >1 million/mm^3), giant platelets, and a hypercellular bone

marrow. Headaches, dizziness, amaurosis fugax, and transient and persistent focal cerebral ischemic symptoms are frequent. Treatment includes myelosuppressive therapy, plateletpheresis, and platelet antiaggregants. Thrombocythemia is common after splenectomy, but does not carry an increased thromboembolic risk. Normalization of platelet counts may occur with hydroxyurea in conjunction with antiplatelet therapy.[240-244]

Polycythemia rubra vera is characterized by increased red blood cell mass and normal arterial oxygen saturation. Patients have splenomegaly, elevated hemoglobin, high hematocrit value, thrombocytosis, leukocytosis, and low erythropoietin levels. A mutation in the JAK2 kinase (V617F) was found to be strongly associated with polycythemia rubra vera.[164,245] Typically, the bone marrow is hypercellular. Cerebral blood flow is reduced in patients with polycythemia. Cerebral hemorrhage and cerebral thrombosis can complicate polycythemia rubra vera. Most intracranial complications in this condition are thrombotic in origin, the larger cerebral arteries being the most frequently involved. The risk of stroke parallels the hemoglobin level: the higher the hemoglobin and hematocrit values, the greater the risk of stroke.

Headaches, dizziness, vertigo, visual disturbances, and carotid and vertebrobasilar transient ischemic attacks are well-recognized features of patients with polycythemia. Spinal cord infarction is rare. Cautious reduction of the hematocrit is a reasonable therapeutic approach. Because of the potential risk of hemorrhagic intracranial complications, aspirin therapy should be used cautiously.[246-257]

Pregnancy

Stroke remains a leading cause of severe complications during pregnancy and puerperium and of maternal morbidity and mortality. Many factors may be responsible for the increased risk of thrombosis during the peripartum period, including hypercoagulable state, peripartum reversible ischemic angiopathy, and peripartum cardiomyopathy. Chapter 10 presents a detailed discussion of stroke in pregnancy.

Oral Contraceptives

Exposure to the effects of OCs may increase the risk of ischemic stroke, particularly venous infarctions (Figs. 9-6 and 9-7). The risk of arterial stroke especially remains controversial.[258-265] Much of the data on increased stroke risk are associated with the use of first-generation OCs containing 50 μg or more of estradiol compared with low-estrogen formulations, although the third-generation OCs seem to confer the same stroke risk.[260,266-273]

The absolute risk remains very small, however, with data predominantly originating from case-control or cohort epidemiologic studies.[258-260,263,269,273-276] Such risk is higher in young women with history of migraine with aura, and its effect is potentiated in the setting of inherited prothrombotic conditions.[273,277-280] Fewer data are available on the association between OC use and hemorrhagic stroke.[263,265,281] Current recommendations are that the use of OCs should be discouraged in women with additional cerebrovascular risk factors such as cigarette smoking and in women with history of migraine, especially with aura; inherited or acquired hypercoagulable states; or prior history of thromboembolic events.[259,263,282]

Ovarian Hyperstimulation Syndrome

The ovarian hyperstimulation syndrome has been reported in women after induction of ovulation with clomiphene, human menopausal gonadotropin, human follicle-stimulating hormone extracted from human pituitary gonadotropin, and human chorionic gonadotropin (see Fig. 9-3). Evidence of body fluid shifts and hypercoagulability has been observed with this syndrome, reflected in thromboembolic events. Stroke is a rare but serious consequence of severe ovarian hyperstimulation syndrome.[283-289]

Nephrotic Syndrome

A child with nephrotic syndrome is at risk for serious complications, including hypovolemia, infections with capsulated organisms (e.g., *Pseudomonas*), hypercholesterolemia,

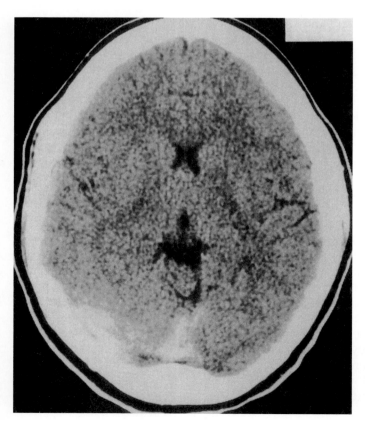

FIGURE 9-6 Non–contrast-enhanced axial CT scan shows abnormal high attenuation along the expected location of the straight sinus and right transverse sinus, suggesting sinus thrombosis, confirmed on angiography. The patient was taking OCs.

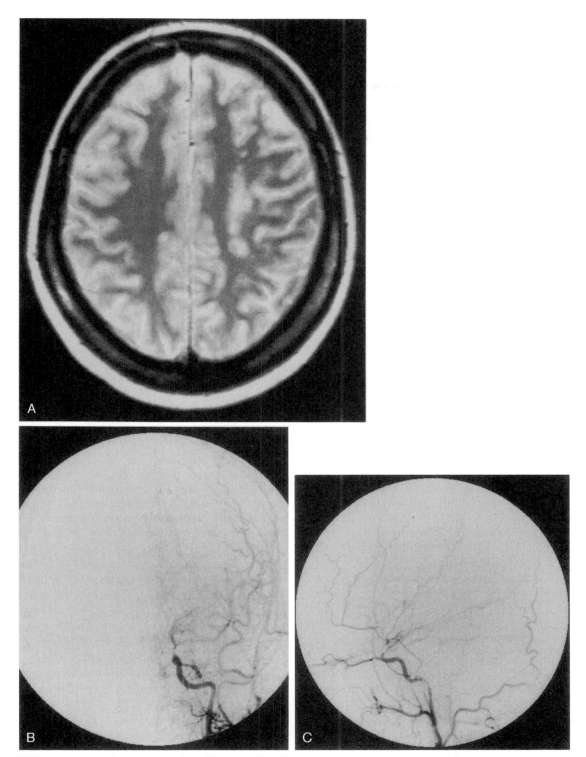

FIGURE 9-7 **A,** Axial fast spin echo (long TR, short TE) MRI shows high signal intensity in the left centrum semiovale consistent with watershed infarction occurring at the peak of estrogenic stimulation in a patient being treated with leuprolide acetate (Lupron), menotropins (Pergonal), metrodin, and progesterone. **B** and **C,** Anteroposterior and lateral views of common carotid angiography show short segment irregular narrowing of the supraclinoid internal carotid artery with poor antegrade filling of the anterior cerebral circulation in the same patient.

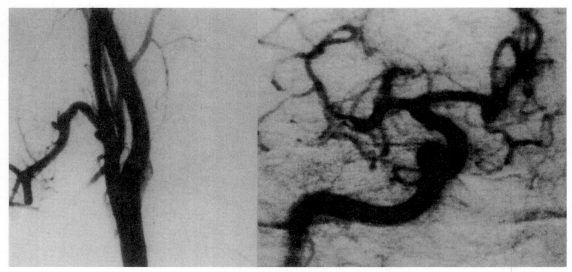

FIGURE 9-8   Common carotid angiography shows filling defects at the level of the carotid bulb and right-middle cerebral artery bifurcation in a patient with nephrotic syndrome.

and thrombosis. Ischemic stroke can be the presenting manifestation of nephrotic syndrome (Fig. 9-8). The mechanism of thromboembolism in nephrotic syndrome is multifactorial. Elevated levels of fibrinogen and of factors V, VII, VIII, and X; thrombocytosis; enhanced platelet aggregation; and reduced levels of AT and protein S have been described in association with the disorder. Elevations in homocysteine levels, plasminogen activator inhibitor type 1, factor VIII, and anticardiolipin antibodies have been reported in patients with thrombotic complications. The exact role of hyperlipidemia, corticosteroid use, and diuretic use is uncertain.

Changes in lipoprotein metabolism are pronounced in patients with nephrotic syndrome, including marked elevation of lipoprotein (a) levels and all apolipoprotein B–containing lipoproteins. Nephrotic syndrome should be considered as a contributing mechanism in any patient with ischemic stroke and preexisting renal disease. Urinalysis is the initial clue to the diagnosis. Treatment of thromboembolism associated with nephrotic syndrome consists of anticoagulants until remission of the renal condition. In addition, low-density lipoprotein apheresis has been shown to decrease urinary albumin excretion and to increase serum levels of albumin in patients with severe hyperlipidemia. In high-risk patients with severe hypoalbuminemia and on diuretics or steroid treatment, prophylactic anticoagulants can be considered to reduce the risk of serious cerebral infarction.[290-297]

Conclusion

Primary and acquired hematologic disorders are associated with increased risk for ischemic stroke, and less commonly intracranial hemorrhage in children and young adults. Although genetic thrombophilias are commonly associated with venous infarctions, arterial strokes also are common. Systematic investigative efforts should be tempered and guided by a relevant family history of venous or arterial thrombosis and a history of unusual, recurrent, or otherwise unexplained thrombotic events. Early diagnosis and management of underlying conditions is key for prevention of a thrombotic event. Although treatment of a first stroke in hypercoagulable state is typically long-term anticoagulation, prospective clinical trial data are needed to support this treatment approach.

REFERENCES

1. Hart RG, Kanter MC. Hematologic disorders and ischemic stroke: a selective review. Stroke 1990;21:1111.
2. Kittner SJ, Stern BJ, Wozniak M, et al. Cerebral infarction in young adults: the Baltimore-Washington Cooperative Young Stroke Study. Neurology 1998;50:890.

3. Matijevic N, Wu KK. Hypercoagulable states and strokes. Curr Atheroscler Rep 2006;8:324.

4. Nagaraja D, Christopher R. Pro-thrombotic states in stroke. Neurol India 2002;50(Suppl):S21.

5. Tatlisumak T, Fisher M. Hematologic disorders associated with ischemic stroke. J Neurol Sci 1996;140(1-2):1.

6. Labauge PM, Bouly S. Thrombotic cocktail in stroke. Neurology 2005;65:781; author reply.

7. Schafer AI. The hypercoagulable states. Ann Intern Med 1985;102:814.

8. Bauer KA, Rosenberg RD. The hypercoagulable state. In Ratnoff OD, Forbes CD, eds. Disorders of Hemostasis, 2nd ed. Philadelphia: WB Saunders, 1991.

9. Bushnell CD, Goldstein LB. Diagnostic testing for coagulopathies in patients with ischemic stroke. Stroke 2000;31:3067.

10. Takano K, Yamaguchi T, Uchida K. Markers of a hypercoagulable state following acute ischemic stroke. Stroke 1992;23:194.

11. Martinez HR, Rangel-Guerra RA, Marfil LJ. Ischemic stroke due to deficiency of coagulation inhibitors: report of 10 young adults. Stroke 1993;24:19.

12. Sastry S, Riding G, Morris J, et al. Young Adult Myocardial Infarction and Ischemic Stroke: the role of paradoxical embolism and thrombophilia (the YAMIS study). J Am Coll Cardiol 2006;48:686.

13. Botto N, Spadoni I, Giusti S, et al. Prothrombotic mutations as risk factors for cryptogenic ischemic cerebrovascular events in young subjects with patent foramen ovale. Stroke 2007;38:2070.

14. Nicolaes GA, Dahlback B. Activated protein C resistance (FV Leiden) and thrombosis: factor V mutations causing hypercoagulable states. Hematol Oncol Clin North Am 2003;17:37.

15. Aparicio C, Dahlback B. Molecular mechanisms of activated protein C resistance: properties of factor V isolated from an individual with homozygosity for the Arg506 to Gln mutation in the factor V gene. Biochem J 1996;313(Pt 2):467.

16. Griffin JH, Heeb MJ, Kojima Y, et al. Activated protein C resistance: molecular mechanisms. Thromb Haemost 1995;74:444.

17. Sheppard DR. Activated protein C resistance: the most common risk factor for venous thromboembolism. J Am Board Fam Pract 2000;13:111.

18. Rees DC, Cox M, Clegg JB. World distribution of factor V Leiden. Lancet 1995;346:1133.

19. Ridker PM, Miletich JP, Hennekens CH, Buring JE. Ethnic distribution of factor V Leiden in 4047 men and women: implications for venous thromboembolism screening. JAMA 1997;277:1305.

20. Zoller B. Familial thrombophilia: clinical and molecular analysis of Swedish families with inherited resistance to activated protein C or protein S deficiency. Scand J Clin Lab Invest Suppl 1996;226:19.

21. Dahlback B, Carlsson M, Svensson PJ. Familial thrombophilia due to a previously unrecognized mechanism characterized by poor anticoagulant response to activated protein C: prediction of a cofactor to activated protein C. Proc Natl Acad Sci U S A 1993;90:1004.

22. Chrobak L, Dulicek P. Resistance to activated protein C as pathogenic factor of venous thromboembolism. Acta Med (Hradec Kralove) 1996;39:55.

23. Dahlback B. Inherited thrombophilia: resistance to activated protein C as a pathogenic factor of venous thromboembolism. Blood 1995;85:607.

24. Jimenez-Zepeda VH, Dominguez-Martinez VJ. Acquired activated protein C resistance and thrombosis in multiple myeloma patients. Thromb J 2006;4:11.

25. Green D, Maliekel K, Sushko E, et al. Activated-protein-C resistance in cancer patients. Haemostasis 1997;27:112.

26. Marchiori A, Mosena L, Prins MH, Prandoni P. The risk of recurrent venous thromboembolism among heterozygous carriers of factor V Leiden or prothrombin G20210A mutation: a systematic review of prospective studies. Haematologica 2007;92:1107.

27. Wu J, Zhou Z, Li X, et al. Activated protein C resistance in antiphospholipid thrombosis syndrome. Chin Med J (Engl) 2000;113:699.

28. Picillo U, De Lucia D, Palatiello E, et al. Association of primary antiphospholipid syndrome with inherited activated protein C resistance. J Rheumatol 1998;25:1232.

29. Aznar J, Villa P, Espana F, et al. Activated protein C resistance phenotype in patients with antiphospholipid antibodies. J Lab Clin Med 1997;130:202.

30. Biousse V, Piette JC, Frances C, et al. Primary antiphospholipid syndrome is not associated with activated protein C resistance caused by factor V Arg 506→Gln mutation. J Rheumatol 1995;22:1215.

31. Standen G, Morse C, Aslam S, Bowron A. Recurrent thrombosis in a patient with pseudohomozygous activated protein C resistance and homozygosity for MTHFR gene polymorphism C677T. Thromb Haemost 1999;81:663.

32. Martinelli I, Landi G, Merati G, et al. Factor V gene mutation is a risk factor for cerebral venous thrombosis. Thromb Haemost 1996;75:393.

33. Girolami A, Simioni P, Girolami B, Radossi P. Homozygous patients with APC resistance may remain paucisymptomatic or asymptomatic during oral contraception. Blood Coagul Fibrinolysis 1996;7:590.

34. Olivieri O, Friso S, Manzato F, et al. Resistance to activated protein C in healthy women taking oral contraceptives. Br J Haematol 1995;91:465.

35. Bokarewa MI, Falk G, Sten-Linder M, et al. Thrombotic risk factors and oral contraception. J Lab Clin Med 1995;126:294.

36. Vandenbroucke JP, Koster T, Briet E, et al. Increased risk of venous thrombosis in oral-contraceptive users who are carriers of factor V Leiden mutation. Lancet 1994;344:1453.

37. Zunker P, Hohenstein C, Plendl HJ, et al. Activated protein C resistance and acute ischaemic stroke: relation to stroke causation and age. J Neurol 2001;248:701.

38. Mohanty S, Saxena R, Behari M. Activated protein C (APC) resistance in young stroke patients. Thromb Haemost 1999;81:465.

39. James RH, O'Dell MW. Resistance to activated protein C as an etiology for stroke in a young adult: a case report. Arch Phys Med Rehabil 1999;80:343.

40. Chaturvedi S, Joshi N, Dzieczkowski J. Activated protein C resistance in young African American patients with ischemic stroke. J Neurol Sci 1999;163:137.

41. Giordano P, Sabato V, Schettini F, et al. Resistance to activated protein C as a risk factor of stroke in a thalassemic patient. Haematologica 1997;82:698.

42. Riikonen RS, Vahtera EM, Kekomaki RM. Physiological anticoagulants and activated protein C resistance in childhood stroke. Acta Paediatr 1996;85:242.

43. Ganesan V, Kelsey H, Cookson J, et al. Activated protein C resistance in childhood stroke. Lancet 1996;347:260.

44. Albucher JF, Guiraud-Chaumeil B, Chollet F, et al. Frequency of resistance to activated protein C due to factor V mutation in young patients with ischemic stroke. Stroke 1996;27:766.

45. Bachmeyer C, Toulon P, Dhote R, et al. Ischemic stroke and activated protein C resistance. JAMA 1995;274:1266.

46. Halbmayer WM, Haushofer A, Schon R, Fischer M. The prevalence of poor anticoagulant response to activated protein C (APC resistance) among patients suffering from stroke or venous thrombosis and among healthy subjects. Blood Coagul Fibrinolysis 1994;5:51.

47. Sallah S, Abdallah JM, Gagnon GA. Recurrent warfarin-induced skin necrosis in kindreds with protein S deficiency. Haemostasis 1998;28:25.

48. Maclean PS, Tait RC. Hereditary and acquired antithrombin deficiency: epidemiology, pathogenesis and treatment options. Drugs 2007;67:1429.

49. Nagaraja D, Christopher R, Tripathi M. Plasma antithrombin III deficiency in ischaemic stroke in the young. Neurol India 1999;47:155.

50. Corral J, Hernandez-Espinosa D, Soria JM, et al. Antithrombin Cambridge II (A384S): an underestimated genetic risk factor for venous thrombosis. Blood 2007;109:4258.

51. Blajchman MA. An overview of the mechanism of action of antithrombin and its inherited deficiency states. Blood Coagul Fibrinolysis 1994;5(Suppl 1):S5.

52. Picard V, Nowak-Gottl U, Biron-Andreani C, et al. Molecular bases of antithrombin deficiency: twenty-two novel mutations in the antithrombin gene. Hum Mutat 2006;27:600.

53. Ernerudh J, Olsson JE, von Schenck H. Antithrombin-III deficiency in ischemic stroke. Stroke 1990;21:967.

54. Hossmann V, Heiss WD, Bewermeyer H. Antithrombin III deficiency in ischaemic stroke. Klin Wochenschr 1983;61:617.

55. Duran R, Biner B, Demir M, et al. Factor V Leiden mutation, deficiency of antithrombin III and elevation of factor VIII in a child with ischemic stroke: a case report. Brain Dev 2006;28:604.

56. Bucur SZ, Levy JH, Despotis GJ, et al. Uses of antithrombin III concentrate in congenital and acquired deficiency states. Transfusion 1998;38:481.

57. Dahlback B, Villoutreix BO. The anticoagulant protein C pathway. FEBS Lett 2005;579:3310.

58. Macias WL, Yan SB, Williams MD, et al. New insights into the protein C pathway: potential implications for the biological activities of drotrecogin alfa (activated). Crit Care 2005;9(Suppl 4):S38.

59. Marlar RA, Mastovich S. Hereditary protein C deficiency: a review of the genetics, clinical presentation, diagnosis and treatment. Blood Coagul Fibrinolysis 1990;1:319.

60. Rappaport ES, Speights VO, Helbert B, et al. Protein C deficiency. South Med J 1987;80:240.

61. Parsi K, Younger I, Gallo J. Warfarin-induced skin necrosis associated with acquired protein C deficiency. Australas J Dermatol 2003;44:57.

62. Oz BS, Asgun F, Oz K, et al. Warfarin-induced skin necrosis after open heart surgery due to protein S and C deficiency. Heart Vessels 2007;22:64.

63. Ng T, Tillyer ML. Warfarin-induced skin necrosis associated with factor V Leiden and protein S deficiency. Clin Lab Haematol 2001;23:261.

64. Makris M, Bardhan G, Preston FE. Warfarin induced skin necrosis associated with activated protein C resistance. Thromb Haemost 1996;75:523.

65. Kurt M, Shorbagi A, Aksu S, et al. Warfarin-induced skin necrosis and leukocytoclastic vasculitis in a patient with acquired protein C and protein S deficiency. Blood Coagul Fibrinolysis 2007;18:805.

66. Anderson DR, Brill-Edwards P, Walker I. Warfarin-induced skin necrosis in 2 patients with protein S deficiency: successful reinstatement of warfarin therapy. Haemostasis 1992;22:124.

67. Tiong IY, Alkotob ML, Ghaffari S. Protein C deficiency manifesting as an acute myocardial infarction and ischaemic stroke. Heart 2003;89:E7.

68. Arkel YS, Ku DH, Gibson D, Lam X. Ischemic stroke in a young patient with protein C deficiency and prothrombin gene mutation G20210A. Blood Coagul Fibrinolysis 1998;9:757.

69. Kennedy CR, Warner G, Kai M, Chisholm M. Protein C deficiency and stroke in early life. Dev Med Child Neurol 1995;37:723.

70. Brown DC, Livingston JH, Minns RA, Eden OB. Protein C and S deficiency causing childhood stroke. Scott Med J 1993;38:114.

71. Camerlingo M, Finazzi G, Casto L, et al. Inherited protein C deficiency and nonhemorrhagic arterial stroke in young adults. Neurology 1991;41:1371.

72. Kohler J, Kasper J, Witt I, von Reutern GM. Ischemic stroke due to protein C deficiency. Stroke 1990;21:1077.

73. Grewal RP, Goldberg MA. Stroke in protein C deficiency. Am J Med 1990;89:538.

74. Israels SJ, Seshia SS. Childhood stroke associated with protein C or S deficiency. J Pediatr 1987;111:562.

75. Simioni P, Battistella PA, Drigo P, et al. Childhood stroke associated with familial protein S deficiency. Brain Dev 1994;16:241.

76. Gomez-Aranda F, Lopez Dominguez JM, Rivera Fernandez V, Martin Garcia E. Stroke and familial protein S deficiency. Stroke 1992;23:299.

77. Wuillemin WA, Demarmels Biasiutti F, Mattle HP, Lammle B. Frequency of protein Z deficiency in patients with ischaemic stroke. Lancet 2001;358:840.
78. Mayer SA, Sacco RL, Hurlet-Jensen A, et al. Free protein S deficiency in acute ischemic stroke: a case-control study. Stroke 1993;24:224.
79. Odegaard OR, Try K, Ly B, et al. [Protein S deficiency, acute phase reaction and thrombosis]. Tidsskr Nor Laegeforen 1993;113:3460.
80. De Stefano V, Chiusolo P, Paciaroni K, et al. Prothrombin G20210A mutant genotype is a risk factor for cerebrovascular ischemic disease in young patients. Blood 1998;91:3562.
81. De Stefano V, Martinelli I, Mannucci PM, et al. The risk of recurrent venous thromboembolism among heterozygous carriers of the G20210A prothrombin gene mutation. Br J Haematol 2001;113:630.
82. Jukic I, Titlic M, Tonkic A, Rosenzweig D. Cerebral venous sinus thrombosis as a recurrent thrombotic event in a patient with heterozygous prothrombin G20210A genotype after discontinuation of oral anticoagulation therapy: how long should we treat these patients with warfarin? J Thromb Thrombolysis 2007;24:77.
83. Zivelin A, Rosenberg N, Faier S, et al. A single genetic origin for the common prothrombotic G20210A polymorphism in the prothrombin gene. Blood 1998;92:1119.
84. Hudaoglu O, Kurul S, Yis U, et al. Basilar artery thrombosis in a child heterozygous for prothrombin gene G20210A mutation. J Child Neurol 2007;22:329.
85. Rosendaal FR, Siscovick DS, Schwartz SM, et al. A common prothrombin variant (20210 G to A) increases the risk of myocardial infarction in young women. Blood 1997;90:1747.
86. Germanakis I, Stiakaki E, Sfyridaki C, et al. Stroke in an infant heterozygous carrier of both factor V G1691A and the G20210A prothrombin mutation. Thromb Haemost 2003;90:760.
87. Lalouschek W, Schillinger M, Hsieh K, et al. Matched case-control study on factor V Leiden and the prothrombin G20210A mutation in patients with ischemic stroke/transient ischemic attack up to the age of 60 years. Stroke 2005;36:1405.
88. Ridker PM, Hennekens CH, Miletich JP. G20210A mutation in prothrombin gene and risk of myocardial infarction, stroke, and venous thrombosis in a large cohort of US men. Circulation 1999;99:999.
89. Rosendaal FR, Doggen CJ, Zivelin A, et al. Geographic distribution of the 20210 G to A prothrombin variant. Thromb Haemost 1998;79:706.
90. Gurgey A, Unal S, Okur H, et al. Prothrombin G20210A mutation in Turkish children with thrombosis and the frequency of prothrombin C20209T. Pediatr Hematol Oncol 2005;22:309.
91. Tollefsen DM. Heparin cofactor II modulates the response to vascular injury. Arterioscler Thromb Vasc Biol 2007;27:454.
92. Akhtar N, Deleu D, Kamran S. Haematologic disorders and cerebral venous thrombosis. J Pak Med Assoc 2006;56:498.
93. Corral J, Aznar J, Gonzalez-Conejero R, et al. Homozygous deficiency of heparin cofactor II: relevance of P17 glutamate residue in serpins, relationship with conformational diseases, and role in thrombosis. Circulation 2004;110:1303.
94. Vicente CP, He L, Tollefsen DM. Accelerated atherogenesis and neointima formation in heparin cofactor II deficient mice. Blood 2007;110:4261.
95. Matsuo T, Kario K, Sakamoto S, et al. Hereditary heparin cofactor II deficiency and coronary artery disease. Thromb Res 1992;65(4-5):495.
96. Simioni P, Lazzaro AR, Coser E, et al. Hereditary heparin cofactor II deficiency and thrombosis: report of six patients belonging to two separate kindreds. Blood Coagul Fibrinolysis 1990;1(4-5):351.
97. Tran TH, Marbet GA, Duckert F. Association of hereditary heparin co-factor II deficiency with thrombosis. Lancet 1985;2:413.
98. Carson NA, Dent CE, Field CM, Gaull GE. Homocystinuria: clinical and pathological review of ten cases. J Pediatr 1965;66:565.
99. de Groot PG, Willems C, Boers GH, et al. Endothelial cell dysfunction in homocystinuria. Eur J Clin Invest 1983;13:405.
100. Newman G, Mitchell JR. Homocystinuria presenting as multiple arterial occlusions. QJM 1984;53:251.
101. Visy JM, Le Coz P, Chadefaux B, et al. Homocystinuria due to 5,10-methylenetetrahydrofolate reductase deficiency revealed by stroke in adult siblings. Neurology 1991;41:1313.
102. Fallon UB, Ben-Shlomo Y. Homocysteine, MTHFR 677C→T polymorphism, and risk of ischemic stroke: results of a meta-analysis. Neurology 2003;60:526; author reply.
103. Casas JP, Bautista LE, Smeeth L, et al. Homocysteine and stroke: evidence on a causal link from mendelian randomisation. Lancet 2005;365:224.
104. Guba SC, Fonseca V, Fink LM. Hyperhomocysteinemia and thrombosis. Semin Thromb Hemost 1999;25:291.
105. Kawamoto R, Kohara K, Oka Y, et al. An association of 5,10-methylenetetrahydrofolate reductase (MTHFR) gene polymorphism and ischemic stroke. J Stroke Cerebrovasc Dis 2005;14:67.
106. Alluri RV, Mohan V, Komandur S, et al. MTHFR C677T gene mutation as a risk factor for arterial stroke: a hospital based study. Eur J Neurol 2005;12:40.
107. Garoufi AJ, Prassouli AA, Attilakos AV, et al. Homozygous MTHFR C677T gene mutation and recurrent stroke in an infant. Pediatr Neurol 2006;35:49.
108. Lalouschek W, Aull S, Serles W, et al. C677T MTHFR mutation and factor V Leiden mutation in patients with TIA/minor stroke: a case-control study. Thromb Res 1999;93:61.
109. McColl MD, Chalmers EA, Thomas A, et al. Factor V Leiden, prothrombin 20210G→A and the MTHFR C677T mutations in childhood stroke. Thromb Haemost 1999;81:690.
110. Panigrahi I, Chatterjee T, Biswas A, et al. Role of MTHFR C677T polymorphism in ischemic stroke. Neurol India 2006;54:48.

111. Pezzini A, Del Zotto E, Archetti S, et al. Plasma homocysteine concentration, C677T MTHFR genotype, and 844ins68bp CBS genotype in young adults with spontaneous cervical artery dissection and atherothrombotic stroke. Stroke 2002;33:664.

112. Pezzini A, Grassi M, Del Zotto E, et al. Migraine mediates the influence of C677T MTHFR genotypes on ischemic stroke risk with a stroke-subtype effect. Stroke 2007;38(12):3145.

113. Sazci A, Ergul E, Tuncer N, et al. Methylenetetrahydrofolate reductase gene polymorphisms are associated with ischemic and hemorrhagic stroke: dual effect of MTHFR polymorphisms C677T and A1298C. Brain Res Bull 2006;71(1-3):45.

114. Szolnoki Z, Somogyvari F, Szabo M, et al. [Interactions between the MTHFR C677T and MTHFR A1298C mutations in ischaemic stroke]. Ideggyogy Sz 2006;59(3-4):107.

115. Ucar F, Sonmez M, Ovali E, et al. MTHFR C677T polymorphism and its relation to ischemic stroke in the Black Sea Turkish population. Am J Hematol 2004;76:40.

116. Brankovic-Sreckovic V, Milic Rasic V, Djordjevic V, et al. Arterial ischemic stroke in a child with beta-thalassemia trait and methylentetrahydrofolate reductase mutation. J Child Neurol 2007;22:208.

117. Choi BO, Kim NK, Kim SH, et al. Homozygous C677T mutation in the MTHFR gene as an independent risk factor for multiple small-artery occlusions. Thromb Res 2003;111(1-2):39.

118. Toole JF, Malinow MR, Chambless LE, et al. Lowering homocysteine in patients with ischemic stroke to prevent recurrent stroke, myocardial infarction, and death: the Vitamin Intervention for Stroke Prevention (VISP) randomized controlled trial. JAMA 2004;291:565.

119. Lonn E, Yusuf S, Arnold MJ, et al. Homocysteine lowering with folic acid and B vitamins in vascular disease. N Engl J Med 2006;354:1567.

120. Matsuo T, Okuno S, Mukaida T, et al. A hereditary dysfibrinogenemia: fibrinogen Awaji. Haemostasis 1987;17(1-2):89.

121. Bithell TC. Hereditary dysfibrinogenemia. Clin Chem 1985;31:509.

122. Bithell TC. Hereditary dysfibrinogenemia—the first 25 years. Acta Haematol 1984;71:145.

123. Carrell N, Gabriel DA, Blatt PM, et al. Hereditary dysfibrinogenemia in a patient with thrombotic disease. Blood 1983;62:439.

124. Schafer AI. Hypercoagulable states: molecular genetics to clinical practice. Lancet 1994;344:1739.

125. Whitlock JA, Janco RL, Phillips JA 3rd. Inherited hypercoagulable states in children. Am J Pediatr Hematol Oncol 1989;11:170.

126. Johansson L, Hedner U, Nilsson IM. A family with thromboembolic disease associated with deficient fibrinolytic activity in vessel wall. Acta Med Scand 1978;203:477.

127. Endler G, Lalouschek W, Exner M, et al. The 4G/4G genotype at nucleotide position -675 in the promotor region of the plasminogen activator inhibitor 1 (PAI-1) gene is less frequent in young patients with minor stroke than in controls. Br J Haematol 2000;110:469.

128. Johansson L, Jansson JH, Boman K, et al. Tissue plasminogen activator, plasminogen activator inhibitor-1, and tissue plasminogen activator/plasminogen activator inhibitor-1 complex as risk factors for the development of a first stroke. Stroke 2000;31:26.

129. Kain K, Young J, Bamford J, et al. Determinants of plasminogen activator inhibitor-1 in South Asians with ischaemic stroke. Cerebrovasc Dis 2002;14:77.

130. Sirgo G, Perez-Vela JL, Morales P, et al. Association between 4G/5G polymorphism of the plasminogen activator inhibitor 1 gene with stroke or encephalopathy after cardiac surgery. Intensive Care Med 2006;32:668.

131. Tsantes AE, Nikolopoulos GK, Bagos PG, et al. Plasminogen activator inhibitor-1 4G/5G polymorphism and risk of ischemic stroke: a meta-analysis. Blood Coagul Fibrinolysis 2007;18:497.

132. Tabrizi P, Wang L, Seeds N, et al. Tissue plasminogen activator (tPA) deficiency exacerbates cerebrovascular fibrin deposition and brain injury in a murine stroke model: studies in tPA-deficient mice and wild-type mice on a matched genetic background. Arterioscler Thromb Vasc Biol 1999;19:2801.

133. Rooth E, Wallen H, Antovic A, et al. Thrombin activatable fibrinolysis inhibitor and its relationship to fibrinolysis and inflammation during the acute and convalescent phase of ischemic stroke. Blood Coagul Fibrinolysis 2007;18:365.

134. Ladenvall C, Gils A, Jood K, et al. Thrombin activatable fibrinolysis inhibitor activation peptide shows association with all major subtypes of ischemic stroke and with TAFI gene variation. Arterioscler Thromb Vasc Biol 2007;27:955.

135. Lichy C, Dong-Si T, Reuner K, et al. Risk of cerebral venous thrombosis and novel gene polymorphisms of the coagulation and fibrinolytic systems. J Neurol 2006;253:316.

136. Santamaria A, Oliver A, Borrell M, et al. Risk of ischemic stroke associated with functional thrombin-activatable fibrinolysis inhibitor plasma levels. Stroke 2003;34:2387.

137. Montaner J, Ribo M, Monasterio J, et al. Thrombin-activable fibrinolysis inhibitor levels in the acute phase of ischemic stroke. Stroke 2003;34:1038.

138. Monasterio J, Bermudez P, Quiroga D, et al. Plasma thrombin-activatable fibrinolytic inhibitor (TAFI) among healthy subjects and patients with vascular diseases: a validation study. Pathophysiol Haemost Thromb 2003;33(5-6):382.

139. McKenzie J, Jaap AJ, Gallacher S, et al. Metabolic, inflammatory and haemostatic effects of a low-dose continuous combined HRT in women with type 2 diabetes: potentially safer with respect to vascular risk? Clin Endocrinol (Oxf) 2003;59:682.

140. Garcia VV, Alberca I, Borrasca AL. Factor VIII-related antigen in cerebrospinal fluid. Thromb Haemost 1983;49:142.

141. Kurekci AE, Gokce H, Akar N. Factor VIII levels in children with thrombosis. Pediatr Int 2003;45:159.

142. Wang TD, Chen WJ, Su SS, et al. Increased levels of tissue plasminogen activator antigen and factor VIII activity in nonvalvular atrial fibrillation: relation to predictors of thromboembolism. J Cardiovasc Electrophysiol 2001;12:877.

143. Catto AJ, Carter AM, Barrett JH, et al. von Willebrand factor and factor VIII:C in acute cerebrovascular disease: relationship to stroke subtype and mortality. Thromb Haemost 1997;77:1104.

144. Chambless LE, Shahar E, Sharrett AR, et al. Association of transient ischemic attack/stroke symptoms assessed by standardized questionnaire and algorithm with cerebrovascular risk factors and carotid artery wall thickness: the ARIC Study, 1987-1989. Am J Epidemiol 1996;144:857.

145. Kosik KS, Furie B. Thrombotic stroke associated with elevated plasma factor VIII. Ann Neurol 1980;8:435.

146. Yang DT, Flanders MM, Kim H, Rodgers GM. Elevated factor XI activity levels are associated with an increased odds ratio for cerebrovascular events. Am J Clin Pathol 2006;126:411.

147. Stibler H, Holzbach U, Tengborn L, Kristiansson B. Complex functional and structural coagulation abnormalities in the carbohydrate-deficient glycoprotein syndrome type I. Blood Coagul Fibrinolysis 1996;7:118.

148. Wilson WA, Gharavi AE. Hypercoagulable states. Ann Intern Med 1997;127:1128–1129.

149. McNeil HP, Chesterman CN, Krilis SA. Anticardiolipin antibodies and lupus anticoagulants comprise separate antibody subgroups with different phospholipid binding characteristics. Br J Haematol 1989;73:506.

150. Brey RL, Hart RG, Sherman DG, Tegeler CH. Antiphospholipid antibodies and cerebral ischemia in young people. Neurology 1990;40:1190.

151. Blohorn A, Guegan-Massardier E, Triquenot A, et al. Antiphospholipid antibodies in the acute phase of cerebral ischaemia in young adults: a descriptive study of 139 patients. Cerebrovasc Dis 2002;13:156.

152. Chandra S, Dutta U, Das R, et al. Mesenteric venous thrombosis causing jejunal stricture: secondary to hypercoagulable states and primary portal hypertension. Dig Dis Sci 2002;47:2017.

153. Nagaraja D, Christopher R, Manjari T. Anticardiolipin antibodies in ischemic stroke in the young: Indian experience. J Neurol Sci 1997;150:137.

154. Kushner MJ. Prospective study of anticardiolipin antibodies in stroke. Stroke 1990;21:295.

155. Anticardiolipin antibodies are an independent risk factor for first ischemic stroke. The Antiphospholipid Antibodies in Stroke Study (APASS) Group. Neurology 1993;43:2069.

156. Devilat M, Toso M, Morales M. Childhood stroke associated with protein C or S deficiency and primary antiphospholipid syndrome. Pediatr Neurol 1993;9:67.

157. Tuhrim S, Rand JH, Wu XX, et al. Elevated anticardiolipin antibody titer is a stroke risk factor in a multiethnic population independent of isotype or degree of positivity. Stroke 1999;30:1561.

158. Tuhrim S, Rand JH, Wu X, et al. Antiphosphatidyl serine antibodies are independently associated with ischemic stroke. Neurology 1999;53:1523.

159. Zielinska J, Ryglewicz D, Wierzchowska E, et al. Anticardiolipin antibodies are an independent risk factor for ischemic stroke. Neurol Res 1999;21:653.

160. Janardhan V, Wolf PA, Kase CS, et al. Anticardiolipin antibodies and risk of ischemic stroke and transient ischemic attack: the Framingham cohort and offspring study. Stroke 2004;35:736.

161. Csepany T, Bereczki D, Kollar J, et al. MRI findings in central nervous system systemic lupus erythematosus are associated with immunoserological parameters and hypertension. J Neurol 2003;250:1348.

162. Provenzale JM, Heinz ER, Ortel TL, et al. Antiphospholipid antibodies in patients without systemic lupus erythematosus: neuroradiologic findings. Radiology 1994;192:531.

163. Bucciarelli S, Espinosa G, Cervera R, et al. Mortality in the catastrophic antiphospholipid syndrome: causes of death and prognostic factors in a series of 250 patients. Arthritis Rheum 2006;54:2568.

164. Levine SR. Hypercoagulable states and stroke: a selective review. CNS Spectr 2005;10:567.

165. Khamashta MA, Cuadrado MJ, Mujic F, et al. The management of thrombosis in the antiphospholipid-antibody syndrome. N Engl J Med 1995;332:993.

166. Finazzi G, Marchioli R, Brancaccio V, et al. A randomized clinical trial of high-intensity warfarin vs. conventional antithrombotic therapy for the prevention of recurrent thrombosis in patients with the antiphospholipid syndrome (WAPS). J Thromb Haemost 2005;3:848.

167. Ruffatti A, Marson P, Pengo V, et al. Plasma exchange in the management of high risk pregnant patients with primary antiphospholipid syndrome: a report of 9 cases and a review of the literature. Autoimmun Rev 2007;6:196.

168. Uthman I, Shamseddine A, Taher A. The role of therapeutic plasma exchange in the catastrophic antiphospholipid syndrome. Transfus Apher Sci 2005;33:11.

169. Erkan D. Therapeutic and prognostic considerations in catastrophic antiphospholipid syndrome. Autoimmun Rev 2006;6:98.

170. Cervera R, Asherson RA, Font J. Catastrophic antiphospholipid syndrome. Rheum Dis Clin North Am 2006;32:575.

171. Rubenstein E, Arkfeld DG, Metyas S, et al. Rituximab treatment for resistant antiphospholipid syndrome. J Rheumatol 2006;33:355.

172. Trappe R, Loew A, Thuss-Patience P, et al. Successful treatment of thrombocytopenia in primary antiphospholipid antibody syndrome with the anti-CD20 antibody rituximab—monitoring of antiphospholipid and anti-GP antibodies: a case report. Ann Hematol 2006;85:134.

173. Merrill JT. Rituximab in antiphospholipid syndrome. Curr Rheumatol Rep 2003;5:381.

174. Ernst E, Hammerschmidt DE, Bagge U, et al. Leukocytes and the risk of ischemic diseases. JAMA 1987;257:2318.

175. Rogers LR. Cerebrovascular complications in cancer patients. Neurol Clin 2003;21:167.

176. Santoro N, Giordano P, Del Vecchio GC, et al. Ischemic stroke in children treated for acute lymphoblastic leukemia: a retrospective study. J Pediatr Hematol Oncol 2005;27:153.

177. Spivak JL, Barosi G, Tognoni G, et al. Chronic myeloproliferative disorders. Hematology Am Soc Hematol Educ Program, 2003, p 200.

178. Caicoya AG, Barco-Nebreda L, Gonzalez-Gutierrez JL, Egido-Herrero JA. [Hashimoto's encephalopathy associated with scleromyxedema: coincidental or the overlapping of two syndromes with a possible autoimmune origin?]. Rev Neurol 2004;39:723.

179. Pavy MD, Murphy PL, Virella G. Paraprotein-induced hyperviscosity: a reversible cause of stroke. Postgrad Med 1980;68:109.

180. Perez-Diaz H, Serrano-Pozo A, Gonzalez-Marcos JR. [Multiple myeloma as a treatable cause of stroke: clinical case and review of the literature]. Neurologia 2007;22:54.

181. Smith BD, La Celle PL. Blood viscosity and thrombosis: clinical considerations. Prog Hemost Thromb 1982;6:179.

182. Lang NP, Wait GM, Read RR. Cardio-cerebrovascular complications from Nd:YAG laser treatment of lung cancer. Am J Surg 1991;162:629.

183. Rogers LR. Cerebrovascular complications in cancer patients. Neurol Clin 1991;9:889.

184. Rogers LR. Cerebrovascular complications in patients with cancer. Semin Neurol 2004;24:453.

185. al-Hakim M, Katirji B, Osorio I, Weisman R. Cerebral venous thrombosis in paroxysmal nocturnal hemoglobinuria: report of two cases. Neurology 1993;43:742.

186. Audebert HJ, Planck J, Eisenburg M, et al. Cerebral ischemic infarction in paroxysmal nocturnal hemoglobinuria report of 2 cases and updated review of 7 previously published patients. J Neurol 2005;252:1379.

187. Poulou LS, Vakrinos G, Pomoni A, et al. Stroke in paroxysmal nocturnal haemoglobinuria: patterns of disease and outcome. Thromb Haemost 2007;98:699.

188. Tejada J, Hernandez-Echebarria L, Sandoval V, Mostaza JL. [Cerebral ischemia as first manifestation of paroxysmal nocturnal hemoglobinuria]. Neurologia 2007;22:471.

189. Zyss J, Cakmak S, Derex L, et al. Danaparoid in the prevention of ischemic stroke in paroxysmal nocturnal hemoglobinuria. Cerebrovasc Dis 2007;23 (5-6):462.

190. Selleng K, Warkentin TE, Greinacher A. Heparin-induced thrombocytopenia in intensive care patients. Crit Care Med 2007;35:1165.

191. LaMonte MP, Brown PM, Hursting MJ. Stroke in patients with heparin-induced thrombocytopenia and the effect of argatroban therapy. Crit Care Med 2004;32:976.

192. Yaguchi H, Mitsumura H, Ozawa R, et al. [A case of heparin-induced thrombocytopenia that worsened preexisting cerebral infarction]. Rinsho Shinkeigaku 2004;44:636.

193. Boon DM, Michiels JJ, Tanghe HL, Kappers-Klunne MC. Heparin-induced thrombocytopenia with multiple cerebral infarctions simulating thrombotic thrombocytopenic purpura: a case report. Angiology 1996;47:407.

194. Cullinan C, Doherty C, Kellett J. Thrombotic stroke as a complication of heparin-induced thrombocytopenia. Ir J Med Sci 1994;163:314.

195. Daneschvar HL, Daw H. Heparin-induced thrombocytopenia (an overview). Int J Clin Pract 2007;61:130.

196. Dang CH, Durkalski VL, Nappi JM. Evaluation of treatment with direct thrombin inhibitors in patients with heparin-induced thrombocytopenia. Pharmacotherapy 2006;26:461.

197. Greinacher A, Farner B, Kroll H, et al. Clinical features of heparin-induced thrombocytopenia including risk factors for thrombosis: a retrospective analysis of 408 patients. Thromb Haemost 2005;94:132.

198. Murphy KD, Galla DH, Vaughn CJ, et al. Heparin-induced thrombocytopenia and thrombosis syndrome. RadioGraphics 1998;18:111.

199. Salehiomran A, Karimi A, Ahmadi H, Yazdanifard P. Delayed-onset heparin-induced thrombocytopenia presenting with multiple arteriovenous thromboses: case report. J Med Case Rep 2007;1:131.

200. Bartholomew JR, Begelman SM, Almahameed A. Heparin-induced thrombocytopenia: principles for early recognition and management. Cleve Clin J Med 2005;72(Suppl 1):S31.

201. Alvarez GF, Bihari D, Collins D. Heparin-induced thrombosis with a normal platelet count. Crit Care Resusc 2007;9:51.

202. Keeling D, Davidson S, Watson H. The management of heparin-induced thrombocytopenia. Br J Haematol 2006;133:259.

203. Badger NO, Butler K, Hallman LC. Excessive anticoagulation and anaphylactic reaction after rechallenge with lepirudin in a patient with heparin-induced thrombocytopenia. Pharmacotherapy 2004;24:1800.

204. Cardenas GA, Deitcher SR. Risk of anaphylaxis after reexposure to intravenous lepirudin in patients with current or past heparin-induced thrombocytopenia. Mayo Clin Proc 2005;80:491.

205. Yeh RW, Jang IK. Argatroban: update. Am Heart J 2006;151:1131.

206. Hovinga JA, Studt JD, Alberio L, Lammle B. von Willebrand factor-cleaving protease (ADAMTS-13) activity determination in the diagnosis of thrombotic microangiopathies: the Swiss experience. Semin Hematol 2004;41:75.

207. Lammle B, Kremer Hovinga JA, Alberio L. Thrombotic thrombocytopenic purpura. J Thromb Haemost 2005;3:1663.

208. Bennett CL, Connors JM, Carwile JM, et al. Thrombotic thrombocytopenic purpura associated with clopidogrel. N Engl J Med 2000;342:1773.

209. Bennett CL, Kim B, Zakarija A, et al. Two mechanistic pathways for thienopyridine-associated thrombotic thrombocytopenic purpura: a report from the SERF-TTP Research Group and the RADAR Project. J Am Coll Cardiol 2007;50:1138.

210. Zakarija A, Bandarenko N, Pandey DK, et al. Clopidogrel-associated TTP: an update of pharmacovigilance efforts conducted by independent researchers, pharmaceutical suppliers, and the Food and Drug Administration. Stroke 2004;35:533.

211. Scheid R, Hegenbart U, Ballaschke O, Von Cramon DY. Major stroke in thrombotic-thrombocytopenic purpura (Moschcowitz syndrome). Cerebrovasc Dis 2004;18:83.

212. Aksay E, Kiyan S, Ersel M, Hudaverdi O. Thrombotic thrombocytopenic purpura mimicking acute ischemic stroke. Emerg Med J 2006;23:e51.

213. Chintagumpala MM, Hurwitz RL, Moake JL, et al. Chronic relapsing thrombotic thrombocytopenic purpura in infants with large von Willebrand factor multimers during remission. J Pediatr 1992;120:49.

214. Greer M. Uncommon causes of stroke, part 2: changes in blood constituents and hemodynamic factors. Geriatrics 1978;33:51.

215. Hirsh LF. Vasculitis, thrombotic thrombocytopenic purpura, and stroke after aneurysm surgery. Surg Neurol 1982;17:426.

216. Ozdogu H, Boga C, Kizilkilic E, et al. A dramatic response to rituximab in a patient with resistant thrombotic thrombocytopenic purpura (TTP) who developed acute stroke. J Thromb Thrombolysis 2007;23:147.

217. Rinkel GJ, Wijdicks EF, Hene RJ. Stroke in relapsing thrombotic thrombocytopenic purpura. Stroke 1991;22:1087.

218. Zakynthinos EG, Vassilakopoulos T, Kontogianni DD, et al. A role for transoesophageal echocardiography in the early diagnosis of catastrophic antiphospholipid syndrome. J Intern Med 2000;248:519.

219. Ahmad A, Aggarwal A, Sharma D, et al. Rituximab for treatment of refractory/relapsing thrombotic thrombocytopenic purpura (TTP). Am J Hematol 2004;77:171.

220. Koulova L, Alexandrescu D, Dutcher JP, et al. Rituximab for the treatment of refractory idiopathic thrombocytopenic purpura (ITP) and thrombotic thrombocytopenic purpura (TTP): report of three cases. Am J Hematol 2005;78:49.

221. Strouse JJ, Hulbert ML, DeBaun MR, et al. Primary hemorrhagic stroke in children with sickle cell disease is associated with recent transfusion and use of corticosteroids. Pediatrics 2006;118:1916.

222. Wang WC. The pathophysiology, prevention, and treatment of stroke in sickle cell disease. Curr Opin Hematol 2007;14:191.

223. Adams RJ. Stroke prevention in sickle cell disease. Curr Opin Hematol 2000;7:101.

224. Adams RJ. Stroke prevention and treatment in sickle cell disease. Arch Neurol 2001;58:565.

225. Mehta SH, Adams RJ. Treatment and prevention of stroke in children with sickle cell disease. Curr Treat Options Neurol 2006;8:503.

226. Adams RJ, Pavlakis S, Roach ES. Sickle cell disease and stroke: primary prevention and transcranial Doppler. Ann Neurol 2003;54:559.

227. Winrow N, Melhem ER. Sickle cell disease and stroke in a pediatric population: evidence-based diagnostic evaluation. Neuroimaging Clin N Am 2003;13:185.

228. Nichols FT, Jones AM, Adams RJ. Stroke prevention in sickle cell disease (STOP) study guidelines for transcranial Doppler testing. J Neuroimaging 2001;11:354.

229. Kirkham FJ. Therapy insight: stroke risk and its management in patients with sickle cell disease. Nat Clin Pract Neurol 2007;3:264.

230. Vernant JC, Buisson GG, Rivierez M, Benyayer P. [Involvement of the large vessels supplying the brain in sickle cell disease: a possible cause of Moya-moya (author's transl)]. Nouv Presse Med 1980;9:25.

231. Dobson SR, Holden KR, Nietert PJ, et al. Moyamoya syndrome in childhood sickle cell disease: a predictive factor for recurrent cerebrovascular events. Blood 2002;99:3144.

232. Ramsewak W, Gill G, Lo R. Moyamoya in sickle cell disease demonstrated by DSA and Hexabrix. J Can Assoc Radiol 1985;36:332.

233. Schmugge M, Frischknecht H, Yonekawa Y, et al. Stroke in hemoglobin (SD) sickle cell disease with moyamoya: successful hydroxyurea treatment after cerebrovascular bypass surgery. Blood 2001;97:2165.

234. Gledhill N, Warburton D, Jamnik V. Haemoglobin, blood volume, cardiac function, and aerobic power. Can J Appl Physiol 1999;24:54.

235. Maguire JL, deVeber G, Parkin PC. Association between iron-deficiency anemia and stroke in young children. Pediatrics 2007;120:1053.

236. Silverberg DS, Wexler D, Blum M, et al. Erythropoietin in heart failure. Semin Nephrol 2005;25:397.

237. Stolz E, Valdueza JM, Grebe M, et al. Anemia as a risk factor for cerebral venous thrombosis? An old hypothesis revisited: results of a prospective study. J Neurol 2007;254:729.

238. Swann IL, Kendra JR. Severe iron deficiency anaemia and stroke. Clin Lab Haematol 2000;22:221.

239. Yager JY, Hartfield DS. Neurologic manifestations of iron deficiency in childhood. Pediatr Neurol 2002;27:85.

240. Alvarez-Larran A, Cervantes F, Bellosillo B, et al. Essential thrombocythemia in young individuals: frequency and risk factors for vascular events and evolution to myelofibrosis in 126 patients. Leukemia 2007;21:1218.

241. Benassi G, Ricci P, Calbucci F, et al. Slowly progressive ischemic stroke as first manifestation of essential thrombocythemia. Stroke 1989;20:1271.

242. Oliveira AS, Miranda MP, Duarte PC, Sarmento JN. [Essential thrombocythemia: apropos a case of cerebrovascular stroke]. Acta Med Port 1993;6:461.

243. Vemmos KN, Spengos K, Tsivgoulis G, Manios E. Progressive stroke due to essential thrombocythemia. Eur J Intern Med 2004;15:390.

244. Arboix A, Besses C, Acin P, et al. Ischemic stroke as first manifestation of essential thrombocythemia: report of six cases. Stroke 1995;26:1463.

245. Baxter EJ, Scott LM, Campbell PJ, et al. Acquired mutation of the tyrosine kinase JAK2 in human myeloproliferative disorders. Lancet 2005;365:1054.

246. Koennecke HC, Bernarding J. Diffusion-weighted magnetic resonance imaging in two patients with polycythemia rubra vera and early ischemic stroke. Eur J Neurol 2001;8:273.

247. Meng R, Zhou J, Ji XM, et al. [The diagnosis and treatment of polycythemia rubra vera manifesting as acute cerebral stroke]. Zhonghua Nei Ke Za Zhi 2006;45:366.

248. Zimmermann C, Walther EU, von Scheidt W, Hamann GF. Ischemic stroke in a 29-year-old man with left atrial spontaneous echoes and polycythemia vera. J Neurol 1999;246:1201.

249. Polycythemia vera: the natural history of 1213 patients followed for 20 years. Gruppo Italiano Studio Policitemia. Ann Intern Med 1995;123:656.

250. Grotta JC, Manner C, Pettigrew LC, Yatsu FM. Red blood cell disorders and stroke. Stroke 1986;17:811.

251. Lahtinen R, Kuikka J. Cerebral blood flow in polycythaemia vera. Ann Clin Res 1983;15(5-6):200.

252. Landolfi R, Marchioli R, Kutti J, et al. Efficacy and safety of low-dose aspirin in polycythemia vera. N Engl J Med 2004;350:114.

253. Najean Y, Mugnier P, Dresch C, Rain JD. Polycythaemia vera in young people: an analysis of 58 cases diagnosed before 40 years. Br J Haematol 1987;67:285.

254. Tartaglia AP, Goldberg JD, Berk PD, Wasserman LR. Adverse effects of antiaggregating platelet therapy in the treatment of polycythemia vera. Semin Hematol 1986;23:172.

255. Berk PD, Goldberg JD, Donovan PB, et al. Therapeutic recommendations in polycythemia vera based on Polycythemia Vera Study Group protocols. Semin Hematol 1986;23:132.

256. Michiels JJ. Aspirin and platelet-lowering agents for the prevention of vascular complications in essential thrombocythemia. Clin Appl Thromb Hemost 1999;5:247.

257. Streiff MB, Smith B, Spivak JL. The diagnosis and management of polycythemia vera in the era since the Polycythemia Vera Study Group: a survey of American Society of Hematology members' practice patterns. Blood 2002;99:1144.

258. Gillum LA, Mamidipudi SK, Johnston SC. Ischemic stroke risk with oral contraceptives: a meta-analysis. JAMA 2000;284:72.

259. Siritho S, Thrift AG, McNeil JJ, et al. Risk of ischemic stroke among users of the oral contraceptive pill: the Melbourne Risk Factor Study (MERFS) Group. Stroke 2003;34:1575.

260. Ischaemic stroke and combined oral contraceptives: results of an international, multicentre, case-control study. WHO Collaborative Study of Cardiovascular Disease and Steroid Hormone Contraception. Lancet 1996;348:498.

261. Haemorrhagic stroke, overall stroke risk, and combined oral contraceptives: results of an international, multicentre, case-control study. WHO Collaborative Study of Cardiovascular Disease and Steroid Hormone Contraception. Lancet 1996;348:505.

262. Lidegaard O, Kreiner S. Contraceptives and cerebral thrombosis: a five-year national case-control study. Contraception 2002;65:197.

263. Chan WS, Ray J, Wai EK, et al. Risk of stroke in women exposed to low-dose oral contraceptives: a critical evaluation of the evidence. Arch Intern Med 2004;164:741.

264. Heinemann LA, Lewis MA, Thorogood M, et al. Case-control study of oral contraceptives and risk of thromboembolic stroke: results from International Study on Oral Contraceptives and Health of Young Women. BMJ 1997;315:1502.

265. Johnston SC, Colford JM Jr, Gress DR. Oral contraceptives and the risk of subarachnoid hemorrhage: a meta-analysis. Neurology 1998;51:411.

266. Kemmeren JM, Tanis BC, van den Bosch MA, et al. Risk of Arterial Thrombosis in Relation to Oral Contraceptives (RATIO) study: oral contraceptives and the risk of ischemic stroke. Stroke 2002;33:1202.

267. Bousser MG, Kittner SJ. Oral contraceptives and stroke. Cephalalgia 2000;20:183.

268. Hannaford PC, Croft PR, Kay CR. Oral contraception and stroke: evidence from the Royal College of General Practitioners' Oral Contraception Study. Stroke 1994;25:935.

269. Lidegaard O. Oral contraception and risk of a cerebral thromboembolic attack: results of a case-control study. BMJ 1993;306:956.

270. Zamorski M. Stroke in users of low-dose oral contraceptives. J Fam Pract 1996;43:343.

271. Petitti DB, Sidney S, Bernstein A, et al. Stroke in users of low-dose oral contraceptives. N Engl J Med 1996;335:8.

272. Carolei A, Marini C. Stroke in users of low-dose oral contraceptives. N Engl J Med 1996;335:1767.

273. Schwartz SM, Siscovick DS, Longstreth WT Jr, et al. Use of low-dose oral contraceptives and stroke in young women. Ann Intern Med 1997;127(8 Pt 1):596.

274. Gillum LA, Johnston SC. Oral contraceptives and stroke risk: the debate continues. Lancet Neurol 2004;3:453.

275. Becker WJ. Use of oral contraceptives in patients with migraine. Neurology 1999;53(4 Suppl 1):S19.

276. Lidegaard O. Oral contraceptives, pregnancy and the risk of cerebral thromboembolism: the influence of diabetes, hypertension, migraine and previous thrombotic disease. Br J Obstet Gynaecol 1995;102:153.

277. Martinelli I, Sacchi E, Landi G, et al. High risk of cerebral-vein thrombosis in carriers of a prothrombin-gene mutation and in users of oral contraceptives. N Engl J Med 1998;338:1793.

278. Zuber M, Toulon P, Marnet L, Mas JL. Factor V Leiden mutation in cerebral venous thrombosis. Stroke 1996;27:1721.

279. Slooter AJ, Rosendaal FR, Tanis BC, et al. Prothrombotic conditions, oral contraceptives, and the risk of ischemic stroke. J Thromb Haemost 2005;3:1213.

280. Schwartz SM, Petitti DB, Siscovick DS, et al. Stroke and use of low-dose oral contraceptives in young women: a pooled analysis of two US studies. Stroke 1998;29:2277.

281. Li Y, Zhou L, Coulter D, et al. Prospective cohort study of the association between use of low-dose

oral contraceptives and stroke in Chinese women. Pharmacoepidemiol Drug Saf 2006;15:726.

282. Bousser MG, Conard J, Kittner S, et al. Recommendations on the risk of ischaemic stroke associated with use of combined oral contraceptives and hormone replacement therapy in women with migraine. The International Headache Society Task Force on Combined Oral Contraceptives & Hormone Replacement Therapy. Cephalalgia 2000;20:155.

283. Di Micco P, D'Uva M, Romano M, et al. Stroke due to left carotid thrombosis in moderate ovarian hyperstimulation syndrome. Thromb Haemost 2003;90:957.

284. Elford K, Leader A, Wee R, Stys PK. Stroke in ovarian hyperstimulation syndrome in early pregnancy treated with intra-arterial rt-PA. Neurology 2002;59:1270.

285. Hwang WJ, Lai ML, Hsu CC, Hou NT. Ischemic stroke in a young woman with ovarian hyperstimulation syndrome. J Formos Med Assoc 1998;97:503.

286. Inbar OJ, Levran D, Mashiach S, Dor J. Ischemic stroke due to induction of ovulation with clomiphene citrate and menotropins without evidence of ovarian hyperstimulation syndrome. Fertil Steril 1994;62:1075.

287. Kermode AG, Churchyard A, Carroll WM. Stroke complicating severe ovarian hyperstimulation syndrome. Aust N Z J Med 1993;23:219.

288. Togay-Isikay C, Celik T, Ustuner I, Yigit A. Ischaemic stroke associated with ovarian hyperstimulation syndrome and factor V Leiden mutation. Aust N Z J Obstet Gynaecol 2004;44:264.

289. Worrell GA, Wijdicks EF, Eggers SD, et al. Ovarian hyperstimulation syndrome with ischemic stroke due to an intracardiac thrombus. Neurology 2001;57:1342.

290. Singhal R, Brimble KS. Thromboembolic complications in the nephrotic syndrome: pathophysiology and clinical management. Thromb Res 2006;118:397.

291. Kronenberg F. Dyslipidemia and nephrotic syndrome: recent advances. J Ren Nutr 2005;15:195.

292. Molino D, De Santo NG, Marotta R, et al. Plasma levels of plasminogen activator inhibitor type 1, factor VIII, prothrombin activation fragment 1+2, anticardiolipin, and antiprothrombin antibodies are risk factors for thrombosis in hemodialysis patients. Semin Nephrol 2004;24:495.

293. Crew RJ, Radhakrishnan J, Appel G. Complications of the nephrotic syndrome and their treatment. Clin Nephrol 2004;62:245.

294. Stenvinkel P, Alvestrand A, Angelin B, Eriksson M. LDL-apheresis in patients with nephrotic syndrome: effects on serum albumin and urinary albumin excretion. Eur J Clin Invest 2000;30:866.

295. Joven J, Arcelus R, Camps J, et al. Determinants of plasma homocyst(e)ine in patients with nephrotic syndrome. J Mol Med 2000;78:147.

296. Citak A, Emre S, Sairin A, et al. Hemostatic problems and thromboembolic complications in nephrotic children. Pediatr Nephrol 2000;14:138.

297. Orth SR, Ritz E. The nephrotic syndrome. N Engl J Med 1998;338:1202.

CHAPTER 10

Stroke and Pregnancy

Rima M. Dafer • José Biller

KEY TERMS	
AVM	arteriovenous malformation
CT	computed tomography
DSA	digital subtraction angiography
HELLP	hemolysis, elevated liver enzymes, and low platelet count
ICH	intracerebral hemorrhage
LMWH	low-molecular-weight heparin
MRI	magnetic resonance imaging
PPCM	peripartum cardiomyopathy
rt-PA	recombinant tissue plasminogen activator
SAH	subarachnoid hemorrhage
VTE	venous thromboembolism

Stroke during pregnancy and the puerperium presents important diagnostic and therapeutic challenges for the obstetrician and the neurologist.[1,2] Despite widespread accessibility to prenatal care, pregnancy-associated stroke remains a major cause of serious morbidity and mortality. Although the mechanisms of stroke during pregnancy remain unclear, pregnancy is considered a procoagulant state because of its physiologic changes. Increased risk of stroke in pregnancy can be determined by hormonally mediated damage to vascular tissue structure, hypercoagulable state, hemodynamic changes, and severe acute arterial hypertension in patients with preeclampsia and eclampsia.

Pregnancy is associated with increased platelet adhesion, increased fibrinogen, increased coagulation factors, and decreased fibrinolysis, with reduced levels of available circulating plasminogen activator. Additionally, pregnancy imposes an added hemodynamic burden with the increase in blood volume, cardiac output, stroke volume, and heart rate; a mild decrease in arterial blood pressure; and a decline in total peripheral and pulmonary vascular resistance.[1-3]

The etiology of stroke in pregnancy and the puerperium is diverse. Pregnancy-associated strokes are roughly evenly divided among hemorrhagic and ischemic strokes. Causes of stroke during pregnancy are listed in Tables 10-1 and 10-2. This chapter reviews the peculiarities of etiology and pathogenesis of pregnancy-associated ischemic and hemorrhagic strokes and discusses the management approach. Table 10-3 outlines the evaluation of a pregnant patient with stroke.

TABLE 10-1 **Etiology of Ischemic Stroke Associated with Pregnancy**

Occlusive arterial disease
  Thrombotic/embolic
Cardioembolic
  Peripartum cardiomyopathy
  Mitral valve prolapse
  Prosthetic heart valves
  Atrial fibrillation
  Rheumatic heart disease
  Infective endocarditis
  Nonbacterial thrombotic endocarditis
  Paradoxical embolism
Rare embolic etiologies
  Amniotic fluid, air, fat
Arterial hypotension
  Border zone infarction
  Sheehan syndrome
Hematologic disorders
  Disseminated intravascular coagulation
  Thrombotic thrombocytopenic purpura
  Sickle cell disease
Arteritis/arteriopathies
  Fibromuscular dysplasia
  Systemic lupus erythematosus
  Takayasu arteritis
  Drugs
  "Isolated" cerebral angiitis
Carotid cavernous fistulas
Dural vascular malformations

TABLE 10-2 **Etiology of Hemorrhagic Stroke Associated with Pregnancy**

Intracerebral Hemorrhage

Eclampsia
Hypertension (unrelated to eclampsia)
Choriocarcinoma
Ruptured vascular malformation
Intracranial venous thrombosis
Vasculitis

Intracranial Venous Thrombosis

Hypercoagulable state
Infectious
Unknown

Subarachnoid Hemorrhage

Aneurysm
  Saccular aneurysm
  Mycotic aneurysm
  Other aneurysm
Arteriovenous malformation
  Cerebral
  Spinal cord
Vasculitis
Eclampsia
Abruptio placentae with disseminated intravascular
  coagulation
Choriocarcinoma
Cerebral venous dural sinus thrombosis

TABLE 10-3 **Evaluation of a Pregnant Patient with Suspected Stroke**

Complete blood count with differential and platelet
  count
Prothrombin time and activated partial
  thromboplastin time
Antiphospholipid antibodies (anticardiolipin
  antibodies, lupus anticoagulant, β_2-glycoprotein
  1 antibodies)
Antithrombin, protein C activity, free and total
  protein S antigen
Activated protein C resistance and factor V Leiden
  mutation
MTHFR mutation
Prothrombin gene (G20210A) mutation
Plasminogen activator inhibitor
Homocysteine
Sickle cell screen
Hemoglobin electrophoresis
Liver function tests
Serum creatinine and blood urea nitrogen
Plasma glucose level
Serum cholesterol and triglycerides
Serum uric acid
Serum electrolytes
Serum VDRL
Serum FTA-ABS
Human immunodeficiency virus serology
Erythrocyte sedimentation rate
Antinuclear antibodies
Blood cultures
Serum and urine human chorionic gonadotropin
Urinalysis with microscopic evaluation
Urine toxicology
Cerebrospinal fluid analysis for human chorionic
  gonadotropin and VDRL (optional)
Chest radiograph
12-lead electrocardiogram
Two-dimensional echocardiography
Cranial CT with abdominal shielding
CT angiography of intracranial vessels
Carotid ultrasound
Transcranial Doppler
MRI
MR angiography
MR venography
DSA with abdominal shielding (optional)

FTA-ABS, fluorescent treponemal antibody absorption; MTHFR, methylene tetrahydrofolate reductase; VDRL, Venereal Disease Research Laboratory.

Epidemiology

Pregnancy increases the risk of stroke by 3-fold to 13-fold; pregnancy-associated strokes are most likely to occur in young patients during late pregnancy and the first postpartum week.[4-8] The incidence of stroke is estimated at 3.5 to 5 per 100,000 pregnancies.[29,10] More recent studies reported an incidence of 69 per 100,000 pregnancies in a tertiary referral. After exclusion of patients referred from smaller hospitals, the incidence decreased to 26 per 100,000 pregnancies, compared with an incidence of 10.7 per 100,000 women-years among nonpregnant women 15 to 44 years old,[11] with a higher incidence reported in African American compared with white populations.[8]

Ischemic Stroke

The mechanism of pregnancy-associated ischemic stroke is unknown. Pregnancy carries a higher risk of arterial and venous stroke owing to accompanying physiologic changes leading to hypercoagulable state, cardiac burden and volume overload, and preeclampsia/ eclampsia.[8,12,13] Common causes of ischemic stroke in young patients are similar in pregnant women compared with nonpregnant women, although most patients with arterial hypertension, diabetes mellitus, hyperlipidemia, or even prosthetic heart valves may have successful pregnancies. Arterial occlusion accounts for 60% to 80% of cerebral ischemic lesions; the carotid and middle cerebral artery territories are most commonly compromised.[7]

Thrombosis of a preexisting arterial stenosis secondary to underlying hypercoagulability is thought to be the main predisposing factor. Other predisposing factors include arterial hypertension, anemia, and hormonal changes. Carotid artery thrombosis is a rare life-threatening complication of the HELLP syndrome (hemolysis, elevated liver enzymes, and low platelet count). Factors other than intrinsic aortic changes directly related to pregnancy are responsible for the increased incidence of aortic dissection in pregnant women; as a result, cerebral and spinal cord ischemia may ensue.[14,15] Other causes include cardioembolism, cardiac arrhythmias, peripartum cardiomyopathy, paradoxical embolism, choriocarcinoma, and cerebral dural venous sinus thrombosis predominantly during late pregnancy and postpartum.[16,17]

Cardiac Causes

Peripartum cardiomyopathy (PPCM) is an uncommon idiopathic congestive cardiomyopathy, affecting previously healthy women in the peripartum period. The incidence of PPCM ranges from 1 in 1300 to 1 in 15,000 pregnancies, and is greatest in African Americans.[18] A review of the National Hospital Discharge Survey from 1990 to 2002 reported an incidence of 1 case per 3189 live births.[19] Risk factors include life in tropical climates, older age, multiparity, twin pregnancy, black race, and pregnancy-associated hypertensive disorders. The diagnosis of PPCM is made when previously healthy pregnant women develop new-onset unexplained heart failure in the last month of pregnancy or in the first 5 months postpartum.

The cause of PPCM remains unknown; viral, autoimmune, and idiopathic causes have been implicated. The clinical syndrome includes dilated cardiomegaly, congestive heart failure, cardiac arrhythmias, and systemic and pulmonary emboli (Fig. 10-1). Early diagnosis and initiation of treatment are essential to optimize pregnancy outcome. Magnetic resonance imaging (MRI) may show late gadolinium enhancement of the left ventricle.[20] Medical management consists of optimization of maternal hemodynamics and prevention of thromboembolism. About half of patients with PPCM recover without complications. The mortality rate is 1.36% to 2.05%.[19,21-23] Persistence of disease after 6 months indicates irreversible cardiomyopathy and poor prognosis.[24,25]

Mitral valve prolapse is present in approximately 6% of the general population and 12% to 17% of women of reproductive age.[26] Most patients are asymptomatic and tolerate pregnancy well. The course of mitral valve prolapse is infrequently complicated by chest pain, severe mitral regurgitation, infective endocarditis, cerebral ischemia, or even sudden death from complex cardiac arrhythmias. The classic auscultatory findings may be attenuated by the physiologic cardiovascular changes seen during pregnancy. Routine endocarditis prophylaxis is not recommended at the time of delivery except in selected cases. Cesarean section is reserved for obstetric indications.[26-31]

Cardiac valve diseases in pregnancy have been considered hazardous with increased risk of fetal and maternal complications. Morbidities are less common after porcine valve

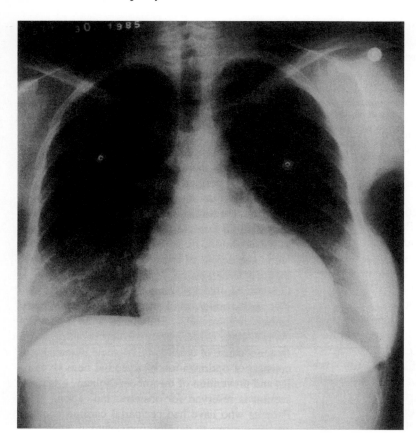

FIGURE 10-1   Anteroposterior chest x-ray shows enlargement of the cardiopericardial silhouette, with mild vascular redistribution in a patient with peripartum cardiomyopathy, complicated by cerebral infarction.

replacement compared with mechanical prostheses, although pregnancy is thought to accelerate the degenerative process and the need for reoperation.[32] Management of a pregnant patient with mechanical heart valve is complex. The hemodynamic load imposed by pregnancy, the increased risk of ineffective endocarditis, cardiac arrhythmias, valve thrombosis, systemic embolization, and the teratogenic effects of warfarin anticoagulation are implicated in higher rates of fetal and maternal morbidities. The optimal anticoagulation strategy during pregnancy remains controversial. Anticoagulation with warfarin derivatives is associated with higher risk of fetal loss and increased bleeding complications; it has been a common practice to switch women to heparin during the first and last trimesters of pregnancy. More recent data showed, however, an increased risk of maternal complications in women on heparin compared with warfarin, supporting the use of warfarin throughout pregnancy except for weeks 6 to 12.[33-37] Routine peripartum

antibiotic prophylaxis is not indicated in patients with cardiac valvulopathies.[37,38]

Pregnancy can precipitate cardiac arrhythmias in previously healthy individuals, with a higher risk during labor and delivery. Direct cardiac electrophysiologic effects of pregnancy, hemodynamic changes, underlying heart disease, and electrolyte imbalance may promote the development of arrhythmias during pregnancy and labor. Management of arrhythmias during pregnancy is similar to that in nonpregnant patients. Caution in antiarrhythmic drug selection should be taken, however, to avoid teratogenic and hemodynamic adverse effects of medications on the fetus, and drugs with the longest safety record should be used as first-line therapy.[39-41]

Paroxysmal supraventricular tachycardia and ventricular premature beats should be managed conservatively with observation and rest. Precipitating factors, such as caffeine use, alcohol consumption, and cigarette smoking, should be avoided. Other potential underlying causes for arrhythmias should be excluded, including endocrine or metabolic disorders. Drug therapy should be avoided during the first trimester of pregnancy. In paroxysmal supraventricular tachycardia, vagal stimulation maneuvers should be attempted first. Intravenous adenosine may be considered in symptomatic patients when vagal maneuvers fail. Cardioselective β-blockers may be considered. Alternatively, calcium channel blockers such as verapamil or diltiazem may be given.[40-43]

Atrial fibrillation carries an increased risk of cardiac failure and thromboembolism. When present in association with rheumatic heart disease and mitral stenosis, atrial fibrillation increases the risk of stroke by approximately 17-fold. In the absence of rheumatic valvular heart disease, the risk of stroke increases more than fivefold in patients with atrial fibrillation.[42,44] Electrical cardioversion should be attempted first to convert to sinus rhythm; if unsuccessful, rate control can be achieved by a cardioselective β-adrenergic blocker drug or digoxin.[40,43]

Ventricular arrhythmias may occur in pregnant women and are associated with a higher rate of fetal loss. Ventricular arrhythmias are more common in patients with preexisting cardiac disorders, such as cardiomyopathy, congenital heart disease, valvular heart disease, and mitral valve prolapse. Electrical cardioversion or treatment with sotalol may be used. Amiodarone should be avoided because of major risks to the fetus.[40,43] In women with long QT segment syndrome, β-blockers must be continued during pregnancy and the postpartum period.[40,43,45]

Infective endocarditis during pregnancy or the puerperium is an exceedingly rare, life-threatening complication of pregnancy, affecting 1 in 4000 to 1 in 8000 pregnancies.[46,47] Although most often a complication of preexisting congenital or rheumatic valvular heart disease, many cases are complications of the use of illicit intravenous drugs, abortion, or uterine curettage; numerous cases occur in patients with prosthetic heart valves. Nonbacterial thrombotic endocarditis is an uncommon cause of stroke in women of childbearing age.[48]

Pregnancy is increasingly common in patients with congenital heart diseases. Women with hypertrophic cardiomyopathy and pulmonary hypertension secondary to septal defects or cyanotic heart diseases should receive prepregnancy counseling and detailed assessment by cardiologists to determine the individual health risks associated with pregnancy. Atrial septal defects are left uncorrected, unless a significant left-to-right shunt or pulmonary hypertension is present. Ventricular septal defects are often corrected in childhood and are rarely encountered in women of childbearing age. Endocarditis prophylaxis is advised at the time of delivery in women with ventricular septal defects.

Thrombo-occlusive Disorders

Hypercoagulability associated with pregnancy results in a marked increase in the incidence of thrombo-occlusive disorders. Other pregnancy-related embolic phenomena include amniotic fluid embolism, air embolism, and trophoblastic embolism.

Pulmonary embolism is a major nonobstetric cause of postpartum maternal mortality. The risk of paradoxical embolism increases during pregnancy and the puerperium because of the increased risk of venous thrombosis in the superficial or deep veins of the lower extremities or in pelvic veins. Patent foramen ovale, alone or together with atrial septal aneurysm, is the most common cardiac defect associated with paradoxical embolism and cryptogenic stroke.[49-51] Percutaneous patent foramen ovale closure with occluder devices has been performed safely in selected patients with recurrent cerebral ischemic stroke secondary to paradoxical embolism during pregnancy.[52,53]

Air embolism is a rare life-threatening complication of obstetric or gynecologic procedures arising as a result of gas bubbles being introduced into the circulation via severed blood vessels. It may follow intrauterine manipulations, uterine rupture, and criminal abortion. Life-threatening acute venous air embolism also may result in air insufflation of the vagina during orogenital sex.[54,55] Extensive brain damage and acute cardiovascular collapse lead to a fatal outcome. A favorable outcome depends on early diagnosis and prompt treatment. Hyperbaric oxygen therapy in addition to supportive care is the first line of treatment for air embolism.[56,57]

Fat embolism may follow long bone fractures, osteoporotic conditions, soft tissue injuries, blood transfusion, pancreatitis, or cardiopulmonary bypass, and can complicate pregnancy in women with hemoglobin SC disease.[58,59] The syndrome is characterized by sudden onset of tachypnea, tachycardia, fever, and encephalopathy. Petechiae are often found in the fundi, conjunctiva, anterior chest, and axilla.

Amniotic fluid embolism is the leading cause of maternal death, with an incidence of 1 in 20,000 to 1 in 80,000 pregnancies. Amniotic fluid embolism is a catastrophic, unpredictable, and rarely preventable obstetric emergency characterized by acute cor pulmonale, nonhemorrhagic primary obstetric shock, and disseminated intravascular coagulation.[60] It is caused by the embolization into the maternal circulation of amniotic fluid debris intrapartum or during the early postpartum period. Warning signs include seizures in the presence of arterial hypotension and bleeding. Management consists of circulatory support, adequate oxygenation, prevention of metabolic acidosis, and correction of associated coagulopathy.[10,61,62] The mortality rate is high.

Strokes resulting from cerebral venous thrombosis represent 10 to 20 per 100,000 deliveries in Western countries.[63,64] Abnormalities in coagulation leading to intravascular clotting in the early puerperium may contribute to venous stasis. Clinical manifestations include focal neurologic signs, seizures, headache, and alterations in consciousness.[63,65,66] Computed tomography (CT) or MRI of the brain with MR venography is essential for the diagnosis. Early administration of heparin may improve outcome.

Arterial Hypotension

Arterial hypotension may result from acute intrapartum blood loss, spinal anesthesia, and embolism of amniotic fluid contents. Severe hypotension can cause watershed infarctions between two main pial artery territories. Sheehan syndrome refers to postpartum panhypopituitarism caused by severe postpartum hemorrhage, leading to ischemia of the territory of the inferior or superior hypophyseal arteries and massive ischemic necrosis of the anterior pituitary.[67-69]

Hematologic Disorders

Hypercoagulable state is a major threat to women during pregnancy, commonly associated with increased risk of intrauterine fetal death and maternal venous and arterial thromboses during the last trimester of gestation and early puerperium.[70-87] The incidence of pregnancy-associated venous thromboembolism (VTE) is approximately 1 in 1500 deliveries, five times higher in a pregnant than in a nonpregnant woman. Women with preexisting hereditary or acquired coagulation disorders should be counseled for the potential increased risk of VTE. Prophylactic use of heparin during pregnancy is recommended in patients with combined coagulation abnormality or prior history of VTE to reduce the risk of recurrent abortions, stillbirth, and preeclampsia. Unfractionated heparin or low-molecular-weight heparin (LMWH) do not cross the placenta and are the anticoagulants of choice. Postpartum prophylaxis should be given to all women with an increased risk for VTE. In patients with recurrent miscarriages associated with antiphospholipid antibody syndrome, treatment with heparin and low-dose aspirin may improve fetal survival compared with aspirin alone.[88-90] Intravenous immunoglobulin therapy may reduce obstetric complications.[91]

Arteritis and Arteriopathies

Fibromuscular dysplasia is an idiopathic disease of small and medium-sized arteries, more commonly occurring in women. The disorder is often an unexpected and asymptomatic finding discovered on arteriographic examination of patients with a variety of neurologic conditions. Cerebral infarction is an infrequent but well-recognized complication of fibromuscular dysplasia of the carotid arteries complicating pregnancy.[92] Other mechanisms of ischemic strokes in pregnancy and the puerperium include dissection of the cervicocerebral arteries, postpartum cerebral angiopathy resulting from cerebral vasospasm, and reversible intimal hyperplasia secondary to the action of female reproductive steroids on the vessel wall.

Postpartum cerebral angiopathy (Call-Fleming syndrome) is a rare cause of ischemic and hemorrhagic strokes in young women. It is characterized by thunderclap-like headache, seizures, focal neurologic deficits, and reversible segmental cerebral vasoconstriction on angiographic studies. MRI may show transient reversible signals resembling the lesions described in patients with reversible posterior ischemic encephalopathy syndrome (Fig. 10-2).[93] The condition is encountered after administration of vasoconstrictive agents, especially in migraine patients.[94,95] Administration of methylprednisolone or cyclophosphamide or both may improve symptoms.[96] Prognosis is favorable.

Management of Ischemic Stroke in Pregnancy

To date, intravenous thrombolysis with recombinant tissue plasminogen activator (rt-PA) is the only pharmacologically approved therapy for ischemic stroke within 3 hours of symptom onset. There are no data from controlled randomized trials in pregnant patients, and historically pregnant women have been excluded from clinical trials. Despite evidence

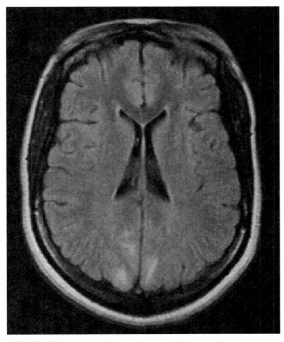

FIGURE 10-2 Axial fluid attenuated inversion recovery MRI shows bilateral occipital hyperintensities in a woman with postpartum cerebral angiopathy.

that rt-PA does not cross the placenta, and in the absence of clinical guidelines, pregnancy remains a relative contraindication for thrombolysis. A series of cases in the literature described administration of thrombolytic therapy with intravenous or intra-arterial rt-PA for ischemic stroke in pregnant women. The complication rate was similar to nonpregnant women, and the fetal fatality rate was estimated at 8%.[97-102]

When administration of platelet antiaggregant therapy is considered for secondary stroke prevention, the risk-to-benefit ratio should be carefully balanced and explained to the patient. Full anticoagulation is necessary but problematic in patients with mechanical heart valve prostheses and other cardioembolic strokes. Warfarin derivatives cross the placenta and may be associated with teratogenic effects, fetal loss, and bleeding complications. Their use is associated, however, with a lower rate of valve thrombosis and maternal complications in patients with high risk of thrombosis, such as patients with prosthetic mitral valve, multiple mechanical valves, and prior history of embolism. Conversely, heparin use during pregnancy is associated with lower risk of embryopathy.

The use of oral anticoagulants should be avoided in the first trimester of pregnancy and in the last 3 weeks before term and should be substituted with unfractionated heparin or LMWH.[103] LMWH is the anticoagulant of choice because of longer half-life and fewer side effects; unfractionated heparin generally is preferred around the time of delivery because of its shorter half-life and ease of monitoring.[104-106] In cases of heparin-induced thrombocytopenia, fondaparinux may be considered.[103,107] More recent data support the use of anticoagulation with warfarin throughout pregnancy in women with artificial heart valves to reduce the risks of maternal complications.[33-37]

Aspirin decreases uterine contractility; may delay labor; increases the risk of prolonged pregnancy; and contributes to fetal complications, antepartum bleeding, and bleeding during delivery. Aspirin is thought to be beneficial in prevention of preeclampsia, however, and has been associated with improved fetal hemodynamic performance and decreased need for intensive neonatal care.[108-110] Low-dose aspirin is safe during the second and third trimesters for the mother and the fetus, and postpartum use by breastfeeding mothers is safe for infants. Aspirin combined with prednisone is the treatment of choice in patients with antiphospholipid syndrome and recurrent miscarriages.[88-90]

Hemorrhagic Stroke

Pregnancy, in particular the puerperium, seems to be associated with an increased risk of intracerebral hemorrhage (ICH). Advanced maternal age, black race, hypertensive diseases, coagulopathies, and tobacco abuse are independent risk factors for pregnancy-related ICH. The rate of pregnancy-related ICH is estimated at 6.1 per 100,000 deliveries.[6-8,111,112] The most common causes of pregnancy-related ICH are eclampsia, ruptured intracranial saccular aneurysms, or vascular malformations (Fig. 10-3). Women with severe preeclampsia may have a reduced number of circulating platelets and increased

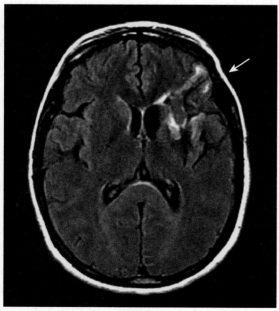

FIGURE 10-3 Axial fluid attenuated inversion recovery MRI shows a small curvilinear area of decreased signal consistent with remote hemorrhage (*arrowhead*). See changes of craniotomy at left convexity (*arrow*). The patient had a primary intracerebral hemorrhage during delivery in the absence of eclampsia.

levels of serum fibrin degradation products. Whether pregnancy increases the risk of rupture of an arteriovenous malformation (AVM) is controversial.[62] Causes of hemorrhagic stroke are listed in Table 10-2.

Less common causes of pregnancy-associated ICH include mycotic (infective) aneurysms, dural AVMs, vasculitides, metastatic choriocarcinoma, cerebral venous thrombosis, anticoagulant therapy, and bleeding diatheses (Fig. 10-4). Depletion of coagulation factors with severe hypofibrinogenemia is the primary cause of hemorrhagic diatheses. Most cases have been associated with abruptio placentae, retained dead fetus syndrome, amniotic fluid embolism, and postpartum hemorrhage. Severe coagulation defects also are seen with intrauterine infection and septic shock, hydatidiform mole, abortion induced with hypertonic solutions, and uterine rupture.

Eclampsia is a hypertensive disease of women in the second half of pregnancy, more common toward term, and characterized by edema, proteinuria, hyperreflexia, convulsions, and coma. The role of eclampsia in the genesis of ICH remains controversial. The onset of eclampsia also may occur in the postpartum period. Maternal death from stroke associated with eclampsia is often due to ICH.[6,10,111,113] Main postmortem neuropathologic lesions include thrombosis; arteriolar fibrinoid necrosis; diffuse microinfarcts; hypoxic-ischemic cerebral changes; cerebral edema; and scattered cortical petechiae, large subcortical hemorrhages, or intraventricular bleeding hemorrhages (Fig. 10-5). Management of eclampsia requires the administration of antihypertensive drugs. Anticonvulsant agents may be needed to prevent or treat eclamptic convulsions.

ICH can complicate many vasculitides, including systemic lupus erythematosus, Wegener granulomatosis, polyarteritis nodosa, rheumatoid arthritis, Henoch-Schönlein purpura, drug abuse, and isolated central nervous system angiitis. Therapy often requires the administration of corticosteroids or other immunosuppressive agents.

Gestational choriocarcinoma is the most malignant, but curable, tumor of gestational trophoblastic neoplasia. Choriocarcinoma may follow hydatidiform mole, miscarriage,

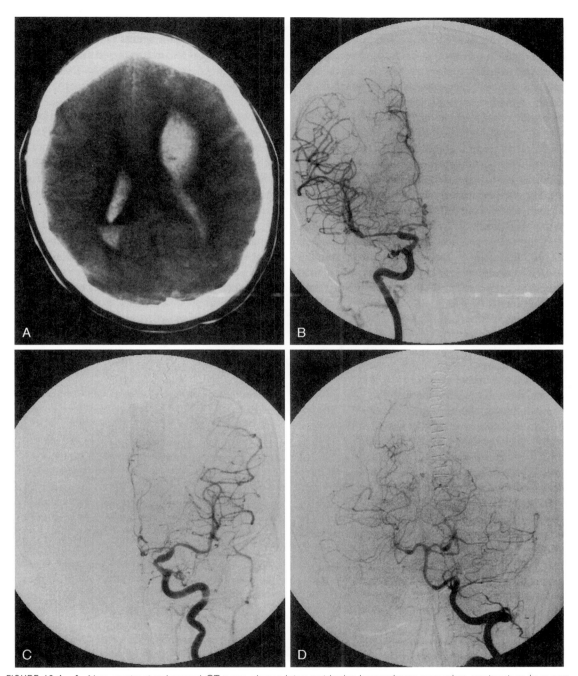

FIGURE 10-4 **A,** Non–contrast-enhanced CT scan shows intraventricular hemorrhage occurring postpartum in a non-eclamptic patient. **B-D,** Anteroposterior right and left internal carotid and anteroposterior vertebrobasilar views on angiography show short segment narrowing of the proximal anterior, middle, and posterior cerebral arteries and basilar artery, consistent with arteritis in the same patient.

ectopic pregnancy, or normal pregnancy. It has been estimated that 300 to 500 women per year have these malignancies in the United States. It grows rapidly and metastasizes to the lung, liver, and, less frequently, the brain. Intracranial metastasis from

choriocarcinoma may manifest as ICH, subarachnoid hemorrhage (SAH), subdural hematoma, and multiple arterial occlusions, and seldom as a neoplastic intracranial aneurysm or neoplastic carotid-cavernous fistula. Treatment of choriocarcinoma metastatic to

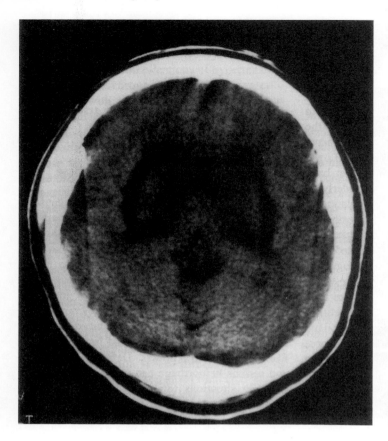

FIGURE 10-5   Axial, non–contrast-enhanced CT scan shows bilateral basal ganglia low densities in a patient with eclampsia.

the brain is craniotomy or stereotactic radio-surgery combined with chemotherapy; whole-brain radiation therapy should be avoided when possible.[88,91,114-120]

Subarachnoid Hemorrhage

SAH resulting from an intracranial aneurysm or AVM is a grave complication of pregnancy, responsible for 5% to 12% of all maternal deaths. Aneurysms are responsible for SAH in three fourths of cases, and AVM in one fourth of cases.[121]

Hemodynamic and endocrine changes in pregnancy may predispose to aneurysm formation, enlargement, and rupture.[122,123] The incidence of ruptured intracranial aneurysm during pregnancy is estimated as 1 to 5 in 10,000 pregnancies, with an associated mortality greater than 40%.[121] Ruptured intracranial aneurysms are most commonly seen in the third trimester of pregnancy, peaking during labor and delivery, or in the early

puerperium. Predisposing factors to aneurysmal rupture include earlier age at menarche, advanced gestational age, and primiparity.[124] The association between parity and risk of SAH is debatable.[125-127] High parity is associated with an increased risk of mortality from vascular complications overall[125]; in contrast, multiparity was shown to confer a moderate long-term protective effect on the risk of SAH.[126,127] Similarly, the risk of SAH is lower in women whose first pregnancy is at an older age and in women who have ever used hormonal replacement therapy.[128]

Intracranial saccular aneurysms generally are located at vascular bifurcations at the base of the brain in the subarachnoid space; most occur in the anterior half of the circle of Willis. The most common sites are the junction of the anterior cerebral–anterior communicating arteries, the junction of the internal carotid–posterior communicating arteries, the main bifurcation of the middle cerebral artery, and the basilar artery bifurcation. After aneurysmal SAH, rebleeding, cerebral vasospasm, and hydrocephalus add to morbidity and mortality.

The evaluation and treatment of aneurysmal SAH during pregnancy should be the same as in a nonpregnant patient, with special consideration for the risk of radiation exposure from digital subtraction angiography (DSA) and coil embolization. Cranial CT and lumbar puncture are diagnostic in most cases. Although CT angiography is preferred to DSA as an initial diagnostic tool, DSA with abdominal shielding can be performed safely. Ruptured cerebral aneurysms should be treated as they would be in patients who are not pregnant with endovascular aneurysmal coiling or clipping.[129,130] The International Subarachnoid Aneurysm Trial showed that endovascular coiling of ruptured intracranial aneurysms was associated with significant reduction in the relative risk of death or dependency compared with neurosurgical clipping.[129,131] Coil embolization may confer radiation risks to the fetus, however.[132] Additionally, partially coiled aneurysm may carry a potential risk of rebleeding, in particular during labor and delivery.[132] On a theoretical basis, surgical clipping may be preferred to coiling in symptomatic ruptured aneurysm during pregnancy.[133] When the aneurysm is successfully clipped or coiled, the pregnancy may be allowed to progress to term, and vaginal delivery is preferred.

Cesarean section is indicated in selected cases or when the aneurysm is diagnosed at term. Emergency cesarean section followed by aneurysmal treatment may be considered in pregnant women with cerebral aneurysmal complications.[134] Unruptured aneurysms should be treated only when symptomatic or rapidly enlarging.[135,136]

Arteriovenous Malformations

AVMs are common causes of lobar intracerebral hemorrhages and are second to ruptured intracranial saccular aneurysms as causes of SAH. AVMs can be located anywhere, but occur with higher frequency in the frontoparietal and temporal regions.[137]

There is controversy regarding the question of whether pregnancy alters the natural tendency of existing cerebrovascular malformations to rupture.[138,139] The New York Islands AVM Study data did not suggest a greatly increased rate of cerebrovascular malformation–related hemorrhage in pregnant women compared with nonpregnant women with ICH (0.50 versus 0.33 per 100,000 person-years).[140] In the same study, pregnancy did not seem to increase the rate of first cerebral hemorrhage from a ruptured AVM. Prospective population-based data on the incidence of cerebral AVM suggest that the natural history risk of unruptured AVMs is significantly lower than the risk of AVMs with rupture.[141,142]

Management guidelines are unavailable; management of AVM rupture during pregnancy should be based primarily on neurosurgical rather than on obstetric considerations. There is a tendency to perform cesarean delivery in patients with prior history of bleeding from an AVM.[143] A Randomized Trial of Unruptured Brain AVMs may shed information on the benefit of invasive versus conservative management in patients with unruptured AVMs.

Dural AVMs are developmental anomalies characterized by an increased number of abnormal blood vessels within the dura mater. They represent approximately 10% of intracranial AVMs. These malformations may cause focal deficits by arterial "steal" or venous congestion, or they may rupture and cause SAH or intracerebral hemorrhage. Pregnancy increases the risk of spontaneous carotid cavernous fistula; it occurs most often in the second half of pregnancy or at childbirth.[144,145] Patients usually present with headaches, chemosis, conjunctival injection, proptosis, and ocular dysmotility (Fig. 10-6).

Conclusion

In patients with symptoms and signs suggestive of stroke, prompt and thorough evaluation and rapid management are key to avoid fetal loss and to prevent maternal complications. Strategies for stroke prevention should take into account the competing risks to the mother and fetus. Although proper counseling is imperative, a history of pregnancy-related stroke should not be a contraindication for subsequent pregnancy.

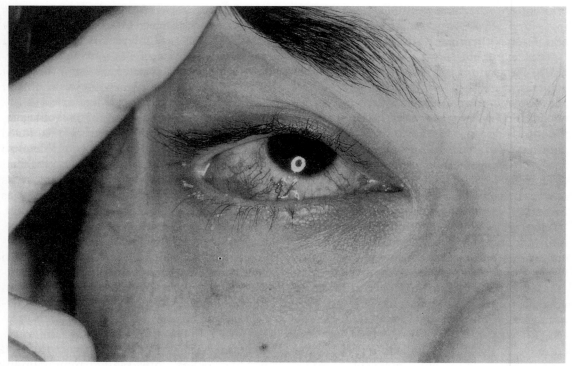

FIGURE 10-6   Chemosis, conjunctival injection, proptosis, and ocular dysmotility in a patient with carotid cavernous fistula.

REFERENCES

1. Donaldson JD. Stroke. In Clinical Obstetrics and Gynecology. Wolters Kluwer Health-Lippincott Williams and Wilkins. Philadelphia. Harper & Row, 1981.
2. Wiebers DO, Whisnant JP. The incidence of stroke among pregnant women in Rochester, Minn, 1955 through 1979. JAMA 1985;254:3055.
3. Brinkman CR. Biologic adaptation to pregnancy. In Creasy RK, Resnik R, eds. Maternal-Fetal Medicine: Principles and Practice. Philadelphia, WB Saunders, 1989.
4. Wiebers DO. Ischemic cerebrovascular complications of pregnancy. Arch Neurol 1985;42:1106.
5. Skidmore FM, Williams LS, Fradkin KD, et al. Presentation, etiology, and outcome of stroke in pregnancy and puerperium. J Stroke Cerebrovasc Dis 2001;10:1.
6. Kittner SJ, Stern BJ, Feeser BR, et al. Pregnancy and the risk of stroke. N Engl J Med 1996;335:768.
7. Jaigobin C, Silver FL. Stroke and pregnancy. Stroke 2000;31:2948.
8. Jeng JS, Tang SC, Yip PK. Incidence and etiologies of stroke during pregnancy and puerperium as evidenced in Taiwanese women. Cerebrovasc Dis 2004;18:290.
9. Cross JN, Castro PO, Jennett WB. Cerebral strokes associated with pregnancy and the puerperium. BMJ 1968;3:214.
10. Sharshar T, Lamy C, Mas JL. Incidence and causes of strokes associated with pregnancy and puerperium: a study in public hospitals of Ile de France. Stroke in Pregnancy Study Group. Stroke 1995;26:930.
11. Petitti DB, Sidney S, Quesenberry CP Jr, Bernstein A. Incidence of stroke and myocardial infarction in women of reproductive age. Stroke 1997;28:280.
12. Lavy S, Kahana E. Cerebral arterial occlusion during pregnancy and puerperium: report of 3 cases. Obstet Gynecol 1970;35:916.
13. Pruitt AB, Mole HW. Middle cerebral artery occlusion in pregnancy: review of the literature and report of a case. Obstet Gynecol 1967;29:545.
14. Goldstein PJ, Stern BJ. Cerebrovascular disease and pregnancy. In Neurological Disorders of Pregnancy, 2nd rev ed. Mount Kisco, NY: Futura Publishing, 1992.
15. Honnorat J. [The neurology of pregnancy]. Rev Neurol (Paris) 2006;162:293.
16. Feske SK. Stroke in pregnancy. Semin Neurol 2007;27:442.
17. Amos DB. The cellular target for lymphocyte-mediated cytotoxicity. Keio J Med 1975;24:261.
18. Brar SS, Khan SS, Sandhu GK, et al. Incidence, mortality, and racial differences in peripartum cardiomyopathy. Am J Cardiol 2007;100:302.
19. Mielniczuk LM, Williams K, Davis DR, et al. Frequency of peripartum cardiomyopathy. Am J Cardiol 2006;97:1765.
20. Kawano H, Tsuneto A, Koide Y, et al. Magnetic resonance imaging in a patient with peripartum cardiomyopathy. Intern Med 2008;47:97.
21. Fett JD. Peripartum cardiomyopathy (PPCM) in both surrogate and biological mother. Hum Reprod 2005;20:2666.

22. Fett JD, Christie LG, Carraway RD, Murphy JG. Five-year prospective study of the incidence and prognosis of peripartum cardiomyopathy at a single institution. Mayo Clin Proc 2005;80:1602.

23. Murali S, Baldisseri MR. Peripartum cardiomyopathy. Crit Care Med 2005;33(10 Suppl):S340.

24. Abboud J, Murad Y, Chen-Scarabelli C, et al. Peripartum cardiomyopathy: a comprehensive review. Int J Cardiol 2007;118:295.

25. Lamparter S, Pankuweit S, Maisch B. Clinical and immunologic characteristics in peripartum cardiomyopathy. Int J Cardiol 2007;118:14.

26. Degani S, Abinader EG, Scharf M. Mitral valve prolapse and pregnancy: a review. Obstet Gynecol Surv 1989;44:642.

27. Wong MC, Giuliani MJ, Haley EC Jr. Cerebrovascular disease and stroke in women. Cardiology 1990;77(Suppl 2):80.

28. Tang LC, Chan SY, Wong VC, Ma HK. Pregnancy in patients with mitral valve prolapse. Int J Gynaecol Obstet 1985;23:217.

29. Chia YT, Yeoh SC, Lim MC, et al. Pregnancy outcome and mitral valve prolapse. Asia Oceania J Obstet Gynaecol 1994;20:383.

30. Cowles T, Gonik B. Mitral valve prolapse in pregnancy. Semin Perinatol 1990;14:34.

31. Jana N, Vasishta K, Khunnu B, et al. Pregnancy in association with mitral valve prolapse. Asia Oceania J Obstet Gynaecol 1993;19:61.

32. Lee CN, Wu CC, Lin PY, et al. Pregnancy following cardiac prosthetic valve replacement. Obstet Gynecol 1994;83:353.

33. Geelani MA, Singh S, Verma A, et al. Anticoagulation in patients with mechanical valves during pregnancy. Asian Cardiovasc Thorac Ann 2005;13:30.

34. Akhtar RP, Abid AR, Zafar H, et al. Anticoagulation in pregnancy with mechanical heart valves: 10-year experience. Asian Cardiovasc Thorac Ann 2007;15:497.

35. Suri V, Sawhney H, Vasishta K, et al. Pregnancy following cardiac valve replacement surgery. Int J Gynaecol Obstet 1999;64:239.

36. Pavankumar P, Venugopal P, Kaul U, et al. Pregnancy in patients with prosthetic cardiac valve: a 10-year experience. Scand J Thorac Cardiovasc Surg 1988;22:19.

37. Bonow RO, Carabello BA, Kanu C, et al. ACC/AHA 2006 guidelines for the management of patients with valvular heart disease: a report of the American College of Cardiology/American Heart Association Task Force on Practice Guidelines (writing committee to revise the 1998 Guidelines for the Management of Patients With Valvular Heart Disease): developed in collaboration with the Society of Cardiovascular Anesthesiologists; endorsed by the Society for Cardiovascular Angiography and Interventions and the Society of Thoracic Surgeons. Circulation 2006;114:e84.

38. Wilson W, Taubert KA, Gewitz M, et al. Prevention of infective endocarditis: guidelines from the American Heart Association: a guideline from the American Heart Association Rheumatic Fever, Endocarditis, and Kawasaki Disease Committee, Council on Cardiovascular Disease in the Young, and the Council on Clinical Cardiology, Council on Cardiovascular Surgery and Anesthesia, and the Quality of Care and Outcomes Research Interdisciplinary Working Group. Circulation 2007;116:1736.

39. Ferrero S, Colombo BM, Ragni N. Maternal arrhythmias during pregnancy. Arch Gynecol Obstet 2004;269:244.

40. Gowda RM, Khan IA, Mehta NJ, et al. Cardiac arrhythmias in pregnancy: clinical and therapeutic considerations. Int J Cardiol 2003;88(2-3):129.

41. Wolbrette D. Treatment of arrhythmias during pregnancy. Curr Women Health Rep 2003;3:135.

42. Kannel WB, Benjamin EJ. Status of the epidemiology of atrial fibrillation. Med Clin North Am 2008;92:17.

43. Flores JR, Marquez MF. [Arrhythmias in pregnancy. How and when to treat?]. Arch Cardiol Mex 2007;77 (Suppl 2):S2–24.

44. Wolf PA, Dawber TR, Thomas HE Jr, Kannel WB. Epidemiologic assessment of chronic atrial fibrillation and risk of stroke: the Framingham study. Neurology 1978;28:973.

45. Seth R, Moss AJ, McNitt S, et al. Long QT syndrome and pregnancy. J Am Coll Cardiol 2007;49:1092.

46. Montoya ME, Karnath BM, Ahmad M. Endocarditis during pregnancy. South Med J 2003;96:1156.

47. Avila WS, Rossi EG, Ramires JA, et al. Pregnancy in patients with heart disease: experience with 1,000 cases. Clin Cardiol 2003;26:135.

48. George J, Lamb JT, Harriman DG. Cerebral embolism due to non-bacterial thrombotic endocarditis following pregnancy. J Neurol Neurosurg Psychiatry 1984;47:79.

49. Webster MW, Chancellor AM, Smith HJ, et al. Patent foramen ovale in young stroke patients. Lancet 1988;2:11.

50. Lechat P, Mas JL, Lascault G, et al. Prevalence of patent foramen ovale in patients with stroke. N Engl J Med 1988;318:1148.

51. Hagen PT, Scholz DG, Edwards WD. Incidence and size of patent foramen ovale during the first 10 decades of life: an autopsy study of 965 normal hearts. Mayo Clin Proc 1984;59:17.

52. Schrale RG, Ormerod J, Ormerod OJ. Percutaneous device closure of the patent foramen ovale during pregnancy. Catheter Cardiovasc Interv 2007;69:579.

53. Daehnert I, Ewert P, Berger F, Lange PE. Echocardiographically guided closure of a patent foramen ovale during pregnancy after recurrent strokes. J Interv Cardiol 2001;14:191.

54. Sanchez JM, Milam MR, Tomlinson TM, Beardslee MA. Cardiac troponin I elevation after orogenital sex during pregnancy. Obstet Gynecol 2008;111:487.

55. Bray P, Myers RA, Cowley RA. Orogenital sex as a cause of nonfatal air embolism in pregnancy. Obstet Gynecol 1983;61:653.

56. Mushkat Y, Luxman D, Nachum Z, et al. Gas embolism complicating obstetric or gynecologic procedures: case reports and review of the literature. Eur J Obstet Gynecol Reprod Biol 1995;63:97.

57. Panni MK, Camann W, Bhavani Shankar K. Hyperbaric therapy for a postpartum patient with prolonged epidural blockade and tomographic evidence of epidural air. Anesth Analg 2003;97:1810.

58. Chmel H, Bertles JF. Hemoglobin S/C disease in a pregnant woman with crisis and fat embolization syndrome. Am J Med 1975;58:563.

59. Jones MB. Pulmonary fat emboli associated with acute fatty liver of pregnancy. Am J Gastroenterol 1993;88:791.

60. Habek D, Habek JC. Nonhemorrhagic primary obstetric shock. Fetal Diagn Ther 2007;23:132.

61. Lamy C, Sharshar T, Mas JL. [Cerebrovascular diseases in pregnancy and puerperium]. Rev Neurol (Paris) 1996;152(6-7):422.

62. Mas JL, Lamy C. Stroke in pregnancy and the puerperium. J Neurol 1998;245(6-7):305.

63. Preter M, Tzourio C, Ameri A, Bousser MG. Long-term prognosis in cerebral venous thrombosis: follow-up of 77 patients. Stroke 1996;27:243.

64. Canhao P, Ferro JM, Lindgren AG, et al. Causes and predictors of death in cerebral venous thrombosis. Stroke 2005;36:1720.

65. Daif A, Awada A, al-Rajeh S, et al. Cerebral venous thrombosis in adults: a study of 40 cases from Saudi Arabia. Stroke 1995;26:1193.

66. Krayenbuhl HA. Cerebral venous and sinus thrombosis. Clin Neurosurg 1966;14:1.

67. Dokmetas HS, Kilicli F, Korkmaz S, Yonem O. Characteristic features of 20 patients with Sheehan's syndrome. Gynecol Endocrinol 2006;22:279.

68. See TT, Lee SP, Chen HF. Spontaneous pregnancy and partial recovery of pituitary function in a patient with Sheehan's syndrome. J Chin Med Assoc 2005;68:187.

69. Sheehan HL, Summers VK. The syndrome of hypopituitarism. QJM 1949;18:319.

70. Maiello M, Torella M, Caserta L, et al. [Hypercoagulability during pregnancy: evidences for a thrombophilic state]. Min Ginecol 2006;58:417.

71. Burneo JG, Elias SB, Barkley GL. Cerebral venous thrombosis due to protein S deficiency in pregnancy. Lancet 2002;359:892.

72. D'Angelo A, Mari G, Della Valle P, et al. Familial protein S deficiency presenting as deep vein thrombosis occurring during pregnancy. Acta Obstet Gynecol Scand 1990;69:537.

73. Funai EF, Klein SA, Lockwood CJ. Successful pregnancy outcome in a patient with both congenital hypofibrinogenemia and protein S deficiency. Obstet Gynecol 1997;89(5 Pt 2):858.

74. Gardiner C, Cohen H, Austin SK, et al. Pregnancy loss, tissue factor pathway inhibitor deficiency and resistance to activated protein C. J Thromb Haemost 2006;4:2724.

75. Gokcil Z, Odabasi Z, Vural O, Yardim M. Cerebral venous thrombosis in pregnancy: the role of protein S deficiency. Acta Neurol Belg 1998;98:36.

76. Hirose M, Kimura F, Wang HQ, et al. Protein S gene mutation in a young woman with type III protein S deficiency and venous thrombosis during pregnancy. J Thromb Thrombolysis 2002;13:85.

77. Martinelli P, Maruotti GM, Coppola A, et al. Pregnancy in a woman with a history of Budd-Chiari syndrome treated by porto-systemic shunt, protein C deficiency and bicornuate uterus. Thromb Haemost 2006;95:1033.

78. Okon MA, Spooner SF. Protein C deficiency and stroke in pregnancy. J Obstet Gynaecol 1998;18:182.

79. Paternoster DM, Simioni P, Girolami A. Protein S deficiency and pregnancy: is there a case for ylaxis? Min Ginecol 1997;49:447.

80. Richards EM, Makris M, Preston FE. The successful use of protein C concentrate during pregnancy in a patient with type 1 protein C deficiency, previous thrombosis and recurrent fetal loss. Br J Haematol 1997;98:660.

81. Rizk N, Toon PG, Watson D, Jones V. Protein S deficiency and factor V Leiden gene in pregnancy. J Obstet Gynaecol 1998;18:178.

82. Tharakan T, Baxi LV, Diuguid D. Protein S deficiency in pregnancy: a case report. Am J Obstet Gynecol 1993;168(1 Pt 1):141.

83. Trauscht-Van Horn JJ, Capeless EL, Easterling TR, Bovill EG. Pregnancy loss and thrombosis with protein C deficiency. Am J Obstet Gynecol 1992;167(4 Pt 1):968.

84. van Heusden AM, Merkus HM, Dullemond-Westland AC. Pregnancy and protein C deficiency. Eur J Obstet Gynecol Reprod Biol 1992;45:207.

85. Vogel JJ, de Moerloose PA, Bounameaux H. Protein C deficiency and pregnancy: a case report. Obstet Gynecol 1989;73(3 Pt 2):455.

86. Wiesli P, Zwimpfer C, Zapf J, Schmid C. Pregnancy-induced changes in insulin-like growth factor I (IGF-I), insulin-like growth factor binding protein 3 (IGFBP-3), and acid-labile subunit (ALS) in patients with growth hormone (GH) deficiency and excess. Acta Obstet Gynecol Scand 2006;85:900.

87. Wilson MR, Hughes SJ. The effect of maternal protein deficiency during pregnancy and lactation on glucose tolerance and pancreatic islet function in adult rat offspring. J Endocrinol 1997;154:177.

88. Inaba H, Kawasaki H, Hamazaki M, et al. A case of metastatic ovarian non-gestational choriocarcinoma: successful treatment with conservative type surgery and myeloablative chemotherapy. Pediatr Int 2000;42:383.

89. Girardi G, Redecha P, Salmon JE. Heparin prevents antiphospholipid antibody-induced fetal loss by inhibiting complement activation. Nat Med 2004;10:1222.

90. Glasnovic M, Bosnjak I, Vcev A, et al. Antibody profile of pregnant women with antiphospholipid syndrome and pregnancy outcome after treatment with low dose aspirin and low-weight-molecular heparin. Coll Antropol 2007;31:173.

91. Farley JH, Heathcock RB, Branch W, et al. Treatment of metastatic gestational choriocarcinoma with oral methotrexate in a combat environment. Obstet Gynecol 2005;105(5 Pt 2):1250.

92. Ezra Y, Kidron D, Beyth Y. Fibromuscular dysplasia of the carotid arteries complicating pregnancy. Obstet Gynecol 1989;73(5 Pt 2):840.

93. Singhal AB. Postpartum angiopathy with reversible posterior leukoencephalopathy. Arch Neurol 2004;61:411.

94. Granier I, Garcia E, Geissler A, et al. Postpartum cerebral angiopathy associated with the administration of sumatriptan and dihydroergotamine—a case report. Intensive Care Med 1999;25:532.

95. Crippa G, Sverzellati E, Pancotti D, Carrara GC. Severe postpartum hypertension and reversible cerebral angiopathy associated with ergot derivative (methergoline) administration. Ann Ital Med Int 2000;15:303.

96. Konstantinopoulos PA, Mousa S, Khairallah R, Mtanos G. Postpartum cerebral angiopathy: an important diagnostic consideration in the postpartum period. Am J Obstet Gynecol 2004;191:375.

97. Wiese KM, Talkad A, Mathews M, Wang D. Intravenous recombinant tissue plasminogen activator in a pregnant woman with cardioembolic stroke. Stroke 2006;37:2168.

98. Murugappan A, Coplin WM, Al-Sadat AN, et al. Thrombolytic therapy of acute ischemic stroke during pregnancy. Neurology 2006;66:768.

99. Leonhardt G, Gaul C, Nietsch HH, et al. Thrombolytic therapy in pregnancy. J Thromb Thrombolysis 2006;21:271.

100. Elford K, Leader A, Wee R, Stys PK. Stroke in ovarian hyperstimulation syndrome in early pregnancy treated with intra-arterial rt-PA. Neurology 2002;59:1270.

101. Johnson DM, Kramer DC, Cohen E, et al. Thrombolytic therapy for acute stroke in late pregnancy with intra-arterial recombinant tissue plasminogen activator. Stroke 2005;36:e53.

102. Flossdorf T, Breulmann M, Hopf HB. Successful treatment of massive pulmonary embolism with recombinant tissue type plasminogen activator (rt-PA) in a pregnant woman with intact gravidity and preterm labour. Intensive Care Med 1990;16:454.

103. Gibson PS, Rosene-Montella K. Drugs in pregnancy: anticoagulants. Best Pract Res Clin Obstet Gynaecol 2001;15:847.

104. Laurent P, Dussarat GV, Bonal J, et al. Low molecular weight heparins: a guide to their optimum use in pregnancy. Drugs 2002;62:463.

105. James AH, Grotegut CA, Brancazio LR, Brown H. Thromboembolism in pregnancy: recurrence and its prevention. Semin Perinatol 2007;31:167.

106. Ghosh K, Shetty S, Vora S, Salvi V. Successful pregnancy outcome in women with bad obstetric history and recurrent fetal loss due to thrombophilia: effect of unfractionated heparin and low molecular weight heparin. Clin Appl Thromb Hemost 2007;14:159.

107. James AH. Prevention and management of venous thromboembolism in pregnancy. Am J Med 2007;120(10 Suppl 2):S26.

108. Louden KA, Broughton Pipkin F, Symonds EM, et al. A randomized placebo-controlled study of the effect of low dose aspirin on platelet reactivity and serum thromboxane B_2 production in non-pregnant women, in normal pregnancy, and in gestational hypertension. Br J Obstet Gynaecol 1992;99:371.

109. Benigni A, Gregorini G, Frusca T, et al. Effect of low-dose aspirin on fetal and maternal generation of thromboxane by platelets in women at risk for pregnancy-induced hypertension. N Engl J Med 1989;321:357.

110. Walsh SW. Low-dose aspirin: treatment for the imbalance of increased thromboxane and decreased prostacyclin in pre-eclampsia. Am J Perinatol 1989;6:124.

111. Simolke GA, Cox SM, Cunningham FG. Cerebrovascular accidents complicating pregnancy and the puerperium. Obstet Gynecol 1991;78:37.

112. James AH, Bushnell CD, Jamison MG, Myers ER. Incidence and risk factors for stroke in pregnancy and the puerperium. Obstet Gynecol 2005;106:509.

113. Gibbs CE. Maternal death due to stroke. Am J Obstet Gynecol 1974;119:69.

114. Verzar Z, Kover E, Doczi T, et al. Successful treatment of FIGO stage IV gestational choriocarcinoma occurring 2 months after delivery. Eur J Obstet Gynecol Reprod Biol 2007.

115. Soper JT, Spillman M, Sampson JH, et al. High-risk gestational trophoblastic neoplasia with brain metastases: individualized multidisciplinary therapy in the management of four patients. Gynecol Oncol 2007;104:691.

116. Sirichand P, Das CM, Hassan N. Postpartum choriocarcinoma. J Coll Physicians Surg Pak 2006;16:489.

117. Nugent D, Hassadia A, Everard J, et al. Postpartum choriocarcinoma presentation, management and survival. J Reprod Med 2006;51:819.

118. Lurain JR, Singh DK, Schink JC. Role of surgery in the management of high-risk gestational trophoblastic neoplasia. J Reprod Med 2006;51:773.

119. Huang CY, Chen CA, Hsieh CY, Cheng WF. Intracerebral hemorrhage as initial presentation of gestational choriocarcinoma: a case report and literature review. Int J Gynecol Cancer 2007;17:1166.

120. Cortes-Charry R, Figueira LM, Garcia-Barriola V, et al. Gestational trophoblastic neoplasia: clinical trends in 8 years at Hospital Universitario de Caracas. J Reprod Med 2006;51:888.

121. Dias MS, Sekhar LN. Intracranial hemorrhage from aneurysms and arteriovenous malformations during pregnancy and the puerperium. Neurosurgery 1990;27:855.

122. Barno A, Freeman DW. Maternal deaths due to spontaneous subarachnoid hemorrhage. Am J Obstet Gynecol 1976;125:384.

123. Barrett JM, Van Hooydonk JE, Boehm FH. Pregnancy-related rupture of arterial aneurysms. Obstet Gynecol Surv 1982;37:557.

124. Okamoto K, Horisawa R, Kawamura T, et al. Menstrual and reproductive factors for subarachnoid hemorrhage risk in women: a case-control study in Nagoya, Japan. Stroke 2001;32:2841.

125. Koski-Rahikkala H, Pouta A, Pietilainen K, Hartikainen AL. Does parity affect mortality among parous women? J Epidemiol Community Health 2006;60:968.

126. Gaist D, Pedersen L, Cnattingius S, Sorensen HT. Parity and risk of subarachnoid hemorrhage in women: a nested case-control study based on national Swedish registries. Stroke 2004;35:28.

127. Yang CY, Chang CC, Kuo HW, Chiu HF. Parity and risk of death from subarachnoid hemorrhage in women: evidence from a cohort in Taiwan. Neurology 2006;67:514.

128. Mhurchu CN, Anderson C, Jamrozik K, et al. Hormonal factors and risk of aneurysmal subarachnoid hemorrhage: an international population-based, case-control study. Stroke 2001;32:606.

129. Molyneux A, Kerr R, Stratton I, et al. International Subarachnoid Aneurysm Trial (ISAT) of neurosurgical clipping versus endovascular coiling in 2143 patients with ruptured intracranial aneurysms: a randomised trial. Lancet 2002;360:1267.

130. Piotin M, de Souza Filho CB, Kothimbakam R, Moret J. Endovascular treatment of acutely ruptured intracranial aneurysms in pregnancy. Am J Obstet Gynecol 2001;185:1261.

131. Molyneux AJ, Kerr RS, Yu LM, et al. International Subarachnoid Aneurysm Trial (ISAT) of neurosurgical clipping versus endovascular coiling in 2143 patients with ruptured intracranial aneurysms: a randomised comparison of effects on survival, dependency, seizures, rebleeding, subgroups, and aneurysm occlusion. Lancet 2005;366:809.

132. Marshman LA, Aspoas AR, Rai MS, Chawda SJ. The implications of ISAT and ISUIA for the management of cerebral aneurysms during pregnancy. Neurosurg Rev 2007;30:177.

133. Selo-Ojeme DO, Marshman LA, Ikomi A, et al. Aneurysmal subarachnoid haemorrhage in pregnancy. Eur J Obstet Gynecol Reprod Biol 2004;116:131.

134. Roman H, Descargues G, Lopes M, et al. Subarachnoid hemorrhage due to cerebral aneurysmal rupture during pregnancy. Acta Obstet Gynecol Scand 2004;83:330.

135. Wiebers DO, Whisnant JP, Huston J 3rd, et al. Unruptured intracranial aneurysms: natural history, clinical outcome, and risks of surgical and endovascular treatment. Lancet 2003;362:103.

136. Unruptured intracranial aneurysms—risk of rupture and risks of surgical intervention. International Study of Unruptured Intracranial Aneurysms Investigators. N Engl J Med 1998;339:1725.

137. Horton JC. Arteriovenous malformations of the brain. N Engl J Med 2007;357:1774.

138. Horton JC, Chambers WA, Lyons SL, et al. Pregnancy and the risk of hemorrhage from cerebral arteriovenous malformations. Neurosurgery 1990;27:867.

139. Robinson JL, Hall CS, Sedzimir CB. Arteriovenous malformations, aneurysms, and pregnancy. J Neurosurg 1974;41:63.

140. Bateman BT, Schumacher HC, Bushnell CD, et al. Intracerebral hemorrhage in pregnancy: frequency, risk factors, and outcome. Neurology 2006;67:424.

141. Stapf C, Mast H, Sciacca RR, et al. The New York Islands AVM Study: design, study progress, and initial results. Stroke 2003;34:e29.

142. Al-Shahi R, Bhattacharya JJ, Currie DG, et al. Scottish Intracranial Vascular Malformation Study (SIVMS): evaluation of methods, ICD-10 coding, and potential sources of bias in a prospective, population-based cohort. Stroke 2003;34:1156.

143. Piotin M, Mounayer C, Spelle L, Moret J. [Cerebral arteriovenous malformations and pregnancy: management of a dilemma.]. J Neuroradiol 2004;31:376.

144. Lin TK, Chang CN, Wai YY. Spontaneous intracerebral hematoma from occult carotid-cavernous fistula during pregnancy and puerperium: case report. J Neurosurg 1992;76:714.

145. Toya S, Shiobara R, Izumi J, et al. Spontaneous carotid-cavernous fistula during pregnancy or in the postpartum stage: report of two cases. J Neurosurg 1981;54:252.

CHAPTER 11

Rare Genetic Disorders Predisposing to Stroke

Betsy B. Love • James F. Meschia • José Biller

KEY TERMS

AVM	arteriovenous malformation
CADASIL	cerebral autosomal dominant arteriopathy with subcortical infarcts and leukoencephalopathy
CT	computed tomography
FMD	fibromuscular dysplasia
HDL	high-density lipoprotein
MELAS	mitochondrial encephalomyopathy, lactic acidosis, and strokelike symptoms
MRI	magnetic resonance imaging
TIA	transient ischemic attack

Despite extensive investigation, approximately 20% to 30% of strokes in children and young adults are classified as stroke of undetermined etiology. In some of these patients, genetic causes of stroke may be overlooked and underdiagnosed.[1] Genetic causes of stroke may be divided into hereditary syndromes leading to early atherosclerosis, inherited syndromes with associated nonatherosclerotic vasculopathies, inherited hematologic disorders, hereditary cardiac disorders, and inherited metabolic syndromes. Table 11-1 lists genetic syndromes associated with stroke.

Inherited Disorders Causing Accelerated Atherosclerosis

In series of stroke in young adults, early atherosclerosis is a common cause of stroke in patients older than 30 years, but is less common in patients younger than 30 years.[2] Although most of these cases of early atherosclerosis are due to secondary causes of hyperlipidemia, such as diabetes, a group of conditions termed "hereditary dyslipoproteinemias" is associated with accelerated atherosclerosis. This is an area that may be overlooked as a potential cause of cerebrovascular disease in young patients. One report indicated that pediatric and young adult patients with unexplained stroke may have familial lipid and lipoprotein abnormalities, such as low levels of high-density lipoprotein (HDL) or high triglyceride levels, or both.[3] In 11 patients who had unexplained stroke after complete investigation, 10 patients had lipid abnormalities and a familial clustering of low HDL cholesterol and elevated triglycerides.[3] Atherosclerotic lesions in children with familial lipid disorders tend to involve the intracranial vessels, rather than typical carotid bifurcation disease.[4] Vessel changes are believed to represent lipoprotein-mediated endothelial damage.[5]

TABLE 11-1 **Genetic Causes of Stroke**

Inherited Diseases Producing Accelerated Atherosclerosis	Hemoglobinopathies (hemoglobin C or S disorders)
Hereditary dyslipoproteinemias	Prekallikrein deficiency
Familial hypercholesterolemia	C_2 deficiency
Familial hypertriglyceridemia	β-thalassemia
Hyperlipoproteinemia (types III and IV)	Plasminogen deficiency or defective release of plasminogen activator
Familial hypoalphalipoproteinemia	Dysfibrinogenemia
Tangier disease	Hereditary polycythemias
Progeria (de Lange, Deckel, Bloom, Cockayne syndromes)	Heparin cofactor II deficiency
	Hereditary platelet defects
Inherited Nonatherosclerotic Vasculopathies	**Inherited Cardiac Disorders**
Ehlers-Danlos (type IV) syndrome	Familial atrial myxomas
Pseudoxanthoma elasticum	Rhabdomyomas (tuberous sclerosis)
Menkes syndrome	Mitral valve prolapse
Marfan syndrome	Cardiac papillary fibroelastoma
Rendu-Osler-Weber syndrome (hereditary hemorrhagic telangiectasia)	Hereditary cardiac conduction disorders
Sturge-Weber syndrome	Hereditary cardiomyopathies
Neurofibromatosis 1	**Inherited Metabolic Disorders**
Tuberous sclerosis complex	Mitochondrial abnormalities
Klippel-Trénaunay-Weber syndrome	MELAS
Polycystic kidney disease	Leigh disease
Fibromuscular dysplasia	Organic acidemia
von Hippel–Lindau syndrome	Methylmalonic acidemia
Bannayan-Zonana syndrome	Propionic acidemia
Moyamoya disease	Isovaleric acidemia
Hereditary amyloidoses	Fabry disease
Migraine	Homocystinuria
Inherited Hematologic Abnormalities	Glutaric aciduria type II
Antithrombin deficiency	Sulfite oxidase deficiency
Protein C and S deficiency	11β-hydroxylase deficiency, 11β-ketoreductase deficiency, 17α-hydroxylase deficiency
Thrombomodulin deficiency	3-Methylcrotonyl-CoA carboxylase 3-hydroxy-3-methylglutaryl-CoA lyase deficiency
Factor V, VII, VIII, IX, X, XI, XII, XIII deficiency	

Familial hypercholesterolemia is an autosomal dominant condition characterized by tendon xanthomas, corneal arcus, coronary artery disease, and, less commonly, stroke. The cause of the condition is a disorder of the low-density lipoprotein (apo B/E) receptor. Familial hypertriglyceridemia was common in pediatric patients with unexplained stroke in one small series of patients.[3] Type III hyperlipoproteinemia is characterized by elevated plasma cholesterol and triglyceride levels. Type IV hyperlipoproteinemia usually is characterized by elevated plasma very-low-density lipoproteins and elevated triglyceride levels.

Some dyslipoproteinemias are characterized by HDL deficiency. Familial hypoalphalipoproteinemia is an autosomal dominant HDL deficiency state that is associated with premature atherosclerosis causing myocardial infarction and stroke. Tangier disease is a much rarer, autosomal recessive disorder characterized by hyperplastic orange tonsils, hepatosplenomegaly, lymphadenopathy, neuropathy, premature atherosclerotic disease, low cholesterol levels, and HDL deficiency.

Finally, some conditions producing progeria may be associated with premature atherosclerosis, such as de Lange, Deckel, Bloom, and Cockayne syndromes. Death may occur from vascular disease in adolescence. These patients may have decreased HDL levels and high low-density lipoprotein and very-low-density lipoprotein bound cholesterol.[6] In patients with certain variants of familial hyperlipidemia, statins may reduce the likelihood of developing intracranial atherosclerosis, although it is unclear that statins have a positive effect on leukoaraiosis.[7]

Inherited Nonatherosclerotic Vasculopathies

Inherited nonatherosclerotic vasculopathies are heterogeneous disorders that typically affect blood vessels by mechanisms other than atherosclerosis. In series of stroke in young adults, these conditions account for approximately 4% of strokes.[8] Ehlers-Danlos syndrome is a group of genetically heterogeneous disorders that in most cases are caused by a defect in collagen synthesis or structure. Patients with this syndrome may have thin, translucent skin with visible veins, variable degrees of cutaneous hyperextensibility, joint hypermobility, easy bruisability, connective tissue fragility, and abnormal scarring. Facial characteristics include large eyes, thin mouth, lobeless ears, and thin scalp hair. Ehlers-Danlos type IV, which is due to mutations in the *COL3A1* gene, is of particular importance because of the prominence of cerebrovascular abnormalities that may be encountered. The inheritance of Ehlers-Danlos type IV may be autosomal dominant or recessive. Patients are predisposed to intracranial aneurysms, carotid-cavernous fistulas, arterial rupture, and artery dissections.[9-13] These unusual complications are attributed to abnormalities in collagen type III.[14] In addition, patients may have mitral valve prolapse as another potential cause of stroke (Figs. 11-1 and 11-2).[15] Patients with Ehlers-Danlos type IV also are at risk for intestinal and uterine rupture. Noninvasive arterial imaging such as Doppler

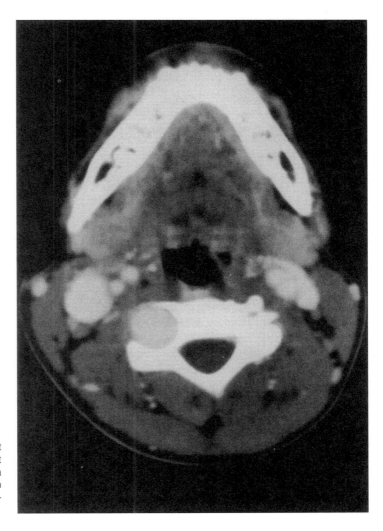

FIGURE 11-1 Axial CT scan after contrast administration shows marked enlargement of the right foramen transversarium by a vertebral artery aneurysm in a patient with Ehlers-Danlos (type IV) syndrome. (Courtesy of Eric Russell, M.D.)

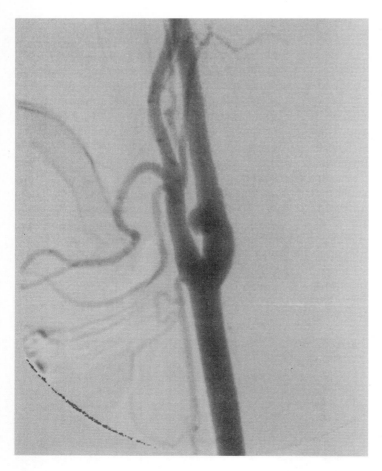

FIGURE 11-2   Common carotid angiogram shows a typical saccular aneurysm of the proximal internal carotid in the same patient shown in Figure 11-1. (Courtesy of Eric Russell, M.D.)

and MRA arteriography is preferred to catheter angiography in patients suspected to have Ehlers-Danlos type IV because of the potential for complications.[16]

Another hereditary connective tissue disorder that is heterogeneous and may be autosomal dominant or recessive is pseudoxanthoma elasticum. Patients with this condition have calcification and degeneration of elastic tissue leading to cutaneous, ocular, and vascular abnormalities.[17] Characteristic findings are angioid streaks of the ocular fundus; skin lesions characterized by a peau d'orange or "plucked chicken" appearance; premature arterial disease of the peripheral vascular, cerebrovascular, and coronary circulations; and gastrointestinal hemorrhage.[18,19] Cerebrovascular complications may be secondary to carotid occlusive disease owing to premature atherosclerosis; vascular abnormalities, including carotid cavernous fistulas, microaneurysms, intracranial aneurysms,

and subarachnoid hemorrhage; or cerebrovascular complications of associated cardiac abnormalities, including coronary artery disease and congestive heart failure.[17,20,21] Of patients, 25% may have associated hypertension, which is an additional potential cause of stroke in this population.[20]

Menkes syndrome (kinky hair or steely hair syndrome) is an X-linked recessive disorder of copper absorption caused by diverse mutations in a copper transport gene, ATP7A. Children rarely survive past the second year of life. There is focal cerebral and cerebellar degeneration; truncal hypotonia; loss of developmental milestones; seizures; and a tendency for tortuosity, elongation, and occlusion of the cerebral and systemic arteries. Early treatment with daily copper injections may improve clinical outcomes.[22]

Marfan syndrome, a common connective tissue disorder, affects approximately 2 to 3 per 10,000 individuals.[23] It is usually an autosomal dominant condition, but it may be sporadic in 15%.[23] Marfan syndrome is caused by mutations in the fibrillin-1 gene (*RBN1*, chromosome 15q21). Individuals with this disorder have skeletal (tall stature with dolichostenomelia [long bone overgrowth], thin body habitus), ocular (lens subluxation), and cardiovascular (mitral valve prolapse, aortic root dilation maximal at the sinus of Valsalva, and aortic dissection) abnormalities (Figs. 11-3, 11-4, and 11-5). Associated conditions that may lead to stroke include aortic dissection, dilated cardiomyopathy, and mitral valve prolapse.[20-26] An increased prevalence of intracranial aneurysms has been questioned more recently.[27]

Rendu-Osler-Weber syndrome (hereditary hemorrhagic telangiectasia) is an uncommon autosomal dominant condition characterized by angiodysplasia of vessels of the skin, mucous membranes, and viscera. It has been estimated that approximately 0.5 million individuals worldwide have Rendu-Osler-Weber disease.[28] Patients can present with bleeding from any site, but most commonly have recurrent epistaxis, hemoptysis, melena, or hematuria. Stroke may be secondary to embolism of air, embolism of septic material, or paradoxical embolism of clots through pulmonary arteriovenous fistula with right-to-left shunting.[29] Patients should be examined carefully for telangiectasias of the skin and mucous membranes, pulmonary bruit, peripheral cyanosis, or digital clubbing. Patients may have cardiac sources of stroke because of high-output heart failure secondary to hepatic arteriovenous fistulas. Polycythemia, secondary to the underlying pulmonary or cardiac disease, could lead to stroke. Cerebral hemorrhages can occur as a result of cerebral arteriovenous malformations (AVMs), mycotic or saccular aneurysms, meningeal telangiectasias, or venous developmental anomalies.[30-32] In some series, brain abscesses are more common than ischemic strokes.[33] Percutaneous embolization or surgical resection or both should be considered for stroke prevention.[34]

Another congenital cutaneous vascular disorder, Sturge-Weber syndrome (encephalofacial angiomatosis), is characterized in its complete form by a trigeminal facial nevus flammeus (port wine stain), hemiparesis with hemiatrophy, hemianopsia, glaucoma, mental retardation, and epilepsy.[35]

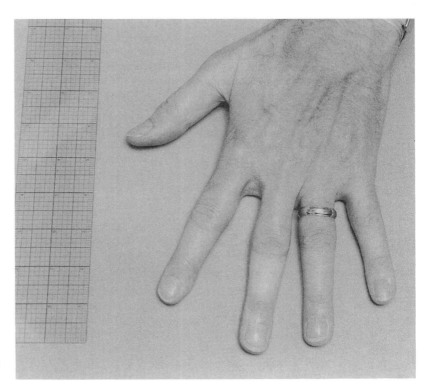

FIGURE 11-3 Arachnodactyly in a patient with Marfan syndrome.

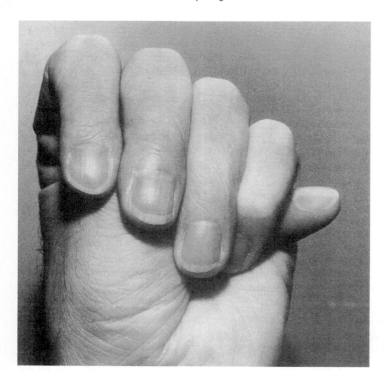

FIGURE 11-4 Steinberg or thumb sign (thumb projects beyond the ulnar border when completely opposed with a clenched hand) in a patient with Marfan syndrome.

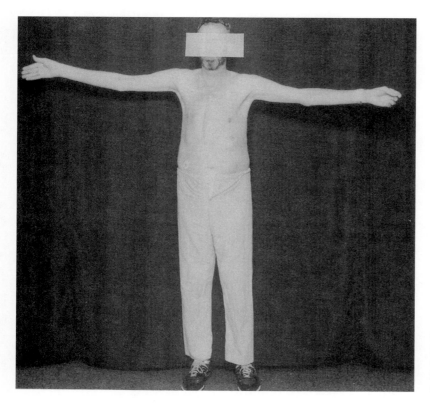

FIGURE 11-5 Dolichostenomelia, pectus carinatum, and arachnodactyly in a patient with Marfan syndrome who underwent aortic valve replacement.

The condition is believed to be sporadic in most individuals, but some investigators have reported a familial tendency, possibly with autosomal dominant inheritance (Figs. 11-6 and 11-7).[36] Cerebrovascular complications may be secondary to recurrent venous occlusion with infarction in the regions of the brain adjacent to leptomeningeal angiomas or, rarely, intracerebral or subarachnoid hemorrhage.[37] Skull x-rays often show the classic "tram line or tram track" calcifications. Described angiographic abnormalities include venous angiomas, AVMs, arterial thromboses, venous and dural sinus anomalies, and anomalies of the external carotid artery.[38,39] Magnetic resonance imaging (MRI) and arterial and venous MR angiography may be helpful in the diagnosis of vascular anomalies associated with this syndrome.[40] Computed tomography (CT) is useful for visualizing the extent of the calcification. Some patients have been described with recurrent thrombotic episodes with gradual neurologic deterioration.[41] Antiplatelet therapy has been beneficial in some of these patients.[41] If antiepileptic drugs are ineffective, surgical treatment must be considered.[42]

Neurofibromatosis 1 is the most common neurocutaneous disorder with a frequency of 1 in 3000 individuals.[43] It is inherited in an autosomal dominant pattern. Cerebrovascular disease is an uncommon complication of neurofibromatosis 1. Stroke occurs by several mechanisms. Patients may have arterial hypertension owing to pheochromocytoma or renal artery stenosis. Hypertension in a child with neurofibromatosis is more likely to be secondary to renal artery stenosis than to be due to a pheochromocytoma.[44] Strokes in childhood caused by severe hypertension associated with neurofibromatosis have been described.[45] Another potential mechanism of stroke is compromise of the cerebral vasculature by neurofibromas.[46] There is an association of neurofibromatosis with moyamoya disease.[47,48] There may be a history in these patients of cranial irradiation for a tumor.[49] Moyamoya disease is discussed later in this chapter, and treatment is addressed in Chapter 6. Finally, there have been several described cases of subarachnoid hemorrhage in patients with neurofibromatosis 1 and a variety of vascular lesions, including arterial stenosis, occlusion, aneurysm, pseudoaneurysm, ectasia, fistula, and arterial rupture.[50]

The triad of adenoma sebaceum, epilepsy, and mental retardation is present in tuberous sclerosis (Fig. 11-8). This condition is transmitted in an autosomal dominant pattern. Patients can have cerebral infarcts owing to embolization from cardiac rhabdomyomas,

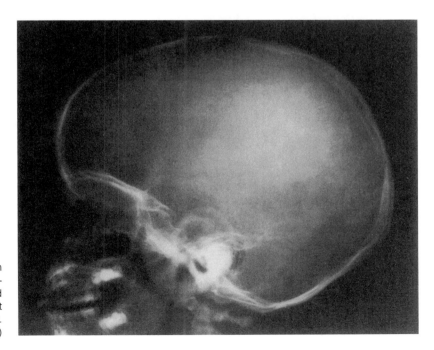

FIGURE 11-6 Lateral skull film shows subtle gyriform calcifications of the left parietal and occipital lobes in a patient with Sturge-Weber syndrome. (Courtesy of Eric Russell, M.D.)

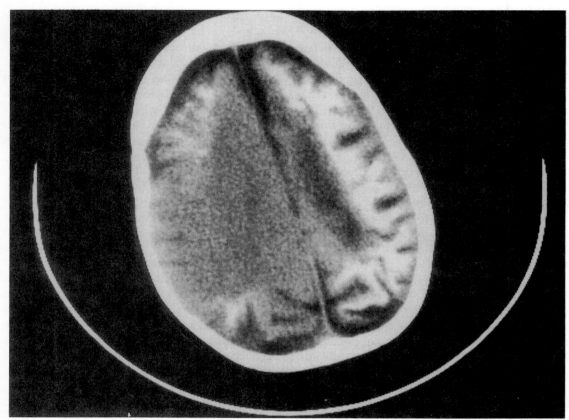

FIGURE 11-7   Axial non–contrast-enhanced CT scan shows extreme cortical calcification involving both cerebral hemispheres, left greater than right, with associated atrophy of the left hemisphere consistent with Sturge-Weber syndrome. (Courtesy of Chris Ellerbroek, M.D.)

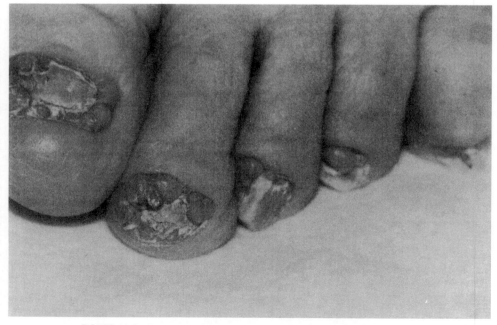

FIGURE 11-8   Toenail hamartomas in a patient with tuberous sclerosis.

cardiac conduction disturbances, intracranial aneurysms, and moyamoya disease.[51-55] Tests that are helpful in diagnosis include Wood lamp examination of the skin to show ash leaf spots; ophthalmologic examination to search for characteristic retinal lesions; echocardiography; and cranial CT or MRI to show associated tumors, subependymal nodules, or heterotopias. Diagnostic criteria for the tuberous sclerosis complex are well detailed in a review of the disorder.[47]

Another neurocutaneous syndrome, Klippel-Trénaunay-Weber syndrome, is characterized by spinal cord vascular malformations, cutaneous vascular nevus, and limb hypertrophy. Rarely, there can be hemorrhagic strokes owing to brain vascular malformations.[56]

Intracranial hemorrhages may be seen with polycystic kidney disease. The adult type is an autosomal dominant condition that may be characterized by intracranial aneurysms, AVMs, hepatic cysts, and renal failure. This condition has been reported to manifest rarely in infancy and early childhood.[57]

In some families, fibromuscular dysplasia (FMD) is believed to be inherited. This disorder is a vasculopathy characterized by fibroblast-like transformation of smooth muscle cells, medial fibroplasia, and microaneurysms. Strokes can occur secondary to arterial stenosis, dissection, or hypertension induced by associated renal FMD. Stroke in relatives of patients with FMD is several times more frequent among females than males. Study of a few pedigrees suggests that there may be an autosomal dominant inheritance with reduced penetrance in males.[58]

von Hippel–Lindau disease is an autosomal dominant condition that rarely may lead to cerebral infarction or cerebellar hemorrhage.[59] The cause of the stroke may be due to polycythemia or due to hypertension secondary to an associated pheochromocytoma. Cerebellar hemangioblastomas may cause either cerebellar hemorrhage or hemorrhagic stroke. Bannayan-Zonana syndrome is a rare condition with macrocephaly; lipomas; and hemangiomas of the skin, viscera, and brain that is associated with intracerebral hemorrhage, particularly in the cerebellum.[60]

Moyamoya disease is a noninflammatory occlusive intracranial vasculopathy; see Chapter 6 for a more detailed description. This condition may be familial in some cases.[61] In addition, moyamoya disease may be associated with other conditions, such as neurofibromatosis, tuberous sclerosis, Sturge-Weber syndrome, FMD, Marfan syndrome, sickle cell anemia, Fanconi anemia, polyarteritis nodosa, cyanotic congenital heart disease, Down syndrome, type I glycogenosis, radiation, vasculitis, and brain tumors.[61] Moyamoya disease tends to produce transient ischemic attacks (TIAs) and ischemic strokes in younger children and hemorrhagic strokes in older children and adults.[62]

Most hereditary amyloidoses that affect the central nervous system have an autosomal dominant mode of inheritance. These conditions may have either intracerebral hemorrhage owing to rupture of weakened amyloid-containing cerebral arteries or hemorrhagic or ischemic stroke owing to occlusion of the abnormal vessels.[63,64] Congophilic angiopathy may be inherited in some families, and the first symptoms of the disorder may manifest in the third decade.[54] Hereditary cerebral amyloid angiopathy is discussed further in Chapter 14.

Migraine is often a familial condition. Familial hemiplegic migraine has an age of onset between 5 and 30 years. One gene linked to familial hemiplegic migraine is the calcium ion gene on chromosome 19p13. Familial hemiplegic migraine also has been linked to chromosome 1. A link to chromosome 19 also has been made for cerebral autosomal dominant arteriopathy with subcortical infarcts and leukoencephalopathy (CADASIL). CADASIL is caused by mutations in the *Notch3* gene. Subcortical infarcts particularly involving the temporal poles begin late in life, often in the fifth or sixth decade. Eosinophilic material within the basement membrane of vascular smooth muscle cells shown on brain or skin biopsy specimens is characteristic of this disease.[65] Pathologic examination shows multiple small, deep cerebral infarcts, leukoencephalopathy, and nonamyloid angiopathy involving the media of small cerebral arteries (Fig. 11-9). Migraine-related stroke is more common in young adults with stroke (16 to 30 years old) than in older stroke patients (31 to 45 years old).[2,66-69] Migraine-related stroke is discussed further in Chapter 8.

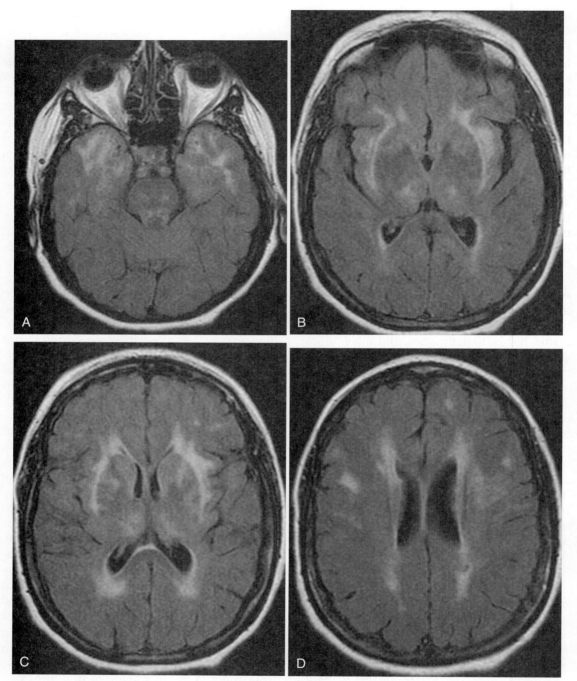

FIGURE 11-9   **A-D,** MRI of the brain shows numerous areas of abnormal T2 and fluid attenuated inversion recovery signal in both corona radiatas and internal capsules, anterior temporal lobes, external and extreme capsules, thalami, and pons in a patient with proven CADASIL.

Migraine-related stroke should be distinguished from hereditary endotheliopathy with retinopathy, nephropathy, and stroke (HERNS) an autosomal-dominant occlusive microangiopathy characterized by progressive visual loss, migraine, focal neurologic deficits, seizures, depression, and dementia. Renal insufficiency and Raynaud phenomenon also are prominent features of this condition.[70]

Inherited Hematologic Abnormalities

Coagulation disturbances may account for 4% of all ischemic strokes in patients younger than 45 years.[71] Heritable thrombophilic conditions are found in approximately 15% of whites, whereas only 0.2% of Taiwan Chinese are heterozygous for factor V Leiden and a similar number for the prothrombin gene *G20210A* mutation. Some of these conditions are inherited disorders that predispose to either thrombosis or hemorrhage.

Antithrombin is a glycoprotein that is an inactivator of circulating thrombin and activated factors IX, X, XI, and XII. Individuals with antithrombin deficiency have venous and arterial thromboses, often at a young age and often during pregnancy because antithrombin III levels decline in early pregnancy.[72] The major clinical manifestations are superficial thrombophlebitis, deep venous thrombosis, and pulmonary emboli. Less commonly, patients have venous thrombosis in other sites, including the cerebral venous sinuses or stroke secondary to cerebral thrombosis.[73] Antithrombin deficiency is inherited as an autosomal dominant gene. The frequency of this defect is 1 per 5000 in the general population.[74] The homozygous state is incompatible with life. Heterozygotes have deficiencies of 35% to 60% of normal. Fetuses of women with a deficiency are stated to have a "high complication rate."[6]

Partial deficiency of protein C or S can be associated with increased incidence of thrombotic disease and recurrent thromboses in young adults.[75-78] Protein C is a vitamin K–dependent factor synthesized in the liver. It circulates in an inactive form until it is activated by endothelial cells. When activated, it is a potent inhibitor of the activated coagulation factors Va and VIIIa, abolishing their activation of prothrombin to thrombin.[79] Protein C has anticoagulant and fibrinolytic properties in its activated form. Hereditary protein C deficiency can be associated with cerebral venous thrombosis, amaurosis fugax, TIAs, and ischemic strokes.[77,80-84] Protein C deficiency is due to an autosomal recessive gene. Parents of affected children have intermediate levels of the protein. There are three clinical forms. The infantile form has very low levels of protein C (<6%). These patients have purpura fulminans, venous and arterial thromboses, and organ infarctions. The juvenile form is a less lethal form that has intermediate protein C levels of 6% to 16%. The adult form has protein C levels of 30% to 60%. These patients may have major venous or arterial infarctions.

Protein S is another vitamin K–dependent plasma protein that is a cofactor for activated protein C. The free form of protein S is the active form. Protein S deficiency has an autosomal dominant mode of inheritance. This deficiency has been associated with cerebral venous thrombosis and, rarely, with ischemic stroke.[85-88]

Deficiencies of factors V, VII, VIII, IX, X, XI, XII, and XIII may be associated with hemorrhagic stroke.[46] Screening with a prothrombin time and activated partial thromboplastin time detects most of these deficiencies.

Hemoglobinopathies can lead to either thrombotic or hemorrhagic strokes. Patients with sickle cell disease have been reported to have stroke in 6% to 9% of cases.[89] Approximately 1 in 10 children with sickle cell disease has a stroke by age 20 years.[90] The peak age for stroke with sickle cell disease is 10 years.[89,91] The incidence of stroke is highest in patients with hemoglobin SS disease and less common in hemoglobin sickle cell disease. Children are more likely to present with cerebral infarction, whereas adults are more likely to have intracerebral hemorrhage or subarachnoid hemorrhage.[92] In addition, patients may have cortical venous or sinus thrombosis. The cause of infarcts in sickle cell disease is probably multifactorial, including a vasculopathy and impaired blood flow. The rate of recurrent stroke can be two thirds in 2 years.[93] Long-term transfusion therapy to decrease levels of hemoglobin S to less than 30% can reduce the risk of recurrent stroke in patients with high-risk values on transcranial Doppler ultrasound studies.[94] Before the Stroke Prevention Trial in Sickle Cell Anemia (STOP) trial proving the efficacy of transcranial Doppler screening and transfusions, the rate of stroke in children in California decreased from 0.88 per 100 person-years to 0.17 per 100 person-years after publication of the study.[95] Patients should be adequately hydrated, have correction of electrolyte imbalance, undergo a thorough search for any associated underlying infection, and have vigorous control of seizures.[96] Before angiography or any contrast load, the concentration of hemoglobin S should be reduced to less than 30%.[94] Strokes have rarely been reported in patients with β-thalassemia[97] and α-thalassemia.[98]

Although most patients with polycythemia have impaired oxygen delivery secondary to nongenetic causes, some familial polycythemias are associated with mutant hemoglobins, abnormal metabolism of 2,3-diphosphoglycerate, or autonomous production of erythropoietin.[46,99] These abnormalities have rarely been associated with stroke. Patients with inappropriate erythropoietin production, such as in von Hippel–Lindau disease, can develop stroke secondary to polycythemia. Suggested initial tests to evaluate for hereditary polycythemia include a complete blood count, arterial blood gas, and hemoglobin electrophoresis.

Hereditary platelet defects can predispose patients to hemorrhagic stroke. These conditions may have qualitative or quantitative defects in platelets. Thrombocytopenia may cause fatal intracranial hemorrhage in infancy in Wiskott-Aldrich syndrome and absent radius syndrome.[46] Hemophilia A and B are sex-linked recessive disorders. Patients with severe hemophilia often have spontaneous joint and muscle bleeds; intracranial bleeding may follow trauma.

Dysfibrinogenemias are rare causes of stroke. Hereditary dysfibrinogenemia is an autosomal dominant condition with mutations in the structure of the fibrinogen molecule. These defects can lead to venous and arterial thrombosis, including stroke. Among the complement deficiency states, an association has been found between C2 deficiency and atherosclerosis. Prekallicrein deficiency, plasminogen deficiency or defective release of plasminogen activator, and heparin cofactor II deficiency are rare inherited conditions possibly associated with hemorrhagic stroke.

Inherited Cardiac Disorders

Intracardiac tumors are a rare cause of stroke in children and young adults. Although most cases of atrial myxomas are sporadic, they can be familial with autosomal dominant or recessive inheritance.[100-103] Left atrial myxomas or right atrial myxomas with an associated right-to-left shunt may be a source

of stroke because of thrombus or tumor embolization. Another cardiac tumor, cardiac rhabdomyoma, may be a source of brain emboli. This tumor is associated with tuberous sclerosis, which was discussed previously.

Mitral valve prolapse affects 5% to 15% of the population and is most common in women. The risk of stroke with mitral valve prolapse is small, approximately 1 per 6000 per year. Mitral valve prolapse may be inherited in an autosomal dominant pattern or may be part of another genetic syndrome, such as osteogenesis imperfecta, Ehlers-Danlos syndrome, Marfan syndrome, Duchenne or Becker muscular dystrophies, myotonic dystrophy, von Willebrand disease, or fragile X syndrome.[46,104] This condition is discussed further in Chapter 6.

Some cardiac conduction disorders may be hereditary. Approximately 2% to 6% of patients with sick sinus syndrome have a familial form that is transmitted in an autosomal dominant fashion.[105] Other rare syndromes with familial sinus node dysfunction have been associated with stroke.[106] Numerous primary disorders of cardiac rhythm and conduction may have autosomal dominant or recessive inheritance.[107] Finally, patients with Kearns-Sayre syndrome may have strokes owing to cardiac conduction disturbances, including complete heart block.

Primary cardiomyopathies include dilated cardiomyopathy, hypertrophic cardiomyopathy, restrictive cardiomyopathy, arrhythmogenic right ventricular cardiomyopathy, and unclassified cardiomyopathy.[108] Some cardiomyopathies may be inherited. Approximately 25% to 30% of dilated cardiomyopathies are familial.[109] Approximately 70% of cases of hypertrophic cardiomyopathy are familial with autosomal dominant inheritance. Hypertrophic obstructive cardiomyopathy may be inherited as a primary familial disorder, or may be part of another genetic syndrome, such as glycogen storage diseases, mitochondrial myopathies, Friedreich's ataxia, or the Turner phenotype.[110]

The incidence of stroke and TIA in patients of all ages with hypertrophic obstructive cardiomyopathy may be 22%.[111] Men have cardiac symptoms at a younger age than women, but the mean age at the time of cardioembolic stroke is similar in men and women (mean 59 years old). Stroke may be the presenting symptom of hypertrophic obstructive cardiomyopathy in approximately 4% of patients.[96] Amyloidoses can have associated cardiomyopathies or arrhythmias that can predispose to stroke. Other conditions, such as hemochromatosis, can lead to restrictive cardiomyopathic heart failure because of a deposition of iron in the myocardium. Arrhythmogenic right ventricular cardiomyopathy can be familial with an autosomal dominant inheritance and incomplete penetrance.

Strokes are a rare complication of inherited neuromuscular diseases, such as Duchenne muscular dystrophy, myotonic dystrophy, Becker muscular dystrophy, and Friedreich ataxia. Stroke occurs especially when there is associated cardiomyopathy or atrial fibrillation or flutter.[112]

Inherited Metabolic Disorders

MELAS (mitochondrial encephalomyopathy, lactic acidosis, and strokelike symptoms) is a non-mendelian, maternally transmitted syndrome (Figs. 11-10 and 11-11). Other features include short stature, nausea, episodic vomiting, headaches, and seizures.[4,98] Diabetes mellitus is seen frequently. Individuals usually have normal early development and subsequently have development of symptoms of MELAS in the first decade or teens. Cerebrovascular involvement may include transient hemiparesis, alternating hemiparesis, hemianopsia, cortical blindness, ataxia, aphasia, or alexia without agraphia.[113]

Neuroimaging studies have been reported to show areas appearing similar to infarcts, which are often bilateral and tend to be located posteriorly.[114] A slowly progressive MRI lesion evolving over weeks has been described.[115] Approximately half of cases have calcification or hypodensities in the basal ganglia.[114] Serum lactate and pyruvate levels are typically elevated. DNA testing can be used to establish the diagnosis. Approximately 80% of patients with MELAS have the 3243 mutation.[116] Increased numbers of giant mitochondria have been described in smooth muscle of cerebral arteries.[117,118] Some investigators have postulated that strokes occur in this syndrome because of impaired oxidative metabolism during stress.[119]

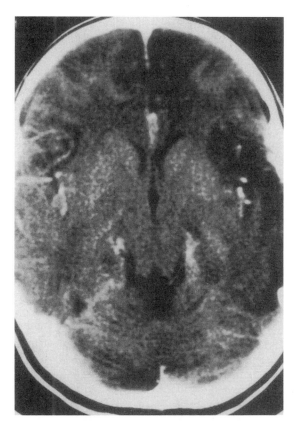

FIGURE 11-10 Postcontrast CT scan shows low attenuation involving predominantly gray matter of the frontal, temporoparietal, and insular cortex consistent with multiple infarctions in a patient with MELAS. (Courtesy of Joel R. Meyer, M.D.)

Leigh disease (subacute necrotizing encephalomyelopathy) is an autosomal recessive or X-linked recessive disorder that typically manifests in infancy or early childhood.[46,120-122] It is characterized by loss of motor control, hypotonia, vomiting, irritability, seizures, respiratory difficulties, ataxia, external ophthalmoplegia, and stroke or strokelike episodes. Neuroimaging studies may show bilateral degeneration of the basal ganglia and brainstem.[123] Several biochemical abnormalities have been described with this disorder, including abnormalities of pyruvate metabolism, cytochrome-c oxidase deficiency, and abnormalities of thiamine metabolism.

Methylmalonic acidemia, propionic acidemia, and isovaleric acidemia are autosomal recessive conditions resulting from inborn errors of branched-chain amino acid catabolism. Strokes may be seen in these conditions

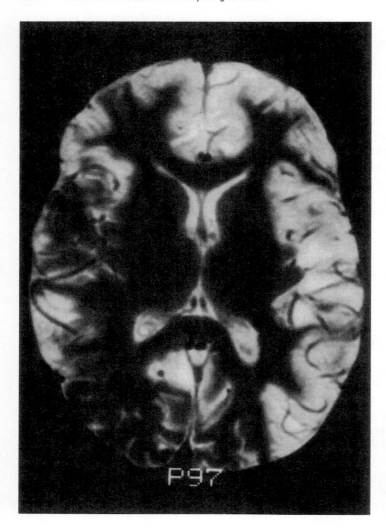

P97

FIGURE 11-11   Axial T2 (long TR, long TE) MR image shows multiple areas of increased signal intensity involving predominantly the gray matter of the frontal, temporoparietal, and insular cortex consistent with multiple infarctions in a patient with MELAS. (Courtesy of Joel R. Meyer, M.D.)

secondary to dehydration and ketoacidosis. Patients with methylmalonic acidemia may have strokes, which have been referred to as "metabolic strokes."[124] Patients may present with acute extrapyramidal signs with lesions of the basal ganglia.[124,125] Cerebellar hemorrhages have rarely been described with methylmalonic, propionic, and isovaleric acidemia.[126,127] Acute treatment is recommended with protein restriction, and cobalamin supplements.[128] Glutaric aciduria is another disorder of amino acid metabolism that may cause stroke. This is an autosomal recessive condition characterized by athetosis, dystonia, and severe mental retardation.[129] Similar to methylmalonic acidemia, there is a tendency for destructive lesions of the basal ganglia, leading to the extrapyramidal disorders.[130]

Fabry disease (angiokeratoma corporis diffusum) is an X-linked recessive disorder that is due to a deficiency of the lysosomal enzyme, α-galactosidase A.[131-133] As a result of this deficiency, glycosphingolipids are deposited in cells, particularly in the vascular endothelium. Stroke may occur in children and young adults as a result of small or large vessel cerebrovascular disease, intracerebral hemorrhage, or aneurysms. Stroke has rarely been the presenting symptom of young men with previously unrecognized Fabry disease.[134] Patients may have cardiac valvular abnormalities, such as mitral valve prolapse,[135,136] cardiomyopathy,[137,138] or conduction disturbances that can increase the risk of cardioembolic stroke. Associated manifestations include renal failure, corneal opacities, angiokeratomas of the skin, and acroparesthesias. Female carriers of the disorder are usually asymptomatic or may have mild ocular or renal manifestations and, rarely, cardiac symptoms.[137] Infusion of agalsidase beta can slow progression of renal, cardiac, and cerebrovascular complications in adults.[139] Although the benefits have not been proven in children, it has been hypothesized that early treatment before end organ damage might be more effective.

Homocystinuria is a group of genetically mediated disorders of methionine metabolism. The most common defect is an autosomal recessive deficiency of cystathionine β-synthase. The prevalence of this disorder is 1 per 80,000 to 200,000 persons.[140,141] It affects males and females equally. Patients have skeletal defects with a marfanoid appearance and lens dislocation. Although these features may lead to some confusion with Marfan syndrome, there may be a difference in the pattern and extent of the lens dislocation. Patients with homocystinuria usually have a dislocation inferiorly or nasally compared with a superior or temporal dislocation in Marfan syndrome.[142] Patients with homocystinuria have a greater incidence of total lens dislocation.[142] Most have mild to moderate developmental delay.[5]

Homocystinuria is associated with severe vascular disease in infants and children.[143] There may be premature cerebrovascular and cardiovascular occlusive disease, peripheral vascular occlusive disease, and renovascular hypertension. Specific cerebrovascular complications observed include sinovenous occlusive disease and ischemic stroke.[144,145] In this condition, there is abnormal accumulation of homocysteine in tissues and blood, which probably initiates premature atherosclerotic vascular disease.[143] Patients with homocystinuria caused by cystathionine β-synthase deficiency may have partial or total correction of the biochemical defects with supplemental vitamin B.[146] Folate may be used successfully in adult patients.[147] Antiplatelet agents are beneficial in reducing the vascular thrombotic tendency.[148,149]

Sulfite oxidase deficiency is a rare, autosomal dominant condition that is a disorder of sulfur metabolism. Patients present at a young age with episodes of acute hemiplegia, seizures, ectopic lens, and mental retardation.

Although the biochemical abnormalities of increased sulfur products in the urine are readily detected, the cause of the ischemic cerebrovascular disease is unknown.

Some rare, inherited enzyme deficiencies such as 11β-hydroxylase deficiency, 11β-ketoreductase deficiency and 17α-hydroxylase deficiency are associated with arterial hypertension and, rarely, with hypertensive strokes. These syndromes may be associated with stroke in any age group, but may manifest in children and young adults if the enzyme defect is severe.

Conclusion

Numerous rare genetic disorders can lead to stroke. It is important to be aware of these conditions and consider them in patients with stroke of apparent unknown etiology. The diagnosis of these conditions has important implications for patients with stroke and their family members.

REFERENCES

1. Pavlakis SG, Kingsley PB, Bialer MG. Stroke in children: genetic and metabolic issues. J Child Neurol 2000;15:308.
2. Bogousslavsky J, Pierre P. Ischemic stroke in patients under age 45. Neurol Clin 1992;10:113.
3. Glueck CJ, Daniels SR, Bates S, et al. Pediatric victims of unexplained stroke and their families: familial lipid and lipoprotein abnormalities. Pediatrics 1982;69:308.
4. Daniels SR, Bates S, Lukin RR, et al. Cerebrovascular arteriopathy (arteriosclerosis) and ischemic childhood stroke. Stroke 1982;13:360.
5. Trescher WH. Ischemic stroke syndromes in childhood. Pediatr Ann 1992;21:374.
6. Shuman RM. The molecular biology of occlusive stroke in childhood. Neurol Clin 1990;8:553.
7. Soljanlahti S, Autti T, Lauerma K, et al. Familial hypercholesterolemia patients treated with statins at no increased risk for intracranial vascular lesions despite increased cholestrol burden and extracranial atherosclerosis. Stroke 2005;36:1572.
8. Schafer AI. The hypercoagulable sites. Ann Intern Med 1985;102:814.
9. Krog M, Almgren B, Eriksson I, Nordstrom S. Vascular complications in the Ehlers-Danlos syndrome. Acta Chir Scand 1982;149:272.
10. Hunter GC, Malone JM, Moore WS, et al. Vascular manifestations in patients with Ehlers Danlos syndrome. Arch Surg 1982;117:495.
11. Schoolman A, Kepes JJ. Bilateral spontaneous carotid-cavernous fistulae in Ehlers-Danlos syndrome. J Neurosurg 1967;26:82.

12. Pretorius ME, Butler IJ. Neurologic manifestations of Ehlers-Danlos syndrome. Neurology 1983;33:1087.

13. Cikrit DF, Glover JR, Dalsing MC, Silver D. The Ehlers Danlos specter revisited. Vasc Endovasc Surg 2002;36:213.

14. Pope FM, Martin GR, Lichtenstein JR, et al. Patients with Ehlers-Danlos syndrome type IV lack type III collagen. Proc Natl Acad Sci U S A 1975;72:1314.

15. Leier CV, Call TD, Fulkerson PK, et al. The spectrum of cardiac defects in the Ehlers-Danlos syndrome, types I and III. Ann Intern Med 1980;92:171.

16. North KN, Whiteman DAH, Pepin MG, Byers PH. Cerebrovascular complications in Ehlers-Danlos syndrome type IV. Ann Neurol 1995;38:960.

17. Rios-Montenegro EN, Behrens MM, Hoyt WF. Pseudoxanthoma elasticum. Arch Neurol 1972;26:151.

18. Altman L, Fialkow PJ, Parker F, Sagebiel RW. Pseudoxanthoma elasticum: an underdiagnosed genetically heterogeneuos disorder with protean manifestations. Arch Intern Med 1974;134:1048.

19. Wolff HH, Stokes JF, Schlesinger BE. Vascular abnormalities associated with pseudoxanthoma elasticum. Arch Dis Child 1952;27:82.

20. Schachner L, Young D. Pseudoxanthoma elasticum with severe cardiovascular disease in a child. Am J Dis Child 1974;127:571.

21. Iqbal A, Alter M, Lee SH. Pseudoxanthoma elasticum: A review of neurological complications. Ann Neurol 1978;4:18-20.

22. Kaler G, Holmes CS, Goldstein DS, et al. Neonatal diagnosis and treatment of Menkes disease. N Engl J Med 2008;358:605.

23. Judge DP, Dietz H. Marfan's syndrome. Lancet 2005;365:1965.

24. Pyeritz RE, McKusick VA. Basic defects in the Marfan syndrome. N Engl J Med 1981;305:1011.

25. ter Berg HWM, Bijlsma JB, Veiga Pires JA, et al. Familial association of intracranial aneurysms and multiple congenital anomalies. Arch Neurol 1986;43:30.

26. Hardin CA. Successful resection of carotid and abdominal aneurysm in two related patients with Marfan's syndrome. N Engl J Med 1962;267:141.

27. Conway JE, Hutchins GM, Tamayo RJ. Marfan syndrome is not associated with intracranial aneurysms. Stroke 1999;30:1632.

28. Marchuk DA, Guttmacher AE, Penner JA, Ganjuly P. Report on the workshop on hereditary hemorrhagic telangiectasia. Am J Med Genet 1998;76:269.

29. Kimura K, Minematsu K, Nakagima M. Isolated pulmonary arteriovenous fistula without Rendu-Osler-Weber disease, as a cause of cryptogenic stroke. J Neurol Neurosurg Psychiatry 2004;75:311.

30. Waller JD, Greenberg JH, Lewis CW. Hereditary hemorrhagic telangiectasia with cerebrovascular malformations. Arch Dermatol 1976;112:49.

31. Peery WH. Clinical spectrum of hereditary hemorrhagic telangiectasia (Osler-Weber-Rendu disease). Am J Med 1987;82:989.

32. Adams HP, Subbiah B, Bosch EP. Neurologic aspects of hereditary hemorrhagic telangiectasia: report of two cases. Arch Neurol 1977;34:101.

33. Cottin V, Chinet T, Lavole A, et al. Pulmonary arteriovenous malformations in hereditary hemorrhagic telangiectasia: series of 126 patients. Medicine 2007;86:1.

34. Maher CO, Piepgras DG, Brown RD, et al. Cerebrovascular manifestations in 321 cases of hereditary hemorrhagic talengiectasia. Stroke 2001;32:877.

35. Alexander GL, Norman RM. The Sturge-Weber Syndrome. Bristol, UK, John Wright & Sons, 1960.

36. Yingkun F, Yinchang Y. Sturge-Weber syndrome. Chin Med J 1980;93:697.

37. Roach ES. Congenital cutaneovascular syndromes. In Toole JF, ed. Handbook of Clinical Neurology, Vascular Disease, Part III. New York: Elsevier Science, 1989.

38. Poser CM, Taveras JM. Cerebral angiography in encephalotrigeminal angiomatosis. Radiology 1957;68:327.

39. Anderson FH, Duncan GW. Sturge-Weber disease with subarachnoid hemorrhage. Stroke 1974;5:509.

40. Vogl TJ, Semmler J, Bergman C, et al. MR and MR angiography of Sturge-Weber syndrome. AJNR Am J Neuroradiol 1993;14:417.

41. Garcia JC, Roach ES, McLean WT. Recurrent thrombotic deterioration in the Sturge-Weber syndrome. Child Brain 1981;8:427.

42. Arzimanoglou AA, Andermann F, Picardin J, et al. Sturge-Weber syndrome: indications and results of surgery on 20 patients. Neurology 2000;55:1472.

43. Riccardi VM. Von Recklinghausen neurofibromatosis. N Engl J Med 1981;305:1617.

44. Kalff V, Shapiro B, Lloyd R, et al. The spectrum of pheochromocytoma in hypertensive patients with neurofibromatosis. Arch Intern Med 1982;142:2092.

45. Pellock JM, Kleinman PK, McDonald BM, Wixson D. Childhood hypertensive stroke with neurofibromatosis. Neurology 1980;30:656.

46. Natowicz M, Kelley RI. Mendelian etiologies of stroke. Ann Neurol 1987;22:175.

47. Roach ES. Neurocutaneous syndromes. Pediatr Clin North Am 1992;39:591.

48. Toboada D, Alonso A, Moreno J, et al. Occlusion of the cerebral arteries in Recklinghausen's disease. Neuroradiology 1979;18:281.

49. Okuno T, Prensky AL, Gado M. The moyamoya syndrome associated with irradiation of an optic glioma in children: report of two cases and review of the literature. Pediatr Neurol 1985;1:311.

50. Rosser TL, Vezina G, Packer RJ. Cerebrovascular complications in a population of children with neurofibromatosis type 1. Neurology 2005;64:553.

51. Blumenkopf B, Huggins MJ. Tuberous sclerosis and multiple intracranial aneurysms: case report. Neurosurgery 1985;17:797.

52. Guttman M, Tanen SM, Lambert CD. Visual loss secondary to a giant aneurysm in a patient with tuberous sclerosis. Can J Neurol Sci 1984;11:472.

53. Kandt RS, Gebarski SS, Goetting MG. Tuberous sclerosis with cardiogenic cerebral embolism: magnetic resonance imaging. Neurology 1985;35:1223.

54. Gomez MR. Strokes in tuberous sclerosis: Are rhabdomyomas a cause? Brain Dev 1989;11:14.

55. Beall S, Delaney P. Tuberous sclerosis with intracranial aneurysm. Arch Neurol 1983;40:826.

56. Djindjian M, Djindjian R, Hurth M, et al. Spinal cord arteriovenous malformations and the Klippel-Trenaunay-Weber syndrome. Surg Neurol 1977;8:229.

57. Proesmans W, Van Damme B, Casaer P, et al. Autosomal dominant polycystic kidney disease in the neonatal period: association with a cerebral arteriovenous malformations. Pediatrics 1982;70:972.

58. Mettinger KL, Ericson K. Fibromuscular dysplasia and the brain: observations on angiographic, clinical and genetic characteristics. Stroke 1982;13:46.

59. Horton WA, Wong V, Eldridge R. Von Hippel–Lindau disease. Arch Intern Med 1976;136:769.

60. Miles JH, Zonana J, MacFarlane JP, et al. Macrocephaly with hamartomas: Bannayan Zonana syndrome. Am J Genet 1984;19:225.

61. Kurokawa T, Chen YJ, Tomita S, et al. Cerebrovascular occlusive disease with and without the moyamoya vascular network in children. Neuropediatrics 1985;16:29.

62. Yonekawa Y, Goto Y, Ogata N. Moyamoya disease: diagnosis, treatment and recent achievements. In Barnett HJM, Mohr JP, Stein BM, Yastu FM, eds. Stroke: Pathophysiology, Diagnosis and Management, 2nd ed. New York: Churchill Livingstone, 1993.

63. Griffiths RA, Mortimer TF, Oppenheimer DR, Spalding JMK. Congophilic angiopathy of the brain: a clinical and pathological report on two siblings. J Neurol Neurosurg Psychiatry 1982;45:396.

64. Gudmundsson G, Hallgrimsson J, Jonasson TA, Bjarnason O. Hereditary cerebral hemorrhage with amyloidosis. Brain 1972;95:387.

65. Chabriat H, Vahedr K, Ba-Zizen MT, et al. Clinical spectrum of CADASIL: a study of 7 families: cerebral autosomal dominant arteriopathy with subcortical infarcts and leukoencephalopathy. Lancet 1995;346:934.

66. Bogousslavsky J, Regli F. Ischemic stroke in adults younger than 30 years of age. Arch Neurol 1987;44:479.

67. Hilton-Jones D, Warlow CP. The cause of stroke in the young. J Neurol 1985;232:137.

68. Spaccavento LI, Solomon GD. Migraine as an etiology of stroke in young adults. Headache 1984;24:19.

69. Snyder BD, Ramirez-Lassepas M. Cerebral infarction in young adults: long term prognosis. Stroke 1980;11:149.

70. Jen J, Cohen Q, Yue JT, et al. Hereditary endotheliopathy with retinopathy, nephropathy, and stroke (HERNS). Neurology 1997;49:1322.

71. Hart RG, Miller VT. Cerebral infarction in young adults: a practical approach. Stroke 1983;14:110.

72. Samson O, Stirling Y, Wolf L. Management of planned pregnancy in a patient with congenital antithrombin III deficiency. Br J Haematol 1984;56:243.

73. Brenner B, Fishman A, Goldsher D, et al. Cerebral thrombosis in a newborn with a congenital deficiency of antithrombin III. Am J Hematol 1988;27:209.

74. Thaler E, Lechner K. Antithrombin III deficiency and thromboembolism. Clin Haematol 1981;10:369.

75. Broekmans AW. Hereditary protein C deficiency. Haemostasis 1985;15:233.

76. Bertina RM. Hereditary protein S deficiency. Haemostasis 1985;15:241.

77. Wintzen AR, Broekmans AW, Bertina RM, et al. Cerebral haemorrhagic infarction in young patients with hereditary protein C deficiency: evidence for "spontaneous" cerebral venous thrombosis. BMJ 1985;290:350.

78. Horellou MH, Conard J, Bertina RM, Samama M. Congenital protein C deficiency and thrombotic disease in nine French families. Br J Med 1984; 289: 1285.

79. Esmon CE, BeBault L, Carroll RC, et al. Biochemical and physiological aspects of protein C. Ricerca Clin Labor 1984;14:455.

80. Smith DB, Ens GE. Protein C deficiency: a cause of amaurosis fugax. J Neurol Neurosurg Psychiatry 1987;50:361.

81. De Stefano V, Leone G, Teofili L, et al. Transient ischemic attack in a patient with congenital protein-C deficiency during treatment with stanozolol. Am J Hematol 1988;29:120.

82. Israels SJ, Sechia SS. Childhood stroke associated with protein C or S deficiency. J Pediatr 1987;111:562.

83. Kohler J, Kasper J, Witt I, Von Reuthern GM. Ischemic stroke due to protein C deficiency. Stroke 1990;21:1077.

84. Haire WD, Newland JR. Protein C deficiency and anticardiolipin antibodies in a family with premature stroke. Am J Hematol 1990;33:61.

85. Koelman JHTM, Bakker CM, Plandsoen WCG, et al. Hereditary protein S deficiency presenting with cerebral sinus thrombosis in an adolescent girl. J Neurol 1992;239:105.

86. Rich C, Gill JC, Wernick S, Konkol RJ. An unusual cause of cerebral venous thrombosis in a four-year-old child. Stroke 1993;24:603.

87. Green D, Otoya I, Oriba H, Rovner R. Protein S deficiency in middle-aged women with stroke. Neurology 1992;42:1029.

88. Sacco RL, Owen I, Mohr JP, et al. Free protein S deficiency: a possible association with cerebrovascular occlusion. Stroke 1989;20:1657.

89. Powars D, Chab LS, Schroeder WA. The variable expression of sickle cell disease is genetically determined. Semin Hematol 1990;27:360.

90. Ohene-Frempong K, Weiner SJ, Sleeper LA, et al. Cerebrovascular accidents in sickle cell disease: rates and risk factors. Blood 1998;91:288.

91. Grotta JC, Manner C, Pettigrew C, et al. Red blood cell disorders and stroke. Stroke 1987;17:811.

92. Sarnaik SA, Lusher JM. Neurological complications of sickle cell anemia. Am J Pediatr Hematol Oncol 1982;4:386.

93. Powars D, Wilson B, Imbus D, et al. The natural history of stroke in sickle cell disease. Am J Med 1978;65:461.

94. Russell MD, Goldberg HI, Hodson A, et al. Effect of transfusion therapy on arteriographic abnormalities and on recurrence of stroke in sickle cell disease. Blood 1984;63:162.

95. Fullerton HJ, Adams RJ, Zaho S, Claiborne Johnston S. Declining stroke rates in California children with sickle cell disease. Blood 2004;104:336.

96. Wood DH. Cerebrovascular complications of sickle cell anemia. Stroke 1978;9:73.
97. Wong V, Yu YL, Liang RHS, et al. Cerebral thrombosis in β-thalassemia/hemoglobin E disease. Stroke 1990;21:812.
98. Miller ST, Rieder RF, Rao SP, Brown AK. Cerebrovascular accidents in children with sickle-cell disease and alpha-thalassemia. J Pediatr 1988;113:847.
99. Prchal JT, Crist WM, Goldwasser E, et al. Autosomal dominant polycythemia. Blood 1985;66:1208.
100. Siltanen P, Tuuteri L, Novio R, et al. Atrial myxoma in a family. Am J Cardiol 1976;38:252.
101. Kleid JM, Klugman J, Haas JM, et al. Familial atrial myxoma. Am J Cardiol 1973;32:361.
102. Farah MG. Familial atrial myxoma. Ann Intern Med 1975;83:358.
103. Sandok BA, von Esstorff I, Guiliani EK. CNS embolism due to atrial myxoma: clinical features and diagnosis. Arch Neurol 1980;37:485.
104. Pavlakis SG, Gould RJ, Zito JL. Stroke in children. Adv Pediatr 1991;38:151.
105. Lehmann H, Kelin UE. Familial sinus node dysfunction with autosomal dominant inheritance. Br Heart J 1978;40:1314.
106. Onat A. Familial sinus node disease and degenerative myopia—a new hereditary syndrome? Hum Genet 1986;72:182.
107. Gunteroth WG, Motulsky AG. Inherited primary disorders of cardiac rhythm and conduction. Prog Med Genet 1983;5:381.
108. Hughes SE, McKenna WJ. New insights into the pathology of inherited cardiomyopathy. Heart 2005;91:257.
109. Grunig E, Tasman JA, Kucherer H, et al. Frequency and phenotypes of familial dilated cardiomyopathy. J Am Coll Cardiol 1998;31:186.
110. Taylor WJ. Genetic aspects of the cardiomyopathies. Prog Med Genet 1983;5:163.
111. Russell JW, Biller J, Hajduczok ZD, et al. Ischemic cerebrovascular complications and risk factors in idiopathic hypertrophic subaortic stenosis. Stroke 1991;22:1143.
112. Biller J, Ionasescu V, Zellweger H, et al. Frequency of cerebral infarction in patients with inherited neuromuscular diseases. Stroke 1987;18:805.
113. Pavlakis SG, Phillips PC, DiMauro S, et al. Mitochondrial myopathy, encephalopathy, lactic acidosis, and stroke-like episodes: A distinctive clinical syndrome. Ann Neurol 1981;16:181.
114. Allard JC, Tilak S, Carter AP. CT and MR of MELAS syndrome. AJNR Am J Neuroradiol 1988;9:1234.
115. Iizuka T, Sakai F, Kan S, Suzuki N. Slowly progressive spread of the stroke-like lesions in MELAS. Neurology 2003;61:1238.
116. McDonnell MT, Schaefer AM, Blakely EL, et al. A mitochondrial DNA mutation using urinary epithelial cells. J Hum Genet 2004;12:778.
117. Hasegawa H, Matsuoka T, Goto Y, Nonaka I. Strongly succinate dehydrogenase-reactive blood vessels in muscles from patients with mitochondrial myopathy, encephalopathy, lactic acidosis, and stroke-like episodes. Ann Neurol 1991; 29:601.
118. Sakuta R, Nonaka I. Vascular involvement in mitochondrial myopathy. Ann Neurol 1989;25:594.
119. Peterson PL, Martens ME, Lee CP. Mitochondrial encephalomyopathies. Neurol Clin 1988;6:529.
120. Plaitakis A, Whetsell WO, Cooper JR, Yahr MD. Chronic Leigh disease: a genetic and biochemical study. Ann Neurol 1980;7:304.
121. Willems JL, Monnens LAH, Trijbels JMF, et al. Leigh's encephalomyelopathy in a patient with cytochrome c oxidase deficiency in muscle tissue. Pediatrics 1977;60:850.
122. Pincus JH. Subacute necrotizing encephalomyelopathy (Leigh's disease): a consideration of clinical features and etiology. Dev Med Child Neurol 1972;14:87.
123. Hall K, Gardner-Medwin D. CT scan appearances in Leigh's disease (subacute necrotizing encephalomyelopathy). Neuroradiology 1978;16:48.
124. Heidenreich R, Natowicz M, Hainline BE, et al. Acute extrapyramidal syndrome in methyl malonic acidemia: "metabolic stroke" involving the globus pallidus. J Pediatr 1988;113:1022.
125. Korf B, Wallman JK, Levy HL. Bilateral lucency of the globus pallidus complicating methylmalonic acidemia. Ann Neurol 1986;20:364.
126. Dave P, Curless RG, Steinman L. Cerebellar hemorrhage complicating methylmalonic and propionic acidemia. Arch Neurol 1984;41:1293.
127. Fischer AQ, Challa VR, Burton BK, McLean WT. Cerebellar hemorrhage complicating isovaleric acidemia: a case report. Neurology 1981;31:746.
128. Matsui SM, Mahoney MJ, Rosenberg LE. The natural history of the inherited methyl malonic acidemias. N Engl J Med 1983;308:857.
129. Goodman SI, Mackey SP, Moe PG, et al. Glutaric aciduria: a "new" disorder of amino acid metabolism. Biochem Med 1975;12:12.
130. Goodman SI, Norenberg MD. Glutaric acidemia as a cause of striatal necrosis in childhood. Ann Neurol 1983; 13:582-583.
131. Rahman AN, Lindenberg R. The neuropathology of hereditary dystopic lipidosis. Arch Neurol 1963;9:373.
132. Lou HOV, Reske-Nielsen E. The central nervous system in Fabry's disease. Arch Neurol 1971;25:351.
133. Morgan SH, d'A Crawford SH. Anderson Fabry disease: a commonly missed diagnosis. BMJ 1988; 297:872.
134. Grewal RP, Barton NW. Fabry's disease presenting with stroke. Clin Neurol Neurosurg 1992;94:177.
135. Goldman ME, Cantor R, Schwartz MF, et al. Echocardiographic abnormalities and disease severity in Fabry's disease. J Am Coll Cardiol 1986;7:1157.
136. Desmick RJ, Blieden LC, Sharp HL, et al. Cardiac valvular anomalies in Fabry disease: clinical, morphologic, and biochemical studies. Circulation 1976;54:818.
137. Broadbent JC, Edwards WD, Gordon H, et al. Fabry cardiomyopathy in the female confirmed by endomyocardial biopsy. Mayo Clin Proc 1981;56:623.
138. Colucci WS, Lorell BH, Schoen FJ, et al. Hypertrophic obstructive cardiomyopathy due to Fabry's disease. N Engl J Med 1982;307:926.

139. Banikazemi M, Bultas J, Woldek S, et al. Agalsidase-beta therapy for advanced Fabry disease: a randomized trial. Ann Intern Med 2007;146:77.
140. Wilcken B. Incidence of homocystinuria. Lancet 1975;1:273.
141. Hladovec J. Experimental homocystinemia, endothelial lesion and thrombosis. Blood Vessel 1979;16:202.
142. Grieco AJ. Homocystinuria. Am J Med Sci 1977; 273:120.
143. Boers GHJ, Smals AGH, Trijbeis FJM. Heterozygosity for homocystinuria in premature peripheral and cerebral occlusive arterial disease. N Engl J Med 1985;313:709.
144. Malinow MR. Hyperhomocyst(e)inemia: a common and easily reversible risk factor for occlusive atherosclerosis. Circulation 1990;81:2004.
145. Schwab FJ, Peyster RG, Brill CB. CT of cerebral venous sinus thrombosis in a child with homocystinuria. Pediatr Radiol 1987;17:244.
146. Mudd SH. Vascular disease and homocysteine metabolism. N Engl J Med 1985;313:751.
147. Brattstrom L, Israelsson B, Jeppson J-O, Hultberg BL. Folic acid—an innocuous means to reduce plasma homocysteine. Scand J Clin Lab Invest 1988;48:215.
148. Hacker LA, Slichter SJ, Scott CR, Ross R. Homocystinemia: vascular injury and arterial thrombosis. N Engl J Med 1974;291:537.
149. Hacker LA, Harlan JM, Ross R. Effect of sulfinpyrazone on homocysteine-induced endothelial injury and arteriosclerosis in baboons. Circ Res 1983;53:731.

CHAPTER **12**

Cerebral Venous Thrombosis

Rima M. Dafer • José Biller

KEY TERMS

AT	antithrombin
CT	computed tomography
CST	cavernous sinus thrombosis
CVT	cerebral venous thrombosis
LMWH	low-molecular-weight heparin
MRI	magnetic resonance imaging
MTHFR	methylene tetrahydrofolate reductase
SLE	systemic lupus erythematosus
SSS	superior sagittal sinus
UFH	unfractionated heparin

Thrombosis of the cerebral venous channels is an uncommon but well-recognized cause of cerebral infarction in children and young adults, accounting for less than 1% of stroke cases. Cerebral venous thrombosis (CVT) affects individuals of any age group. CVT was first described by Ribes in 1825[1] in a 45-year-old man with disseminated malignancy associated with superior sagittal sinus (SSS) thrombosis. Kalabag and Woolf[2] in a monograph on CVT stated that aseptic CVT is common, especially among children, elderly patients, and women in the puerperium. The diagnosis of CVT is often difficult and requires a mixture of high clinical awareness and objective tests. CVT has a heterogeneous clinical presentation with variable outcome. CVT often is underrecognized, and opportunities for early therapeutic intervention are often missed. With the advent of modern neuroimaging techniques, computed tomography (CT) and magnetic resonance imaging (MRI), CVT is more easily diagnosed, and treatment is instituted early in the course of the disease.

Incidence

The true incidence of CVT is unknown. Most incidence estimates of CVT in the pre-angiography, pre-CT era were based on retrospective autopsy studies. Towbin[3] in a prospective autopsy series of 182 patients with CVT reported an incidence of 8.3% among patients younger than 50 years, and of 9.3% among patients older than 50 years. The study did not include patients younger than age 23 years.[3] In the pre-CT and pre-MRI era, cerebral angiographic studies reported an incidence of 3.3% among children older than 18 months.[4] The incidence of CVT is seemingly higher in some Asian countries, approximately

233

10 times more common, than in developed countries.[5] The prevalence of CVT in a series of 40 patients 16 to 40 years old from Saudi Arabia was 7 per 100,000 patients.[6] The Canadian Pediatric Ischemic Stroke Registry, which included newborns to children up to 18 years, found an incidence of 0.67 case per 100,000 per year.[7] With the advent of newer imaging techniques, in particular, MR venography, the incidence of CVT is likely to be much higher than previously reported.[8]

Anatomy of the Cerebral Sinovenous System

The intracranial venous anatomy is complex, and anatomic variations of important intracranial venous structures are common. Knowledge of the anatomy of the cerebral sinovenous system is particularly important today with the many imaging modalities available. Cerebral lesions and clinical syndromes resulting from CVT occur in patterns directly related to the venous anatomy, and infarctions usually cross a particular arterial distribution, often with hemorrhagic transformation.

Constant features of the intracranial venous systems are a superficial sinovenous system, also called the dural venous sinuses, and a deep venous system. These systems are contiguous and have a rich network of anastomoses.[9] Thrombosis of these intracranial venous channels may be limited to one system, resulting in a distinct clinical syndrome; however, often there is involvement of both systems with a more variable clinical presentation. The SSS is the most commonly involved dural sinus, followed by the lateral sinus.

The SSS drains the superficial surface of the cerebral hemispheres. It runs from the crista galli along the convex margin of the falx cerebri, receiving blood from the superior cerebral veins, and ends at the confluence of sinuses or torcular Herophili. The lateral sinus extends laterally from the confluence of sinuses in the tentorium cerebelli and travels ventrally to become the sigmoid sinus, which continues into the internal jugular. The tributaries of the major cerebral sinuses and veins are outlined in Table 12-1. Figures 12-1 and 12-2 depict normal cerebral venous anatomy.

TABLE 12-1 **Cerebral Sinovenous Structures and Their Tributaries**

Venous Structure(s)	Tributaries
Superior sagittal sinus	Cortical veins (frontal/parietal/occipital)
	Trolard vein
	Parietal emissary veins
	Frontal diploic veins
Inferior sagittal sinus	Callosal veins
	Cingulate veins
	Medial frontal veins
	Medial parietal veins
Straight sinus	Inferior sagittal sinus
	Great cerebral vein of Galen
	Superior cerebellar veins
	Basal veins
	Tentorial veins
Torcular Herophili	Superior sagittal sinus
	Straight sinus
	Occipital sinus
	Occipital emissary veins
	Occipital diploic veins
Transverse sinuses	Torcular Herophili
	Superior sagittal sinus
	Straight sinuses
	Inferior cerebral veins
	Labbé vein
	Cerebellar veins
	Mastoid and occipital emissary veins
	Parietal and occipital diploic veins
Sigmoid sinuses	Transverse sinuses
	Superior petrosal sinuses
	Cerebellar veins
	Pontine veins
	Veins of the medulla oblongata
	Condyloid emissary veins
	Occipital diploic veins
Internal jugular veins	Sigmoid sinuses
	Inferior petrosal sinuses
Cavernous sinuses	Facial veins
	Ophthalmic veins
	Retinal veins
	Middle cerebral veins
	Meningeal veins
	Intercavernous (circular) sinus
Superior petrosal sinuses	Cavernous sinuses
	Inferior cerebral veins
	Superior cerebellar veins
	Mesencephalic veins
Inferior petrosal sinuses	Cavernous sinuses
	Inferior cerebellar veins
	Brainstem veins
	Internal auditory veins
Great cerebral vein of Galen	Internal cerebral veins
	Basal vein of Rosenthal
	Pericallosal veins
	Occipital veins
	Mesencephalic veins
	Superior cerebellar veins

TABLE 12-1 **Cerebral Sinovenous Structures and Their Tributaries—Cont'd**

Venous Structure(s)	Tributaries
Internal cerebral veins	Septal veins
	Thalamostriate veins
	Thalamic veins
	Caudate veins
	Choroidal veins
	Atrial veins
	Habenular veins
	Callosal veins
Basal vein of Rosenthal	Anterior cerebral veins
	Olfactory veins
	Striate veins
	Inferior frontal veins
	Deep middle cerebral veins
	Inferior thalamic veins
	Thalamogeniculate veins
	Hypothalamic veins
	Inferior ventricular veins
	Peduncular veins
	Lateral mesencephalic veins
	Hippocampal veins
	Inferior temporo-occipital veins
	Internal occipital veins

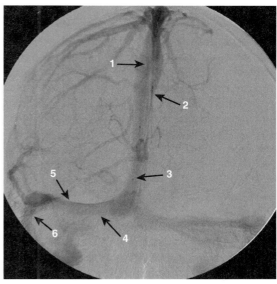

FIGURE 12-2 Left internal carotid angiogram (venous phase, anteroposterior view). *1,* superior sagittal sinus; *2,* inferior sagittal sinus; *3,* straight sinus; *4,* torcular Herophili; *5,* lateral sinus; *6,* sigmoid sinus.

Clinical Presentation

The clinical spectrum of CVT varies and is largely determined by the venous channel involved, etiology, age, and time interval between onset of disease and clinical presentation. Onset of symptoms may be acute, subacute, or chronic. The most common presentation is headache, often associated with lethargy and papilledema (Table 12-2). Headaches are often gradual in onset, although rarely patients with CVT may present with thunderclap headaches.

Increased intracranial pressure occurs in about 20% of patients with CVT as a direct result of venous occlusion with increased venous pressure, and consequent interference with venous drainage and

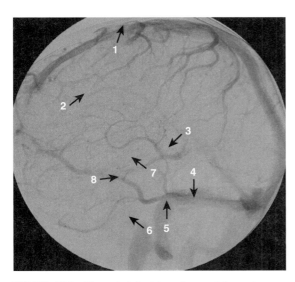

FIGURE 12-1 Normal left internal carotid angiogram (venous phase, lateral view). *1,* superior sagittal sinus; *2,* inferior sagittal sinus; *3,* straight sinus; *4,* torcular Herophili; *5,* lateral sinus; *6,* sigmoid sinus; *7,* vein of Galen; *8,* vein of Labbé.

TABLE 12-2 **Common Clinical Manifestations of Cerebral Venous Thrombosis**

Symptoms and Signs	%
Headaches	88.8
Seizures	39.3
Focal motor deficits	37.2
Papilledema	28.3
Mental status changes	22
Aphasia	19.1
Stupor or coma	13.9
Diplopia	13.5
Visual loss	13.2

Adapted from Ferro JM, Canhao P, Stam J, et al. Prognosis of cerebral vein and dural sinus thrombosis: results of the International Study on Cerebral Vein and Dural Sinus Thrombosis (ISCVT). Stroke 2004;35:664.

cerebrospinal fluid absorption.[10,11] Signs and symptoms of increased intracranial pressure may occur in isolation, making it difficult to discern CVT from idiopathic intracranial hypertension (IIH). In a retrospective study by Lin and colleagues,[12] CVT accounted for 9.4% of patients with presumed IIH in three tertiary care neuro-ophthalmology services.[12] Hydrocephalus is rare in CVT, but clinically important in infants with open sutures and among patients with CVT involving the deep cerebral venous system.[11,13,14]

Headache is the most common initial presenting symptom of CVT, occurring in more than 80% of patients.[8,10,15] More than half of children and adults have papilledema. Depressed level of consciousness or confusion is encountered in one fourth of patients, usually indicating deep cerebral venous system involvement.[6,7,10,15,16] Other possible symptoms of CVT referable to intracranial pressure include nausea, vomiting, transient visual obscurations, horizontal binocular diplopia owing to sixth cranial nerve (abducens) palsy, and pulsatile tinnitus.

Focal or generalized seizures occur in approximately one fourth of patients,[10] predominantly among patients with focal deficits and patients with focal edema and ischemic or hemorrhagic changes on CT or MRI of the brain. Seizures may be a predictor for poor outcome or death or both.[17] The variable clinical presentation of CVT reflects the extensive anatomic communications of the intricate intracranial venous network. Edema, infarction, and hemorrhage may involve the cerebral cortex and deep white matter in cases associated with thrombosis of cortical veins.[18] Focal neurologic signs, such as hemiparesis with lower limbs more severely involved than the upper limbs, hemisensory disturbances, homonymous hemianopsia, aphasia, agnosia, apraxia, and cortical blindness, may occur in more than one third of older children and adults with dural sinus thrombosis.[10,15,18-20] Bilateral symptoms occur frequently, with the legs more affected than the arms.

Thrombosis of the deep cerebral venous system is an extremely rare cause of stroke.[21] The deep cerebral venous system drains the dorsal thalamus, basal ganglia, choroid plexus, and periventricular white matter via thalamostriate, septal, and choroid veins, which form the internal cerebral veins on the roof of the third ventricle. The basal vein of Rosenthal drains the ventral thalamus, midbrain pons, and medulla from its anterior and posterior perforating veins. The two internal cerebral veins and two basal veins of Rosenthal form the great vein of Galen inferior to the splenium of the corpus callosum, which feeds into the straight sinus with the inferior sagittal sinus eventually draining into the internal jugular vein. Clinically, deep cerebral venous thrombosis manifests with headache, nausea and vomiting, alteration of consciousness, and corticospinal tract signs, often with rapid clinical deterioration and death.[22] Seizures and papilledema are more frequent with dural sinus involvement. In cases of thrombosis of the deep cerebral venous system, thalamic edema, infarction, or hemorrhage also may result in a predominantly transcortical sensory aphasia, hemisensory loss, and "thalamic dementia."[18,23] With basal ganglia involvement, choreoathetosis and akathisia may be predominant features.[24]

Cavernous sinus thrombosis (CST) is usually the result of a late complication of bacterial infection of the midface or facial or paranasal sinuses. Signs and symptoms of CST occur either as a result of disruption of venous drainage from orbital and periorbital tissues or as a result of compression of intracavernous structures, such as the carotid artery and cranial nerves III, IV, and VI, and the first two divisions of cranial nerve V. Rarely, involvement of the intracavernous carotid artery by direct compression, inflammation, or extension of the septic process may result in a carotid-cavernous fistula or carotid internal occlusion and ipsilateral hemispheric infarction. Thrombosis may propagate via the petrosal sinuses to the lateral sinuses, resulting in intracranial hypertension.

Clinical Presentations in Neonates and Infants

Neonatal CVT is an extremely rare but devastating condition, occurring in 0.6 per 100,000 population per year.[7] Most common risk factors include ear infections (mainly mastoiditis), persistent pulmonary hypertension, cardiac disorders (predominantly cyanotic congenital heart disease), dehydration, nutritional disorders, and hereditary hypercoagulability disorders.[16,25-28] The clinical presentation of neonates and infants with CVT may be similar to that seen in older children and young adults, but has certain unique features. Children often present with fever, headache, anorexia, vomiting, lethargy, and respiratory distress. Seizures are the most prominent symptom, occurring in 80% of neonates with CVT. Seizures may occur 1 hour after birth, and most commonly occur within the first week of life.[29-31] Other clinical features reported to occur in neonates and older infants include dilated scalp veins, scalp edema, bulging fontanelles, hydrocephalus, macrocephaly, difficulty walking, opisthotonos, vomiting, high-pitched cry, failure to thrive, anorexia, weight loss, and developmental delay. As with older children and young adults, focal signs are common.[16,25] Death may rarely occur.[7]

Predisposing Conditions

"Thrombophilias" (prothrombotic state) is the term used to describe a tendency toward thrombosis. Although infections remain a major cause in developing countries, prothrombotic state is the most common risk factor for CVT in industrialized countries. Other precipitating factors include dehydration, hyperviscosity particularly in the peripartum period, low-flow states, head injuries, birth-related injuries, invasion by cancer, and use of oral contraceptives (Table 12-3).

Hypercoagulable States

Prothrombotic disorders associated with CVT include deficiencies of the natural anticoagulants antithrombin (AT),[7,32,33] protein C,[26,34] protein S,[35,36] and dysfibrinogenemia.[37] Deficiencies of natural anticoagulants are hereditary, with homozygous states most commonly associated with veno-occlusive disease in neonates, whereas such complications have been recognized in heterozygous deficiencies in children and young adults, especially when associated with other comorbid thrombotic conditions. Acquired deficiencies of AT,

TABLE 12-3 **Causes of Cerebral Venous Thrombosis**

Idiopathic
Prothrombotic state
  Protein C or S deficiency
  Antithrombin deficiency
  Factor V Leiden mutation
  Activated protein C resistance
  Prothrombin G20210A mutation
  Mutations in thrombomodulin
  Platelet glycoprotein IIIa (β_3) mutation
  Heparin cofactor II deficiency
  Mutations in plasminogen gene
  MTHFR C677 mutation
  Dysfibrinogenemia
  Elevated plasminogen activator inhibitor
  Tissue plasminogen activator deficiency
  Increased factors VIII, IX, X, von Willebrand factor
  Mutations in tissue factor pathway inhibitor
  Sickle cell disease and trait
  Reactive thrombocytosis and essential
    thrombocythemia
  Pregnancy and puerperium
Postoperative state
Antiphospholipid antibody syndrome
Hyperhomocysteinemia
Homocystinuria
Cancer
Inflammatory bowel diseases
Dehydration
Congestive heart failure
Paroxysmal nocturnal hemoglobinuria
Marasmus
Iron deficiency anemia
Nephrotic syndrome
Thrombocytopenia
Essential thrombocythemia
Disseminated intravascular coagulation
Thrombotic microangiopathies
Polycythemia vera and secondary polycythemia
Hyperlipidemia
Familial histidine-rich glycoprotein deficiency

Drugs
Asparaginase
Estrogen and oral contraceptives
Androgen
ε-aminocaproic acid
Cisplatin and etoposide
Medroxyprogesterone
Heparin (heparin-induced thrombocytopenia)
IgG (intravenous immunoglobulin)

Infections
Herpes zoster virus
Myeloidosis
Mucormycosis
Aspergillosis
Pneumococcal meningitis
Syphilis
Human immunodeficiency virus
Otitis

Continued

TABLE 12-3   **Causes of Cerebral Venous Thrombosis—Cont'd**

Infections (cont'd)
Mastoiditis
Sinusitis
Peritonsillar abscess
Endotoxemia
Trichinosis
Sepsis

Vasculitides
Behçet disease
Sarcoidosis
Wegener granulomatosis
Systemic lupus erythematosus
Polyarteritis nodosa

Trauma
Head trauma
Neurosurgical procedures
Strangulation
Intravenous catheters
Cardiac pacemakers

Others
Osteopetrosis
Malignant atrophic papulosis (Kohlmeier-Degos disease)
Chronic lung disease
Diabetes mellitus
Budd-Chiari syndrome
Arteriovenous malformation
Sturge-Weber syndrome
Cerebral arterial occlusions
Neoplasm (meningioma, metastasis, glomus tumors)

protein C, and protein S are mainly encountered in inflammatory bowel diseases, nephrotic syndrome, and disseminated infection and disseminated intravascular coagulation. SSS thrombosis has been associated with primary hematologic disorders, including essential thrombocythemia,[38-40] and in infants with primary thrombocytopenia without any identifiable thrombophilic risk factors.[41] Other hypercoagulable conditions associated with CVT include factor V Leiden mutation,[26,33,42-44] prothrombin G20210A mutation,[26,45,46] methylenetetrahydrofolate reductase (MTHFR) deficiency,[26,42,43,47] hyperhomocystinemia, and elevated lipoprotein (a).[26]

Antiphospholipid antibody syndrome is a common cause of arterial and venous thrombosis. Lupus anticoagulant and anticardiolipin antibodies have been associated with CVT, especially in young women taking oral contraceptives.[33,36,43,48-51] Antiphospholipid antibodies occur in approximately one third of patients with systemic lupus erythematosus (SLE), but also are found in patients with rheumatoid arthritis, patients with sickle cell disease, and a small percentage of healthy individuals.[52]

CVT also has been reported in children with the idiopathic hypereosinophilic syndrome[53] and young adults with Graves disease and markedly elevated factor VIII.[54] CVT and other thromboembolic events are well-described complications of nephrotic syndrome in children and young adults. A hypercoagulable state is often believed to be the cause, with urinary loss of natural anticoagulants such as AT and proteins C and S, in addition to thrombocytosis, increased platelet aggregation, increased levels of clotting factors, and hemoconcentration owing to hypoalbuminemia.[55-58] Corticosteroids used during the active stages also may contribute to the hypercoagulable state.[56]

Paroxysmal nocturnal hemoglobinuria, caused by somatic mutation of hematopoietic cells, is associated with complement-mediated hemolysis and a hypercoagulable state and should be considered in patients with unexplained CVT.[59-63] Platelet dysfunction, including reactive thrombocytosis secondary to anemia, and heparin-induced thrombocytopenia are secondary causes of hypercoagulable state associated with CVT.[64,65]

Infections

Chronic otitis media and mastoiditis are common causes of transverse sinus thrombosis. Infections are a common cause of CVT in India, especially among women of childbearing age during the puerperium. Orbital or basal furuncles and infections of the midface are common causes of CST. The most common pathogen is *Staphylococcus aureus,* but other organisms, including fungal infections, are especially common in diabetics and immunocompromised individuals.

Inflammatory Conditions

Inflammatory multisystem vasculitides, such as Behçet disease, SLE, Wegener granulomatosis, and sarcoidosis, have been associated with CVT. Behçet disease, a chronic inflammatory disorder clinically characterized by multisystemic vasculitis, is associated with recurrent venous thrombosis of the dural sinus, with the treatment directed toward controlling the primary inflammatory process.[66-70] The mechanism of venous thrombosis in SLE is multifactorial, with the presence of lupus anticoagulant being the most common cause. Necrotizing cerebral thrombophlebitis may complicate Wegener granulomatosis, the cause of which is unknown.

Low-Flow State

Hypotension, dehydration, anemia, and low cardiac output are associated with CVT. Neonates with gastroenteritis and diarrhea are particularly prone, mainly as a result of loss of natural anticoagulant and hyperviscosity, as well as infants with congenital cyanotic heart disease by causing high venous pressure and low perfusion pressure.

Drugs

CVT is a well-recognized complication of asparaginase therapy in patients with acute lymphocytic leukemia. The disorder is usually reversible on discontinuation of the drug. The use of oral contraceptives, especially in patients who are known carriers of a hereditary prothrombotic condition and in smokers, increases the risk and interacts in a multiplicative way in the development of CVT.[71] Such risk is much lower among users of the oral contraceptive patch.[72] Transverse sinus thrombosis also has been described in patients receiving intravenous immunoglobulin therapy[73] and oxymetholone, a synthetic androgen analogue, for the treatment of aplastic anemia.[74]

Trauma

Head injury, including closed or open and depressed skull fractures, is a rarely recognized but important cause of dural sinus thrombosis, especially in children. Children presenting with persistent giddiness and vomiting after minor head injury should be screened for

CVT. This vigilant approach may unmask an unrecognized subclinical hypercoagulable state.[75-87] Birth trauma with direct injury to the dural sinuses may be a common cause of CVT in neonates. Other uncommon causes include strangulation, jugular venous compressions, and a negative-pressure support ventilator.

Invasion by Cancer

Direct compression or invasion of intracranial venous sinus walls by malignant cells from dural or calvarial metastasis may cause sinus thrombosis in patients with acute leukemia or solid tumors.[88-91]

Diagnostic Procedures

Despite the variable clinical presentation, CVT should be suspected on clinical grounds in children and young adults presenting with new-onset headaches and focal neurologic deficits even in the absence of risk factors for stroke, and in neonates and infants presenting with lethargy, respiratory distress, and seizures. Special attention should be paid to patients with an IIH-like picture, especially in patients not fitting the stereotypic pattern of the disease, such as young men or patients who are not overweight. Noninvasive brain imaging studies, such as CT with venography or MRI with MR venography, are necessary to exclude an intracranial mass as part of the differential diagnosis and to identify CVT. An extensive laboratory workup is required to determine the underlying cause of the thrombosis.

Neuroimaging

MRI with diffusion-weighted imaging in combination with MR venography is the preferred imaging modality for the detection of CVT, especially CST and CVT involving the deep venous system. MRI and diffusion-weighted imaging are particularly useful techniques for detecting cerebral venous and brain parenchymal changes that may be related to thrombosis, with infarction usually not following classic arterial boundaries. An abnormal hyperintense signal in a thrombosed sinus on T1-weighted and T2-weighted MRI corresponding with absence of flow on MR venography is diagnostic. Elliptic centric ordered three-dimensional MR venography technique is a new imaging modality that has been shown more recently to be superior to time-of-flight MR venography for the diagnosis or exclusion of CVT.[92]

If MRI is unavailable, CT is useful in showing hemorrhagic infarction, intraparenchymal hemorrhage, or subarachnoid hemorrhage resulting from CVT. The delta sign (also referred to as the empty delta sign) and the cord sign are classic signs of intracranial venous sinus thrombosis on cranial CT scanning. The delta sign appears on contrast-enhanced CT and MRI (Fig. 12-3). It represents the cross section appearance of hypodense thrombus within the hyperdense, contrast-enhanced SSS or straight sinus. The cord sign is a hyperdense superficial lesion seen on non–contrast-enhanced scans, representing a thrombosed cortical vein. CT venography is a promising new technique for visualization of the cerebral venous system with high sensitivity for detecting CVT. MR venography or CT venography findings should be interpreted with caution, especially findings of the transverse sinus, because

hypoplasia of one of the sinuses is a common anatomic variation. Cerebral angiography provides better details of cerebral veins and cavernous sinus and remains the gold standard in the diagnosis of CVT, and should be considered in highly suspect patients with normal MRI or CT venography.

Laboratory Studies

When imaging studies reveal CVT, further workup should be directed toward determining the cause. Investigations should be individualized, keeping in mind the previously mentioned conditions that may be associated with CVT. Because it is common for patients to have more than one risk factor for thrombosis, detailed investigations should be done even if one risk factor is readily apparent by history or examination. Attention should be given to special hereditary thrombophilic disorders in patients with a family history of repeated episodes of thromboembolism, venous or arterial thrombosis at unusual sites, or cases of thrombosis occurring before age 45.

Visual Field Testing

Regular visual field testing and optic coherence tomography, which measures nerve fiber layer thickness, are useful follow-up tools in patients with intracranial hypertension and papilledema.[93]

Management

Management of CVT is usually directed toward treatment of the underlying cause of thrombosis. Various treatments include steroids, antiepileptic drugs, diuretics, osmotherapy, antiplatelet agents, anticoagulants, thrombolytic therapy, repeated lumbar punctures, and surgical intervention. Primary treatment is aimed at the underlying responsible condition. Infections should be treated with antimicrobials and, when appropriate, surgical drainage of abscesses. Patients with sickle cell disease with a sickling crisis should receive exchange transfusion and vigorous hydration. Iatrogenic agents,

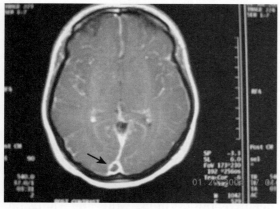

FIGURE 12-3 Empty delta sign (*arrow*) on MRI with gadolinium in a 19-year-old woman who presented with severe headaches, papilledema, and right abducens palsy. She was taking oral contraceptive pills.

such as oral contraceptives and asparaginase, should be discontinued. Seizures should be treated aggressively; prophylactic use of antiepileptic drugs is unnecessary.

When venous cerebral infarction results in hemorrhage, attention should be directed toward preventing cerebral edema and herniation. Osmotherapy with intravenous mannitol should be administered in patients with imminent herniation or in patients with rapid mental shifts. Surgical intervention may be lifesaving in rapidly deteriorating patients, with evacuation of the hematoma or decompressive hemicraniectomy.[94-96]

In patients with persistent increased intracranial hypertension and papilledema, optic nerve sheath fenestration may be required to salvage visual function. Ventriculoperitoneal and lumboperitoneal shunts should be avoided. Shunts should be considered only in selective patients with persistent increased intracranial pressure and papilledema who fail to respond to medical management.

Anticoagulation Therapy

Anticoagulation is thought to reduce the risk of thrombus progression and prevent further neurologic decline. The frequent association of hemorrhagic infarction tempers its use, however. The effect of anticoagulation with heparins has been examined in three small randomized, controlled clinical trials.[97-99]

de Bruijn and Stam[97] compared the effect of a fixed dose of subcutaneous low-molecular-weight heparin (LMWH), nadroparin, with placebo in 60 patients with CVT, and showed a favorable outcome for patients treated with nadroparin. The difference was not statistically significant, however. This study excluded patients with intracranial hemorrhage at enrollment. The second trial compared the effect of intravenous unfractionated heparin (UFH) with that of placebo in 20 patients, 10 in each treatment group. The study showed a significant benefit of anticoagulation with dose-adjusted intravenous unfractionated heparin.[99] The third study compared the effect of intravenous

unfractionated heparin with that of placebo in 57 women diagnosed with CVT in the puerperium.[98] The study showed decreased risk of dependence and death in patients who received anticoagulation.

Combining the results of these three trials in a pooled meta-analysis showed a nonsignificant decreased risk of dependence or death (relative risk [RR] 0.46, 95% confidence interval [CI] 0.17 to 1.28) from CVT in patients who received anticoagulation. Additionally, anticoagulation showed a nonsignificant decreased risk of death (RR 0.32, 95% CI 0.09 to 1.15), a nonsignificant decreased risk of pulmonary embolism (RR 0.43, 95% CI 0.06 to 2.91), and a nonsignificant decreased risk of intracranial or major extracranial hemorrhage (RR 0.74, 95% CI 0.11-4.85). The power of these combined studies was insufficient, however, to exclude an important benefit of anticoagulation relative to survival, independence, and complete recovery, or to exclude an important increased risk of hemorrhage from anticoagulation.[100] A large prospective multinational, multicenter, cohort observational study collected information on 624 patients with CVT with a median follow-up of 16 months. In this study, most patients (83.3%) were treated with anticoagulants, and the prognosis of CVT was better than previously reported trials, with recovery achieved in 79% and death observed only in 8% of patients.[10]

There is no good experience with anticoagulation treatment in neonates, and the experience in older children is limited. In a study by Sebire and coworkers,[25] patients with CVT receiving anticoagulation were more likely to have a good cognitive outcome, with a statistical trend of borderline significance, and a non–statistically significant reduction in mortality. In a retrospective review of 17 pediatric patients with CVT (15 of which received anticoagulation), anticoagulation was associated with clinical improvement without an increase in bleeding complications.[101]

Despite the absence of evidence-based medicine to support its use, anticoagulation with heparin (UFH or LMWH) seems safe and potentially beneficial in patients with CVT. Treatment should be initiated as soon as the diagnosis of CVT is confirmed, even in the presence of hemorrhagic infarcts at baseline. No studies have compared the effect of LMWH with that of UFH in the treatment of CVT. A possible useful extrapolation regarding duration of anticoagulant therapy may be found in the guidelines proposed by the consensus conference of the American College of Chest Physicians.[102] Unless a contraindication exists, oral anticoagulant therapy with warfarin (target international normalized ratio 2.5) is continued for several months. The optimal duration of oral anticoagulant treatment for CVT is unknown. Measurement of D-dimer may be useful because subjects with venous thromboembolism and normal D-dimer after discontinuation of oral anticoagulants have a low risk of recurrence.[103-105] After the transition from heparins (UFH or LMWH) to warfarin, a decision must be made regarding the duration of oral anticoagulation.

Thrombolytic Therapy

The use of endovascular thrombolysis into the dural sinuses has been attempted in isolation or in combination with mechanical thrombectomy with promising results in case reports and uncontrolled studies,[106-118] with limited data in the pediatric population.[110] A more recent review of the literature by Canhao and colleagues[119] identified 72 case reports in the literature pertinent to thrombolytic therapy for CVT. Urokinase was the thrombolytic agent most frequently administered into the occluded sinus. Intracranial hemorrhages occurred in 17% of cases, clinical deterioration in 7%, and death in 5% of patients.

It is unknown whether this treatment method is superior to anticoagulation with heparins in the absence of randomized controlled trials to compare the two forms of treatment. Until further data are available, endovascular thrombolysis should be limited to high-risk patients with rapidly progressive symptoms.

Others

Rheolytic catheter thrombectomy may be considered in conjunction with thrombolysis in selected patients with rapidly progressive symptoms.[120,121] Surgical decompressive craniotomy and evacuation of intracerebral hematoma are potential lifesaving approaches in patients with signs of brain herniation.[94-96]

Prognosis

CVT has a variable prognosis. Although most cases (>80%) are associated with complete recovery, a fatal outcome may occur in less than 10% of patients.[122] Focal neurologic deficits, coma, baseline intracerebral hemorrhage, advanced age, and involvement of the deep venous system are predictors for poor outcome.[123-127] Recurrent thrombosis is seen in 2% of patients, and extracranial thrombotic events occur in 4% of patients within 1 year.[122]

Conclusion

CVT is a potentially treatable cause of stroke in children and young adults. CVT should be included in the differential diagnosis of lethargy and respiratory distress in neonates, and headaches, seizures, or focal neurologic symptoms in children and young adults. Women complaining of headaches in the early puerperium warrant special attention. A detailed history and extensive laboratory workup often reveal the underlying cause of CVT. Newer imaging technologies, including CT angiography, MRI, and MR venography, play an important role in early detection of CVT (Figs. 12-4 through 12-7).

Management includes treatment of the underlying cause, seizure control, and management of increased intracranial pressure. Despite the lack of clinical evidence, the use of anticoagulation is common in CVT, and its use is not contraindicated in patients with hemorrhagic changes. Local thrombolysis, mechanical thrombectomy, and decompressive hemicraniectomy may be required in rapidly deteriorating patients who fail adequate anticoagulation.

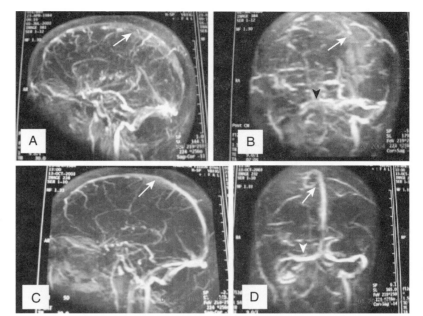

FIGURE 12-4 **A** and **B,** Serial MR venography of a young woman with CVT showing acute thrombus of the SSS (*arrow*) and lateral sinus (*arrow*) on midsagittal (**A**) and coronal (**B**) views. **C** and **D,** Two months later, there is return of a normal hypointense flow void in the SSS midsagittal (**C**) and coronal (**D**) images.

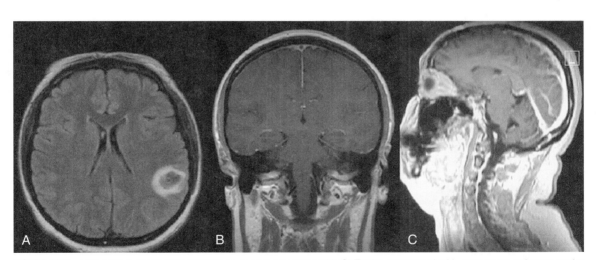

FIGURE 12-5   MRI shows acute hemorrhage in a young woman with CVT who presented with new-onset seizures and a history of anemia secondary to metromenorrhagia and MTHFR deficiency. **A,** Subacute hemorrhage in the left parietal cortex. **B,** Clot visualized in the torcula Herophili on coronal view. **C,** Anterior two thirds of the SSS is poorly visualized.

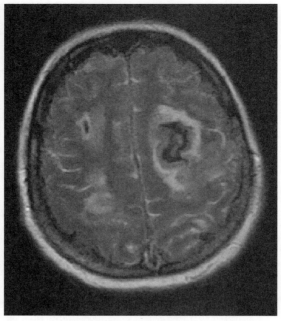

FIGURE 12-6 T2 MRI sequence of a young woman with CVT shows bilateral cerebral infarctions crossing anatomic arterial distributions with hemorrhagic transformation.

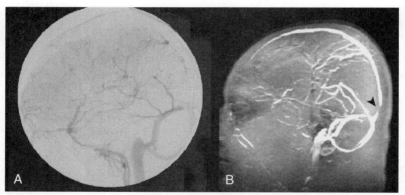

FIGURE 12-7 Cerebral angiogram (lateral view) of a young woman with new-onset headache, seizures, and right hemiparesis. The patient was taking oral contraceptive pills and had factor V Leiden mutation. **A,** The SSS, great vein of Galen, straight sinus, and lateral sinus are not visualized. **B,** MR venography performed after local thrombolytic therapy into the dural sinuses shows recanalization of the sinuses with persistent filling defect in the straight sinus as it drains into the torcula Herophili (*arrowhead*).

REFERENCES

1. Ribes MF. Des recherches faites sur la phlebite. Revue Medicale Francaise et Etrangere et Journal de Clinique de l'Hotel Dieu et de la Charite de Paris 1825;3:5.
2. Kalabag RM, Woolf AL. Cerebral Venous Thrombosis, Vol 1. London: University Press, 1967.
3. Towbin A. The syndrome of latent cerebral venous thrombosis: its frequency and relation to age and congestive heart failure. Stroke 1973;4:419.
4. Scotti LN, Goldman RL, Hardman DR, Heinz ER. Venous thrombosis in infants and children. Radiology 1974;112:393.
5. Siddiqui FM, Kamal AK. Incidence and epidemiology of cerebral venous thrombosis. J Pak Med Assoc 2006;56:485.
6. Daif A, Awada A, al-Rajeh S, et al. Cerebral venous thrombosis in adults: a study of 40 cases from Saudi Arabia. Stroke 1995;26:1193.
7. deVeber G, Andrew M, Adams C, et al. Cerebral sinovenous thrombosis in children. N Engl J Med 2001;345:417.
8. Bousser MG, Russel RRW. Cerebral Venous Thrombosis. London: WB Saunders, 1997.
9. Capra NF, Anderson KV. Anatomy of the cerebral venous system. In Kapp JP, Schmidek HH, eds. The Cerebral Venous System and Its Disorders. Orlando, FL: Grune & Stratton, 1984.
10. Ferro JM, Canhao P, Stam J, et al. Prognosis of cerebral vein and dural sinus thrombosis: results of the International Study on Cerebral Vein and Dural Sinus Thrombosis (ISCVT). Stroke 2004;35:664.
11. Weidauer S, Marquardt G, Seifert V, Zanella FE. Hydrocephalus due to superior sagittal sinus thrombosis. Acta Neurochir (Wien) 2005;147:427.
12. Lin A, Foroozan R, Danesh-Meyer HV, et al. Occurrence of cerebral venous sinus thrombosis in patients with presumed idiopathic intracranial hypertension. Ophthalmology 2006;113:2281.
13. Andeweg J. Concepts of cerebral venous drainage and the aetiology of hydrocephalus. J Neurol Neurosurg Psychiatry 1991;54:830.
14. Goldberg AL, Rosenbaum AE, Wang H, et al. Computed tomography of dural sinus thrombosis. J Comput Assist Tomogr 1986;10:16.
15. Stam J. Thrombosis of the cerebral veins and sinuses. N Engl J Med 2005;352:1791.
16. Carvalho KS, Bodensteiner JB, Connolly PJ, Garg BP. Cerebral venous thrombosis in children. J Child Neurol 2001;16:574.
17. Ferro JM, Correia M, Rosas MJ, et al. Seizures in cerebral vein and dural sinus thrombosis. Cerebrovasc Dis 2003;15:78.
18. Haley ECJr, Brashear HR, Barth JT, et al. Deep cerebral venous thrombosis: clinical, neuroradiological, and neuropsychological correlates. Arch Neurol 1989;46:337.
19. Patronas NJ, Argyropoulou M. Intravascular thrombosis as a possible cause of transient cortical brain lesions: CT and MRI. J Comput Assist Tomogr 1992;16:849.
20. Buccino G, Scoditti U, Patteri I, et al. Neurological and cognitive long-term outcome in patients with cerebral venous sinus thrombosis. Acta Neurol Scand 2003;107:330.
21. Krayenbuhl HA. Cerebral venous and sinus thrombosis. Clin Neurosurg 1966;14:1.
22. Crawford SC, Digre KB, Palmer CA, et al. Thrombosis of the deep venous drainage of the brain in adults: analysis of seven cases with review of the literature. Arch Neurol 1995;52:1101.
23. Nakazato Y, Sonoda K, Senda M, et al. [Case of straight sinus venous thrombosis presenting as depression and disorientation due to bilateral thalamic lesions]. Rinsho Shinkeigaku 2006;46:652.
24. Lopez-Trabada Gomez JR, Pascual Arriazu J, Rubio Valladolid G, et al. [Psychic symptomatology in thrombosis of the upper longitudinal sinus: apropos of a case]. Actas Luso Esp Neurol Psiquiatr Cienc Afines 1987;15:115.
25. Sebire G, Tabarki B, Saunders DE, et al. Cerebral venous sinus thrombosis in children: risk factors, presentation, diagnosis and outcome. Brain 2005;128:477.
26. Kurnik K, Kosch A, Strater R, et al. Recurrent thromboembolism in infants and children suffering from symptomatic neonatal arterial stroke: a prospective follow-up study. Stroke 2003;34:2887.
27. Lee AC, Li CH, Szeto SC, Ma ES. Symptomatic venous thromboembolism in Hong Kong Chinese children. Hong Kong Med J 2003;9:259.
28. Farstad H, Gaustad P, Kristiansen P, et al. Cerebral venous thrombosis and *Escherichia coli* infection in neonates. Acta Paediatr 2003;92:254.
29. Draaisma JM, Rotteveel JJ, Meekma R, Geven WB. [Neonatal dural sinus thrombosis]. Tijdschr Kindergeneeskd 1991;59:64.
30. Shevell MI, Silver K, O'Gorman AM, et al. Neonatal dural sinus thrombosis. Pediatr Neurol 1989; 5:161.
31. Hurst RW, Kerns SR, McIlhenny J, et al. Neonatal dural venous sinus thrombosis associated with central venous catheterization: CT and MR studies. J Comput Assist Tomogr 1989;13:504.
32. Enevoldson TP, Russell RW. Cerebral venous thrombosis: new causes for an old syndrome? QJM 1990;77:1255.
33. Deschiens MA, Conard J, Horellou MH, et al. Coagulation studies, factor V Leiden, and anticardiolipin antibodies in 40 cases of cerebral venous thrombosis. Stroke 1996;27:1724.
34. De Lucia D, Napolitano M, Di Micco P, et al. Benign intracranial hypertension associated to blood coagulation derangements. Thromb J 2006;4:21.
35. Dzialo AF, Black-Schaffer RM. Cerebral venous thrombosis in young adults: 2 case reports. Arch Phys Med Rehabil 2001;82:683.
36. De Schryver EL, Hoogenraad TU, Banga JD, Kappelle LJ. Thyrotoxicosis, protein C deficiency and lupus anticoagulant in a case of cerebral sinus thrombosis. Neth J Med 1999;55:201.
37. Chan AK, deVeber G. Prothrombotic disorders and ischemic stroke in children. Semin Pediatr Neurol 2000;7:301.

38. Arai M, Sugiura A. [Superior sagittal sinus thrombosis as first manifestation of essential thrombocythemia]. Rinsho Shinkeigaku 2004;44:34.

39. Walther EU, Tiecks FP, Haberl RL. Cranial sinus thrombosis associated with essential thrombocythemia followed by heparin-associated thrombocytopenia. Neurology 1996;47:300.

40. McDonald TD, Tatemichi TK, Kranzler SJ, et al. Thrombosis of the superior sagittal sinus associated with essential thrombocytosis followed by MRI during anticoagulant therapy. Neurology 1989;39:1554.

41. Alper G, Berrak SG, Ekinci G, et al. Sagittal sinus thrombosis associated with thrombocytopenia: a report of two patients. Pediatr Neurol 1999;21:573.

42. Dindagur N, Kruthika-Vinod TP, Christopher R. Thrombophilic gene polymorphisms in puerperal cerebral veno-sinus thrombosis. J Neurol Sci 2006;249:25.

43. Uthman I, Khalil I, Sawaya R, Taher A. Lupus anticoagulant, factor V Leiden, and methylenetetrahydrofolate reductase gene mutation in a lupus patient with cerebral venous thrombosis. Clin Rheumatol 2004;23:362.

44. Ludemann P, Nabavi DG, Junker R, et al. Factor V Leiden mutation is a risk factor for cerebral venous thrombosis: a case-control study of 55 patients. Stroke 1998;29:2507.

45. Jukic I, Titlic M, Tonkic A, Rosenzweig D. Cerebral venous sinus thrombosis as a recurrent thrombotic event in a patient with heterozygous prothrombin G20210A genotype after discontinuation of oral anticoagulation therapy: how long should we treat these patients with warfarin? J Thromb Thrombolysis 2007;24:77.

46. Reuner KH, Ruf A, Grau A, et al. Prothrombin gene G20210→A transition is a risk factor for cerebral venous thrombosis. Stroke 1998;29:1765.

47. Wermes C, Fleischhack G, Junker R, et al. Cerebral venous sinus thrombosis in children with acute lymphoblastic leukemia carrying the MTHFR TC677 genotype and further prothrombotic risk factors. Klin Padiatr 1999;211:211.

48. Marietta M, Bertesi M, Simoni L, et al. Cerebral vein thrombosis and lupus anticoagulant antibodies. Clin Appl Thromb Hemost 2001;7:238.

49. Carhuapoma JR, Mitsias P, Levine SR. Cerebral venous thrombosis and anticardiolipin antibodies. Stroke 1997;28:2363.

50. Christopher R, Nagaraja D, Dixit NS, Narayanan CP. Anticardiolipin antibodies: a study in cerebral venous thrombosis. Acta Neurol Scand 1999;99:121.

51. Brey RL, Escalante A. Neurological manifestations of antiphospholipid antibody syndrome. Lupus 1998;7(Suppl 2):S67.

52. Greaves M. Antiphospholipid antibodies and thrombosis. Lancet 1999;353:1348.

53. Sakuta R, Tomita Y, Ohashi M, et al. Idiopathic hypereosinophilic syndrome complicated by central sinovenous thrombosis. Brain Dev 2007;29:182.

54. Kasuga K, Naruse S, Umeda M, et al. [Case of cerebral venous thrombosis due to Graves' disease with increased factor VIII activity]. Rinsho Shinkeigaku 2006;46:270.

55. Fofah O, Roth P. Congenital nephrotic syndrome presenting with cerebral venous thrombosis, hypocalcemia, and seizures in the neonatal period. J Perinatol 1997;17:492.

56. Laversuch CJ, Brown MM, Clifton A, Bourke BE. Cerebral venous thrombosis and acquired protein S deficiency: an uncommon cause of headache in systemic lupus erythematosus. Br J Rheumatol 1995;34:572.

57. Nishi H, Abe A, Kita A, et al. Cerebral venous thrombosis in adult nephrotic syndrome due to systemic amyloidosis. Clin Nephrol 2006;65:61.

58. Sung SF, Jeng JS, Yip PK, Huang KM. Cerebral venous thrombosis in patients with nephrotic syndrome—case reports. Angiology 1999;50:427.

59. Alfaro A. Cerebral venous thrombosis in paroxysmal nocturnal haemoglobinuria. J Neurol Neurosurg Psychiatry 1992;55:412.

60. Hassan KM, Varadarajulu R, Sharma SK, et al. Cerebral venous thrombosis in a patient of paroxysmal nocturnal haemoglobinuria following aplastic anaemia. J Assoc Physicians India 2001;49:753.

61. Hauser D, Barzilai N, Zalish M, et al. Bilateral papilledema with retinal hemorrhages in association with cerebral venous sinus thrombosis and paroxysmal nocturnal hemoglobinuria. Am J Ophthalmol 1996;122:592.

62. Rafalowska J, Dziewulska D, Szyluk B, Wieczorek J. Morphological picture in paroxysmal nocturnal hemoglobinuria: case report. Folia Neuropathol 1994;32:161.

63. Sharma A, Itha S, Baijal SS, et al. Superior sagittal sinus thrombosis and Budd-Chiari syndrome due to paroxysmal nocturnal hemoglobinuria managed with transjugular intrahepatic portosystemic shunt: a case report. Trop Gastroenterol 2005;26:146.

64. Merz S, Fehr R, Gulke C. [Sinus vein thrombosis: a rare complication of heparin-induced thrombocytopenia type II]. Anaesthesist 2004;53:551.

65. Schill D. [Sinus thrombosis in heparin-induced thrombocytopenia type II]. Med Monatsschr Pharm 2005;28:253.

66. Chaloupka K, Baglivo E, Hofer M, et al. [Cerebral sinus thrombosis in Behçet disease: case report and review of the literature]. Klin Monatsbl Augenheilkd 2003;220:186.

67. Yazici H, Fresko I, Yurdakul S. Behçet's syndrome: disease manifestations, management, and advances in treatment. Nat Clin Pract Rheumatol 2007;3:148.

68. Bir LS, Sabir N, Kilincer A, et al. Aseptic meningitis, venous sinus thrombosis, intracranial hypertension and callosal involvement contemporaneously in a young patient with Behçet's disease. Swiss Med Wkly 2005;135:684.

69. Saltik S, Saip S, Kocer N, et al. MRI findings in pediatric neuro-Behçet's disease. Neuropediatrics 2004;35:190.

70. Alper G, Yilmaz Y, Ekinci G, Kose O. Cerebral vein thrombosis in Behçet's disease. Pediatr Neurol 2001;25:332.

71. de Bruijn SF, Stam J, Koopman MM, Vanden-broucke JP. Case-control study of risk of cerebral sinus thrombosis in oral contraceptive users and in [correction of who are] carriers of hereditary prothrombotic conditions: The Cerebral Venous Sinus Thrombosis Study Group. BMJ 1998;316:589.

72. Jick SS, Jick H. Cerebral venous sinus thrombosis in users of four hormonal contraceptives: levonor-gestrel-containing oral contraceptives, norgesti-mate-containing oral contraceptives, desogestrel-containing oral contraceptives and the contraceptive patch. Contraception 2006;74:290.

73. Evangelou N, Littlewood T, Anslow P, Chapel H. Transverse sinus thrombosis and IVIg treatment: a case report and discussion of risk-benefit assessment for immunoglobulin treatment. J Clin Pathol 2003;56:308.

74. Chu K, Kang DW, Kim DE, Roh JK. Cerebral venous thrombosis associated with tentorial subdural hematoma during oxymetholone therapy. J Neurol Sci 2001;185:27.

75. Brors D, Schafers M, Schick B, et al. Sigmoid and transverse sinus thrombosis after closed head injury presenting with unilateral hearing loss. Neuroradiology 2001;43:144.

76. Ferrera PC, Pauze DR, Chan L. Sagittal sinus thrombosis after closed head injury. Am J Emerg Med 1998;16:382.

77. Hesselbrock R, Sawaya R, Tomsick T, Wadhwa S. Superior sagittal sinus thrombosis after closed head injury. Neurosurgery 1985;16:825.

78. Kabatas S, Civelek E, Sencer A, et al. [A case of superior sagittal sinus thrombosis after closed head injury]. Ulus Travma Derg 2004;10:208.

79. Kumar GS, Chacko AG, Chacko M. Superior sagittal sinus and torcula thrombosis in minor head injury. Neurol India 2004;52:123.

80. Muthukumar N. Cerebral venous sinus thrombosis and thrombophilia presenting as pseudo-tumour syndrome following mild head injury. J Clin Neurosci 2004;11:924.

81. Muthukumar N. Uncommon cause of sinus thrombosis following closed mild head injury in a child. Childs Nerv Syst 2005;21:86.

82. Satoh H, Kumano K, Ogami R, et al. Sigmoid sinus thrombosis after mild closed head injury in an infant: diagnosis by magnetic resonance imaging in the acute phase—case report. Neurol Med Chir (Tokyo) 2000;40:361.

83. Sousa J, O'Brien D, Bartlett R, Vaz J. Sigmoid sinus thrombosis in a child after closed head injury. Br J Neurosurg 2004;18:187.

84. Stringer WL, Peerless SJ. Superior sagittal sinus thrombosis after closed head injury. Neurosurgery 1983;12:95.

85. Taha JM, Crone KR, Berger TS, et al. Sigmoid sinus thrombosis after closed head injury in children. Neurosurgery 1993;32:541.

86. Tamimi A, Abu-Elrub M, Shudifat A, et al. Superior sagittal sinus thrombosis associated with raised intracranial pressure in closed head injury with depressed skull fracture. Pediatr Neurosurg 2005;41:237.

87. Yuen HW, Gan BK, Seow WT, Tan HK. Dural sinus thrombosis after minor head injury in a child. Ann Acad Med Singapore 2005;34:639.

88. Raizer JJ, DeAngelis LM. Cerebral sinus thrombosis diagnosed by MRI and MR venography in cancer patients. Neurology 2000;54:1222.

89. Sigsbee B, Deck MD, Posner JB. Nonmetastatic superior sagittal sinus thrombosis complicating systemic cancer. Neurology 1979;29:139.

90. Packer RJ, Rorke LB, Lange BJ, et al. Cerebrovascular accidents in children with cancer. Pediatrics 1985;76:194.

91. Ali L, Biller J, Mattson D, Roos K. Case report: sagittal sinus thrombosis as the first clinical manifestation of metastatic breast cancer. Semin Cereb Dis Stroke 2003;3:246.

92. Klingebiel R, Bauknecht HC, Bohner G, et al. Comparative evaluation of 2D time-of-flight and 3D elliptic centric contrast-enhanced MR venography in patients with presumptive cerebral venous and sinus thrombosis. Eur J Neurol 2007;14:139.

93. Sanchez-Tocino H, Bringas R, Iglesias D, et al. [Utility of optic coherence tomography (OCT) in the follow-up of idiopathic intracranial hypertension in childhood.]. Arch Soc Esp Oftalmol 2006;81:383.

94. Stefini R, Latronico N, Cornali C, et al. Emergent decompressive craniectomy in patients with fixed dilated pupils due to cerebral venous and dural sinus thrombosis: report of three cases. Neurosurgery 1999;45:626.

95. Keller E, Pangalu A, Fandino J, et al. Decompressive craniectomy in severe cerebral venous and dural sinus thrombosis. Acta Neurochir Suppl 2005; 94:177.

96. Weber J, Spring A. [Unilateral decompressive craniectomy in left transverse and sigmoid sinus thrombosis]. Zentralbl Neurochir 2004;65:135.

97. de Bruijn SF, Stam J. Randomized, placebo-controlled trial of anticoagulant treatment with low-molecular-weight heparin for cerebral sinus thrombosis. Stroke 1999;30:484.

98. Nagaraja D, Rao BSS, Taly AB, Subhash MN. Randomized controlled trial of heparin in puerperal cerebral venous/sinus thrombosis. Nimhans J 1995;1:111.

99. Einhaupl KM, Villringer A, Meister W, et al. Heparin treatment in sinus venous thrombosis. Lancet 1991;338:597.

100. Dafer RM. Anticoagulants for cerebral vein thrombosis. Presented at American Academy of Neurology 59th Annual Meeting, Boston, 2007.

101. Johnson MC, Parkerson N, Ward S, de Alarcon PA. Pediatric sinovenous thrombosis. J Pediatr Hematol Oncol 2003;25:312.

102. Buller HR, Agnelli G, Hull RD, et al. Antithrombotic therapy for venous thromboembolic disease: the Seventh ACCP Conference on Antithrombotic and Thrombolytic Therapy. Chest 2004;126:401S.

103. Palareti G, Legnani C, Cosmi B, et al. Risk of venous thromboembolism recurrence: high negative predictive value of D-dimer performed after oral anticoagulation is stopped. Thromb Haemost 2002;97:7.

104. Eichinger S, Minar E, Bialonczyk C, et al. D-dimer levels and risk of venous thromboembolism. JAMA 2003;290:1071.

105. Cosmi B, Palareti G. D-dimer, oral anticoagulation, and venous thromboembolism recurrence. Semin Vasc Med 2005;5:365.

106. Yang YH, Liu CK, Shih MC, Chou MS. Fibrin-nonspecific agents in the direct thrombolytic treatment of venous sinus thrombosis. QJM 2002;95:763.

107. Tsai FY, Higashida RT, Matovich V, Alfieri K. Acute thrombosis of the intracranial dural sinus: direct thrombolytic treatment. AJNR Am J Neuroradiol 1992;13:1137.

108. Takami T, Suzuki T, Tokuno H, et al. [A case report of dural sinus thrombosis: direct thrombolytic therapy using endovascular surgery]. No Shinkei Geka 1995;23:321.

109. Sztriha LK, Voros E, Vecsei L. Endovascular thrombolytic treatment of extensive dural sinus thrombosis in a heterozygous carrier of prothrombin gene G20210A mutation. Eur J Neurol 2004;11:214.

110. Niwa J, Ohyama H, Matumura S, et al. Treatment of acute superior sagittal sinus thrombosis by t-PA infusion via venography—direct thrombolytic therapy in the acute phase. Surg Neurol 1998;49:425.

111. Kim SY, Suh JH. Direct endovascular thrombolytic therapy for dural sinus thrombosis: infusion of alteplase. AJNR Am J Neuroradiol 1997;18:639.

112. Khoo KB, Long FL, Tuck RR, et al. Cerebral venous sinus thrombosis associated with the primary antiphospholipid syndrome: resolution with local thrombolytic therapy. Med J Aust 1995;162:30.

113. Higashida RT, Helmer E, Halbach VV, Hieshima GB. Direct thrombolytic therapy for superior sagittal sinus thrombosis. AJNR Am J Neuroradiol 1989;10:S4.

114. Gurley MB, King TS, Tsai FY. Sigmoid sinus thrombosis associated with internal jugular venous occlusion: direct thrombolytic treatment. J Endovasc Surg 1996;3:306.

115. Barnwell SL, Higashida RT, Halbach VV, et al. Direct endovascular thrombolytic therapy for dural sinus thrombosis. Neurosurgery 1991;28:135.

116. Bagley LJ, Hurst RW, Galetta S, et al. Use of a microsnare to aid direct thrombolytic therapy of dural sinus thrombosis. AJR Am J Roentgenol 1998;170:784.

117. Aoki N, Uchinuno H, Tanikawa T, et al. Superior sagittal sinus thrombosis treated with combined local thrombolytic and systemic anticoagulation therapy. Acta Neurochir (Wien) 1997;139:332.

118. Prasad RS, Michaels LA, Roychowdhury S, et al. Combined venous sinus angioplasty and low-dose thrombolytic therapy for treatment of hemorrhagic transverse sinus thrombosis in a pediatric patient. J Pediatr Hematol Oncol 2006;28:196.

119. Canhao P, Falcao F, Ferro JM. Thrombolytics for cerebral sinus thrombosis: a systematic review. Cerebrovasc Dis 2003;15:159.

120. Kirsch J, Rasmussen PA, Masaryk TJ, et al. Adjunctive rheolytic thrombectomy for central venous sinus thrombosis: technical case report. Neurosurgery 2007;60:E577.

121. Dowd CF, Malek AM, Phatouros CC, Hemphill JC 3rd. Application of a rheolytic thrombectomy device in the treatment of dural sinus thrombosis: a new technique. AJNR Am J Neuroradiol 1999;20:568.

122. Ameri A, Bousser MG. Cerebral venous thrombosis. Neurol Clin 1992;10:87.

123. Preter M, Tzourio C, Ameri A, Bousser MG. Long-term prognosis in cerebral venous thrombosis: follow-up of 77 patients. Stroke 1996;27:243.

124. Canhao P, Ferro JM, Lindgren AG, et al. Causes and predictors of death in cerebral venous thrombosis. Stroke 2005;36:1720.

125. Girot M, Ferro JM, Canhao P, et al. Predictors of outcome in patients with cerebral venous thrombosis and intracerebral hemorrhage. Stroke 2007;38:337.

126. Breteau G, Mounier-Vehier F, Godefroy O, et al. Cerebral venous thrombosis 3-year clinical outcome in 55 consecutive patients. J Neurol 2003;250:29.

127. Ferro JM, Canhao P, Bousser MG, et al. Cerebral vein and dural sinus thrombosis in elderly patients. Stroke 2005;36:1927.

CHAPTER 13

Neonatal Intracranial Hemorrhage

Eugene R. Schnitzler • Marc G. Weiss

Despite advances in obstetric care, intracranial hemorrhage remains a significant management problem in the neonatal intensive care unit. The etiology of intracranial hemorrhage varies with gestational age. Birth trauma and asphyxia, often in combination, are still the primary etiologic factors, however. Although traumatic intracranial hemorrhages continue to decline in incidence, intraventricular hemorrhages (IVH) are still seen frequently.[1,2] This situation is partly due to the increasing rate of preterm delivery and improved survival rates of very-low-birth-weight premature infants.[3] Neurology consultation is often requested for neonates with intracranial hemorrhages because neonatal seizures may be an early symptom.[4]

Etiology

Trauma to the head during labor and delivery can result in extracranial, epidural, subdural, subarachnoid, intraventricular, or intracerebellar hemorrhage. Traumatic deliveries most commonly occur in primiparous mothers with large term infants. Obstetric complications that predispose to trauma include cephalopelvic disproportion with prolonged labor, breech position, precipitous delivery, vacuum extraction, and use of forceps.[5] Forceps, in particular, have been implicated in depressed skull fractures, which can be associated with epidural and subdural bleeding.[6]

Rarely, intracranial hemorrhage in a neonate is due to other factors, such as congenital arteriovenous malformation, aneurysms, or vascular neoplasms.[7-9] Hypertension associated with coarctation of the aorta also has been reported to cause intracranial bleeding.[10] In addition, inherited and acquired coagulopathies occasionally can increase susceptibility to intracranial hemorrhage.[11,12] Vitamin K deficiency in particular can cause hemorrhagic disease of the newborn with resultant intracranial hemorrhages. Early hemorrhagic disease is an occasional complication of maternal treatment with anticonvulsants.[13] This condition is prevented by prophylactic administration of vitamin K after birth. Extracorporeal membrane oxygenation also has been linked to a high risk of intracranial hemorrhages presumably related to heparinization, increased cerebral blood flow, and increased central venous pressure.[14]

Cerebrospinal Fluid Findings

Abnormal findings on cerebrospinal fluid (CSF) analysis may be the first indication of intracranial hemorrhage in a newborn. Abnormalities most commonly seen are increase of red blood cells, elevated protein content, and xanthochromia. These abnormalities should not automatically be assumed to be due to a traumatic tap. Volpe[15] found a greater than 90% correlation between grossly bloody CSF and intracranial hemorrhages on computed tomography (CT) scan. In his sample of 76 infants with grossly bloody CSF and elevated CSF protein, 22 were found to have subarachnoid hemorrhage (SAH), and 48 had IVH. Normal CSF protein values average 90 mg/dL in term neonates and 115 mg/dL in preterm infants.[16,17] These values are significantly higher than values in older children and adults. After intracranial hemorrhage, protein values may double or triple. Conversely, CSF glucose levels are commonly decreased after intracranial hemorrhage[18,19]; this may persist for several weeks. CSF pleocytosis also often accompanies intracranial hemorrhage and may cause concerns about meningitis. CSF xanthochromia has been cited as a reliable early indicator of intracranial hemorrhage in adults and older children. Xanthochromia may be a less consistent observation in the neonatal period, however, and may be more difficult to interpret if hyperbilirubinemia is present.[20]

Extracranial Hemorrhages

Extracranial hemorrhages include caput succedaneum, subgaleal hemorrhage, and cephalhematoma. Caput occurs in one third of vaginal deliveries, especially with vacuum extraction, and is recognized by soft swelling of the scalp at the vertex that crosses suture lines. Caput is considered benign and resolves over several days without treatment.

Subgaleal hemorrhage refers to bleeding beneath the scalp. It also is seen more frequently after vacuum extraction and requires observation for jaundice and anemia. Large subgaleal hemorrhages suggest the possibility of comorbid coagulopathy. Subgaleal hemorrhages cross suture lines and may enlarge after birth. Large subgaleal hemorrhages may lead to hypovolemic shock with a mortality rate of nearly 25%.[21]

Cephalhematoma is a unilateral hemorrhage in the subperiosteal space, usually of the parietal bone. A cephalhematoma is unilateral and does not cross suture lines, although it can enlarge after birth. Cephalhematomas usually are not associated with significant blood loss and do not cause neurologic sequelae.

Epidural hematomas are the equivalent of cephalhematomas, but occur on the inner surface of the skull between the bone and the periosteum. Epidural hemorrhages are rare in the neonatal period. They often are associated with cephalhematomas and linear skull fractures after a difficult labor and delivery.[22] Bleeding arises from venous sinuses or from tears in the meningeal arteries. An infant with an epidural hemorrhage may present with seizures and increased intracranial pressure. The lesion generally requires emergency surgical evacuation or aspiration, although smaller epidural hematomas may be managed conservatively.[23]

Subdural Hemorrhage

Subdural hemorrhages usually are complications of difficult traumatic labor and deliveries.[24] Factors predisposing to subdural hemorrhages include cephalopelvic disproportion, particularly in a primiparous mother with a rigid pelvis and a large infant. Precipitous or prolonged labor may result in excessive molding of the head. Atypical presentations, including breech, face, or brow, also increase the chance of subdural bleeding. Instrumentation with forceps, vacuum extraction, or rotation during delivery are additional risk factors.[5] Breech delivery, in particular, can result in occipital diastasis, which is a separation of the squamous and lateral portions of the occipital bone.[25] Catastrophic posterior fossa subdural hemorrhage may occur with contusion or actual tearing of the cerebellum (Fig. 13-1).

Subdural hemorrhages tend to occur in several locations. Laceration of the tentorium usually results in infratentorial subdural hemorrhage, which can lead to rapid compression of the posterior fossa and brainstem.[26] Such infants typically begin to show deterioration immediately after delivery. As the hemorrhage enlarges, the infant may become comatose. Nuchal rigidity and opisthotonos may be present. Eye muscle imbalance with unequal pupils may be noted. Apnea and bradycardia may be followed by respiratory arrest and death. Smaller posterior fossa subdural hemorrhages may result in a less fulminant course, but can cause increased intracranial pressure, irritability, lethargy, seizures, hydrocephalus, and cranial nerve palsies.[27]

Infants with supratentorial subdural hemorrhages usually present with milder clinical signs and symptoms. The underlying pathophysiology consists of tears of the bridging veins over the cerebral convexities and lacerations at the junction of the falx and tentorium. The infant may have minimal findings, and the bleeding may be visualized as an incidental finding on CT scan. Irritability also has been reported. Unilateral subdural hematomas may result in contralateral hemiparesis, focal seizures, and a unilateral dilated pupil if tentorial herniation has occurred.[24] Milder subdural hemorrhages resolve over time, resulting in chronic subdural effusions. These benign subdural collections[28] subsequently may lead to a condition known as "external hydrocephalus" (Fig. 13-2). This condition is characterized by accelerated head growth in infancy. CT and magnetic resonance imaging (MRI) show enlargement of the subarachnoid and subdural spaces and mild to moderate prominence of the ventricles.[29]

Treatment of subdural hematomas varies with location and severity of the bleeding. Rapidly expanding hematomas, especially in the posterior fossa, require emergency surgical evacuation. Smaller hemorrhages over the cerebral convexities may be managed conservatively.

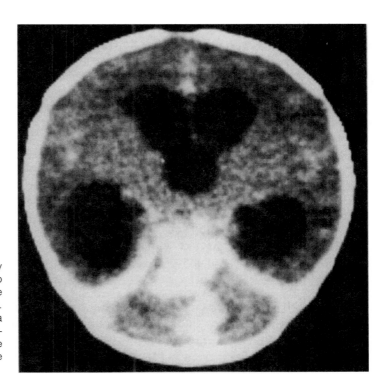

FIGURE 13-1 This infant was delivered by cesarean section because of failure to progress. At 8 hours of age, he became acutely lethargic. CSF was grossly bloody. CT scan done at 32 hours of age reveals a posterior fossa hemorrhage and hydrocephalus. At surgery, there was a large subdural hematoma and a clot in the cerebellum.

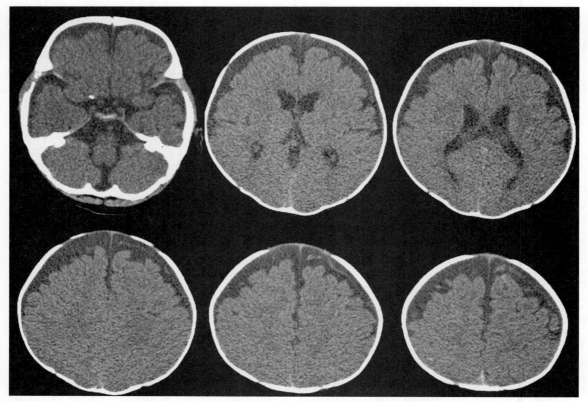

FIGURE 13-2   CT scan of a 6-month-old boy with a history of bilateral small subdural hematomas at birth. There are bilateral subdural collections and mild enlargement of the ventricles. This condition also is referred to as benign subdural collections or external hydrocephalus.

Primary Subarachnoid Hemorrhage

Primary SAH is bleeding in the subarachnoid space that is not the result of subdural, intraventricular, or intraparenchymal hemorrhage. SAH probably results from combinations of trauma and hypoxic-ischemic encephalopathy.[30] Bleeding is thought to occur from bridging veins or involution of anastomoses of leptomeningeal arteries.[31] Primary SAH is a common variant of neonatal intracranial bleeding. Minor degrees of SAH may be clinically asymptomatic. Seizures may be another presentation, usually on the first or second day of life in a full-term infant. A more fulminant course may be seen with SAH, but these neonates usually have associated hypoxic-ischemic encephalopathy. Diagnosis of SAH requires CT scan because cranial ultrasound does not visualize the hemorrhage. Treatment is supportive and symptomatic.

Intracerebral Hemorrhage and Cerebellar Hemorrhage

Intracerebral hemorrhages occur in term infants who appear normal. The hemorrhage is often heralded by focal or multifocal seizure activity during the first week of life. There may be an underlying aneurysm, arteriovenous malformation, or coagulopathy, which may be visualized on CT (Fig. 13-3). or MRI, or the etiology may be idiopathic.[32] Hemiplegia, developmental delays, and epilepsy are common sequelae. Cerebellar hemorrhage occurs more often in premature infants and may be associated with hypoxic-ischemic encephalopathy and traumatic delivery.[33] These patients present with apnea, bradycardia, cranial nerve palsies, and flaccid quadriparesis owing to brainstem compression. Survivors often develop hydrocephalus. Diagnosis is confirmed by CT or MRI. Treatment ranges from

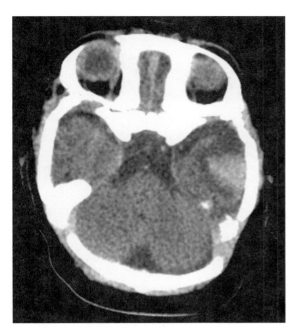

FIGURE 13-3 A 38-week newborn girl with birth asphyxia and extremely low Apgar scores. Multifocal clonic seizure activity was noted on day 1 of life. CT scan on day 8 of life shows a left temporal hematoma.

surgical decompression to conservative measures. Survivors often develop hydrocephalus, and most patients have neurodevelopmental sequelae.[34]

Intraventricular Hemorrhage in a Term Neonate

IVH in a term infant is uncommon. Bleeding can occur from the choroid plexus and the subependymal germinal matrix.[35,36] Thalamic hemorrhagic infarction has been postulated as another site, particularly in late-onset hemorrhages.[37] Birth trauma and asphyxia are contributing factors in at least half of IVH in term neonates. In about one fourth of cases, no obvious pathogenetic cause can be identified. Term infants with IVH show early symptoms soon after birth or a delayed presentation of up to 4 weeks. Symptoms include seizures, apnea, irritability, and lethargy. Posthemorrhagic ventricular dilation and hydrocephalus are common sequelae, and ventriculoperitoneal shunting may be necessary. Prognosis varies with gradation of the hemorrhage and the presence of comorbid trauma, asphyxia, or both.[38]

Germinal Matrix Intraventricular Hemorrhage in a Premature Infant

Germinal matrix IVH occurs almost uniquely in premature infants and is the most common type of intracranial hemorrhage seen in newborns. The incidence of IVH in very-low-birth-weight infants (<1500 g) varies directly with prematurity and low birth weight. The overall incidence of IVH has decreased over the past 3 decades from approximately 40% to 15%.[27] The increased survival of extremely premature infants has significantly offset these statistics, however, in terms of prevalence.[39]

The pathophysiology of IVH is complex and multifactorial. These hemorrhages occur in the subependymal germinal matrix (Fig. 13-4). This is a highly vascular region composed of a gelatinous network of neuronal and glial precursor cells.[40] The microvasculature is fragile, consisting of thin-walled, immature, endothelial-lined vessels that lack supporting structural elements. As such, this region is highly vulnerable to hemorrhages secondary to hypoxic-ischemic, metabolic, and blood pressure changes. Normally, the germinal matrix undergoes a physiologic involution in the last trimester and is absent in term infants,[41] which is why germinal matrix IVH is seen almost exclusively in premature infants.

Hemorrhage in the germinal matrix leads to a predictable sequence of neuropathologic outcomes. Invariably, even the smallest hemorrhage (Fig. 13-5). results in destruction of the germinal matrix with possible negative long-term neurodevelopmental effects. Larger hemorrhages can result in periventricular hemorrhagic infarction, which is seen after approximately 15% of IVH.[27] One third of extremely-low-birth-weight infants (<1000 g) may be affected.[42] These parenchymal lesions are usually unilateral and consist of hemorrhagic necrosis in the white matter adjacent to the lateral ventricle.[43] Studies by Gould and colleagues[44] and Takashima and associates[45] suggest that periventricular hemorrhagic infarction is secondary to obstruction of blood flow in the terminal and medullary veins after ipsilateral germinal matrix hemorrhages, rather than extension of bleeding from the ventricle.

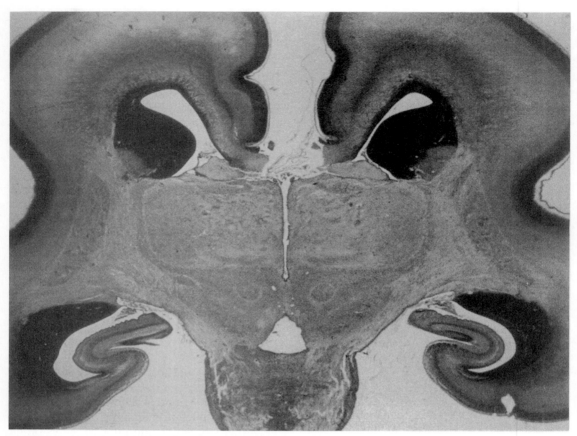

FIGURE 13-4   Normal germinal matrices are apparent in this section through a premature infant brain as dark, symmetric periventricular structures.

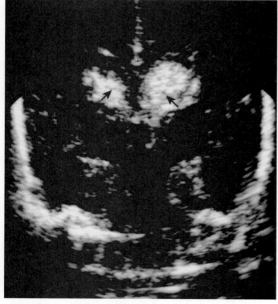

FIGURE 13-5   A 26-week preterm infant with mild hyaline membrane disease. Screening sonogram on day 7 of life shows bilateral grade I IVH (*arrows*).

Periventricular leukomalacia (PVL) is another neuropathologic lesion commonly associated with prematurity. PVL is believed to be associated with antecedent hypoxic-ischemic injuries. PVL is generally symmetric and nonhemorrhagic, although one fourth of PVL cases also may have associated hemorrhages. Because hypoxic-ischemic encephalopathy is a common precursor of IVH, PVL is a common correlative finding in those infants.[46,47] Although the IVH is not a direct cause of PVL, venous obstruction from IVH could lead to hemorrhagic exacerbation of PVL lesions.

IVH also can lead to posthemorrhagic ventricular dilation and hydrocephalus.[48,49] The degree of dilation is related to the severity of the hemorrhage. More severe hemorrhages can result in acute hydrocephalus with ventricular enlargement occurring within a few days.[50] Slower ventricular enlargement over several weeks may follow smaller hemorrhages. The presence of blood clot and breakdown products in the ventricles is thought to result in mechanical obstruction of the foramen of Monro. This debris also may impair CSF absorption by the arachnoid villi. An additional mechanism seems to be a reactive arachnoiditis in the posterior fossa, which, over time, obstructs the outflow of the fourth ventricle.[51]

Papile and coworkers[52] classified four grades of IVH as follows:

Grade I—subependymal germinal matrix hemorrhage

Grade II—subependymal hemorrhage with bleeding into normal-sized ventricles

Grade III—subependymal hemorrhage with bleeding into dilated ventricles

Grade IV—same as grades I, II, and III with involvement of adjacent brain parenchyma

Examples of grade II, grade III, and grade IV IVH are shown in Figures 13-6, 13-7, and 13-8.

Alternatively, Volpe's[27] classification consists of three gradations as follows:

Grade I—germinal matrix hemorrhage with absent or minimal IVH (<10% of ventricle involved)

Grade II—IVH involving 10% to 50% of the ventricles

Grade III—IVH involving greater than 50% of the ventricles, usually accompanied by dilation of the lateral ventricles.

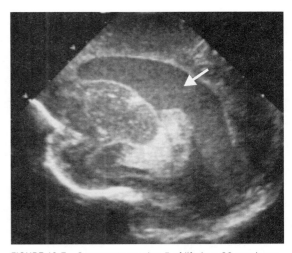

FIGURE 13-7 Sonogram on day 5 of life in a 30-week preterm infant with hyaline membrane disease. An acute decrease in hematocrit had occurred on day 2. There are low-level echoes consistent with debris from evolving grade III IVH in the dilated lateral ventricle (*arrow*).

Volpe[27] included a separate category of hemorrhagic involvement of the brain parenchyma.

Clinical Features

IVH typically occurs in premature infants with respiratory distress syndrome on ventilatory support in the first 3 days of life. Less than 10% occur beyond 7 days of age.[53] The pathogenetic mechanisms involved include variable cerebral blood flow and increased cerebral venous pressure, which can lead to tears of the weakened germinal matrix capillaries. Bleeding is enhanced further by impaired coagulation and excessive fibrinolysis in the germinal matrix.

Volpe[27] described three clinical IVH syndromes. Fifty percent of patients are classified with the "clinically silent" syndrome. These infants present with no obvious clinical signs or at most an unexplained decrease in hematocrit. The "saltatory syndrome" is another common clinical presentation and is characterized by altered consciousness, decreased spontaneous movements, abnormal eye movements, hypotonia, and possible respiratory irregularities. Infants who present with the "catastrophic syndrome" rapidly become comatose, often with accompanying tonic seizures or decerebrate

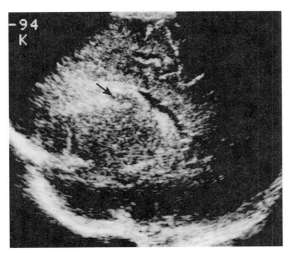

FIGURE 13-6 A 32-week preterm infant, briefly intubated at delivery. Screening sonogram on day 6 of life shows a grade II IVH (*arrow*).

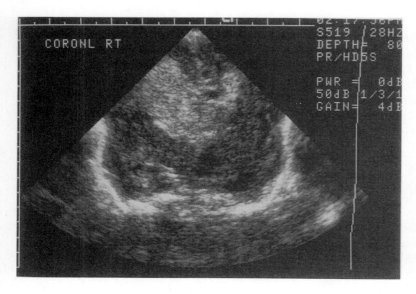

FIGURE 13-8 Large parenchymal hemorrhage and grade IV IVH in a 710-g infant born at 28 weeks' gestation, with Apgar scores of 1 at 1 minute and 4 at 5 minutes. The pregnancy was complicated by preeclampsia. This infant died at 11 days of age.

posturing. Additional signs include fixed, nonreactive pupils, absent oculovestibular reflexes, bulging fontanelle, arterial hypotension, bradycardia, and acidosis.

Diagnosis

Diagnosis of IVH can be accomplished by routine cranial ultrasound through the anterior fontanelle. Routine screening on day 5 to 7 of life would be expected to diagnose 90% of these hemorrhages.[54] Cranial ultrasound also can detect periventricular hemorrhagic infarction, PVL, porencephalic cysts, and posthemorrhagic ventricular dilation.[55] Cranial ultrasound is particularly advantageous because of portability, affordability, and safety of the procedure. CT and MRI also are useful techniques, but require transport of the patient to the scanner and potential exposure to radiation and problems with metallic equipment in magnetic fields. In addition, CSF analysis may show corroborative findings, such as elevated red blood cells and protein, xanthochromia, and persistent hypoglycorrhachia.

Treatment Options

Prevention of IVH is crucial for improvement of survival and neurodevelopmental outcomes. Prevention of premature birth and transport of high-risk infants in utero to

perinatal centers are logical first steps in achieving this goal. In addition, various prenatal medications have been suggested to reduce the risk of IVH. Trials of prenatal phenobarbital, magnesium sulfate, and vitamin K have yielded mixed results.[56-58] Administration of antenatal corticosteroids seems to result in a diminished incidence of subsequent IVH, however.[59] The mechanism is probably primarily due to improved cardiovascular function, rather than reduced severity of respiratory distress syndrome, which also occurs after prenatal corticosteroids.[60] Early elective cesarean section also may reduce the severity of IVH in extremely premature infants.[61]

After birth, prevention of IVH may be enhanced by prompt resuscitation of a premature infant to reduce hypoxia and hypercapnia and to protect autoregulatory mechanisms of cerebral blood flow. Perlman and colleagues[62,63] showed a significant decrease in the incidence of IVH in infants who were paralyzed with pancuronium bromide. Muscle paralysis in ventilated infants resulted in a marked improvement in variability of cerebral blood flow velocities. Paralysis has significant risks, however, and other measures to synchronize ventilation and stabilize blood pressure are currently employed.

It also is recommended that routine procedures in the neonatal intensive care unit be modified to minimize handling and avoid variations in cerebral blood flow. Examples include avoiding procedures that cause crying, minimizing tracheal suctioning, and close monitoring for pneumothorax.[64,65] Blood pressure should be carefully controlled. Overhydration and rapid infusions of colloid, blood, or hypertonic solutions (e.g., sodium bicarbonate or hypertonic saline) should be avoided.

Several medications have been suggested for prevention of IVH, including phenobarbital, indomethacin, vitamin E, and ethamsylate. Although indomethacin and vitamin E have shown some efficacy, results are too variable and inconsistent to consider routine use of these drugs. Even when shown to decrease IVH rates, indomethacin has not shown improved long-term benefits.[66]

When the diagnosis of IVH is established, treatment efforts are primarily supportive. Seizures may be associated with IVH and should be recognized and treated promptly. Tonic seizures, in particular, have been observed in infants with IVH. These seizures may be confused with decerebrate posturing, however, which also can accompany IVH.[67]

The grade of hemorrhage and degree of posthemorrhagic ventricular dilation should be monitored by cranial ultrasound on a weekly basis. Posthemorrhagic hydrocephalus can be managed by several interventions depending on the rate of ventricular dilation. These interventions include serial lumbar punctures, external ventriculotomy drainage, and ventricular peritoneal shunts.[68-70] Medications including acetazolamide, furosemide, and glycerol have been tried to reduce CSF production, but serious potential complications preclude their routine use in treating IVH.[71,72]

Prognosis of IVH varies with gradation of the hemorrhage and comorbid periventricular hemorrhagic infarction and PVL.[73] Higher grades of hemorrhage, particularly with periventricular hemorrhagic infarction, have mortality rates of 50% with neurologic sequelae rates of 90%. In grade I hemorrhages, the mortality rates are only 5%, but milder developmental problems still may be observed at follow-up.[27] Survival and neurodevelopmental outcomes may vary with early recognition and management of the IVH.

Conclusion

Neonatal intracranial hemorrhages occur at multiple locations and vary with risk factors, such as gestational age, trauma, asphyxia, and occasionally vascular malformations, neoplasms, and coagulopathies. Improvements in obstetric care can enhance prevention by reducing the incidence of trauma, asphyxia, and prematurity. Prompt recognition and clinical management of intracranial hemorrhages can lead to optimization of survival and neurodevelopmental outcomes. Care of an infant with intracranial hemorrhage is multidisciplinary and requires the vigilance and cooperative efforts of neonatologists, neurosurgeons, and pediatric neurologists. The current shortage of pediatric neurologists suggests a need for general neurologists to become familiar with the diagnosis and management of these infants as well.

REFERENCES

1. Hannigan WC, Morgan AM, Stahlberg LK, et al. Tentorial hemorrhage associated with vacuum extraction. Pediatrics 1950;85:534.
2. Sheth RD. Trends in incidence and severity of intraventricular hemorrhage. J Child Neurol 1998; 13:261.
3. Hamilton BE, Minino AM, Martin JA, et al. Annual summary of vital statistics: 2005. Pediatrics 2007;119:345.
4. Tekgul H, Gauvreau K, Soul J, et al. The current etiologic profile and neurodevelopmental outcome of seizures in term new born infants. Pediatrics 2006;117:1270.
5. Gardella C, Taylor M, Benedetti T, et al. The effect of sequential use of vacuum and forceps for assisted vaginal delivery on neonatal and maternal outcomes. Am J Obstet Gynecol 2001;185:896.
6. Dupuis O, Silveira R, Dupont C, et al. Comparison of "instrument-associated" and "spontaneous" obstetric depressed skull fractures in a cohort of 68 neonates. Am J Obstet Gynecol 2005;192:165.
7. Hayashi N, Endo S, Oka N, et al. Intracranial hemorrhage due to rupture of an arteriovenous malformation in a full-term neonate. Childs Nerv Syst 1994;10:344.
8. Zee CS, Segall HD, McComb G, et al. Intracranial arterial aneurysms in childhood: more recent considerations. J Child Neurol 1986;1:99.
9. Ernestus RI, Schroder R, Klug N. Intracerebral hemorrhage from an unsuspected ependymoma in early infancy. Childs Nerv Syst 1992;8:357.
10. Young RSK, Liberthson RR, Zalneraitis EL. Cerebral hemorrhage in neonates with coarctation of the aorta. Stroke 1992;13:491.

11. Matthay KK, Koerper MA, Ablin AR. Intracranial hemorrhage in congenital factor VII deficiency. J Pediatr 1979;94:413.
12. Volpe JJ, Manica JP, Land VJ, et al. Neonatal subdural hematoma associated with severe hemophilia A. J Pediatr 1976;88:1023.
13. Kohler HG. Haemorrhage in the newborn of epileptic mothers. Lancet 1966;1:267.
14. Cilley RE, Zwischengerger JB, Andrews AF, et al. Intracranial hemorrhage during extracorporeal membrane oxygenation in neonates. Pediatrics 1986;78:699.
15. Volpe JJ. Intracranial hemorrhage: Subdural, primary subarachnoid, intracerebellar, intraventricular (term infant) and miscellaneous. In Neurology of the Newborn, 2nd ed. Philadelphia: WB Saunders, 1987.
16. Sarff LD, Platt LH, McCracken GH. Cerebrospinal fluid evaluation in neonates: comparison of high risk infants with and without meningitis. J Pediatr 1976;88:473.
17. Escobedo M, Barton LL, Volpe JJ. Cerebrospinal fluid studies in an intensive care nursery. J Perinat Med 1975;3:204.
18. Nelson RM, Bucciarelli RL, Nagel JW. Hypoglycorrhachia associated with intracranial hemorrhage in newborn infants. J Pediatr 1979;94:800.
19. Troost B, Walker T, Cherington M. Hypoglycorrhachia associated with subarachnoid hemorrhage. Arch Neurol 1968;19:438.
20. Roost KT, Pimstone NR, Diamond I, et al. The formation of cerebrospinal fluid xanthochromia after subarachnoid hemorrhage: enzymatic conversion of hemoglobin to bilirubin by the arachnoid and choroid plexus. Neurology 1972;22:973.
21. Plauche WC. Subgaleal hematoma: a complication of instrumental delivery. JAMA 1980;244:1597.
22. Gama CH, Fenichel GM. Epidural hematoma of the newborn due to birth trauma. Pediatr Neurol 1985;1:52.
23. Negishi H, Lee Y, Itoh K, et al. Nonsurgical management of epidural hematoma in neonates. Pediatr Neurol 1989;5:52.
24. Hayashi T, Hashimoto T, Fakuda D, et al. Neonatal subdural hematoma secondary to birth injury. Child Nerv Syst 1987;3:23.
25. Wigglesworth JS, Husemeyer RP. Intracranial birth trauma in vaginal breech delivery: the continued importance of injury to the occipital bone. Br J Obstet Gynaecol 1977;88:684.
26. Huang CC, Shen EY. Tentorial subdural hemorrhage in term newborns: ultrasonographic diagnosis and clinical correlates. Pediatr Neurol 1991;7:171.
27. Volpe JJ. Intracranial hemorrhage: subdural, primary subarachnoid, intracerebellar, intraventricular (term infant) and miscellaneous. In Neurology of the Newborn, 4th ed. Philadelphia: WB Saunders, 2001.
28. Robertson WC Jr, Chun RW, Orrison WW, et al. Benign subdural collections of infancy. J Pediatr 1979;94:382.
29. Azais A, Echenne B. Idiopathic subarachnoid space enlargement (benign external hydrocephalus) in infants. Ann Pediatr 1992;39:550.
30. Fenichel GM, Webster DL, Wong WKT. Intracranial hemorrhage in the term newborn. Arch Neurol 1984;41:30.
31. DeReuck JL. Cerebral angioarchitecture and perinatal brain lesions in mature and full-term infants. Acta Neurol Scand 1984;70:391.
32. Meidell R, Marinelli PV, Randall V, et al. Intracranial parenchymal hemorrhage in a full-term infant. Clin Pediatr 1983;22:780.
33. Grunnet ML, Shields WD. Cerebellar hemorrhage in the premature infant. J Pediatr 1976;89:605.
34. Muller H, Beedgen B, Schenk JP, et al. Intracerebellar hemorrhage in premature infants: sonographic detection and outcome. J Perinat Med 2007; 35:67.
35. Scher MS, Wright FS, Lockman LA, et al. Intraventricular hemorrhage in the full-term neonate. Arch Neurol 1982;39:769.
36. Hayden CK Jr, Shattuck KE, Richardson CJ, et al. Subependymal germinal matrix hemorrhage in full-term neonates. Pediatrics 1985;75:714.
37. Roland EH, Flodmark O, Hill A. Thalamic hemorrhage with intraventricular hemorrhage in the full-term newborn. Pediatrics 1990;85:737.
38. Jocelyn LJ, Casiro OG. Neurodevelopmental outcome of term infants with intraventricular hemorrhage. Am J Dis Child 1992;146:194.
39. Horbar JD, Badjer GJ, Carpenter JH, et al. Trends in mortality and morbidity for very low birth weight infants. Pediatrics 2002; 110:143.
40. Ballabh P, Braun A, Nedergaard M. Anatomic analysis of blood vessels in germinal matrix, cerebral cortex, and white matter in developing infants. Pediatr Res 2004;56:117.
41. Szymonowicz W, Schafler K, Cussen LJ, et al. Ultrasound and necropsy study of periventricular haemorrhage in preterm infants. Arch Dis Child 1984;59:637.
42. Fanaroff AA, Wright LL, Stevenson DK, et al. Very low birth weight outcomes of the National Institute of Child Health and Human Development Neonatal Research Network, May 1991 through December 1992. Am J Obstet Gynecol 1995;173:1141.
43. Guzetta F, Shackelford GD, Volpe S, et al. Periventricular intraparenchymal echodensities in the premature newborn: critical determinant of neurologic outcome. Pediatrics 1986;78:995.
44. Gould SJ, Howard S, Hope PL, et al. Periventricular intraparenchymal cerebral haemorrhage in preterm infants: the role of venous infarction. J Pathol 1987;151:197.
45. Takashima S, Mito T, Ando Y. Pathogenesis of periventricular white matter hemorrhages in preterm infants. Brain Dev 1986;8:25.
46. Van den Broeck C, Himpens E, Vanhaesebrouck P, et al. Influence of gestational age on the type of brain injury and neuromotor outcome in high-risk neonates. Eur J Pediatr 2007;166:1261.
47. Rushton DI, Preston PR, Durbin GM. Structure and evolution of echodense lesions in the neonatal brain: a combined ultrasound and necropsy study. Arch Dis Child 1985;60:798.
48. Allan WC, Holt PJ, Sawyer LR, et al. Ventricular dilation after neonatal periventricular-intraventricular

hemorrhage: natural history and therapeutic implications. Am J Dis Child 1982;136:589.

49. Dykes FD, Dunbar B, Lazarra A, et al. Posthemorrhagic hydrocephalus in high-risk pre-term infants: natural history, management and long-term outcome. J Pediatr 1989;114:611.

50. Levy ML, Masri LS, McComb JG. Outcome for preterm infants with germinal matrix hemorrhage and progressive hydrocephalus, Neurosurgery 1997; 41:1111.

51. Pukumizu M, Takashima S, Becker LE. Glial reaction in periventricular areas of the brainstem in fetal and neonatal posthemorrhagic hydrocephalus and congenital hydrocephalus. Brain Dev 1996;18:40.

52. Papile LA, Burstein J, Burstein R, Koffler H. Incidence and evolution of subependymal and intraventricular hemorrhage: a study of infants with birth weights less than 1,500 gm. J Pediatr 1978; 92:529.

53. Partridge JC, Babcock DS, Steichen JJ, et al. Optimal timing for diagnostic cranial ultrasound in low-birth-weight infants: detection of intracranial hemorrhage and ventricular dilation. J Pediatr 1983; 102:281.

54. Bowerman RA, Donn SM, Silver TM, et al. Natural history of neonatal periventricular/intraventricular hemorrhage and its complications: sonographic observations. AJR Am J Roentgenol 1984; 143:1041.

55. Rumack CM, Johnson ML. Perinatal and Infant Brain Imaging. Chicago: Mosby, 1984.

56. Kaempf JW, Porreco R, Molina R, et al. Antenatal phenobarbital for the prevention of periventricular and intraventricular hemorrhage: a double-blind, randomized, placebo-controlled, multihospital trial. J Pediatr 1990;117:933.

57. Leviton A, Peneth N, Susser M, et al. Maternal receipt of magnesium sulfate does not seem to reduce the risk of neonatal white matter damage. Pediatrics 1997;99:1.

58. Morales WJ, Angel JL, O'Brien WF, et al. The use of antenatal vitamin K in the prevention of early neonatal intraventricular hemorrhage. Am J Obstet Gynecol 1988;159:774.

59. Wright LL, Verter J, Younes N, et al. Antenatal corticosteroid administration and neonatal outcome in very low birth weight infants: the NICHD Neonatal Research Network. Am J Obstet Gynecol 1995; 173:269.

60. Moise AA, Wearden ME, Kozinetz CA, et al. Antenatal steroids are associated with less need for blood pressure support in extremely premature infants, Pediatrics 1995;95:845.

61. Anderson GD, Bada HS, Shaver DC, et al. The effect of cesarean section on intraventricular hemorrhage in the preterm infant. Am J Obstet Gynecol 1992; 166:1091.

62. Perlman JM, McMenamin JB, Volpe JJ. Fluctuating cerebral blood-flow velocity in respiratory-distress syndrome: relation to the development of intraventricular hemorrhage. N Engl J Med 1983;309:204.

63. Perlman JM, Goodman S, Kreusser KL, et al. Reduction in intraventricular hemorrhage by elimination of fluctuating cerebral blood-flow velocity in preterm infants with respiratory distress syndrome. N Engl J Med 1985;312:1353.

64. Panconi S, Due G. Intratracheal suctioning in sick preterm infants: prevention of intracranial hypertension and cerebral hypoperfusion by muscle paralysis. Pediatrics 1987;79:538.

65. Hill A, Perlman JM, Volpe JJ. Relationship of pneumothorax to occurrence of intraventricular hemorrhage in the premature newborn. Pediatrics 1982;69:144.

66. Schmidt B, Davis P, Moddeman D, et al. Long-term effects of indomethacin prophylaxis in extremely-low-birth-weight infants. N Engl J Med 2001; 344:1966.

67. Seay AR, Bray PF. Significance of seizures in infants weighing less than 2,500 grams. Arch Neurol 1977;34:381.

68. Papile LA, Koffler H, Burstein R, et al. Non-surgical treatment of acquired hydrocephalus: evaluation of serial lumbar puncture. Pediatr Res 1978;12:445.

69. Kreusser KL, Tarby TJ, Taylor D, et al. Rapidly progressive posthemorrhagic hydrocephalus: treatment with external ventricular drainage. Am J Dis Child 1984;138:633.

70. Sasidharan P, Marquez E, Dizon E, et al. Developmental outcome of infants with severe intracranial-intraventricular hemorrhage and hydrocephalus with and without ventriculoperitoneal shunt. Childs Nerv Syst 1986;2:149.

71. International PHVD Drug Trial Group. International randomized controlled trial of acetazolamide and furosemide in posthemorrhagic ventricular dilation in infancy. Lancet 1998;352:433.

72. Taylor DA, Hill A, Fishman MA, et al. Treatment of posthemorrhagic hydrocephalus with glycerol. Ann Neurol 1981;10:297.

73. Vohr BR, Wright LL, Dusick AM, et al. Neurodevelopmental and functional outcomes of extremely low birth weight infants in the National Institute of Child Health and Human Development Neonatal Research Network, 1993–1994. Pediatrics 2000; 105:1216.

CHAPTER 14

Spontaneous Intracerebral Hemorrhage

José Biller • Michael J. Schneck

Epidemiology

Spontaneous intracerebral hemorrhage (ICH) accounts for approximately 15% of all strokes and is about twice as prevalent as subarachnoid hemorrhage (SAH).[1-4] Spontaneous ICH occurs more frequently in men, and in Hispanics, African Americans, East Asians, and Pacific Islanders.[5-7] The Brain Attack Surveillance in Corpus Christi, Texas, project showed an increased overall stroke incidence among Mexican-Americans compared with non-Hispanic whites, and an increased risk of ICH and SAH, adjusted for age.[8] The risk of ICH is increased further by arterial hypertension. The rate of ICH in the United States is predicted to double in the ensuing decades because of the aging of the population and changes in racial demographics.[4]

Age is an important risk factor for ICH, and the ICH rate increases with advanced age. The relative frequency of ICH versus ischemic stroke is increased, however, among children and young adults. In addition, the average age for ICH is increasing. In Rochester, Minnesota, the median age for intracranial hemorrhages occurring in the 1945 to 1952 period was 65 years, and 71 years for hemorrhages occurring in the 1969 to 1976 period.[9] In Cincinnati, Ohio, patients older than 70 years had seven times the risk compared with patients younger than 70 years.[6] In the Pilot Stroke Data Bank, the median age of patients with ICH was 56 years.[10] In Florence, Italy, the incidence of ICH was 1.4 per 100,000 for patients 15 to 34 years old, and 2.7 per 100,000 for patients 35 to 44 years old.[11] Matsumoto and colleagues[3] found that ICH accounted for only 1% to 2% of strokes among individuals younger than 45 years. Conversely, Lin and coworkers[12] found the proportion of hemorrhage to infarction decreased from 1:1.5 in patients 35 to 44 years old to 1:5.4 in patients older than 75 years. In a separate 5-year Italian stroke registry of 4353 patients, 89 young adult patients were identified. In this registry, the prevalence of SAH and ICH was 42.7% in young adults compared with 15.7% in older patients.[13]

In the Italian stroke registry,[13] more than half (52.6%) of the hemorrhagic strokes were due to cerebral aneurysms or arteriovenous malformations (AVMs). The proportion with good outcome was highest for patients with SAH (60%), whereas patients with ischemic stroke had the highest proportion of severe disability (47%). Mortality rates in this small young adult cohort were highest for patients with ICH (44%), but with a lower proportion of severely disabled patients (17%).[13]

Long-term administration of anticoagulants also is a risk factor for ICH.[14-16] Patients with liver cirrhosis are at increased risk for ICH.[17] Alcohol consumption, independently of arterial hypertension or other risk factors, also increases the risk of hemorrhagic stroke.[18] Likewise, very low levels of cholesterol have been associated with intracranial hemorrhage,[19] and lower levels of low-density lipoprotein cholesterol, regardless of statin use, have been associated with hemorrhagic conversion after thrombolytic therapy for ischemic stroke.[20]

The Stroke Prevention by Aggressive Reduction in Cholesterol Levels (SPARCL) study[21,22] showed a decrease in recurrent ischemic stroke and cardiac events among adult patients enrolled with either ischemic or hemorrhagic stroke treated with atorvastatin to reduce serum lipid levels. A post-hoc analysis showed, however, a two thirds increase in the relative risk of hemorrhagic stroke among patients in the atorvastatin arm of the trial. The absolute event rate remained low; of the 88 of 4371 patients who had a hemorrhagic stroke, 55 were in the atorvastatin group, and 33 were in the placebo group. A preliminary report from secondary analyses of the SPARCL study did not identify a relationship between brain hemorrhage and reduction of low-density lipoprotein cholesterol among these adult patients.[23]

Pregnancy also is associated with an increased risk of ICH. The Baltimore-Washington Cooperative Young Stroke Study reported a 2.4 increased risk in women during pregnancy and the postpartum period compared with nonpregnant women.[24] During pregnancy, ischemic stroke risk was not increased, but the ICH risk was 2.5. In the 6-week postpartum period, ischemic stroke risk was 8.7, but the ICH relative risk increased to 28.3.[24] Similar observations were reported in a Swedish database.[25]

Circadian rhythms also have been reported for ICH, with onset of symptoms more common in the morning, and greater occurrence during winter months.[26,27] Overall, ICH is more frequent in temperate climates and in winter.[28]

Etiology

ICH accounts for approximately 40% of stroke cases in young adults.[29-36] The most commonly reported causes of spontaneous ICH in children and young adults are intracranial vascular malformations, intracranial aneurysms, arterial hypertension, and abuse of sympathomimetic illicit drugs.[37] Brain hemorrhage associated with bleeding diatheses, cerebral venous thrombosis, eclampsia, brain tumors, vasculitides, moyamoya disease, infectious disorders, or following surgical procedures, is less frequent but well recognized (Table 14-1).[38-40]

Vascular Malformations

Central nervous system (CNS) vascular malformations include AVMs (Fig. 14-1), capillary telangiectasias, cavernous malformations (Fig. 14-2), and developmental venous anomalies (Fig. 14-3).[41,42] AVMs are slightly more prevalent in men. Familial cases have been reported. AVMs account for 30% to 50% of hemorrhagic strokes in children.[36-41] Among children with known AVMs, the annual risk of bleeding is about 2% to 4% with a high cumulative bleeding risk. Children are more likely to present with hemorrhages, have a greater risk of recurrence after treatment, and have a higher overall morbidity

TABLE 14-1   **Causes of Spontaneous Intracerebral Hemorrhage in Young Adults**

Vascular malformations
  AVMs
  Capillary telangiectasias
  Cavernous malformations
  Developmental venous anomalies
Aneurysms
  Saccular
  Infective
  Traumatic
  Neoplastic
Arterial hypertension
  Secondary
  Primary
Bleeding diatheses
  Leukemia
  Thrombocytopenia
  Disseminated intravascular
    coagulation
  Polycythemia
  Hyperviscosity syndromes
  Hemophilia
  Hypoprothrombinemia
  Afibrinogenemia
  Selective factor deficiencies
  von Willebrand disease
  Sickle cell anemia
  Antiplatelet therapy
  Anticoagulant therapy
  Thrombolytic therapy
Icelandic form of CAA
Arteritis/arteriopathies
  Infectious vasculitides
  Multisystem vasculitides
  Isolated CNS angiitis
  Moyamoya disease
Drug related
  Amphetamines
  Cocaine
  Phenylpropanolamine
  Pentazocine-pyribenzamine
  Phencyclidine
  Heroin
  Monoamine oxidase inhibitor
  Other drugs
Intracranial tumors
  Primary malignant or benign
  Metastatic
Cerebral venous occlusive disease
Miscellaneous
  Post carotid endarterectomy
  Post selective neurosurgical procedures
  Post spinal anesthesia
  Post myelography
  Cold related
  Post painful dental procedures
  Protracted migraine
  Methanol intoxication

and mortality compared with adults. Children also have more deep-seated lesions and a greater risk of bleeding when the AVMs are located in the posterior fossa.[43-52]

AVMs can be pial, dural, or mixed pial-dural. Most AVMs are pial and predominate supratentorially. Less frequent are dural AVMs, in which the vascular shunt is between meningeal branches of the external carotid, internal carotid, or vertebral arteries and veins. Dural AVMs are less likely to bleed than pial AVMs except for AVMs involving the tentorial incisura and the anterior fossa.[53-57]

Children and young adults with AVMs most frequently present with intracranial hemorrhage or seizures. Intracranial hemorrhage is usually parenchymatous or subarachnoid in location. Intraventricular hemorrhage (IVH) may occur at the time of rupture. Subdural hemorrhage is uncommon. Other symptoms, such as periodic headaches and progressive neurologic deficits, occur less frequently.

CNS vascular malformations occasionally are associated with mucocutaneous telangiectasias, other cutaneous vascular nevi, or cirsoid aneurysms of the scalp.[58] Hereditary hemorrhagic telangiectasia (Rendu-Osler-Weber syndrome) is an autosomal dominant disorder characterized by fibrovascular dysplasia of mucous membranes, skin, and viscera. Neurologic manifestations include cerebral infarction, intracranial or spinal hemorrhage, brain abscess, and encephalopathy. Approximately 15% to 20% of patients have a pulmonary AVM that may be the source of either septic or nonseptic cerebral embolism. Cerebrovascular malformations also have been reported in patients with this condition.[59-61]

Klippel-Trénaunay-Weber syndrome is characterized by varicose veins, cutaneous hemangioma, and hypertrophy of the involved limb. Neurovascular anomalies are uncommon. Spinal cord AVMs and cerebral arteriovenous fistula have been reported with this congenital anomaly (Fig. 14-4).[62,63]

AVMs of the great vein of Galen are infrequent high-flow midline vascular lesions that drain into and dilate the vein of Galen. Symptoms depend on patient age. Affected

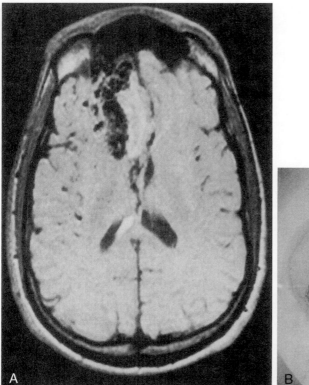
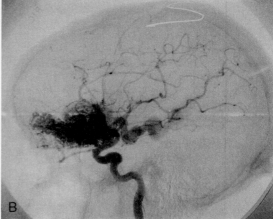

FIGURE 14-1 **A,** Axial T1 (short TR, short TE) MR image of the brain shows hemorrhage in the medial right frontal lobe associated with serpentine flow voids suggestive of an AVM. **B,** Right internal carotid angiogram shows a large frontal AVM with prominent draining vein. (Courtesy of Joel R. Meyer, M.D.)

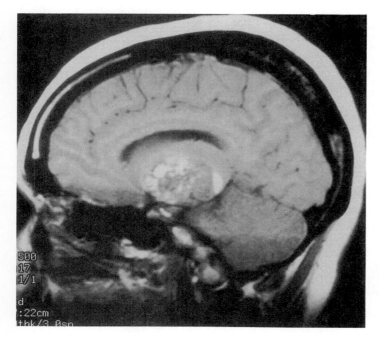

FIGURE 14-2 Sagittal T1 (short TR, short TE) MR image of the brain with heterogeneous signal abnormality in the thalamus representing a surgically proven cavernous malformation.

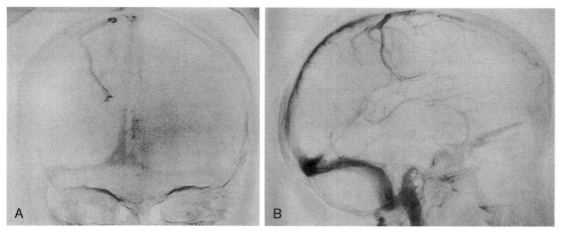

FIGURE 14-3 **A** and **B,** Anteroposterior and lateral carotid angiography (venous phase) shows the classic caput medusa appearance of a developmental venous anomaly. (Courtesy of Joel R. Meyer, M.D.)

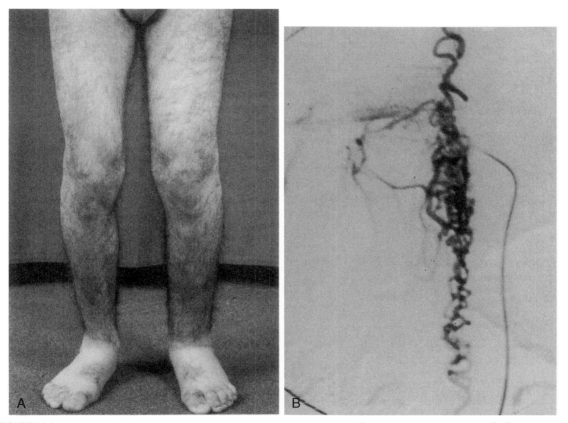

FIGURE 14-4 **A,** Hypertrophic left lower extremity in a patient with Klippel-Trénaunay-Weber syndrome. **B,** Spinal angiogram shows midthoracic AVM in the same patient. (Courtesy of Eric Russell, M.D.)

patients present with symptoms of high-output heart failure in the neonatal period. Older infants usually have seizures or progressive hydrocephalus owing to obstruction of the aqueduct of Sylvius. Older children and adolescents present with headaches, ICH, or SAH.[64-72]

Cryptic cerebrovascular malformations are small (usually <2 to 3 cm) and angiographically occult. They are an important cause of spontaneous ICH and seizures. ICH is more commonly associated with cryptic AVMs and developmental venous anomalies, and less frequently with cavernous malformations. Familial cases have been reported. The risk of rupture is unknown, but is believed to be 3% per year.[73-79]

Cerebral cavernous malformations (CCMs) are developmental or acquired vascular malformations with heterogeneous presentations depending on the size and location of the associated hemorrhage. Frequently, these lesions are found incidentally by magnetic resonance imaging (MRI) of the brain obtained for other indications. These lesions are discrete circumscribed lobular lesions containing hemorrhages of varying age.[80,81] Pathologically, CCMs are characterized by thin-walled, simple endothelial layered vessels that lack an internal elastic layer; have a very thin collagen ring; and, as opposed to capillary telangiectasias, have no intervening neural tissue.[80] There are familial forms, which typically manifest with multiple CCMs, and sporadic cases, which are usually solitary and may occur after trauma, infection, or radiation therapy.[80,81] At least three different genetic loci have been identified: the *CCM1*

gene on chromosome 7 at band 7q11.2-q21, the *CCM2* gene on chromosome 7 at band p15-p13, and the *CCM3* gene on chromosome 3 at band 3q 25.2-27.[82] There also is an association of CCM with developmental venous anomalies.[80]

Intracranial Aneurysms

Approximately 2% of adults without risk factors have an intracranial aneurysm.[83] Intracranial saccular aneurysms rarely occur in children.[83-89] The Cooperative Aneurysm Study found only 41 patients younger than 19 years among a total of 6368 cases of intracranial aneurysms,[95] whereas Patel and Richardson[86] in their report of 3000 aneurysms found only 16 patients younger than age 15. Besides SAH, rupture of an intracranial aneurysm may cause ICH (Fig. 14-5). Intracranial aneurysms are classified as saccular, mycotic, traumatic, neoplastic, arteritic, luetic, arteriosclerotic, or dissecting. The saccular type is most common. These aneurysms arise at branching points around the circle of Willis.[96] In children, there is a predilection for posterior circulation and internal carotid bifurcation aneurysms. Giant aneurysms also are more

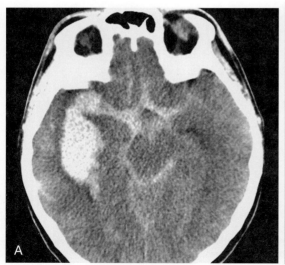
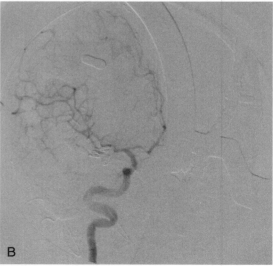

FIGURE 14-5   A, Non–contrast-enhanced head CT scan shows an acute parenchymal hematoma within the deep right temporal lobe extending into the right frontoparietal and lateral right basal ganglia regions. There also is extensive SAH most prominent in the right sylvian fissure. The patient was taken emergently to the operating room, where she was found to have two right middle cerebral artery aneurysms near the trifurcation of the middle cerebral artery. The hematoma was evacuated, and the aneurysm was clipped. **B,** Intraoperative cerebral angiogram shows the clipped aneurysm with filling of the right internal carotid, middle cerebral, and anterior cerebral arteries, but no residual aneurysm filling of the clipped aneurysms.

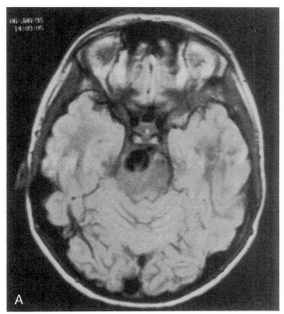 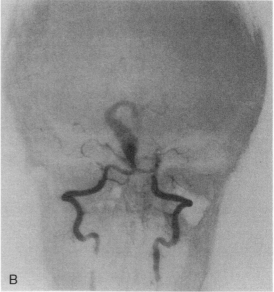

FIGURE 14-6   **A,** Axial T1 (short TR, short TE) MR image of the brain shows a 1-cm flow void posterior to the basilar artery in the interpeduncular cistern, causing compression of the brainstem in a 14-year-old boy. **B,** Anteroposterior view of a vertebrobasilar angiogram shows a large fusiform aneurysmal dilation of the basilar artery in the same patient.

common in children compared with adults (Fig. 14-6). Multiple aneurysms are present in approximately 5% of children versus 20% in adults. Intracranial aneurysms are more common in boys and young men, whereas after 40 years of age they are more common in women.[83-94]

Intracranial aneurysms have been described in association with autosomal dominant polycystic kidney disease, Ehlers-Danlos syndrome type IV, pseudoxanthoma elasticum, Marfan syndrome, type III collagen deficiency, coarctation of the aorta, fibromuscular dysplasia, moyamoya disease, sickle cell disease (SCD), AVMs, glucocorticoid remediable aldosteronism, and pituitary tumors.[97-104] Several studies have shown the existence of familial cases of intracranial aneurysms.[105-108]

ICH associated with aneurysms is most often caused by rupture of middle cerebral artery, anterior communicating artery, or internal carotid artery aneurysms. Aneurysms arising from the middle cerebral artery often cause hematomas within the anterior temporal lobe or insula. Hematomas originating from aneurysms of the anterior communicating artery complex or more distal branches of the anterior cerebral artery involve the septum and inferior frontal lobe. Blood may penetrate through the lamina terminalis into the third ventricle or directly into the hypothalamus. Distal anterior cerebral artery aneurysms are more prone to cause hematomas of the anterior superior corpus callosum. Hematomas arising from intracranial internal carotid artery bifurcation aneurysms also may be the source of IVHs.[109]

Rupture of infective (mycotic) aneurysms is a rare cause of ICH or SAH. Mycotic aneurysms, most often found with infective endocarditis, result from septic embolization of the vasa vasorum of a major intracranial artery. They tend to occur on distal branches of major cerebral vessels.[110,111]

Arterial Hypertension

Arterial hypertension in children is defined as blood pressure (measured on at least three separate occasions) greater than the 95th percentile for the child's age, gender, and height. Despite reports of disagreement, arterial hypertension is a common cause of ICH.[112,113] In the Regional Stroke Program at the University of Mississippi, 78.2% of patients 15 to 50 years old with ICH had arterial hypertension preceding their vascular event.[114] Hypertension is a less common cause of ICH in children because overall hypertensive cardiovascular disease is reported to occur in only 1% to 2% of children. Secondary causes of arterial hypertension always should be investigated in young patients.

Causes that should be considered include renal parenchymal (e.g., glomerulonephritis, polycystic kidneys, reflux nephropathy) and renal vascular (e.g., neurofibromatosis, Williams syndrome) diseases, congenital renal malformations, endocrinopathies (e.g., Cushing disease or corticosteroid therapy, pheochromocytoma, Conn syndrome, thyroid abnormalities, congenital adrenal hyperplasia, glucocorticoid-remediable aldosteronism, apparent mineralocorticoid excess), coarctation of the aorta, and bronchopulmonary dysplasias. ICH associated with pheochromocytoma is uncommon. Although only 0.5% of hypertensive patients have pheochromocytomas, early diagnosis is crucial to prevent devastating complications.[115] Guidelines have been established for the diagnosis of hypertension in children of various ages.[116]

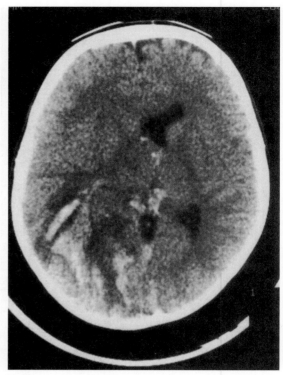

FIGURE 14-7   Non–contrast-enhanced CT scan shows a large area of hemorrhagic infarction with associated mass effect in a patient with acute lymphocytic leukemia. (Courtesy of Eric Russell, M.D.)

Bleeding Diatheses

Leukemia affects children at all ages. Intracranial hemorrhage as a result of leukemia is often a terminal event.[117-119] In many instances, stasis of leukemic cells may lead to microinfarctions and hemorrhages (Fig. 14-7). Intracranial hemorrhage is more frequent with acute lymphoblastic leukemia and acute nonlymphocytic leukemia. Bleeding may occur into the brain substance, subdural space, or subarachnoid space. Hemorrhages are often multifocal and predominate in the cerebral white matter. Intracranial bleeding is often associated with severe thrombocytopenia or hyperleukocytosis.

ICH is the most serious neurologic complication of thrombocytopenia.[120-125] The risk of bleeding depends on the platelet count. Bleeding may be intracerebral, subarachnoid, or subdural. Thrombocytopenia also may result in petechiae, purpura, bruisability, mucosal bleeding, hematuria, and severe gastrointestinal bleeding. Hemorrhage is unusual if the platelet count is greater than 20,000/mm³. Idiopathic thrombocytopenic purpura is the most common cause of thrombocytopenia in children. Intracranial bleeding occurs in less than 2% of cases. The risk of spontaneous ICH in patients with idiopathic thrombocytopenic purpura is usually associated with severe thrombocytopenia. ICH also has been reported in thrombotic thrombocytopenic purpura. Various degrees of thrombocytopenia and microangiopathic schistocytic hemolytic anemia are caused by thrombotic thrombocytopenic purpura.

Patients may present with a variety of focal or diffuse neurologic manifestations, including intracranial hemorrhage (Fig. 14-8). ICH also has been reported in aplastic anemia, acute myelofibrosis, angioimmunoblastic lymphadenopathy, post-transfusion purpura, dysmyelopoietic syndromes, paraproteinemias, hyperviscosity states, and infectious mononucleosis. Hemorrhage in the CNS is

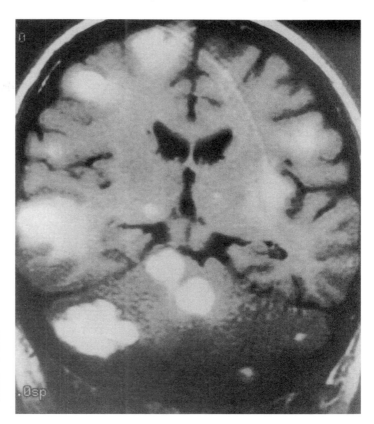

FIGURE 14-8 Coronal T1 (short TR, short TE) MR image of the brain shows multiple areas of high signal intensity in the supratentorial and infratentorial compartments, consistent with multiple hemorrhages in a patient with thrombotic thrombocytopenic purpura. (Courtesy of Joel R. Meyer, M.D.)

occasionally seen in patients with thrombocytopenia associated with viral hemorrhagic fevers.

Disseminated intravascular coagulation is a multifaceted syndrome seen in various pathologic states,[125,126] including malignancies, infections, sepsis (e.g., meningococcal septicemia), obstetric complications, trauma, burns, shock, heatstroke, liver and renal disease, transfusion reactions, and many other disorders (Fig. 14-9). Disseminated intravascular coagulation yields to a spectrum of abnormalities ranging from a hypercoagulable state causing ischemic change to tissues and organs on one hand, to severe bleeding tendencies from depletion of clotting factors and platelets, and activation of fibrinolysis on the other hand. Intracranial bleeding is rare. Hemorrhages tend to be multiple and predominate in the cerebral cortex. ICH also may result from the defibrination effects of snake envenomization and from the hypofibrinogenemic effects of asparaginase chemotherapy.

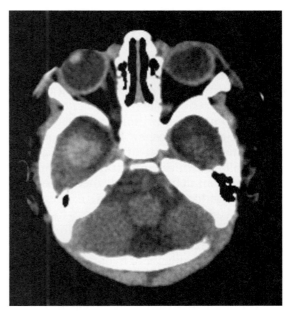

FIGURE 14-9 Non–contrast-enhanced head CT scan of a 2-week-old boy with neonatal streptococcal meningitis and septic shock who subsequently developed a 1.3-cm intraparenchymal hemorrhage in the right anterior temporal lobe.

ICH is an infrequent complication of polycythemia vera.[127,128] Most cases of polycythemia in children are secondary to chronic arterial oxygen desaturation. Bleeding may involve the brain substance, subdural space, or subarachnoid space. Bleeding is probably related to defective platelet function, defective clot formation, and engorgement of veins and capillaries. Chronic myelogenous leukemia and other myeloproliferative disorders are otherwise rare in pediatric patients.

Most patients with hemophilia have factor VIII deficiency (hemophilia A), whereas the remainder are deficient in factor IX (hemophilia B). Most children present with recurrent spontaneous bleeding into joints and muscles. Both disorders have an X-linked recessive inheritance pattern. Neonatal bleeding may occur after circumcision. CNS hemorrhage is a leading cause of death among hemophiliacs. The reported incidence of intracranial hemorrhage ranges from 2.2% to 13%. Most hemorrhages occur in children and youngsters. The location of intracranial bleeding is equally common in the brain substance, subarachnoid space, and subdural space. Posterior fossa bleeding, IVHs, and cranial and spinal epidural hematomas occur less frequently. Intracranial hemorrhage in hemophiliacs may be spontaneous, especially among patients severely affected. Delayed intracranial bleeding after trauma is common.[129-134]

Hypoprothrombinemia may result in ICH. It has been found in association with hemorrhagic disease of the newborn owing to vitamin K deficiency; dietary deficiency states; total parenteral nutrition; tropical sprue; short bowel and other fat malabsorption syndromes (e.g., cystic fibrosis, celiac disease, biliary atresia, obstructive jaundice); α_1-antitrypsin deficiency; advanced liver disease; megadoses of vitamin E; systemic lupus erythematosus associated with lupus anticoagulants; and the administration of warfarin anticoagulants, salicylates, broad-spectrum antibiotics, and hydantoins. Infants born to mothers taking antiepileptic drugs (e.g., phenobarbital, phenytoin, primidone) sometimes bleed, apparently because of a reduction of vitamin K–dependent (II, VII, IX, X) coagulation factors.[135-137] Intracranial hemorrhage has been attributed less often to congenital afibrinogenemia, factor XIII deficiency, factor V deficiency, and von Willebrand disease.[138,139]

Various neurologic complications have been documented in patients with SCD. CNS complications are among the leading causes of death in SCD. Cerebral infarction is the most common neurologic complication and occurs most often in children younger than 15 years old.[140-144] Intracranial bleeding is uncommon in children. Intracranial hemorrhagic complications include hemorrhagic infarction, ICH, and SAH.[143,144] IVH is unusual, but may be associated with moyamoya disease in patients with SCD. Massive intracranial hemorrhage also may be confined to the subdural space, and there are reports of epidural hematoma in the absence of major head trauma. ICH also may occur as a result of cerebral venous sinus thrombosis in patients with SCD.

ICH in adults with sickle cell anemia is likely to be intracerebral or subarachnoid, whereas children are more prone to SAH. The probable pathogenesis is related to a large vessel cerebral vasculopathy secondary to the abnormal rheologic features of sickled erythrocytes. Hemorrhage related to SCD vasculopathy also may occur as a result of an acquired form of moyamoya disease.[145,146] Although there is a theoretical risk that the hypertonic contrast medium can cause sickling, cerebral angiography can be performed safely. Exchange transfusion to decrease the relative level of hemoglobin S to less than 30% is recommended.[147,148] Stroke, either ischemic or hemorrhagic, has rarely been reported in association with β-thalassemia major. Rapid large blood transfusions should be avoided in these patients.[149]

CNS hemorrhage is a well-known complication of anticoagulant therapy.[10-13,150,151] The long-term use of oral anticoagulants increases the risk of ICH by approximately eightfold compared with a control population.[152] Patients may bleed intracranially, into the spinal cord, and into the peripheral nervous system. The most common intracranial sites of bleeding in decreasing order of frequency are the subdural space, brain parenchyma, subarachnoid space, and epidural space. Anticoagulant-related parenchymal hemorrhages tend to be larger and have a worse prognosis than hemorrhages of patients without anticoagulation. Anticoagulant-related ICH may result from underlying arterial hypertension, preceding cerebral infarction, older age, supratherapeutic international normalized ratio, or excessive prolongation of the activated partial thromboplastin time.

Thrombolytic therapy is another cause of intracerebral bleeding. Most of the hemorrhages are lobar or multilobar and are associated with a high mortality. The risk of ICH in patients with acute myocardial infarction has been reported to be 1.3% in patients treated with 150 mg of recombinant tissue plasminogen activator (rt-PA), whereas the risk was 0.4% in patients treated with only 100 mg of rt-PA. The risk of ICH in adult patients treated with intravenous rt-PA for acute ischemic stroke is around 6% among patients treated according to established guidelines.[153] The pathogenesis of thrombolytic-related ICH is not well established. Arterial hypertension, advanced age, previous strokes, and excessive prolongation of the activated partial thromboplastin time by concomitant use of intravenous heparin have been implicated as possible risk factors.[147-150,154-157] Severe uremia and deficiencies of factor V, VII, XII, and XIII also may result in ICH.[159,160]

Cerebral Amyloid Angiopathy

Cerebral amyloid angiopathy (CAA) is characterized by localized amyloid deposits in the media and adventitia of small arteries and arterioles of the cerebral cortex and leptomeninges. CAA is not associated with systemic amyloidosis. The affected vessels stain positive with Congo red, with yellow-green birefringence under polarized light. CAA predominantly affects elderly normotensive individuals as opposed to children and young adults. It is often associated with large, often multiple and recurrent lobar subcortical white matter cerebral hemorrhages. The parieto-occipital areas are most frequently involved.[161-165] A rare familial form, inherited as autosomal dominant and leading to ICHs in the third and fifth decades of life, is the Icelandic variety of CAA. In this condition, an abnormal microprotein known as gamma-trace or cystatin C, a cysteine protease inhibitor, is deposited in the blood vessels. Diagnosis can be made on the basis of reduced levels of cerebrospinal fluid cystatin C.[166-168] The Dutch form of CAA, another autosomal dominant form, affects older individuals in their fifth and sixth decades of life.[169]

Vasculitides and Vasculopathies

Cerebral involvement with infectious or inflammatory vasculitides may become evident because of either hemorrhagic or ischemic complications.[170-173] Luetic arteritis is far more frequently followed by cerebral infarction than by cerebral hemorrhage. Punctate cerebral hemorrhages may be seen with a variety of rickettsial diseases. Infectious causes of ICH are common in tropical climates.[173] Strokes can result from tuberculous endarteritis; cerebral hemorrhages are rare. Small, punctate brain hemorrhages can result from cerebral malaria. Candidiasis, rhinocerebral mucormycosis, aspergillosis, typhoid fever, African trypanosomiasis, amebic (*Naegleria fowleri*) meningoencephalitis, and filariasis also can cause hemorrhagic brain lesions. Acquired immunodeficiency syndrome (AIDS) seldom causes hemorrhagic strokes.[174,175] Spontaneous ICH in hemophiliacs with AIDS has been reported.

Hemorrhagic strokes also can be a complication of severe multisystem vasculitides. Cerebral hemorrhages have been described in patients with polyarteritis nodosa, systemic lupus erythematosus, rheumatoid arthritis, Wegener granulomatosis, Sjögren syndrome, Kohlmeier-Degos syndrome (malignant atrophic papulosis), Takayasu arteritis, and isolated CNS vasculitis (Fig. 14-10).[175] Moyamoya disease, a noninflammatory arteriopathy, also should be considered as a potential cause of parenchymal hemorrhage or SAH.[176]

Illicit Drug Use

ICH is being recognized with increasing frequency among users of illicit drugs.[177,178] With the increasing use of cocaine, amphetamines, and other designer drugs, substance abuse may supplant the more traditional risks of arterial hypertension or CNS vascular malformations as the cause of ICH in young adults (Fig. 14-11).[179]

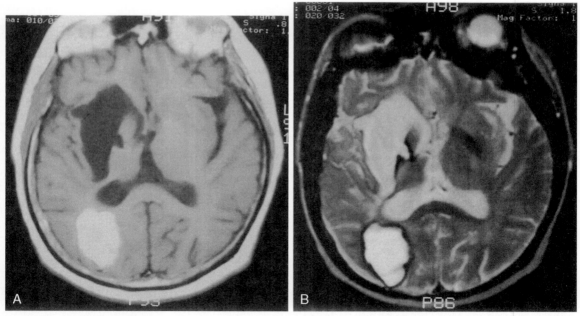

FIGURE 14-10   **A,** Non–contrast-enhanced axial T1 (short TR, short TE) MR image of the brain shows subacute hemorrhage in the right lateral occipital lobe and encephalomalacia in the right basal ganglia consistent with prior hemorrhage in a patient with systemic lupus erythematosus. **B,** Axial T2 (long TR, long TE) MR image shows hemosiderin along the periphery of both lesions in the same patient.

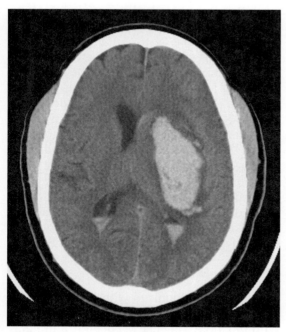

FIGURE 14-11   Non–contrast-enhanced head CT scan of a young man with no prior medical history that shows a large left basal ganglionic hemorrhage with intraventricular extension. The urine toxicology screen was positive for cocaine metabolites.

Most commonly, the implicated substances are amphetamines,[180-184] cocaine (freebase or crack),[185-189] phenylpropanolamine,[190-193] Talwin in combination with pyribenzamine ("T's and blues"),[194] and phencyclidine.[176] ICH also has been reported after the administration of intravenous heroin,[195] and use of monoamine oxidase inhibitors,[196] ephedrine,[197,198] and pseudoephedrine.[199] Heroin is usually associated with stroke in the setting of infective endocarditis. Hemorrhagic strokes complicating illicit drug use have been attributed to drug-induced sympathomimetic pressor effects, vasospasm, or drug-induced vasculitis. Vasculitis is probably a rare phenomenon with illicit drug use, especially with cocaine.[200] Acute drug-induced hypertension is the most likely cause of ICH. In addition, many patients with intracranial hemorrhage in the setting of cocaine use have preexisting intracranial aneurysms or AVMs.[200]

Intracranial Tumors

Most brain tumors in children are almost always primary malignancies, and about two thirds are infratentorial. Although almost every tumor known to affect the CNS has been implicated as a cause of intracranial hemorrhage, most are malignant, either primary or metastatic.[201-204] Primary CNS tumors with a propensity to bleed include glioblastoma multiforme, oligodendrogliomas, medulloblastomas, and ependymomas (Fig. 14-12). Intracranial hemorrhage also may result from a pituitary adenoma or

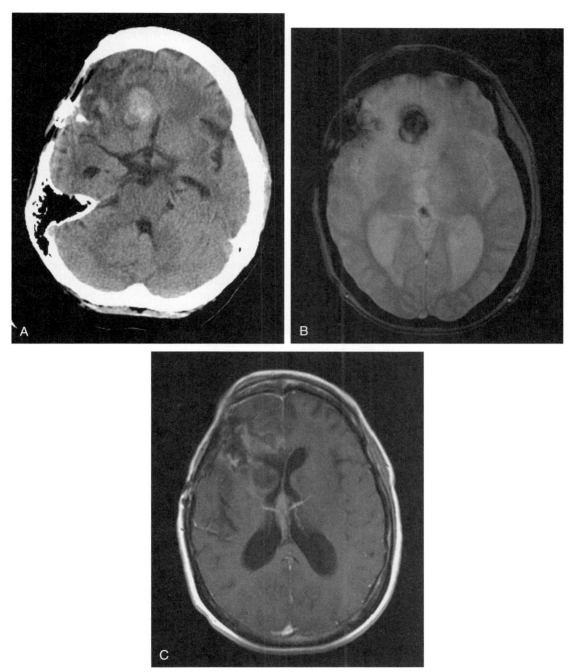

FIGURE 14-12 **A,** Non–contrast-enhanced head CT scan of a young woman with a recent history of recurrent oligoastrocytoma status post resection of tumor. CT scan reveals a new area of hemorrhage in the region of recurrent tumor in the medial frontal lobe. **B,** Gradient echo axial MR image shows the area of acute hemorrhage within the tumor bed. **C,** Postcontrast axial T1-weighted MR image shows the extent of this tumor. The tumor has caused mass effect on the right lateral ventricle with only minimal midline shift.

meningioma. von Hippel–Lindau disease is an autosomal dominant condition characterized by retinal angiomatosis; hemangioblastoma of the cerebellum, of the medulla, and of the spinal cord; visceral angiomatosis; adenomas of the kidneys; renal cell carcinoma; pheochromocytoma; and cystic lesions of the pancreas, kidney, and epididymis. Intracranial hemorrhage is a potential complication of metastatic tumors that are highly vascular, such as choriocarcinoma, melanoma, and renal cell carcinoma. Commonly in pediatric patients, hemorrhage also may occur in patients with leukemic infiltrates. Metastatic bronchogenic carcinoma also is known to cause hemorrhage into the brain parenchyma.

Cerebral Venous Occlusive Disease

Cerebral venous thrombosis should be considered a potential cause for intracranial hemorrhage.[205,206] Bleeding may be parenchymatous, subarachnoid, or subdural. Hemorrhages involve the white matter to a greater extent than the cortex and are often bilateral and parasagittal. Cerebral venous thrombosis may occur at any time from infancy to old age, although women of childbearing age are disproportionately affected during pregnancy and the puerperium or while taking oral contraceptives. Chief complaints are headaches, vomiting, lethargy, and seizures. Papilledema is common. There may be hemiparesis or paraparesis, or other focal neurologic manifestations according to the location of the venous structure involved. Cerebral venous thrombosis is discussed in detail in Chapter 12.

Miscellaneous

ICH rarely follows carotid endarterectomy,[207,208] extracranial-intracranial artery bypass anastomosis,[209] cardiac catheterization, and cardiac surgery.[210,211] Postoperative ICH also is a rare complication of the use of subarachnoid bolts for intracranial pressure (ICP) monitoring and ventriculoperitoneal shunting (Fig. 14-13).[212-214] Hemorrhagic cerebrovascular disease in pregnancy commonly manifests as ICH or SAH and is discussed in Chapter 9. Lightning stroke and heatstroke are rare causes of ICH.[215] ICH associated with prolonged painful dental work,[216] protracted migrainous attacks,[217] maintenance hemodialysis[218] and ingestion of methanol[219] are unusual causes. ICH rarely complicates spinal anesthesia and myelography.[220]

Clinical Features

Neurologic manifestations of ICH vary with location, size, direction of spread, and rate of development of the intracranial bleeding.[221-223] Hematoma growth occurs in approximately three quarters of all patients with ICH.[224] Significant hematoma growth within the first 24 hours after symptom onset may occur in one third of patients with growth of hematoma.[222-227] Percentage of hematoma growth, initial hemorrhage volume, and presence of IVH are predictors of mortality and, along with age, predict disability outcomes. There are several clinical grading scores for prediction of post-ICH morbidity and mortality.[225-227] Predictors of outcome in these scales include age (<60 years or <80 years depending on the scale), hematoma volume (<30 mL or >30 mL), presence of IVH, location of ICH (infratentorial versus supratentorial), and severity of clinical deficit as measured by Glasgow Coma Scale or National Institutes of Health Stroke Scale scores.[225-227] Separately, percentage of hematoma growth also has been reported as a predictor of mortality and disability outcomes.[224]

Depending on the location and size, approximately half of patients complain of headaches, nausea, and vomiting. Patients may have a variable level of alertness. Seizures are common with lobar hemorrhages. The structures most likely to be involved by spontaneous ICH are the putamen, the lobar subcortical white matter, the thalamus, the cerebellum, and the pons.

Putaminal Hemorrhage

The putamen is the most common site for hypertensive ICH.[228] Hemorrhages may remain localized to the putamen; enlarge to involve the internal capsule, corona radiata,

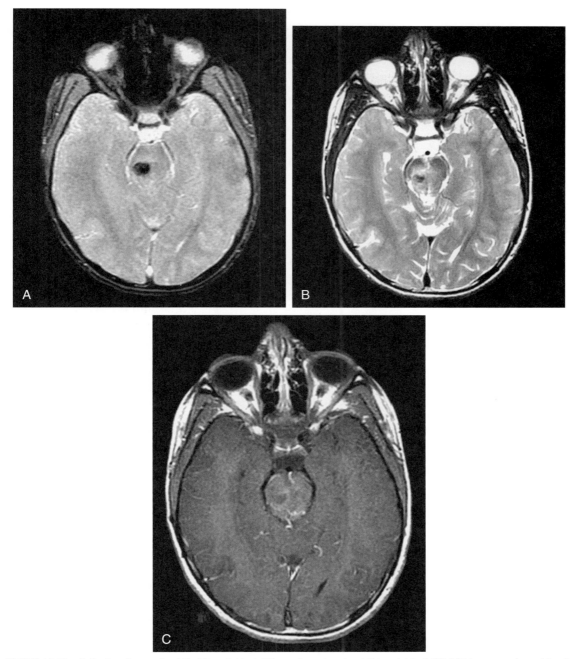

FIGURE 14-13   **A-C,** Gradient echo (**A**), T2-weighted (**B**), and postcontrast T1-weighted (**C**) MR images of a midbrain hemorrhage in an 8-year-old patient with a prior history of hydrocephalus status post ventriculoperitoneal shunt. The diagnostic evaluation did not show any other cause for this hemorrhage.

centrum semiovale, or temporal lobe; or rupture into the ventricular system (Fig. 14-14). The clinical picture is characterized by contralateral hemiparesis or hemiplegia, accompanied by conjugate preference to the side of the hematoma. There may be less severe contralateral hemisensory loss. Left putaminal hemorrhages result in aphasia; right putaminal hemorrhages produce apractagnosia, left visual field neglect, and constructional apraxia. Homonymous hemianopsia may be present.

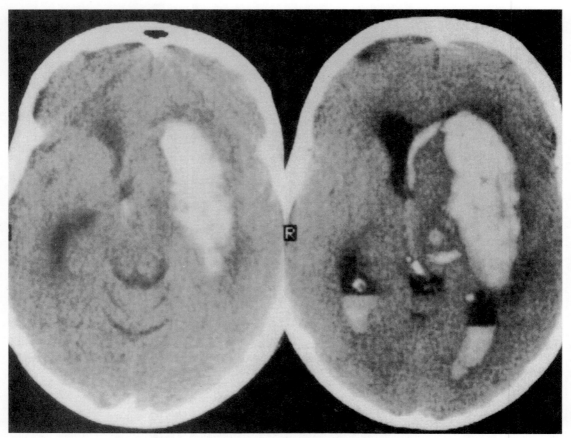

FIGURE 14-14 Non–contrast-enhanced axial CT scans show large left basal ganglia hemorrhage with associated intraventricular extension and significant mass effect.

Lobar Hemorrhages

Lobar hemorrhages occurring within the subcortical white matter are frequent in children and young adults (Fig. 14-15). They can arise from any cause, with structural lesions being more common than arterial hypertension.[229] Frontal lobe hemorrhages may result in contralateral hemiparesis and abulia. Conjugate deviation toward the hematoma may be found. Parietal hemorrhages may cause contralateral hemianesthesia and a variety of disorders of tactile function, disorders of body image, and neglect of the contralateral visual field. Dominant temporal lobe hemorrhages can result in Wernicke aphasia. Right temporal hematomas may result in variable degrees of visual field deficits. Occipital lobe hemorrhages are characterized by ipsilateral orbital pain and contralateral homonymous hemianopsia.

Thalamic Hemorrhage

Thalamic hemorrhages are often hypertensive, but may be secondary to an underlying structural lesion.[230] They may be confined to the thalamus or extend laterally to involve the internal capsule, inferomedially to compromise the subthalamus and midbrain, or medially to involve the third ventricle. Thalamic hemorrhages are characterized by contralateral pan-hemisensory loss. Hemiparesis develops if the internal capsule becomes involved. Compromise of the ascending reticular activating system may account for decreased level of consciousness and hypersomnolence. Inferomedial extension accounts for restriction of vertical gaze, convergence retraction nystagmoid movements, pupillary light-near dissociation, and disconjugate gaze with impaired abduction of one or both eyes. The eyes become tonically deviated

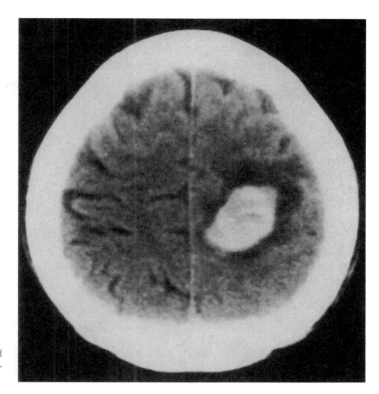

FIGURE 14-15   Non–contrast-enhanced axial CT scan shows a hematoma at the left frontoparietal junction with associated edema.

downward and slightly abducted. They may be tonically deviated away from the thalamic hematoma, or there may be a conjugate gaze deviation as seen in putaminal hemorrhages. Left thalamic hemorrhages can cause a transient aphasia. Right thalamic hematomas may account for visuospatial abnormalities and anosognosia.

Cerebellar Hemorrhage

Variations in location, size, and development of the hematoma; brainstem compression; fourth ventricular penetration; and development of hydrocephalus result in variations in the mode of presentation of cerebellar hemorrhage.[231] The history is typically that of a sudden onset of occipital or frontal headaches, nausea, vomiting, dizziness or vertigo, and inability to stand or walk. Patients often have truncal or limb ataxia, ipsilateral gaze palsy, and small reactive pupils. Horizontal gaze, paretic nystagmus, and facial weakness also are frequent. Frank hemiparesis is absent. Progression occurs because of hydrocephalus or edema. Not all patients present such a dramatic picture. Patients with small

(usually <3 cm in diameter) cerebellar hematoma may present with vomiting and with no headaches, gait instability, or limb ataxia.

Pontine Hemorrhage

Massive pontine hematomas cause coma, decerebrate rigidity, quadriparesis, absent horizontal eye movements, and miotic pupils (Fig. 14-16). Ocular bobbing may be present. Partial damage to the lateral basis pontis may cause pure motor hemiparesis.[232] Hemorrhages originating in the lateral pontine tegmentum may account for an ipsilateral internuclear ophthalmoplegia, one-and-a-half syndrome, and ocular bobbing. Laterally placed tegmental hemorrhages may produce ipsilateral hemiataxia with contralateral hemiparesis and hemisensory deficits.[233]

Paraclinical Evaluation

Initial history and cardiopulmonary and neurologic assessment are obtained in all patients before proceeding with radiographic and imaging techniques. Several blood tests are regularly obtained. Blood dyscrasias are

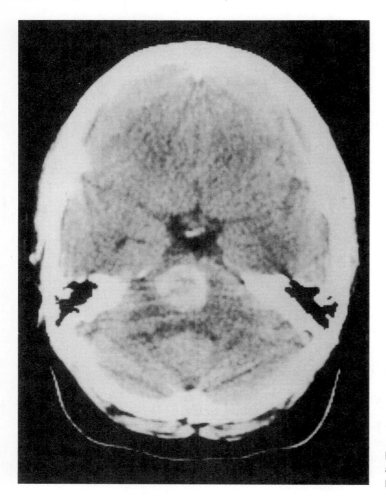

FIGURE   14-16 Non–contrast-enhanced axial CT scan shows a hematoma in the pons.

identified by appropriate blood investigations. When ICH is suspected, computed tomography (CT) is mandatory. Because of its widespread availability and speed, non–contrast-enhanced CT is still the safest, most effective method currently available to diagnose an acute ICH accurately. CT determines the size and location, and suggests possible causes of the ICH. A contrast-enhanced CT scan rarely is required to exclude the possibility of a primary or metastatic brain tumor. MRI is more sensitive to delayed hemorrhages associated with infarction and is highly sensitive to the presence of occult vascular malformations and cerebral venous thrombosis (Fig. 14-17).

Because of the ease and widespread availability of CT in the acute setting, MRI has not yet supplanted CT in the early evaluation of ICH. Gradient echo MRI is sensitive to the paramagnetic effects of blood breakdown products and can be used to identify local heterogeneities caused by hemosiderin. As such, this sequence is particularly useful in identifying microhemorrhages. With diffusion-weighted and gradient echo sequences, MRI can supplant head CT for the evaluation of even hyperacute stroke, and provide a perspective regarding microbleeds and delayed hemorrhages.[234]

Repeat imaging of patients in the acute phase is crucial because an ICH can expand significantly within the first several hours after the initial bleed. Repeat imaging should be performed for all acute ICHs within the first 6 hours and again within the ensuing 24 hours to assess possible expansion of hemorrhage.

Arteriography should be part of the evaluation in most young patients with spontaneous ICH. CT angiography and MR angiography may be useful adjuncts that sometimes

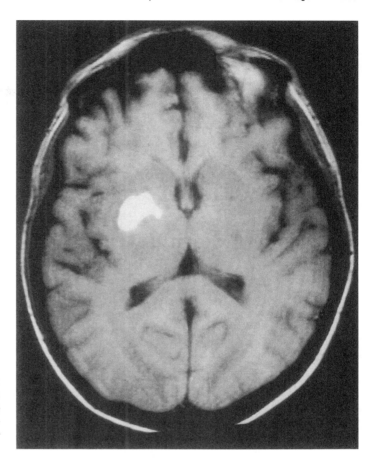

FIGURE 14-17 Non–contrast-enhanced axial T1 (short TR, short TE) MR image of the brain shows abnormal high signal intensity in the globus pallidus and putamen owing to methemoglobin associated with a subacute hemorrhage. (Courtesy of Joel R. Meyer, M.D.)

obviate the need for catheter cerebral angiography. MR angiography can be limited by susceptibility artifacts, and a small vascular malformation or tumor may not be visible on initial MR angiography in the presence of a large hemorrhage. The diagnostic yield for angiography is greater in lobar hemorrhages compared with brainstem or basal ganglia bleeds. A normal angiogram does not exclude a "cryptic" AVM, neoplasm, or vasculopathy associated with abuse of illicit drugs. Ultrasound is useful in the infant with an open fontanelle.[38,235,236] Paraclinical investigations recommended as part of the evaluation of patients with ICH are listed in Tables 14-2 and 14-3.

Treatment

Treatment of ICH emphasizes controlling complications, including cerebral edema and increased ICP, and maintaining adequate cerebral perfusion pressure. At present, much of the care surrounding a patient with ICH is supportive, including control of blood pressure, glucose, temperature, nutrition, and oxygenation. Blood pressure targets of mean

TABLE 14-2 **Routine Paraclinical Evaluation in Intracerebral Hemorrhage**

Complete blood count with platelet count
Prothrombin time (PT) with INR Activated partial
  thromboplastin time (aPTT)
Erythrocyte sedimentation rate (ESR)
Blood glucose
Serum alkaline phosphatase, serum aspartate
  transaminase
Serum calcium
Serum
Complete metabolic panel (CMP)
Urinalysis
Chest radiograph
Electrocardiogram
Unenhanced CT scan

INR, International Normalized Ratio
CMP includes: glucose, calcium, albumin, total protein, sodium, potassium, CO2 (carbon dioxide, bicarbonate), chloride, BUN (blood urea nitrogen), creatinine, alkaline phosphatase (ALP), alanine aminotransferase (ALT), aspartate aminotransferase (AST), and bilirubin.

TABLE 14-3 **Selective Paraclinical Evaluation in Intracerebral Hemorrhage**

Plasma level of factors V, VIII, IX, and XI
Fibrinogen
Fibrin degradation products
Thrombin time
Blood culture
Drug screen
Antinuclear antibodies
Sickle cell screen
Hemoglobin electrophoresis
Serum fibrinogen, fibrinogen split products, serum viscosity
HIV serology
Contrast-enhanced CT scan
CT angiography
MRI of the brain with Gd-DTPA
MR angiography
Sonography (carotid duplex, transcranial Doppler, cranial ultrasound)
Catheter cerebral angiography
Brain/leptomeningeal biopsy
Biopsy of hematoma wall

Gd-DTPA, gadolinium-diethylene-triamine-pentaacetic acid; HIV, human immunodeficiency virus.

arterial pressures less than 130 mm Hg with consideration of cerebral perfusion pressure greater than 70 mm Hg in patients with elevated ICP have been recommended by the American Heart Association guidelines, but firm parameters regarding the optimal agents and target blood pressures are unclear at this time.[237,238] In patients without elevated ICP, and systolic blood pressure greater than 180 mm Hg or mean arterial blood pressure greater than 130 mm Hg, a target mean arterial blood pressure of 110 mm Hg seems reasonable. As noted in the American Heart Association guidelines on spontaneous ICH, potential treatments focus on decreasing the initial bleeding and removing blood from the brain and ventricles to decrease mass effect ("mechanical" factors) and irritation ("chemical" factors).[237]

Before a patient with a presumed ICH arrives at a critical care unit, basic medical and neurologic evaluation and, if necessary, stabilization should be performed in the emergency department. Management of the airway and maintenance of adequate ventilation and oxygenation must be accomplished immediately. When signs of increased ICP

and herniation exist, endotracheal intubation, hyperventilation, and intravenous osmotherapy are indicated. The patient's head is elevated to more than 30 degrees to prevent an increase in ICP; excessive flexion or rotation is avoided.[38]

Corticosteroids are not routinely used except in cases associated with primary or metastatic brain tumors or intracranial vasculitis. The blood pressure should be monitored continuously during the first 48 to 72 hours after ICH. If the mean arterial pressure is persistently greater than 130 mm Hg, and there is evidence of end organ damage, a very cautious lowering seems justified.[38]

Prophylactic antiepileptic drugs are not routinely used. Our current approach is not to use them, even in cases of subcortical or lobar white matter hemorrhages. Hemostatic defects, if present, should be corrected. Appropriate factor replacement should be initiated immediately. In patients with hemophilia, a minimum level of 30% to 50% factor VIII or IX should be maintained for at least 10 to 14 days.[131]

Oral anticoagulant–related hemorrhages require discontinuation of the offending drug and administration of vitamin K, fresh frozen plasma, or prothrombin complex concentrate.[237,239,240] Additionally, recombinant activated factor VII can be used to correct the coagulopathy in nonhemophiliac patients. Infusion of recombinant factor VIIa was thought to be promising in a phase IIb clinical trial for ICH patients treated within 4 hours of symptom onset.[241] A more recent phase III clinical trial of recombinant factor VIIa was disappointing, however, because it failed to confirm the findings of the earlier trial (Mayer SA, personal communication).

ICH in a patient receiving heparin sodium is an indication for immediate discontinuation of the drug and the slow administration of intravenous protamine sulfate.[151] Similarly, intracranial hemorrhage in patients receiving thrombolytic therapy requires prompt discontinuation of the thrombolytic agent and the administration of fresh frozen plasma, platelets, and cryoprecipitate.[158] Patients with profound thrombocytopenia who develop intracranial hemorrhage should be treated immediately with platelet transfusions. Additional measures in patients with idiopathic thrombocytopenic purpura may include the administration of corticosteroids, plasmapheresis, or emergency splenectomy.[122]

The indications for surgical treatment of spontaneous ICH have been debated for decades.[237,242-247] A large trial in Europe failed to confirm benefit.[237,248] Ongoing clinical trials are investigating whether stereotactic catheter–directed clot aspiration with assisted thrombolytic lysis of clot of either IVH or ICH would have benefit. Preliminary reports have anecdotally described dramatic reduction of clot burden with this approach (Fig. 14-18)[237,248]; whether this would result in significant reduction in disability remains to be determined. Despite continued controversy, most investigators agree that surgery is of no benefit in moribund patients with massive hemorrhages, and that fully conscious patients with small intracerebral hematomas, regardless of location, rarely need surgical therapy. The debate remains as to whether patients with intermediate-sized hemorrhages are better managed surgically or medically.

A review suggests that surgery should be considered in deteriorating patients with lobar hematomas and cerebellar hematomas.[247] Surgery seems rarely indicated in cases of thalamic or brainstem hemorrhages. Particular emphasis must be placed on cases of cerebellar hemorrhage for which emergency surgery may be indicated. Cerebellar hemorrhage is a potentially lethal but often completely reversible condition when compression of the brainstem is released promptly. Patients with cerebellar hemorrhages greater than 3 cm in diameter, even if fully conscious, should be referred for surgery. Medical management under strict and careful observation has been recommended for small (<3 cm in diameter) cerebellar hemorrhages. If there is any evidence of deterioration, surgery should be undertaken immediately (Fig. 14-19).[38,248]

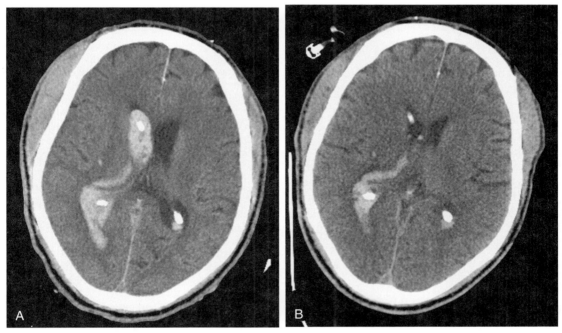

FIGURE 14-18 **A,** Non–contrast-enhanced head CT scan shows IVH. The IVH filled the right lateral ventricle and third ventricle with some leakage of blood into the left lateral ventricle and fourth ventricle. Note the extraventricular drainage catheter in the tip of the right frontal horn. **B,** The patient received tPA via the intraventricular catheter as part of a research protocol. Non–contrast-enhanced head CT scan, performed 2 days after admission, shows the dissolution of clot in the right frontal horn and third ventricle with decrease in size of the remaining clot in the lateral compartment and posterior horn of the right ventricle.

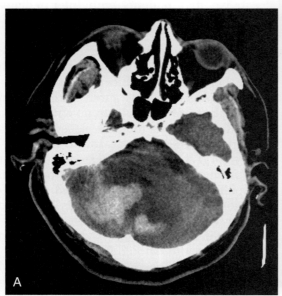
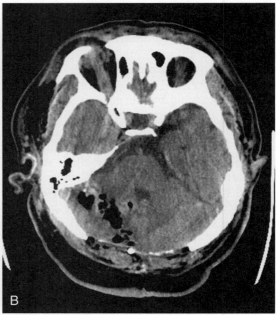

FIGURE 14-19 **A,** Non–contrast-enhanced head CT scan of a young man with a cerebellar hemorrhage observed in the intensive care unit with worsening mental status 4 days post bleed. There is a large acute intraparenchymal hematoma involving much of the right cerebellar hemisphere with a component of adjacent subdural and subarachnoid blood. The fourth ventricle is significantly effaced with local mass effect and midline shift among infratentorial structures and mass effect and effacement of brainstem structures. **B,** The patient was taken to the operating room for a suboccipital craniectomy with evacuation of the hematoma. Note the decrease in mass effect and shift on the fourth ventricle and brainstem.

Conclusion

ICH must be considered as a possible diagnosis in every patient with acute onset of focal cerebral dysfunction, even in the absence of headache. Although stroke is much less common in children and young adults, the ratio of hemorrhagic to ischemic stroke is higher in this population than in older patients. Young patients with ICH represent a heterogeneous group. Lobar hemorrhages are frequent. A cause can be found in most patients. The prognosis for recovery depends on the cause, site, and size of the hemorrhage, and the patient's neurologic status.

REFERENCES

1. Mohr JP, Caplan LR, Melski J, et al. The Harvard Cooperative Stroke Registry: a prospective registry. Neurology 1978;28:754.
2. Whisnant JP, Fitzgibbons JP, Kurland LT, et al. Natural history of stroke in Rochester, Minnesota, 1945 through 1954. Stroke 1971;2:11.
3. Matsumoto N, Whisnant JP, Kurland LT, et al. Natural history of stroke in Rochester, Minnesota, 1955 through 1969: an extension of a previous study, 1945 through 1954. Stroke 1973;4:20.
4. Qureshi AI, Tuhrim S, Broderick JP, et al. Spontaneous intracerebral hemorrhage. N Engl J Med 2001;344:1450.
5. Gross CR, Kase CS, Mohr JP, et al. Stroke in South Alabama: incidence and diagnostic features: a population-based study. Stroke 1986;15:249.
6. Brott T, Thalinger K, Hertzberg V. Hypertension as a risk factor for spontaneous intracerebral hemorrhage. Stroke 1986;17:1078.
7. Rosamond W, Flegal K, Friday G, et al. AHA heart disease and stroke statistics—2007 update. Circulation 2007;115:69.
8. Morganstern LB, Smith MA, Lisabeth LD, et al. Excess stroke in Mexican Americans compared with non-Hispanic whites: the Brain Attack Surveillance in Corpus Christi Project. Am J Epidemiol 2004;160:376.
9. Furlan AJ, Whisnant JP, Elveback LR. The decreasing incidence of primary intracerebral hemorrhage: a population study. Ann Neurol 1979;5:367.
10. Kunitz SC, Gross CR, Heyman A, et al. Pilot Stroke Data Bank: definition, design, and data. Stroke 1984;15:740.
11. Nencini P, Inzitari D, Baruffi MC, et al. Incidence of stroke in young adults in Florence, Italy. Stroke 1988;19:977.
12. Lin CH, Shimizu Y, Kato H, et al. Cerebrovascular diseases in a fixed population of Hiroshima and

Nagasaki, with special reference to relationship between type and risk factors. Stroke 1984;15:653.

13. Marini C, Totaro R, De Santis F, et al. Stroke in young adults in the community-based L'Aquila registry: incidence and prognosis. Stroke 2001;32:52.

14. Silverstein A. Neurological complications of anticoagulation therapy: a neurologist's review. Arch Intern Med 1979;139:217.

15. Wintzen AR, de Jonge H, Loeliger EA, Bots GTAM. The risk of intracerebral hemorrhage during oral anticoagulant treatment: a population study. Ann Neurol 1984;16:553.

16. Kase CS, Robinson RK, Stein RW, et al. Anticoagulant-related intracerebral hemorrhage. Neurology 1985;35:943.

17. Calandre L, Arnal C, Ortega JF, et al. Risk factors for spontaneous cerebral hematomas: case-control study. Stroke 1986;17:1126.

18. Donahue RP, Abbott RD, Reed DM, et al. Alcohol and hemorrhagic stroke. The Honolulu Heart Program. JAMA 1986;255:2311.

19. Iso H, Jacobs DR Jr, Wenworth D, et al. Serum cholesterol levels and six year mortality from stroke in 350,977 men screened for the multiple risk factor intervention trial. N Engl J Med 1989;320:904.

20. Bang OY, Saver JL, Liebeskind DS, et al. Cholesterol level and symptomatic hemorrhagic transformation after ischemic stroke thrombolysis. Neurology 2007;68:737.

21. The Stroke Prevention by Aggressive Reduction in Cholesterol Levels (SPARCL) Investigators. High-dose atorvastatin after stroke or transient ischemic attack. N Engl J Med 2006;355:549.

22. Welch KMA; for the SPARCL Investigators. Statin therapy after stroke or transient ischemic attack (letters to the editor). N Engl J Med 2006;355:2368.

23. Woo D, Kissela BM, Khoury JC, et al. Hypercholesterolemia, HMG-CoA reductase inhibitors and risk of intracerebral hemorrhage: a case-control study. Stroke 2004;35:1360.

24. Sloan MA, Price TR, Foulkes MA, et al. Circadian rhythmicity of stroke onset: intracerebral and subarachnoid hemorrhage. Stroke 1992;23:1420.

25. Galleranti M, Trappella G, Manfredini R, et al. Acute intracerebral hemorrhage: circadian and circannual patterns of onset. Act Neurol Scand 1994;89:280.

26. Kittner SJ, Stern BJ, Feeser BR, et al. Pregnancy and the risk of stroke. N Engl J Med 1996;335:768.

27. Ros H, Lichtenstein P, Bellocco R, et al. Increased risk of circulatory diseases in late pregnancy and puerperium. Epidemiology 2001;12:456.

28. Biller J, Jones MP, Bruno A, et al. Seasonal variation of stroke: does it exist? Neuroepidemiology 1988;7:89.

29. Jolly SS, Rai B, Singh N, et al. Cerebrovascular accidents in young adults (15-40 years): a study of 253 cases. Indian J Med Sci 1971;25:518.

30. Chopra JS, Prabhakar S. Clinical features and risk factors in stroke in young. Acta Neurol Scand 1979;60:289.

31. Lacy JR, Filley CM, Earnest MP, Graff-Radford NR. Brain infarction and hemorrhage in young and middle-aged adults. West J Med 1984;141:329.

32. Hilton-Jones D, Warlow CP. The causes of stroke in the young. J Neurol 1985;232:137.

33. Hachinski V, Norris JW. The young stroke. In Idem, ed. The Acute Stroke. Philadelphia: FA Davis, 1985.

34. Radhakrishnan K, Ashok PP, Sridharan R, Mousa ME. Stroke in the young: Incidence and pattern in Benghazi, Lybia. Acta Med Scand 1986;73:344.

35. Gautier JC, Pradat-Diehl P, Loron PH, et al. Accidents vasculaires cerebraux de sujets ans. Rev Neurol 1989;6-7:437.

36. Bevan H, Sharma K, Bradley W. Stroke in young adults. Stroke 1990;21:382.

37. Toffol GJ, Biller J, Adams HP Jr. Nontraumatic intracerebral hemorrhage in young adults. Arch Neurol 1987;44:483.

38. Adams HP Jr, Biller J. Hemorrhagic intracranial vascular disease. In Joynt RJ, ed. Clinical Neurology. Philadelphia: JB Lippincott, 1988.

39. Caplan L. Intracerebral hemorrhage revisited. Neurology 1988;38:624.

40. Adams HP Jr, Marsh EE. Intraparenchymal hemorrhage. Curr Opin Neurol Neurosurg 1989;2:52.

41. McCormick WF. The pathology of vascular ("arteriovenous") malformations. J Neurosurg 1966;24:865.

42. Stein BM, Wolpert SM. Arteriovenous malformations of the brain, I: current concepts and treatment. Arch Neurol 1980;37:1.

43. Kelly JJ Jr, Mellinger JF, Sundt TM Jr. Intracranial arteriovenous malformations in childhood. Ann Neurol 1978;3:338.

44. Snead OC, Acker JD, Morawetz R. Familial arteriovenous malformation. Ann Neurol 1979;5:585.

45. Brunelle FOS, Harwood-Nash DCF, Fitz CR, Chuang SH. Intracranial vascular malformations in children: computed tomographic and angiographic evaluation. Radiology 1983;149:455.

46. Celli P, Ferrante L, Palma L, Cavedon G. Cerebral arteriovenous malformations in children: clinical features and outcome of treatment in children and in adults. Surg Neurol 1984;22:43.

47. Fong D, Chan S. Arteriovenous malformations in children. Child Nerv Syst 1988;4:199.

48. Malik GM, Sadasivan B, Knighton RS, Ausman JI. The management of arteriovenous malformations in children. Child Nerv Syst 1991;7:43.

49. Smith ER, Butler WE, Ogilvy CS. Surgical approaches to vascular anomalies of the child's brain. Clin Opin Neurol 2002;15:165.

50. Kondzioka D, Humphreys RP, Hoffman HJ, et al. Arteriovenous malformations of the brain in children: a forty year experience. Can J Neurol Sci 1992;19:40.

51. Bristol RE, Albuquerque FC, Spetzler RF, et al. Surgical management of arteriovenous malformations in children. J Neurosurg 2006;105(2 suppl Pediatrics):88.

52. Cohen-Gadol AA, Pollock BE. Radiosurgery for arteriovenous malformations in children. J Neurosurg 2006;104:388.

53. Aminoff MJ. Vascular anomalies in the intracranial dura mater. Brain 1973;6:601.

54. Aminoff MJ, Kendall BE. Asymptomatic dural vascular anomalies. Br J Radiol 1973;46:662.

55. Kosnik EJ, Hunt WE, Miller CA. Dural arteriovenous malformations. J Neurosurg 1974;40:322.
56. Albright AL, Latchaw RE, Price RA. Posterior dural arteriovenous malformations in infancy. Neurosurgery 1983;13:129.
57. Awad IA, Little JR, Akrawi WP, et al. Intracranial dural arteriovenous malformations: factors predisposing to an aggressive neurological course. J Neurosurg 1990;72:839.
58. Pascual-Castroviejo I. The association of extra-cranial and intracranial vascular malformations in children. Can J Neurol Sci 1985;12:139.
59. Waller JD, Greenberg JH, Lewis CW. Hereditary hemorrhagic telangiectasia with cerebrovascular malformations. Arch Dermatol 1976;112:49.
60. Adams HP Jr, Bosch EP. Neurologic aspects of hereditary hemorrhagic telangiectasia: report of two cases. Arch Neurol 1977;34:101.
61. Roman G, Fisher M, Perl DP, et al. Neurological manifestations of hereditary hemorrhagic telangiectasia (Rendu-Osler-Weber disease): Report of two cases and review of the literature. Ann Neurol 1978;4:130.
62. Djindjian M, Djindjian R, Hurth M, et al. Spinal cord arteriovenous malformations and the Klippel-Trenaunay-Weber syndrome. Surg Neurol 1977;8:229.
63. Benhaiem-Sigaux N, Zerah M, Gherardi R, et al. A retromedullary arteriovenous fistula associated with the Klippel-Trenaunay-Weber syndrome: a clinicopathologic study. Acta Neuropathol (Berl) 1985;66:318.
64. Silverman BK, Brekz T, Craig J, et al. Congestive failure in the newborn caused by cerebral AV fistula. Am J Dis Child 1959;89:539.
65. Watson DG, Smith RR, Brann AW Jr. Arteriovenous malformation of the vein of Galen. Am J Dis Child 1976;130:520.
66. Diebler C, Dulac O, Renier D, et al. Aneurysms of the vein of Galen in infants aged 2 to 15 months: diagnosis and natural evolution. Neuroradiology 1981;21:185.
67. Hoffman HJ, Chuang S, Hendrick EB, et al. Malformations of the vein of Galen: experience at The Hospital for Sick Children, Toronto. J Neurosurg 1982;57:316.
68. Moodie DS, Sterba R, Rothner AD, et al. Great vein of Galen malformations in infancy. Cleve Clin Q 1983;50:295.
69. Grossman RI, Bruce DA, Zimmerman RA, et al. Vascular steal associated with vein of Galen aneurysm. Neuroradiology 1984;26:381.
70. Mickle JP, Quisling RG. The transtorcular embolization of vein of Galen aneurysms. J Neurosurg 1986;64:731.
71. Johnston IH, Whittle IR, Besser M, Morgan MK. Vein of Galen malformation: diagnosis and management. Neurosurgery 1987;20:747.
72. King WA, Wackym A, Viñuela F, Peacock WJ. Management of vein of Galen aneurysms: combined surgical and endovascular approach. Child Nerv Syst 1989;5:208.
73. Becker DH, Townsend JJ, Kramer RA, Newton TH. Occult cerebrovascular malformation: a series of
74. 18 histologically verified cases with negative angiography. Brain 1979;102:249.
74. Wharen RE, Scheithauer BW, Laws ER Jr. Thrombosed arteriovenous malformations of the brain: an important entity in the differential diagnosis of intractable focal seizures. J Neurosurg 1982;57:520.
75. Cohen HCM, Tucker WS, Humphreys RP, Perrin RJ. Angiographically cryptic histologically verified cerebrovascular malformations. Neurosurgery 1982;10:704.
76. Vaquero J, Leunda G, Martinez R, Bravo G. Cavernomas of the brain. Neurosurgery 1983;12:208.
77. Hayman LA, Evans RA, Ferrell RE, et al. Familial cavernous angiomas: natural history and genetic study over a 5-year period. Am J Med Genet 1982;11:147.
78. Gomori JM, Grossman RI, Goldberg HI, et al. Occult cerebral vascular malformation: high-field MR imaging. Radiology 1986;158:707.
79. King WA, Martin NA. Intracerebral hemorrhage due to arteriovenous malformations and fistulae. Neurosurg Clin North Am 1992;3:577.
80. Brown RD Jr, Flemming KD, Meyer FB, et al. Natural history, evaluation and management of intracranial vascular malformations. Mayo Clin Proc 2005;80:269.
81. Zambraski J, Henn J, Coons S. Pathology of cerebral vascular malformations. Neurosurg Clin North Am 1999;10:395.
82. Dashti SR, Hoffer A, Hu YC, Selman WR. Molecular genetics of familial cerebral cavernous malformations. Neurosurg Focus 2006;21:E2.
83. Vernooij MW, Ikram MA, Tanghe HL, et al. Incidental findings on brain MRI in the general population. N Engl J Med 2007;357:1821.
84. Newcomb AL, Munns GF. Rupture of aneurysm of the circle of Willis in the newborn. Pediatrics 1949;3:769.
85. Matson DD. Intracranial arterial aneurysms in childhood. J Neurosurg 1965;23:578.
86. Patel AN, Richardson AE. Ruptured intracranial aneurysms in the first two decades of life. J Neurosurg 1971;35:571.
87. Sedzimir CB, Robinson J. Intracranial hemorrhage in children and adolescents. J Neurosurg 1973;38:269.
88. Shucart WA, Wolpert SM. Intracranial arterial aneurysms in childhood. Am J Dis Child 1974;127:288.
89. Almeida GM, Pindaro J, Plese P, et al. Intracranial arterial aneurysms in infancy and childhood. Child Brain 1977;3:193.
90. Lee YJ, Kandall SR, Ghali VS. Intracranial arterial aneurysm in a newborn. Arch Neurol 1978;35:171.
91. Gerosa M, Licata C, Fiore D, Iraci G. Intracranial aneurysms of childhood. Child Brain 1980;6:295.
92. Keren G, Barzilay Z, Cohen BE. Ruptured intracranial arterial aneurysm in the first year of life. Arch Neurol 1980;37:392.
93. Storrs BB, Humphreys RP, Hendrick EB, Hoffman HJ. Intracranial aneurysms in the pediatric age-group. Child Brain 1982;9:358.
94. Ito M, Yoshihara M, Ishii M, et al. Cerebral aneurysms in children. Brain Dev 1992;14:263.
95. Locksley HB. Report of the Cooperative Study of Intracranial Aneurysms and Subarachnoid

Hemorrhage. Section V, part I: natural history of subarachnoid hemorrhage, intracranial aneurysms and arteriovenous malformations. J Neurosurg 1966;25:219.

96. Stehbens WE. Aneurysms and anatomical variations of cerebral arteries. Arch Pathol 1963;75:45.

97. Kontusaari R, Tromp G, Kuivaniemi H, et al. Inheritance of an RNA splicing mutation (G $+^{IIVS20}$) in the type III Procollagen gene (COL3AI) in a family having aortic aneurysms and easy bruisability: phenotypic overlap between familial arterial aneurysms and Ehlers Danlos syndrome type IV. Am J Hum Genet 1990;47:112.

98. Finney HL, Roberts TS, Anderson RE. Giant intracranial aneurysm associated with Marfan's syndrome. J Neurosurg 1976;45:342.

99. ter Berg HWM, Bijlsma JB, Pires JAV, et al. Familial association of intracranial aneurysms and multiple congenital anomalies. Arch Neurol 1986;43:30.

100. Neil-Dwyer G, Bartlett JR, Nicholls AC, et al. Collagen deficiency and ruptured cerebral aneurysms: a clinical and biochemical study. J Neurosurg 1983;59:16.

101. Bigelow NH. The association of polycystic kidneys with intracranial aneurysms and other related disorders. Am J Med Sci 1953;325:485.

102. Ditlefsen EML, Tonjum AM. Intracranial aneurysms and polycystic kidneys. Acta Med Scand 1960;168:51.

103. Chapman AB, Rubinstein D, Hughes R, et al. Intracranial aneurysms in autosomal dominant polycystic kidney disease. N Engl J Med 1992;327:916.

104. Natowicz M, Kelley RI. Mendelian etiologies of stroke. Ann Neurol 1987;22:175.

105. Bannerman RM, Ingall GB, Graf CJ. The familial occurrence of intracranial aneurysms. Neurology 1970;20:283.

106. Brisman R, Abbassioun K, Brisman R. Familial intracranial aneurysms. J Neurosurg 1971;34:678.

107. Halal F, Mohr G, Toussi T, Martinez SN. Intracranial aneurysms: a report of a large pedigree. Am J Med Genet 1983;15:89.

108. Dippel DWJ, ter Berg JWM, Habbema JDF. Screening for unruptured familial intracranial aneurysms: a decision analysis. Acta Neurol Scand 1992;86:381.

109. Benoit BG, Cochrane DD, Durity F, et al. Clinical-radiological correlates in intracerebral hematomas due to aneurysmal rupture. Can J Neurol Sci 1982;9:409.

110. Bohmfalk GL, Story JL, Wissinger JP, Brown WE. Bacterial intracranial aneurysms. J Neurosurg 1978;48:369.

111. Morawetz RB, Acker JD, Harsh GR III. Management of mycotic (bacterial) intracranial aneurysms. Contemp Neurosurg 1981;3:1-6.

112. McCormick WF, Rosenfield DB. Massive brain hemorrhage. Stroke 1973;4:946.

113. Brott T, Thalinger K, Hertzberg V. Hypertension as a risk factor for spontaneous intracerebral hemorrhage. Stroke 1986;17:1078.

114. Haerer AF, Smith RR. Cerebrovascular disease of young adults in a Mississippi teaching hospital. Stroke 1970;1:466.

115. Scardigli K, Biller J, Brooks M, et al. Pontine hemorrhage in a patient with pheochromocytoma. Arch Intern Med 1985;145:343.

116. The Fifth Report of the Joint National Committee on Detection, Evaluation, and Treatment of High Blood Pressure (JNC V). National High Blood Pressure Education Program, National Heart, Lung, and Blood Institute. Bethesda, MD, National Institutes of Health, 1992.

117. Groch SN, Sayre GP, Heck FJ. Cerebral hemorrhage in leukemia. Arch Neurol 1960;2:439.

118. Pochedly C. Neurologic manifestations in acute leukemias, I: symptoms due to increased cerebrospinal fluid pressure and hemorrhage. N Y State J Med 1975;75:575.

119. Davies-Jones GAB, Preston FE, Timperley WR. Neurological Complications in Clinical Haematology. Oxford: Blackwell Scientific Publications, 1980.

120. Humphreys RP, Hockley AD, Freedman MH, Saunders EF. Management of intracerebral hemorrhage in idiopathic thrombocytopenic purpura. J Neurosurg 1976;45:700.

121. Woerner SI, Abildgaard CF, French BN. Intracranial hemorrhage in children with idiopathic thrombocytopenic purpura. Pediatrics 1981;67:453.

122. Krivit W, Tate D, White JG, Robison LL. Idiopathic thrombocytopenic purpura and intracranial hemorrhage. Pediatrics 1981;67:570.

123. Almaani WS, Awidi AS. Spontaneous intracranial bleeding in hemorrhagic diathesis. Surg Neurol 1982;17:137.

124. Marcus AL. Platelets and their disorders. In Ratnoff OD, Forbes CD, eds. Disorders of Hemostasis, 2nd ed. Philadelphia: WB Saunders, 1991.

125. Schwartzman RJ, Hill JB. Neurologic complications of disseminated intravascular coagulation. Neurology 1982;32:791.

126. Ratnoff OD. Disseminated intravascular coagulation. In Ratnoff OD, Forbes CD, eds. Disorders of Hemostasis, 2nd ed. Philadelphia: WB Saunders, 1991.

127. Silverstein A, Gilbert H, Wasserman LR. Neurologic complications of polycythemia. Ann Intern Med 1962;6:909.

128. Grotta JC, Manner C, Pettigrew LC, Yatsu FM. Red blood cell disorders and stroke. Stroke 1986;17:811.

129. Silverstein A. Intracranial bleeding in hemophilia. Arch Neurol 1960;3:141.

130. Baehner RL, Strauss HS. Hemophilia in the first year of life. N Engl J Med 1966;275:524.

131. Eyster ME, Gill FM, Blatt PM, et al. Central nervous system bleeding in hemophiliacs. Blood 1978; 51:1179.

132. Petterson H, McClure P, Fitz C. Intracranial hemorrhage in hemophilic children: CT follow-up. Acta Radiol 1984;25:161.

133. Kasper CK, Boylen AL, Ewing NP, et al. Hematologic management of hemophilia A for surgery. JAMA 1985;253:1279.

134. Martinowitz U, Heim M, Tadmor R, et al. Intracranial hemorrhage in patients with hemophilia. Neurosurgery 1986;18:538.

135. Sutherland JM, Glueck H, Gleser G. Hemorrhagic disease of the newborn: breast feeding is a

necessary factor in the pathogenesis. Am J Dis Child 1967;113:524.

136. Evans AR, Forrester RM, Discombe C. Neonatal hemorrhage following maternal anticonvulsant therapy. Lancet 1970;1:517.

137. Payne NR, Hasegawa DK. Vitamin K deficiency in newborns: a case report in α -1 antitrypsin deficiency and a review of factors predisposing to hemorrhage. Pediatrics 1984;73:712.

138. Chalgren WS. Neurologic complications of the hemorrhagic diseases. Neurology 1953;3:126.

139. Osenbach R, Loftus CM, Menezes A, et al. Management of intraventricular hemorrhage secondary to ruptured arteriovenous malformation in a child with von Willebrand's disease. J Neurol Neurosurg Psychiatry 1989;52:1452.

140. Portnoy BA, Herron JC. Neurological manifestations of sickle cell disease with a review of the literature and emphasis on the prevalence of hemiplegia. Ann Intern Med 1972;76:643.

141. Wood DH. Cerebrovascular complications of sickle cell anemia. Stroke 1978;9:73.

142. Powers D, Wilson B, Imbus C, et al. The natural history of stroke in sickle cell disease. Am J Med 1978;65:461.

143. Van Hoff J, Ritchey AK, Shaywitz BA. Intracranial hemorrhage in children with sickle cell disease. Am J Dis Child 1985;139:1120.

144. Ohene-Frempong K. Stroke in sickle cell disease: demographic, clinical, and therapeutic considerations. Semin Hematol 1991;28:213.

145. Steen RG, Helton KJ, Horwitz EM, et al. Moyamoya in children with sickle cell anemia and cerebrovascular occlusion. J Pediatr 1978;92:808.

146. Dobson SR, Holden KR, Nietert PJ, et al. Moyamoya syndrome in childhood sickle cell disease: a predictive factor for recurrent cerebrovascular events. Blood 2002; 99:3144.

147. Cheatham ML, Brackett CE. Problems in management of subarachnoid hemorrhage in sickle cell anemia. J Neurosurg 1965;23:488.

148. Russell MD, Goldberg HI, Hodson A, et al. Effect of transfusion therapy on arteriographic abnormalities and on recurrence of stroke in sickle cell disease. Blood 1984;63:162.

149. Sinniah D, Ekert H, Bosco J, et al. Intracranial hemorrhage and circulating coagulation inhibitor in β-thalassemia major. J Pediatr 1981;99:700.

150. Kase CS. Intracerebral hemorrhage: non-hypertensive causes. Stroke 1986;17:590.

151. Forsting M, Mattle HP, Huber P. Anticoagulation-related intracerebral hemorrhage. Cerebrovasc Dis 1991;1:97.

152. Forfar JC. Prediction of hemorrhage in patients on long-term oral coumarin anticoagulation by excessive prothrombin ratio. Am Heart J 1982; 102:445.

153. Adams HP Jr, del Zoppo G, Alberts MJ, et al. Guidelines for the early management of adults with ischemic stroke. Stroke 2007;38:1655.

154. Marder VJ. The use of thrombolytic agents: choice of patient, drug, administration, laboratory monitoring. Ann Intern Med 1979;90:802.

155. Kase CS, O'Neal AM, Fisher M, et al. Intracranial hemorrhage after use of tissue plasminogen activator for coronary thrombolysis. Ann Intern Med 1990;112:17.

156. Gore JM, Sloan M, Price TR, et al. Intra cerebral hemorrhage, cerebral infarction, and subdural hematoma after acute myocardial infarction and thrombolytic therapy in the Thrombolysis in Myocardial Infarction study: Thrombolysis in Myocardial Infarction, phase II, pilot and clinical data. Circulation 1991;83:448.

157. Kase CS, Pessin MS, Zivin JA, et al. Intracranial hemorrhage after coronary thrombolysis with tissue plasminogen activator. Am J Med 1992;92:384.

158. Eleff SM, Borel C, Bell WR, Long DM. Acute management of intracranial hemorrhage in patients receiving thrombolytic therapy: case reports. Neurosurgery 1990;26:867.

159. Matthay KK, Koerper MA, Ablin AR. Intracranial hemorrhage in congenital factor VII deficiency. J Pediatr 1979;94:413.

160. Kovalainen S, Myllyla VV, Tolonen U, Hokkanen E. Recurrent subarachnoid hemorrhages in patients with Hageman factor deficiency. Lancet 1979;1:1035.

161. Kitchens C, Newcomb T. Factor XIII. Medicine 1979;58:413.

162. Jellinger K. Cerebrovascular amyloidosis with cerebral hemorrhage. J Neurol 1977;214:195.

163. Tomonaga M. Cerebral amyloid angiopathy in the elderly. J Am Geriatr Soc 1981;29:151.

164. Vinters HV, Gilbert JJ. Cerebral amyloid angiopathy: incidence and complications in the aging brain, II: the distribution of amyloid vascular changes. Stroke 1983;14:924.

165. Vinters HV. Cerebral amyloid angiopathy: a critical review. Stroke 1987;18:311.

166. Levy E, Lopez-Otin C, Ghiso J, et al. Stroke in Icelandic patients with hereditary amyloid angiopathy is related to a mutation in the cystatin C gene, an inhibitor of cysteine proteases. J Exp Med 1989;169:1771.

167. Grubb A, Jensson O, Gudmundsson G, et al. Abnormal metabolism of γ-trace alkaline microprotein: the basic defect in hereditary cerebral hemorrhage with amyloidosis. N Engl J Med 1984;311:1547.

168. Jennson O, Palsdothir A, Thorsteinsson A, Arnason A. The saga of cystatin C gene mutation causing amyloid angiopathy and brain hemorrhage—clinical genetics in Iceland. Clin Genet 1989;36:368.

169. Van Duinen SG, Castaflo EM, Prelli F, et al. Hereditary cerebral hemorrhage with amyloidosis in patients of Dutch origin is related to Alzheimer disease. Proc Natl Acad Sci U S A 1987;84:5991.

170. Moore PM, Cupps TR. Neurological complications of vasculitis. Ann Neurol 1983;14:155.

171. Cohen BA, Biller J. Hemorrhagic stroke due to cerebral vasculitis and the role of immunosuppressive therapy. Neurosurg Clin North Am 1992;3:611.

172. Biller J, Sparks LH. Diagnosis and management of cerebral vasculitis. In Adams HP Jr, ed. Handbook of Cerebrovascular Diseases. New York: Marcel Dekker, 1993.

173. Schneck MJ, Biller J. Hemorrhagic stroke in the tropics. Semin Neurol 2005;25:300.
174. Ferris EJ, Levine HL. Cerebral arteritis: classification. Neuroradiology 1973;109:326.
175. Edwards KR. Hemorrhagic complications of cerebral arteritis. Arch Neurol 1977;34:549.
176. Suzuki J, Takaku A. Cerebrovascular "Moyamoya" disease. Arch Neurol 1969;20:288.
177. Caplan LR, Hier DB, Banks G. Current concepts of cerebrovascular disease: stroke and drug abuse. Stroke 1982;13:869.
178. Kaku DA, Lavenstein DH. Emergence of recreational drug abuse as a major risk factor for stroke in young adults. Ann Intern Med 1990;113:821.
179. McEvoy AW, Kitchen ND, Thomas DGT. Intracerebral hemorrhage and drug abuse in young adults. Br J Neurosurg 2000;14:449.
180. Citron BP, Halpern M, McCaroon L, et al. Necrotizing angiitis associated with drug abuse. N Engl J Med 1970;283:1003.
181. Margolis MT, Newton TH. Methamphetamine ("speed") arteritis. Neuroradiology 1971;2:179.
182. Delaney P, Estes M. Intracranial hemorrhage with amphetamine abuse. Neurology 1980;30:1125.
183. Harrington H, Heller A, Dawson D, et al. Intracerebral hemorrhage and oral amphetamine. Arch Neurol 1983;40:503.
184. Lukes SA. Intracerebral hemorrhage from an arteriovenous malformation after amphetamine injection. Arch Neurol 1983;40:60.
185. Nalls G, Disher A, Daryabagi J, et al. Subcortical cerebral hemorrhage associated with cocaine abuse: CT and MR findings. J Comput Assist Tomogr 1989;13:1.
186. Klonoff DC, Andrews BT, Obana WG. Stroke associated with cocaine use. Arch Neurol 1989; 46:989.
187. Mercado A, Johnson G, Calver D, Sokol RJ. Cocaine, pregnancy, and postpartum intracerebral hemorrhage. Obstet Gynecol 1989;73:467.
188. Green RM, Kelly KM, Gabrielsen T, et al. Multiple intracerebral hemorrhages after smoking "crack" cocaine. Stroke 1990;21:957.
189. Levine SR, Brust JCM, Futrell N, et al. Cerebrovascular complications of the use of "crack" form of alkaloidal cocaine. N Engl J Med 1990;323:699.
190. Bernstein E, Diskant BM. Phenylpropanolamine: a potentially hazardous drug. Ann Emerg Med 1982;11:311.
191. Mueller SM, Muller J, Asdell SM. Cerebral hemorrhage associated with phenylpropanolamine in consumption with caffeine. Stroke 1984;15:119.
192. Fallis RJ, Fisher M. Cerebral vasculitis and hemorrhage associated with phenylpropanolamine. Neurology 1985;35:405.
193. Kase CS, Foster TE, Reed JE, et al. Intracerebral hemorrhage and phenylpropanolamine use. Neurology 1987;37:399.
194. Caplan LR, Thomas C, Banks G. Central nervous system complications of addiction to T's and blues. Neurology 1982;32:623.
195. King J, Richards M, Tress B. Cerebral arteritis associated with heroin abuse. Med J Aust 1978;2:444.
196. Shapiro R, Biller J. Pure motor hemiplegia associated with phenelzine use. Ill Med J 1983;16:278.
197. Wooten MR, Khangure MS, Murphy MJ. Intracerebral hemorrhage and vasculitis related to ephedrine abuse. Ann Neurol 1983;13:337.
198. Yin P-A. Ephedrine induced intracerebral hemorrhage and central nervous system vasculitis. Stroke 1990;21:1641.
199. Loizou LA, Hamilton JG, Tsementzis SA. Intracranial hemorrhage in association with pseudoephedrine overdosage. J Neurol Neurosurg Psychiatry 1982;45:471.
200. Aggarwal SK, Williams V, Levine SR, et al. Cocaine associated intracranial hemorrhage: absence of vasculitis in 14 cases. Neurology 1996;46:1741.
201. Scott M. Spontaneous intracerebral hematoma caused by cerebral neoplasms: report of eight verified cases. J Neurosurg 1975;42:338.
202. Little JR, Dial B, Bellenger G, Carpenter S. Brain hemorrhage from intracranial tumor. Stroke 1979;10:283.
203. Wakai S, Yamakawa K, Manaka S, Takakura K. Spontaneous intracranial hemorrhage caused by brain tumor: its incidence and clinical significance. Neurosurgery 1982;10:437.
204. Bitoh S, Hasegawa H, Ohtsuki H, et al. Cerebral neoplasms initially presenting with massive intracerebral hemorrhage. Surg Neurol 1984;22:57.
205. Barnett HJM, Hyland HH. Noninfective intracranial venous thrombosis. Brain 1953;76:36.
206. Bousser MG, Chiras J, Bones J, Castaigne P. Cerebral venous thrombosis—a review of 38 cases. Stroke 1985;16:199.
207. Caplan LR, Skillman J, Ojemann R, Fields WS. Intracerebral hemorrhage following carotid endarterectomy: a hypertensive complication? Stroke 1978;9:457.
208. Solomon RA, Loftus CM, Quest DO, Correll JW. Incidence and etiology of intracerebral hemorrhage following carotid endarterectomy. J Neurosurg 1986;64:29.
209. Heros RC, Nelson PB. Intracerebral hemorrhage after microsurgical cerebral revascularization. Neurosurgery 1980;6:371.
210. Humphreys RP, Hoffman HJ, Mustard WT, Trusier GA. Cerebral hemorrhage following heart surgery. J Neurosurg 1975;43:671.
211. Anderson DE, Biller J, Schreiber RR. Spontaneous cerebellar hemorrhage after coronary artery bypass surgery. Eur Neurol 1985;24:145.
212. Vaquero J, Cabezudo JM, DeSola G, Nombela L. Intratumoral hemorrhage in posterior fossa tumors after ventricular drainage: report of two cases. J Neurosurg 1981;54:406.
213. Waga S, Shimosaka S, Sakakura M. Intracerebral hemorrhage remote from the site of the initial surgical procedure. Neurosurgery 1983;13:662.
214. Snow RB, Zimmerman RD, Devinsky O. Delayed intracerebral hemorrhage after ventriculoperitoneal shunting. Neurosurgery 1986;19:305.
215. Stanley LD, Suss RA. Intracerebral hematoma secondary to lightning stroke: case report and review of the literature. Neurosurgery 1985;16:686.

216. Barbas N, Caplan LR, Baquis G, et al. Dental chair intracerebral hemorrhage. Neurology 1987;37:511.
217. Shuaib A, Metz L, Hing T. Migraine and intracerebral hemorrhage. Cephalalgia 1989;9:59.
218. Onoyama K, Ibayashi S, Nanishi F, et al. Cerebral hemorrhage in patients on maintenance hemodialysis. Eur Neurol 1987;26:171.
219. Phang PT, Passerini L, Mielke B, et al. Brain hemorrhage associated with methanol poisoning. Crit Care Med 1988;16:137.
220. Van de Kelft E, Bosmans J, Parizel PM, et al. Intracerebral hemorrhage after lumbar myelography with iohexol: report of a case review of the literature. Neurosurgery 1991;28:570.
221. Fisher CM. Clinical sydromes in cerebral hemorrhage. In Fields WS, ed. Pathogenesis and Treatment of Cerebrovascular Disease. Springfield, IL: Charles C Thomas, 1961.
222. Gebel JM, Broderick JP. Intracerebral hemorrhage. Neurol Clin 2000;18:419.
223. Brott T, Broderick J, Kothari R, et al. Early hemorrhage growth in patients with intracerebral hemorrhage. Stroke 1997;28:1.
224. Davis SM, Broderick J, Hennerici M, et al. Hematoma growth is a determinant of mortality and poor outcome after intracerebral hemorrhage. Neurology 2005;66:1175.
225. Hemphill JC 3rd, Bonovich DC, Besmertis L, et al. The ICH score: a simple reliable grading scale for intracerebral hemorrhage. Stroke 2001;32:891.
226. Cheung RT, Zou LY. Use of the original modified or new intracerebral hemorrhage score to predict mortality and morbidity after intracerebral hemorrhage. Stroke 2003;34:1717.
227. Weimar C, Benemann J, Diener HC. German Stroke Study Collaboration. Development and validation of the Essen Intracerebral Haemorrhage Score. J Neurol Neurosurg Psychiatry 2006;77:601.
228. Hier DB, Davis KR, Richardson EP, Mohr JP. Hypertensive putaminal hemorrhage. Ann Neurol 1977;1:152.
229. Ropper AH, Davis KR. Lobar cerebral hemorrhage: acute clinical syndromes in 26 cases. Ann Neurol 1980;8:141.
230. Weisberg LA. Thalamic hemorrhage: clinical-CT correlations. Neurology 1986;36:1382.
231. Fisher CM, Picard EH, Polak A, et al. Acute hypertensive cerebellar hemorrhage: diagnosis and surgical treatment. J Nerv Ment Dis 1966;140:38.
232. Goto N, Kaneko M, Hosaka Y, Koga H. Primary pontine hemorrhage: clinicopathological correlations. Stroke 1980;11:84.
233. Caplan LR, Goodwin J. Lateral tegmental brainstem hemorrhages. Neurology 1980;32:252.
234. Schellinger PD, Jansen O, Fiebach JB, et al. Standardized MRI stroke protocol : comparison with CT in hyperacute intracerebral hemorrhage. Stroke 1999;30:765.
235. Jinkins JR. Current neuroradiological investigations of spontaneous hemorrhage into the craniospinal axis. Neurosurgery 1986;18:664.
236. Frank JI, Biller J. Laboratory evaluation of intracerebral hemorrhage. In Feldman E, ed. Intracerebral Hemorrhage. Mt. Kisco, NY: Futura Publishing, 1994.
237. Broderick J,Connolly S, Feldmann E, et al. Guidelines for the management of spontaneous intracerebral hemorrhage in adults: 2007 update. Stroke 2007;38:2001.
238. Qureshi AI, Harris-Lane P, Kirmani JF, et al. Treatment of acute hypertension in patients with intracerebral hemorrhage using American Heart Associate guidelines. Crit Care Med 2006;34:1975.
239. Cartmill M, Dolan G, Byrne JL, Byrne PO. Prothrombin complex concentrate for oral anticoagulant reversal in neurosurgical emergencies. Br J Neurosurg 2000;14:458.
240. Vigue B, Ract C, Tremey B, et al. Ultra-rapid management of oral anticoagulant therapy-related surgical intracranial hemorrhage. Intensive Care Med 2007;33:721.
241. Mayer SA, Brun NC, Begtrup K, et al. Recombinant activated factor VII for acute intracerebral hemorrhage. N Engl J Med 2005;352:777.
242. McKissock W, Richardson A, Taylor J. Primary intracerebral hemorrhage: a controlled trial of surgical and conservative treatment in 180 unselected cases. Lancet 1961;2:221.
243. Kammo T, Sano H, Shinomiya Y, et al. Role of surgery in hypertensive intracerebral hematoma: a comparative study of 305 nonsurgical and 154 surgical cases. J Neurosurg 1984;61:1091.
244. Juvela S, Heiskanen O, Poranen A, et al. The treatment of spontaneous intracerebral hemorrhage: a prospective randomized trial of surgical and conservative treatment. J Neurosurg 1989;70:755.
245. Auer LM, Deisberger W, Niederkorn K, et al. Endoscopic surgery versus medical treatment for spontaneous intracerebral hematoma: a randomized study. J Neurosurg 1989;70:530.
246. Batjer HH, Reisch JS, Allen BC, et al. Failure of surgery to improve outcome in hypertensive putaminal hemorrhage. Arch Neurol 1990;47:1103.
247. Fewel ME, Thompson BG Jr, Hoff JT. Spontaneous intracerebral hemorrhage: a review. Neurosurg Focus 2003;15:1-16.
248. Hsieh PC, Awad IA, Getch CC, et al. Current updates in perioperative management of intracerebral hemorrhage. Neurol Clin 2006;24:745.

CHAPTER 15

Subarachnoid Hemorrhage in Young Adults

Lotfi Hacein-Bey • Thomas C. Origitano • José Biller

Etiology, Epidemiology, and Risk Factor Modification

Subarachnoid hemorrhage (SAH) is defined as the abnormal presence of blood in the subarachnoid space, which is normally filled only by cerebrospinal fluid (CSF). Most instances of SAH encountered in young patients result from head injury from mechanical trauma, usually in relation to motor vehicle collisions. This chapter deals only with nontraumatic or "spontaneous" SAH.

Causes of Nontraumatic Subarachnoid Hemorrhage in Young Patients

Most (70% to 80%) cases of SAH in young patients (as in older patients) are due to a ruptured intracranial aneurysm.[1,2] Most cerebral aneurysms are saccular, although other types of aneurysms are present in younger patients and are discussed in detail in this chapter. Approximately 10% of young patients whose clinical presentation is more favorable, whose SAH is confined to posterior fossa cisterns, and in whom investigations fail to show an aneurysm, have a benign and self-limiting cause of SAH, termed "perimesencephalic hemorrhage." Other causes of SAH in young patients include ruptured arteriovenous malformations (AVMs), which may be pial, dural, or located at the spinal cord level; arterial hypertension (usually in association with intraparenchymal hemorrhage); use of illicit drugs, such as cocaine; primary or secondary brain tumors; vasculitides; hemoglobinopathies and coagulation disorders; arterial dissections; and dural sinus thrombosis (Table 15-1).[1,2]

TABLE 15-1   **Causes of Spontaneous Subarachnoid Hemorrhage in Young Adults**

Cerebral aneurysm rupture
Perimesencephalic hemorrhage
Vascular malformation rupture (AVM, arteriovenous
   fistula, cavernous malformations)
Other
   Congenital disorders
      Coarctation of the aorta
      Pseudoxanthoma elasticum
      Menkes kinky hair syndrome
      Sturge-Weber syndrome
      Tuberous sclerosis complex
      Neurofibromatosis 1
         (von Recklinghausen disease)
      Hereditary hemorrhagic telangiectasia
         (Rendu-Osler disease)
      Ehlers-Danlos syndrome
      Klinefelter syndrome
      Autosomal dominant polycystic kidney disease
   Systemic vascular disease
      Hypertension
      Cerebral embolism
      Moyamoya disease
      Cerebral venous occlusive disease
      Eclampsia
   Hematologic disorders
      Hemophilia
      Aplastic anemia
      Sickle cell anemia
      Leukemias
      Thrombocytopenic purpura
      Anticoagulant therapy
      Thrombolytic therapy
   Infectious diseases
      Infective endocarditis
      Tubercular meningitis
      Luetic meningoencephalitis
      Fungal central nervous system infections
      Infectious mononucleosis
      Tick-borne relapsing fever

Autoimmune disorders
   Systemic lupus erythematosus
   Polyarteritis nodosa
   Henoch-Schönlein purpura
   Poststreptococcal glomerulonephritis
   Kawasaki disease
Other systemic diseases
   Heatstroke
   Conn syndrome
   Thyrotoxicosis
   Wolman disease
   Spinal endometriosis
Neoplasms
   Gliomas
   Meningiomas
   Acoustic neuromas
   Choroid plexus papillomas
   Pituitary adenomas
   Pineocytomas
   Chordomas
   Subependymomas
   Metastatic carcinoma
   Intraspinal neoplasms
Drugs
   Amphetamines
   Cocaine
   Ephedrine
   Monoamine oxidase inhibitors
   Oral contraceptive pills
   Phencyclidine
   Alcohol
Miscellaneous
   α-galactosidase deficiency
   α_1-antitrypsin deficiency
   Cystic fibrosis
   Klippel-Trénaunay-Weber syndrome
   Parry-Romberg syndrome
   3-M syndrome

Epidemiology of Subarachnoid Hemorrhage

Nontraumatic SAH accounts for 4% to 7% of all strokes, although in young patients, SAH is proportionally more represented than ischemic stroke and intracerebral hemorrhage (ICH).[3] The incidence of SAH in North America and Western Europe is 6 to 8 per 100,000 per year and has remained stable for the past 3 decades[3]; this translates into 15,000 to 30,000 new episodes each year in the United States.[4] There are regional variations in the incidence of SAH. A more recent worldwide meta-analysis reported rates of 22.7 per 100,000 per year in Japan, 19.7 per 100,000 per year in Finland, 4.2 per 100,000 per year in South and Central America, and 9.1 per 100,000 per year in the rest of the world. A female predominance has not been found in young subjects, although a 1.24 higher incidence was noted over men after age 55.[5] The same study confirmed an average worldwide decline in SAH of 0.6% per year since 1996.[5]

A study from Iowa[1] found that greater than 30% of strokes in patients 15 to 45 years old were due to SAH, whereas in Finland, reported rates of SAH between the ages of 25 and 45 were 45% in men and 42% in women.[6] Reported percentages of aneurysmal SAH in young adults versus the whole population vary with the population studied. A study from the northern United Kingdom[7] reported that 18.4% of 1609 SAH patients seen over a 9-year period were 18 to 39 years old, whereas another study from Japan of 2493 patients over a 13-year period found that only 5% of all patients were in their third and fourth decades.[8]

Patients with SAH may develop several complications, including rebleeding, hydrocephalus, seizures, vasospasm with or without resulting permanent infarcts, hyponatremia, stunned myocardium and cardiac arrhythmias, pulmonary edema, and other complications. Mortality rates from SAH have been at least stable for the last 30 years and have even been reported by some to have steadily decreased by an average of 0.5% per year owing to major advances in the diagnosis and management of aneurysmal SAH and its complications.[9] Currently, the prognosis for this lethal disease remains dismal, however, with average case-fatality rates ranging from 41% to 51%,[9,10] and only one third of survivors living independently.[9]

Evidence-based Risk Factor Modification Recommendations

Reported nonmodifiable risk factors for aneurysmal SAH include female gender, advancing age, and black race.[10,16] A relatively lower SAH rate in whites compared with non-whites has been challenged,[11] as has been the concept that SAH is more frequent in patients on hormone replacement therapy, patients with hypercholesterolemia, or patients with diabetes.[11] Smoking, hypertension, illicit drugs, and excessive alcohol intake remain the most important modifiable risk factors for SAH. Associations between common cardiovascular risk factors and risk of SAH are not thought to differ much worldwide; a study of Asian and Australasian regions found cigarette smoking and systolic blood pressure to be the most important risk factors for SAH in the Asia-Pacific region, as is the case in Western countries.[12]

More recent studies of prognosis for outcome after aneurysmal SAH have failed to show a difference in mortality after SAH between blacks and other ethnic groups, highlighting the appropriateness of primary prevention programs aimed at modifying risk factors.[13,14] It has been suggested, however,

that certain factors, other than the severity of the initial hemorrhagic event, have a negative impact on outcomes in survivors of SAH; hyperglycemia on admission, excess weight, and hypertension all were found to elevate the risk of cerebral infarction after SAH.[15]

Risk factor modification has been suggested as a means to reduce the frequency of, and the morbidity from, SAH, similar to what has already been shown for intracerebral hemorrhage (ICH).[16,17] Some investigators believe that aneurysmal SAH in young patients is largely preventable by pharmacologic (blood pressure control) or behavioral (cigarette smoking, alcohol use, and recreational drug use) methods.[16] Lifestyle behavioral changes are particularly important to stress because more than one third of prior smokers who are SAH survivors continue to use nicotine products.[17]

Diagnosis
Clinical Diagnosis

The typical clinical manifestations of SAH are headache, nausea, vomiting, nuchal rigidity, and transient alteration in mental status. Most of the time, the diagnosis is straightforward, and the patient is immediately admitted for the appropriate investigations and treatment. A sentinel headache and other warning signs also may be present in some patients (around 10%), and may not be acknowledged by the patient or recognized by physicians. Such "warning leaks" are increasingly considered to be true hemorrhagic episodes, which has management implications on issues such as hydrocephalus and timing of vasospasm.[18]

The headache is classically described as "the worst ever" in the patient's life and commonly localizes to the occipital region before generalizing rapidly. The headache, however, may be subtle; atypically localized; referred as facial, ocular, or low back pain; or even absent. Nuchal rigidity, which is related to meningeal irritation, may be variable or absent, depending on the amount and distribution of blood in the subarachnoid space. There may or may not be a positive Kernig sign, associated vomiting, photophobia, or phonophobia. Likewise, the patient's level of consciousness may vary from normal to a comatose state. Occasionally, a focal neurologic deficit is present at the time of presentation, such as a cranial nerve palsy (particularly the third nerve, adjacent to the posterior communicating artery) or a hemiparesis, which may offer clues to the diagnosis, although it also may wrongly orient the physician toward other diagnoses, such as an ischemic stroke or other pathology.

Failure to recognize and treat SAH promptly may have major clinical and possibly legal implications, particularly because it results in delayed treatment during the period patients are at highest risk for recurrent hemorrhage and death.[4] In young patients at the prime of their lives, one also has to take into account economic loss. SAH survivors whose warning headache is ignored have a worse prognosis than patients treated early.[19] A population-based study in the province of Ontario, Canada, revealed that of 1507 patients admitted with SAH within a 3-year period at all types of medical facilities ranging from large emergency departments to small community hospitals, the rate of misdiagnosis was 5.4%.[20] The risk of misdiagnosis was greater in nonteaching hospitals, although unrelated to annual volumes of SAH seen or access to computed tomography (CT), and greater in emergency departments in patients triaged as low-acuity patients.[20]

Conversely, numerous conditions may be mistaken for SAH (Table 15-2). The most common mimics of SAH are migraine headache,[21] acute viral illness, and acute sinusitis. A particularly painful and recurrent form of headache in young patients has been identified more recently as benign thunderclap headache, which may be associated with cerebral arterial spasm, without evidence of hemorrhage.[22] Benign thunderclap headache is likely associated with generalized abnormal vasoreactivity, similar to preeclampsia, in which circulating "vascular injurants" have been identified, and has been reported to herald acute myocardial infarction.[23] Other conditions that may be mistaken for SAH include tension headache; viral meningitis; seizure; ischemic stroke or transient ischemic attack; systemic bacterial illness; hypertensive encephalopathy[21]; and cervicocephalic arterial dissection, which may involve the carotid, middle cerebral, or vertebral artery, mimicking migraine or cluster headache.[24,25] Very rarely, in young patients, acute disseminated encephalomyelitis or multiple sclerosis may cause an acute severe pain syndrome (i.e., hemicrania and trigeminal neuralgia), which may be mistaken for SAH.[26]

The clinical diagnosis of SAH is greatly aided by CT, which has reported accuracy rates of greater than 98%. Lumbar puncture should be performed in equivocal cases; it has a very low risk in patients whose CT does not show herniation or diffuse cerebral edema. Lumbar puncture can falsely suggest a diagnosis of SAH, however, in patients with an intracerebral hematoma or in patients with a traumatic tap.[27] From 8 to 12 hours of the hemorrhagic event on, the presence of xanthochromia is considered by many authors to be the primary criterion for the diagnosis of SAH in patients with negative CT scans,[2,21,27] although some authors assert that the presence of erythrocytes, even in the absence of xanthochromia, is more accurate.[28]

TABLE 15-2 **Differential Diagnosis of Subarachnoid Hemorrhage**

Tension headache
Migraine headache
Acute sinusitis
Acute viral illness
Systemic infectious illness
Hypertensive encephalopathy
Arterial dissection (carotid, middle cerebral, vertebral artery) mimicking migraine or cluster headache
Viral meningitis
Thunderclap headache
Seizures
Ischemic stroke or transient ischemic attack
Acute demyelinating disease

Radiologic Evaluation

Pathophysiology of Subarachnoid Hemorrhage

Hemorrhage into the subarachnoid space results in the rapid spread of red blood cells (RBCs) into the whole subarachnoid compartment (Fig. 15-1). Often, a hematoma forms at the bleeding site, most commonly a traumatized vessel or a ruptured aneurysm, offering clues as to the site of hemorrhage (Fig. 15-2). The hematoma immediately becomes the target of physiologic fibrinolysis, mostly as a result of the action of plasmin, so that, a few

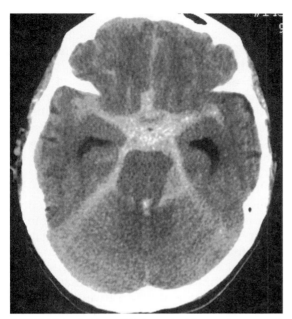

FIGURE 15-1   **SAH on CT.** There is diffuse subarachnoid blood appearing as hyperdense fluid involving most basal cisterns. The temporal horns of the lateral ventricles are enlarged, indicating early hydrocephalus. This patient had a ruptured left superior cerebellar artery, although the offending aneurysm could be in numerous locations.

days after the initial bleed, and barring repeat hemorrhage, there is a gradual decrease in its size. RBCs that are circulating in the subarachnoid space do not usually penetrate the ventricular system early in the absence of direct transependymal hemorrhage, mostly because of the outward pattern of CSF flow exiting the fourth ventricle through the foramina of Magendie and Luschka. Intraventricular hemorrhage (IVH) commonly soon follows SAH, however, owing to saturation of the convexity arachnoid villi, which become trapped and ineffective, and to the increase in circulating RBCs in the subarachnoid space from lysis of the initial hematoma. This situation may cause communicating hydrocephalus, which usually takes a few days to set in, although it can be hyperacute, requiring vigilant management.

The clearance of RBCs in the subarachnoid space is limited compared with other compartments owing to the lack of capillaries in the subarachnoid space; macrophages must reach their sites by diapedesis through capillaries and veins, so their action

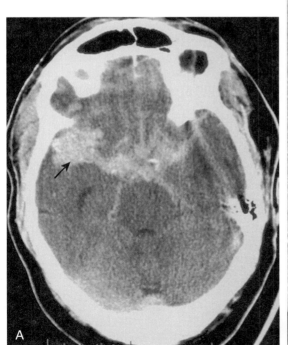

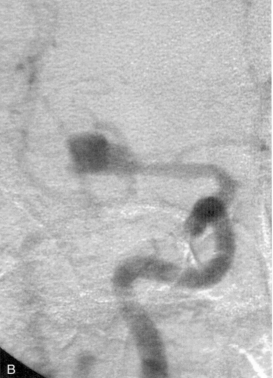

FIGURE 15-2   **A,** SAH outlines middle cerebral artery aneurysm (*arrow*) in right sylvian fissure, which is the site of the highest concentration of subarachnoid blood. **B,** Cerebral angiogram confirms the presence of a large right middle cerebral artery bifurcation aneurysm.

is limited to a very small part of the sub-arachnoid space. Most of the clearance of blood in CSF relies on the flushing of free hemoglobin and RBC debris by the flow of CSF, after completion of cell lysis. This clearance mechanism is efficient, as long as CSF production and drainage remain within physiologic limits.

Hemoglobin degradation is followed by the deposition of iron products hemosiderin and ferritin on the arachnoid trabeculae, pia mater, cranial nerves, and spinal cord, easily identified by MRI, and resulting in a condition called hemosiderosis. Repeated hemorrhages may result in severe and symptomatic hemosiderosis because iron has marked toxic effects on cranial nerves, particularly the cochleovestibular complex, causing progressive and irreversible sensorineural hearing loss, pulsatile tinnitus, ataxia, nystagmus, pyramidal signs, and other signs.

Computed Tomography and Computed Tomography Angiography

CT is currently the diagnostic method of reference for SAH, and is considered by some authors to be the only reliable marker for SAH in epidemiologic studies owing to the false-positive results of lumbar puncture, and the lack of angiographic data in many poor grade patients.[3] CT relies on differences in electronic attenuation between acute blood and the surrounding parenchyma (see Fig. 15-1) and has reported accuracy rates of 98% to 99%,[27] and even 100% for fifth-generation scanners.[29] SAH may be subtle and restricted to the sylvian or the interhemispheric fissure or the basal cisterns. It may be abundant, in which case the location of the thickest clot may point to the offending aneurysm (see Fig. 15-2). In addition to showing subarachnoid blood, and suggesting the location of the bleeding lesion, CT allows the clinician to evaluate the ventricular system, which may be dilated (see Fig. 15-1), and the status of the brain parenchyma, which could harbor a hematoma (Fig. 15-3) or diffuse cerebral edema.

Fisher and others[30,31] have determined that the thickness, location, and distribution of subarachnoid blood on CT correlate with the likelihood of subsequent vasospasm. Their four-level grading system is widely used as part of the initial assessment of patients and in decision making regarding hemodynamic management.

There are very few pitfalls related to the presence of SAH on CT. One condition that may cause severe headaches in young patients and hyperdense basal cisterns from spontaneous enhancement of thickened meninges is spontaneous intracranial hypotension.[32]

CT angiography, which is performed on multidetector row scanners using spiral techniques, is increasingly used for the detection of vascular lesions, including intracranial aneurysms.[33-37] Although some investigators claim that CT angiography may replace conventional angiography to detect intracranial aneurysms in SAH,[36] most agree that, for the time being, it is not sensitive enough to replace digital subtraction angiography.[37] CT angiography has the capacity to detect most intracranial aneurysms 3 mm or larger, and allows evaluation of the osseous anatomy at the same time as the three-dimensional rendering of vessels (see Fig. 15-3), which most neurosurgeons find extremely helpful.

Magnetic Resonance Imaging and Magnetic Resonance Angiography

MRI is used much less frequently than CT to detect acute SAH because it is less widely available, and it is generally considered less effective than CT. Fluid attenuated inversion recovery and gradient echo techniques allow the clinician to detect subtle differences in signal in the subarachnoid space, which makes MRI suitable for the early diagnosis of SAH.[38] MRI may have a role in rare situations, in which CT and CSF analysis are inconclusive or equivocal.

MR angiography is widely used as a screening method to detect aneurysms in patients with a family history or warning signs.[39] The three-dimensional time-of-flight technique is the most widely accepted one because it provides good spatial resolution, is minimally sensitive to signal loss caused by turbulent flow, and has acceptable acquisition times.[39,40] Major technical limitations of MR angiography in acute SAH include artifacts from signal changes caused by paramagnetic blood breakdown products

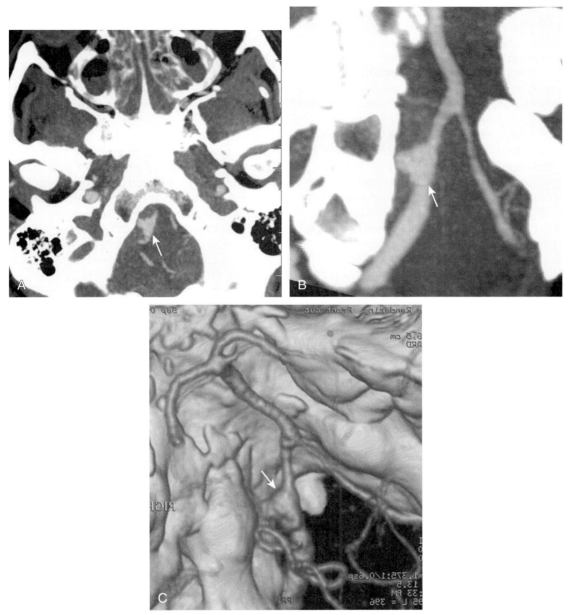

FIGURE 15-3   A 38-year-old man with SAH from a dissecting aneurysm of the right intracranial vertebral artery. **A,** Axial contrast-enhanced CT scan shows outpouching (*arrow*) of the intracranial right vertebral artery immediately distal to the posterior inferior cerebellar artery. **B,** Two-dimensional coronal reconstruction shows increased detail of the aneurysm (*arrow*). **C,** Three-dimensional reconstruction shows exquisite detail of the aneurysm (*arrow*), the vasculature, and the bony anatomy.

(particularly severe with intracerebral hematomas), which may affect the visualization of lesions, and decreased visibility of arteries in case of vasospasm because of signal loss. Several technical improvements, such as magnetization transfer saturation, the use of a large imaging matrix, and variable flip-angle excitation, may improve the technique significantly; MR angiography has been reported to detect ruptured aneurysms accurately in patients with SAH.[40]

Catheter Angiography

Despite the increasing number of noninvasive techniques used to evaluate the intracranial circulation, and their increasing accuracy (see earlier), catheter angiography remains the gold standard to study a patient with SAH. In most programs where neuroendovascular care is available, aneurysm therapy may be performed at the same time as the angiographic study, if indicated. Angiography requires complex equipment, consisting of an angiographic table, a high power x-ray tube, and an image intensifier with rapid filming capability. Catheters are introduced into the vascular system via the femoral artery, and contrast medium is injected during image acquisition. The digital subtraction angiography technique used has the highest spatial resolution of all currently available. The addition of three-dimensional rotational angiography has enhanced further the usefulness and accuracy of catheter angiography, particularly regarding aneurysm neck evaluation, so that it remains the gold standard.[37,41]

Angiography is an invasive test that can cause neurologic and other complications, with an overall reported incidence of 0.5% to 4%, although permanent complications do not exceed 0.5%.[42,43] The potential nephrotoxicity of angiographic contrast media and the risks of radiation, particularly in lengthy procedures, also have to be factored in.

A "negative angiogram" in a young patient with SAH should trigger subsequent angiographic evaluation because the consequences of missing a previously ruptured aneurysm are serious and far outweigh the risk of angiography. Reasons for missing an aneurysm include thrombosis (self-extinction), vasospasm involving the aneurysm neck, and inadequate angiographic technique. It is customary to obtain a second angiogram 1 week after the initial study, and if negative again, a third study may be repeated 2 to 3 weeks later, with a low threshold to study cervical and spinal cord arteries in patients with a non-perimesencephalic hemorrhagic pattern.[44-46] The reported yield of subsequent angiograms is 5% to 18%.[44-46]

Also, two or more aneurysms may be discovered in 15% to 25% of patients, particularly patients with familial aneurysms, which may complicate clear identification of the ruptured one. Other identified risk factors predisposing to multiple aneurysms are hypertension, cigarette smoking, a family

history of cerebrovascular disease, female sex, and postmenopausal state in female patients.[47]

Management of Aneurysmal Subarachnoid Hemorrhage

Intracranial aneurysms most commonly bleed from either the dome or a daughter lobule. Natural immediate protective factors include the formation of a thrombin-fibrin plug at the bleeding site, and an increase in intracranial pressure (ICP). Recurrent bleeding is common, estimated at a maximum of 4% on day 0, and 1.5% per day for subsequent days for a total of 27% in the first 2 weeks.[48] Recurrent hemorrhage is the main preventable complication of SAH. It is often fatal or severely disabling, with reported morbidities of 48% to 78%.[49,50] A crucial part of treatment is obliterating the offending aneurysm as early as possible.

Rarely, a patient with a ruptured aneurysm may present without SAH, which could be related to aneurysm location, timing of CT, and physiologic factors. Young patients presenting with intracerebral hemorrhage, especially involving the temporal lobe, or with IVH should be fully evaluated for a possible ruptured aneurysm, even in the absence of diffuse SAH.[51]

Aneurysm Obliteration

The goal of aneurysm treatment is total exclusion of the aneurysm and preservation of parent and neighboring arteries. Surgical clipping and endovascular therapy (most commonly using detachable coils) are currently the two available options.[52-57] A large international study found that SAH patients whose aneurysms were treated by endovascular means fared better than patients whose aneurysms were treated surgically.[52,53] Because aneurysms vary greatly in their physical features, however, a multidisciplinary evaluation produces the best results,[54-56] particularly because incompletely treated lesions by whichever method pose significant subsequent challenges.[55,57]

Saccular Aneurysms

Saccular aneurysms, also called berry aneurysms, are thought to be present in at least 1% of the general population and possibly

2%.[58] These aneurysms are considered congenital and degenerative because it is currently believed that both a preexisting weakness in the tunica media and wear and tear over a long time (i.e., shear stress to arteries from turbulent blood flow, high blood pressure, cigarette smoking, and other factors) are necessary.

Saccular aneurysms tend to occur at sites of arterial branching, but may occur at other locations. Most cerebral aneurysms are found at predictable locations around the circle of Willis; the three most common are the junction of the anterior communicating artery with the anterior cerebral artery (30% to 35%), the posterior communicating artery at the junction with the internal carotid artery (30% to 35%), and the middle cerebral artery bifurcation (20%). About 15% of aneurysms involve the posterior circulation, most commonly the basilar apex and the origin of the posterior inferior cerebellar artery.

Saccular aneurysms may be categorized according to their size: small (≤15 mm), large (15 to 25 mm), and giant (25 to 50 mm). Super-giant aneurysms (>50 mm) are rarely encountered. The annual risk of hemorrhage is estimated at 2%, assuming an incidence of SAH of 10 per 100,000 per year and a maximum prevalence of rupture of 0.5% in unruptured aneurysms. Two or more aneurysms may be discovered in 15% to 25% of patients. Useful criteria to help identify the offending aneurysm include the amount of blood on CT and aneurysm size (the larger, the more likely) and shape (presence of a "daughter sac" or "nipple" indicating the area of rupture [Fig. 15-4]).

Numerous conditions have been reported to be associated with intracranial saccular aneurysms, suggesting a genetic origin (see Table 15-1).[59] All these disorders combined account for less than 1% of all aneurysms in the population, however, and cannot explain most aneurysms. Nevertheless, there is a familial predisposition to some aneurysms.

Familial Aneurysms

Clinical observations have long suggested a familial pattern to SAH, with hemorrhagic episodes at a young age; a predilection for aneurysms to involve the middle cerebral artery bifurcation; and variable modes of

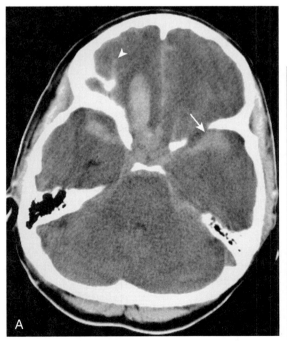
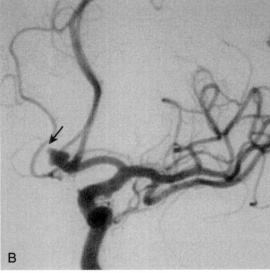

FIGURE 15-4 A 40-year-old woman with severe SAH. **A,** CT scan shows diffuse SAH (*arrow*) and a right frontal intracerebral hematoma (*arrowhead*). **B,** Angiography shows the offending aneurysm, with a right-pointing daughter sac (*arrow*).

inheritance, including autosomal dominant.[60] Also, autopsy studies have shown in these patients a diffuse arteriopathic pattern of the tunica media affecting intracranial and extracranial arteries.[61]

A genetic origin to intracranial aneurysms has long been sought by analyzing genes with a possible contribution to aneurysm predisposition. So far, genes that have been studied include genes that participate in type III collagen coding and that code for α_1-antitrypsin, apolipoprotein E, lipoprotein lipase, and elastin, with no convincing evidence of linkage. To date, the only identified genetic regions with a possible link to a familial predisposition to aneurysms are chromosome 19[62] in a Finnish population and chromosome 1p.[63] Because cerebral aneurysms are known to have an increased incidence in several rare mendelian conditions, such as polycystic kidney disease and Ehlers-Danlos syndrome, and because aneurysms have obvious phenotypic features that can be accurately studied with imaging, genetic analyses are expected to shed significant light on the mechanism of aneurysm formation, particularly if environmental covariates, such as cigarette smoking, are incorporated in the design of studies.[64]

Dissecting Aneurysms

Dissecting aneurysms characteristically affect young or middle-aged men and are associated with a high rebleeding rate and a very high morbidity.[65,66] Typical locations for dissecting aneurysm include the intracranial vertebral artery around the origin of the posterior inferior cerebellar artery (see Fig. 15-3) and, less commonly, the basilar artery (Fig. 15-5). Although dissecting aneurysms typically appear as fusiform dilations of the parent vessel, other patterns, such as lateral outpouching, and focal stenosis also are possible and should raise concern. Mortality rates of 80% have been reported with these lesions. Treatment uncommonly permits the preservation of the parent artery, which may contribute further to total morbidity, although stent-based endovascular techniques may increasingly allow parent vessel–sparing therapy (see Fig. 15-5).[67]

Aneurysms Associated with Arterial Fenestrations

Arterial fenestrations are divisions of the arterial lumen with resulting separate channels, each with its own endothelial layer and muscularis tunica, whereas the adventitial layer may or may not be shared between channels. These divisions are due to incomplete or absent fusion between primitive neural arteries. At most, a fenestration results in multiplication, usually duplication of the vessel. Duplications involve the anterior communicating artery, where spider-like connections have been shown in 19% of autopsy specimens; the vertebrobasilar system; the anterior cerebral artery; and, extremely rarely, other cerebral arteries.[68] Fenestrations of the cerebral arteries are rare, and there is a significant discrepancy between their reported angiographic (0.03% to 1%)[69,70] and postmortem incidence (1.3% to 5.3%).[68] Factors that contribute to saccular aneurysm formation include the presence of defects in the medial layer with a decrease in smooth muscle and collagen content at the proximal and distal edges of the duplicated segment, more severe at the medial and ventral walls of the proximal juncture,[71] and flow phenomena at the proximal end of fenestrations, where hemodynamic stress and increased turbulence are present.[72] Most reported fenestration-related aneurysms have been treated surgically, although successful transvascular therapy has been reported using Guglielmi detachable coils (Fig. 15-6).[73]

Blood Blister Aneurysms

"Blood blister aneurysms," also called "blister-like" aneurysms, have been recognized more recently as having unique pathologic and clinical features. These aneurysms are located at nonbranching sites of the parent artery, usually the supraclinoid internal carotid artery, although they may be found in the posterior circulation (Fig. 15-7).[74] Most patients are female and hypertensive.[74,75]

These aneurysms are best treated surgically, although success often requires adjustments to the standard clip placement maneuver, including clipping combined with wrapping,[74-76] or the use of an encircling clip graft,[77] in addition to generous brain relaxation techniques,

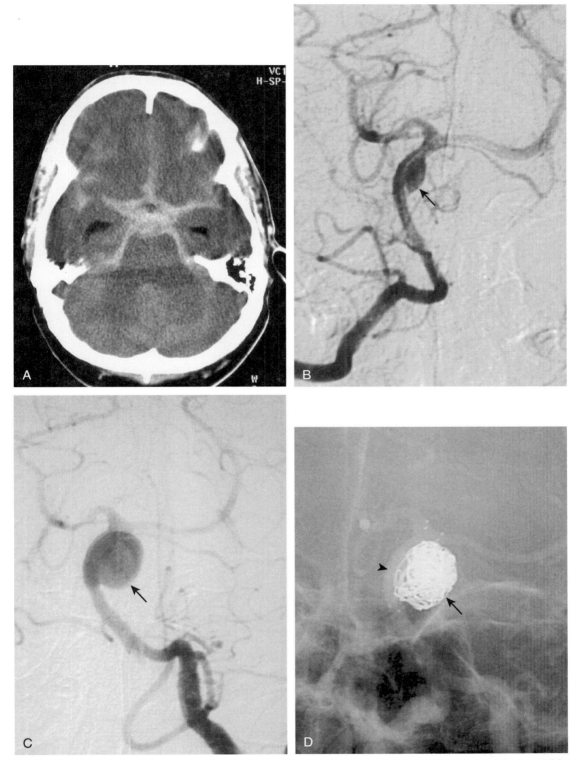

FIGURE 15-5   **A,** A 36-year-old man with diffuse SAH on CT and progressive left hemiparesis and cranial nerve palsies. **B,** A dissecting aneurysm of the basilar artery is found (*arrow*). **C,** Two days later, after referral to a tertiary institution for treatment, the aneurysm has grown significantly (*arrow*). **D,** Endovascular therapy allows preservation of the basilar artery with a stent (*arrowhead*) in the true lumen and aneurysm obliteration with coils (*arrow*) in the false lumen.

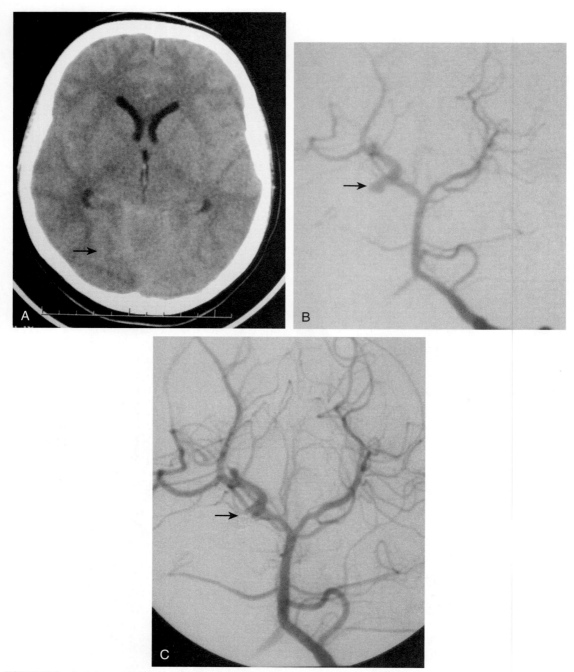

FIGURE 15-6 **A,** A 1-year-old boy with SAH localized to the vermian region (*arrow*). **B** and **C,** Angiography shows a small aneurysm at the proximal end of a fenestration of the right posterior cerebral artery (*arrow* on **B**), which was fully obliterated with detachable coils (*arrow* on **C**).

such as draining CSF, gentle subpial dissection, anterior clinoidectomy, and exposure of the cervical internal carotid artery. A subgroup of these lesions, also encountered in younger female patients and labeled "subclinoid aneurysms," involves the lateral surface of the carotid artery, proximal to its dural ring and adjacent to the anterior clinoid process, which may cover the aneurysm partially or completely at surgery.[76] Occasionally, blood blister aneurysms may be treated by endovascular techniques (see Fig. 15-7).[78]

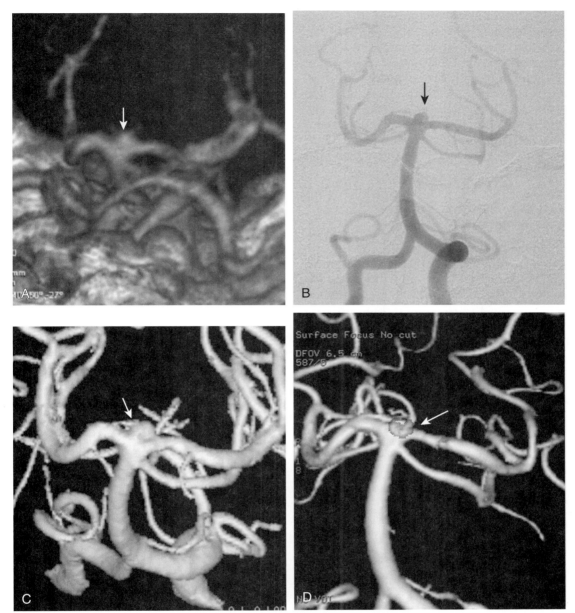

FIGURE 15-7   A 32-year-old man with SAH. **A,** Three-dimensional CT angiography suggests a "bleb" in the basilar apex (*arrow*). **B-D,** Conventional angiography (*arrow* on **B**) with three-dimensional rotational imaging (*arrow* on **C**) confirms a blood blister aneurysm, which was treated with small detachable coils (*arrow* on **D**).

Traumatic Aneurysms

Although this chapter deals with nontraumatic SAH, mention must be made of traumatic aneurysms. These lesions are extremely rare, estimated to constitute less than 1% of all intracranial aneurysms.[79] Although traumatic cerebral aneurysms are commonly associated with significant prior injury (including penetrating injury), skull fractures, cerebral contusions, and a history of coma in many, in some patients only minor injury can be elicited from the history. Most are false aneurysms, although true or mixed lesions also are seen. The interval between the causative initial trauma and rebleeding from the aneurysm varies from hours to years, with a median of 2 to 3 weeks. Reported locations include the distal or proximal middle cerebral artery, the basal internal carotid artery (including the petrous segment),[80] the anterior cerebral artery, the anterior choroidal artery, and rarely the posterior circulation. Untreated after SAH, these aneurysms have a very high mortality because the disrupted wall of the lesion is consistent only with an organized hematoma. Despite significant reported morbidities in the 20% range, treatment is highly recommended, whether surgery or endovascular therapy.[81,82]

Neurologic Intensive Care Management

The clinical condition of the patient at the time of admission correlates largely with the chances of recovery and the outcome, as indicated in the Hunt and Hess grading system (Table 15-3).[83] In addition, SAH is a severe event that sets off a cascade of several ensuing problems, which requires a methodical and aggressive management plan, as shown in Table 15-4. The critical care of a patient with SAH is of utmost importance to maximize the chances of a good recovery. These patients should be managed in an

TABLE 15-3 **Hunt and Hess Grading and Predicted Mortality from Subarachnoid Hemorrhage**

Hunt and Hess Grade	Mortality (%)
0—unruptured aneurysm without symptoms	0
1—asymptomatic or minimal headache and slight nuchal rigidity	1
1a—no acute meningeal or brain reaction, but with fixed neurologic deficit	1
2—moderate-to-severe headache, nuchal rigidity, no neurologic deficit other than cranial nerve palsy	5
3—drowsy, confused, or mild focal deficit	19
4—stupor, moderate-to-severe hemiparesis, possible early decerebrate rigidity, and vegetative disturbances	42
5—deep coma, decerebrate rigidity, moribund	77

From Hunt WE, Hess RM: Surgical risk as related to time of intervention in the repair of intracranial aneurysms. J Neurosurg 1968;28:14.

TABLE 15-4 **Management of Subarachnoid Hemorrhage**

Early (Days 0-3)

Stabilization of patient (hemodynamic, neurologic, cardiac, pulmonary)
Prevention of rebleeding (surgical/endovascular)
Control of ICP (hyperventilation, mannitol, ventricular drain, removal of mass lesion)

Later (Days 3-20)

Prevention of vasospasm (calcium channel blockers, hypervolemic-hypertensive-hemodilution (HHH) therapy
Treatment of vasospasm (intra-arterial vasodilators, i.e., calcium channel blockers, angioplasty)
Control of ICP (hyperventilation, mannitol, ventricular drain, mass lesion removal)
Treatment of symptomatic hydrocephalus (drainage, shunting)
Prevention and treatment of endocrine complications
Prevention and treatment of seizures
Prevention and treatment of systemic complications
Prevention and treatment of venous thromboembolism

Late (Post Intensive Care Unit)

Early and aggressive rehabilitation
Recognition and management of psychiatric manifestations (i.e., depression)

intensive care unit (ICU), where many require airway support and ventilatory assistance. A dedicated neurosciences unit with a team of specialized physicians, nurses, and social workers is preferable.

General Principles of Medical Management

Patients with SAH are admitted to an ICU to receive continuous hemodynamic and neurologic monitoring. Patients are kept at bed rest, are given analgesics and stool softeners, and are started on deep venous thrombosis prophylactic measures. In a patient with an unsecured aneurysm, blood pressure reduction seems logical, particularly if the patient is hypertensive. Induced hypotension does not prevent repeat hemorrhage, however, and can cause or aggravate ischemia. Early aneurysm obliteration is the goal and should be possible in most young patients. Uncommonly, in patients whose aneurysms cannot be secured early for whatever reason, antifibrinolytic therapy using aminocaproic acid may be considered to offer temporary protection.[84]

Prevention of Major Complications of Subarachnoid Hemorrhage

Other than rebleeding, the most feared neurosurgical complications of SAH are hydrocephalus and vasospasm. Many potential neurologic and medical complications require a high level of attention and specialized care.[85]

Hydrocephalus is rarely acute and, if untreated, may be rapidly fatal. Many patients who present with a poor initial Hunt and Hess grade and evidence of hydrocephalus on CT show clinical improvement after ventriculostomy. Most commonly, however, hydrocephalus is progressive, causing gradual obtundation correlating with enlarged ventricles on CT, and ventriculostomy allows simultaneous immediate decompression and continuous ICP monitoring. Later, patients are weaned over a period of days. Patients (20% to 46%) who do not tolerate shunt clamping may require a ventriculoperitoneal shunt after blood has cleared from the CSF.[86]

It has been claimed that intraoperative fenestration of the lamina terminalis in patients treated surgically for ruptured anterior communicating artery aneurysms decreased the need for a permanent ventriculoperitoneal shunt,[87] although that was not verified by other investigators.[88] There does not seem to be a significant difference in shunt dependency between patients treated surgically and patients treated by endovascular means.[89]

IVH in the context of SAH is considered a predictor of poor outcome and has a mortality of 33% to 65%.[90,91] Pathophysiologic mechanisms contributing to worsening in outcomes include ventricular enlargement, obstructive hydrocephalus, increased ICP and decreased cerebral perfusion pressure, ventricular dilation with local ischemia, periventricular edema and inflammation, delayed cerebral ischemia, and delayed communicating hydrocephalus.[92] IVH is managed with intraventricular catheters and external ventricular drainage to drain the hemorrhagic CSF and to decrease ventricular pressure. This approach is frequently ineffective because of clotting of the catheter, requiring frequent replacement. Intraventricular instillation of thrombolytics has shown some success in eliminating IVH in SAH patients[93,94] and may be used increasingly in the future,

particularly if newer, safer thrombolytic drugs are used.

Intracerebral hematoma may accompany SAH (see Fig. 15-3). Although most hematomas do not cause significant increases in ICP, surgical evacuation is occasionally indicated in patients who have evidence of mass effect causing clinical deterioration despite maximum medical therapy. Hematoma evacuation may provide access to the surgical treatment of the offending aneurysm, particularly aneurysms involving the middle cerebral artery bifurcation.

Vasospasm is an important cause of morbidity and mortality after SAH, with estimated 30% to 46% of additional disability or death before modern hemodynamic management. When abundant, subarachnoid blood infrequently lyses naturally and has a tendency to become caked around vessels at the base of the brain, which causes morphologic changes in arterial walls and major interference with vascular smooth muscle contraction. Numerous blood factors have been incriminated in vasospasm, particularly oxyhemoglobin and deoxyhemoglobin, which may induce an increase in the activity of vasoactive peptides (endothelins) that are localized to vascular smooth muscle and endothelial cells.[95] More recently discovered arachidonic acid derivatives, which serve as a second messenger in the myogenic response of vascular smooth muscle by regulating K^+ channel activity, have been implicated in vasospasm as strong potentiators of endothelins.[96,97] Reversal of severe vasospasm has been shown following enzymatic blockade of these arachidonic acid derivatives.[98,99]

Vasospasm is uncommon before day 3 of SAH, peaks around day 7, and becomes infrequent after day 14.[95,100,101] Numerous pharmacologic agents directed at preventing or dulling the vasospastic response after SAH have been and continue to be investigated. To date, only nimodipine, a calcium channel blocker, has shown a consistent, albeit moderate protective effect,[102] which justifies its routine use at the usual dose of 60 mg every 4 hours by mouth or nasogastric tube.

In addition to vasoactive phenomena, SAH triggers a severe inflammatory response in the meninges, the ventricles, and the arterial walls, and markedly elevated eicosanoids (prostaglandins and thromboxanes) are found in cisternal and lumbar CSF.[103] The use of steroids has been proposed in SAH patients on the basis that vasospasm and SAH-related cerebral ischemia have a significant inflammatory component. In one study, a group of patients with SAH who were treated with high-dose intravenous methylprednisolone (30 mg/kg for 72 hours, progressively tapered) showed a decrease in mortality and delayed cerebral ischemia and a higher rate of "excellent outcomes" compared with matched controls not receiving steroids.[104] Other studies, however, have suggested only minimal benefit from steroids on severe vasospasm, at the costs of an increased risk of gastrointestinal bleeding[105] and infection.[106] A study of 242 patients divided by grade on admission suggested that patients treated with high-dose dexamethasone (at least 12 mg/day for 5 days) versus low-dose dexamethasone had a lower incidence of rebleeding and hydrocephalus, and better outcome scores at 6 months, although the rate of vasospasm was not affected.[107]

Steroids, particularly fludrocortisone, a mineralocorticoid, also have been used to treat successfully excessive natriuresis, which is common after SAH.[108] Tirilizad, a 21-aminosteroid, and magnesium no longer are used.[102]

There is increasing suggestion that statins may also have a moderate protective role.[109,110] In patients treated surgically, removal of large subarachnoid clots and intracisternal thrombolytic therapy during surgery have also been thought to protect against vasospasm.

The advent of hypervolemic-hypertensive-hemodilution (triple-H) therapy has reduced the incidence and morbidity of clinically manifest vasospasm, but without eliminating it.[111,112] Modest hemodilution results in increased cerebral blood flow mainly via a decrease in blood viscosity, hypervolemia causes volume expansion, and deliberate hypertension results in improved perfusion.[111,112] A high level of suspicion must be constantly present within 2 weeks of SAH (≤20 days) in patients with a sudden, otherwise unexplained, new neurologic deficit because vasospasm that is refractory to triple-H therapy may cause severe morbidity.

Daily assessment with transcranial Doppler of intracranial arterial blood flow is useful and standard in most practices.

Management of Neurologic and Medical Complications

Increased ICP commonly follows SAH, resulting from hemorrhage, mass effect from a localized hematoma, hydrocephalus, cerebral edema, or cerebral ischemia secondary to vasospasm. Alert patients are unlikely to have elevated ICP, but progressive stupor should raise major concern. Hydrocephalus must be managed with external drainage, and mass lesions must be surgically evacuated. Medical measures to reduce ICP elevation include restriction of free water, steroid therapy, moderate hyperventilation, and diuretics, especially mannitol (an osmotic diuretic). Mannitol is given in 20% solution; its effect lasts 4 to 6 hours, and administration may be repeated.

Seizures after SAH occur in 6% to 8% of patients[113,114] and may be generalized, focal, or complex partial. Electroencephalogram changes are common after SAH, generally consistent with slow waves, although spikes are common. Middle cerebral artery bifurcation aneurysms are significantly more epileptogenic than other locations, particularly if SAH is associated with an intracerebral hematoma. Prophylactic use of antiepileptic drugs after SAH has been justified as a protector from rebleeding during a seizure in patients with yet unsecured aneurysms. More recent studies suggest, however, that the administration of antiepileptic drugs may be associated with worse neurologic and cognitive outcomes after SAH.[115] Phenytoin is often the standard drug used in the United States, given as a loading intravenous dose of 1000 mg and a daily maintenance dose of 300 mg. There is increasing evidence that the phenytoin burden[115] from clinical and subclinical side effects may have an independent impact in lowering functional outcomes in SAH patients. Newer drugs, such as levetiracetam, may have neuroprotective effects in SAH animal models.[116]

Electrolyte abnormalities are common after SAH. Hyponatremia is frequent, affecting more than one third of patients. Hyponatremia results from a salt-wasting syndrome caused by a centrally produced atrial natriuretic factor[117]; it is no longer thought to be related to inappropriate antidiuretic hormone secretion. Along with low sodium levels, there is a reduction in total blood volume with resultant hemoconcentration and low blood pressure. Hyponatremia should be corrected with sodium-containing fluid solutions or colloid solutions (5% albumin). A sodium level less than 115 mEq/L should be corrected by the careful administration of a 3% saline solution, which may aggravate preexisting cardiac disease and hypertension. Hypernatremia also may occur from diabetes insipidus. In patients treated surgically, postoperative mobilization of intraoperative venous fluids may mimic diabetes insipidus. Consequently, before giving vasopressin, the diagnosis should be seriously considered in patients with polyuria (>250 mL for 2 consecutive hours), with polydipsia, whose serum osmolarity exceeds 320 mOsm/kg, and whose urine osmolarity is less than 1 mOsm/kg. Hypernatremic diabetes insipidus is rare and most often seen after SAH from and surgery on ruptured anterior communicating artery aneurysms.[118]

Cardiac complications are a known occurrence after SAH; they were present in 50% of patients in one series, in whom the complications were defined as abnormal electrocardiogram, echocardiography, or cardiac troponin I, which is released in the bloodstream and has been associated with a neurogenic form of myocardial injury.[119] Subendocardial ischemia is common after SAH, owing to circulating catecholamines (primarily norepinephrine), and is benign and reversible in most cases. Myocardial infarctions with documented serial enzyme and electrocardiogram changes are frequent. Myocardial stunning is common, particularly with posterior circulation aneurysms.[120] Pathologic studies also have amply shown numerous cardiac changes with SAH, which has been coined "myocytolysis," ranging from focal myocardial edema, necrosis, and hemorrhage to massive infarction.

Electrocardiographic changes are extremely common, consisting of prolonged Q-T intervals, T wave and ST changes, and U waves. Cardiac arrhythmias also are very common, affecting virtually all patients in the first 48 hours of SAH; one third of patients have severe arrhythmias, such as ventricular tachycardia.[121]

Hypertension also is common after SAH and has been attributed to catecholamine release, requiring control in unsecured aneurysms. In most patients, sedation provides control of hypertension. In a few patients, control of malignant hypertension requires the use of sodium nitroprusside, which must be cautiously manipulated to avoid cerebral ischemia.

Pulmonary complications are very common after SAH. Patients with a decreased level of consciousness are at risk for hypoxia, atelectasis, aspiration, pneumonia, and pulmonary edema; the last-mentioned may be neurogenic in origin. Pulmonary dysfunction results in hypoxia, hypercarbia, and acidosis, which may contribute to decreasing cerebral perfusion and increasing ICP. Obtunded patients must be intubated because only controlled ventilation maintains oxygenation in these patients. Hypocarbia in the range of 30 mm Hg may help control ICP, although lower levels may decrease cerebral perfusion and precipitate ischemia. Pulmonary edema is common after SAH[122] and may result from increased ICP, increased fluid administration (i.e., from hypervolemic hemodilution therapy), or a neurogenic response to SAH secondary to circulating catecholamines, in which case α-adrenergic antagonists may be useful. Frequent pulmonary care and diuretics are useful. Pneumonia also is very common after SAH, requiring frequent evaluation of chest x-rays and sputum.

Infectious complications are frequent in comatose and surgical patients and must be searched for systematically; unexplained rashes are particularly suspicious. Infections may be insidious and severe owing to the use of steroids, and can have severe consequences in these patients who harbor many potential sources of bacterial entry (i.e., ventricular catheters, intravenous and arterial lines, bladder catheters, and craniotomy wounds or femoral punctures).

Venous thrombosis is common in bedridden patients, particularly patients with stroke. Pneumatic compression stockings and early mobilization are the rule. Subcutaneous unfractionated heparin and low-molecular-weight heparin are useful and seem to be safe after the aneurysm has been secured.

Gastrointestinal hemorrhage from erosive and ulcerative gastric and duodenal abnormalities are frequent after SAH and can be exacerbated by the use of steroids. These problems are more frequent in patients with a prior history of gastrointestinal bleeding, and justify the routine use of antacids and H_2 blockers. Other ICU complications after SAH include fever, anemia, and hyperglycemia, all of which may worsen outcomes further.[123]

Management of Symptomatic Vasospasm

Despite aggressive triple-H therapy, which is feasible in most young adults with acceptable cardiovascular and pulmonary functions, rapidly evolving and clinically manifest vasospasm is encountered in some patients (5% to 15% of aneurysmal SAH admissions). As mentioned, only thorough and continuous monitoring of these patients allows identification of the problem at a time reversal can be expected. A new neurologic deficit that cannot be explained should be attributed to vasospasm until otherwise proven and should prompt immediate evaluation by CT, to ensure that a large completed infarction is not present, which could become hemorrhagic after reperfusion. Commonly, the velocity profile of cerebral flow in these patients either has not been assessed because of technical limitations or shows recent consistent increase. Emergent imaging of the intracranial circulation needs to be obtained, either by CT angiography[124] or preferably with angiography, which not only is more reliable, but also permits treatment at the same time. Intra-arterial vasodilators (calcium channel blockers or papaverine) and balloon angioplasty (Fig. 15-8) are the available options, and their timely use can clearly reverse ischemic deficits.[125-128]

Exceptionally, diffuse vasospasm may be extremely malignant, refractory to repeated and aggressive endovascular therapy. For those situations, the use of an intra-aortic balloon pump[129] or hypothermia[130] has been suggested.

Nontraumatic Nonaneurysmal Subarachnoid Hemorrhage

Perimesencephalic Hemorrhage

Perimesencephalic hemorrhage occurs in approximately 10% of all patients with SAH.[131,132] In nonaneurysmal perimesencephalic hemorrhage, subarachnoid blood accumulates around the midbrain. These patients have distinct clinical and radiologic characteristics, which suggest a venous origin to the hemorrhage. Clinically, they are in a much better grade than expected for the amount of blood in the CSF compared with patients with aneurysmal SAH. Radiographically, CT shows the so-called perimesencephalic hemorrhage pattern, in which blood is confined to the cisterns around the midbrain (Fig. 15-9),[131-133] as opposed to the more common aneurysmal or non-perimesencephalic SAH pattern.[134]

An abnormal pattern of venous drainage, which would promote venous rupture and hemorrhage in these patients, has been suggested. van der Schaaf and colleagues[135] studied the venous drainage in 55 patients with perimesencephalic hemorrhage and 42 patients with SAH secondary to posterior circulation aneurysm rupture and found three patterns: (1) normal continuous, with continuity of the basal vein of Rosenthal with the deep middle cerebral vein, draining into the vein of Galen; (2) normal discontinuous, with basal vein of Rosenthal drainage anterior to uncal veins and posterior to the vein of Galen; and (3) primitive variant, with basal vein of Rosenthal drainage to the dural sinuses instead of the vein of Galen. These authors found that the primitive drainage variant was present in more than half of their patients, and determined that in all patients with perimesencephalic hemorrhage and a unilateral primitive drainage variant, blood was found only on the side of the abnormal drainage.

These patients often have a history of physical exertion. It has been speculated that increased intrathoracic pressure during physical exercise impairs jugular return, which results in increased intracranial venous pressures that promote venous or capillary breakage.[136]

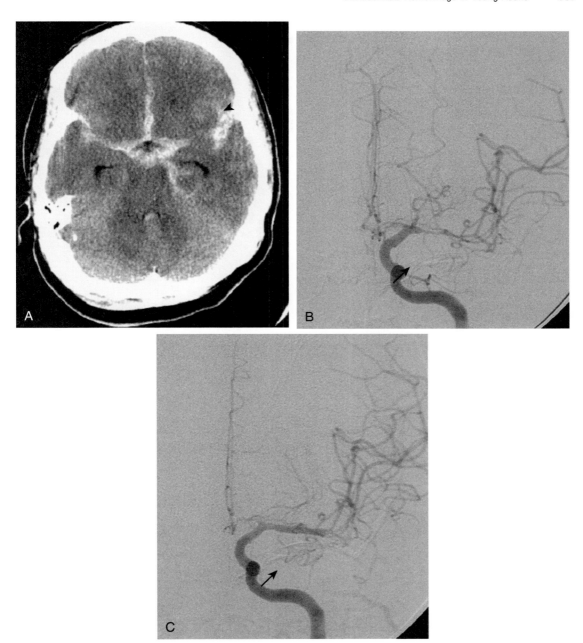

FIGURE 15-8   A 40-year-old woman with diffuse SAH after cocaine use. **A,** A large clot is present in the left sylvian fissure (*arrowhead*). No aneurysm was found. **B,** On day 7 post-SAH, the patient had symptomatic vasospasm, causing right hemiparesis and motor aphasia, correlating with severe left middle cerebral artery vasospasm (*arrow*). **C,** After angioplasty, there is restoration of the left middle cerebral artery lumen and flow (*arrow*) with immediate improvement of the patient's neurologic status.

A full initial diagnostic workup is warranted in these patients, including arteriography, although it has been suggested by some investigators to use CT and CT angiography only in these patients.[132] During hospitalization, some patients with particularly abundant perimesencephalic hemorrhage may go on to develop symptomatic vasospasm despite aggressive hemodynamic and fluid therapy, which may require endovascular therapy. Most do well during their hospital stay, however, and require neither aggressive management beyond standard ICU care nor repeat angiography,[137] although symptomatic vasospasm requiring

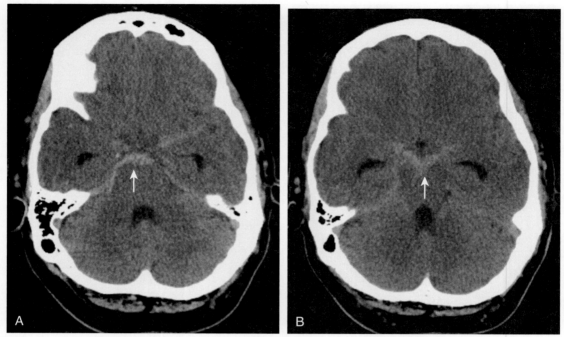

FIGURE 15-9 A 39-year-old man with SAH and mild headache. **A** and **B,** CT shows the typical pattern for perimesencephalic hemorrhage, mainly concentrated in the prepontine (*arrow* on **A**) and interpeduncular (*arrow* on **B**) cisterns. The patient presented in Hunt and Hess grade 1, and had a benign hospital course.

treatment has been reported after perimesencephalic hemorrhage.[138] On discharge, these patients need not be subjected to the same restrictions in activities as for patients with aneurysmal SAH. Life expectancy in these patients is the same as in the general population. Recurrence of hemorrhage does not occur, and no special restrictions should be applied to these patients.[139]

Drug-related Subarachnoid Hemorrhage

The use of drugs for recreational purposes is so widespread that toxicologic screening of urine and serum has become part of the routine assessment of patients admitted with any stroke, including SAH.[11,140] Cocaine and its alkaloid variants known as "crack"[140] are the most commonly used drugs. In these patients, multidrug use, including alcohol, tobacco, marijuana, and heroin, is common.[16,141,142]

In addition, drugs, in particular, cocaine, have been shown to affect adversely the presentation of and the outcome in patients with aneurysmal SAH owing to the vasoactive properties of the drug, which aggravate cerebral hemodynamics, including cerebral vasospasm.[142] The general mechanism of action of cocaine, amphetamines, and related drugs is to increase the amount of circulating catecholamines by blocking reuptake and increasing receptor sensitivity, with resultant sympathetic hyperstimulation and hypertension.[141,143] Also, these drugs have been shown to induce apoptosis in vascular smooth muscle cells, causing diffuse spasm and thrombotic occlusions.[144] A direct neurotoxic effect also has been elicited, as cocaine upregulates the expression of stress proteins in the endoplasmic reticulum of striatal neurons via glutamate and dopamine receptors.[145] Lastly, the effects of adulterants and impurities found in cocaine and other drugs should not be underestimated. Arsenic, a common contaminant of recreational drugs, is linked to thromboangiitis obliterans, which is an important part of the spectrum of vascular derangements in these patients.[146]

Heavy drug users have been shown to experience aneurysmal rupture at a much earlier age than patients in the general population and to have smaller aneurysms.[141] The management of these patients is the same as management of patients with aneurysmal SAH and should be aggressive. Contrary to a commonly held belief, good outcomes may be obtained in these patients with aggressive management.[143]

Alcohol, including occasional use and heavy drinking, was reported to increase twofold the risk of aneurysmal rupture and SAH in a Finnish population of young adults.[147] Alcohol and cigarette smoking are often used concomitantly and are known predisposing factors to SAH.[11]

Phenylpropanolamine, used in nasal decongestants and appetite-reducing drugs, has been incriminated in cerebral hemorrhage in young adults, including SAH, and banned from over-the-counter medications by the U.S. Food and Drug Administration. A study in Mexico failed to elicit an association between phenylpropanolamine and SAH, however.[148]

Arteriovenous Malformations and Fistulas

Most ruptured cerebral AVM ruptures cause intracerebral hemorrhage or IVH. In one study of 23 ruptured cerebral AVMs, no SAH was encountered.[149] SAH is rarely seen after rupture of a cerebral or spinal AVM or fistula,[150] however, and may be due to aneurysmal rupture. Aneurysms associated with AVMs may be intranidal, perinidal, or seated on parent arteries, either incidental saccular aneurysms or "flow-related," with a low hemorrhagic risk. The management of ruptured cerebral or spinal AVMs is best handled by multidisciplinary teams that can offer the highest level of comprehensive surgical, radiosurgical, and endovascular therapy.

Puerperal and Postpartum Hemorrhage

SAH in pregnancy and the postpartum period is usually caused by aneurysm rupture or severe hypertension, usually but not always related to eclampsia. During pregnancy, these problems need to be managed the same way as with nonpregnant patients. Patients with postpartum eclampsia may be normotensive, and yet have SAH. Angiographic evaluation may show diffuse vessel narrowing, consistent with postpartum angiopathy.[151]

Because SAH may recur in this patient population,[152] caution is advised, and careful observation in an ICU is recommended. Chapter 10 contains a more comprehensive review of puerperal and postpartum cerebrovascular pathology.

Rare Causes of Subarachnoid Hemorrhage

Spontaneous dissection of intracranial arteries that run in the subarachnoid space, such as the intracranial carotid artery of the middle cerebral artery, has been reported to cause SAH.[153,154] A thorough investigation is necessary; management of these patients is challenging because anticoagulation may be indicated. Takayasu arteritis[155] and other vasculitides and moyamoya disease[156] also have been reported to cause SAH.

Some cerebral lesions that are located close to, or on the surface of, the brain or spinal cord, such as cavernous angiomas,[157] primary glial tumors,[158] other tumors such as hemangioblastomas,[159] and diffuse meningeal metastatic disease, also rarely may cause SAH.[160] Infective endocarditis with or without demonstrable cerebral mycotic aneurysms[161] and pituitary apoplexy[162] have been reported to cause SAH in young patients. Lastly, patients with the 3–M syndrome, a rare autosomal recessive disorder that causes dwarfism, unusual facial features, and skeletal abnormalities, and first identified by Miller, McKussick and Malvaux, may be at an increased risk of having intracranial aneurysms.[163]

Conclusion

SAH accounts for a significant percentage of strokes in young adults at the prime of their productive lives, causing significant morbidity and loss. Most of these patients have aneurysms of various kinds. Although considerable advances have been made in the management of aneurysmal SAH and the epidemiology, with significant expected benefit, the prognosis remains poor in many patients. SAH resulting from drug abuse is particularly severe. Perimesencephalic hemorrhage is a specific entity associated with excellent outcomes.

REFERENCES

1. Biller J, Toffol GJ, Kassell NF, et al. Spontaneous subarachnoid hemorrhage in young adults. Neurosurgery 1987;21:664.
2. Salcman M. Subarachnoid hemorrhage. In Salcman M, ed. Neurologic Emergencies: Recognition and Management, 2nd ed. New York: Raven Press, 1990.
3. Linn FH, Rinkel GJ, Algra A, van Gijn J. Incidence of subarachnoid hemorrhage: role of region, year, and rate of computed tomography: a meta-analysis. Stroke 1996;27:625.
4. Mayberg MR, Batjer HH, Dacey R, et al. Guidelines for the management of aneurysmal subarachnoid hemorrhage. A statement for healthcare professionals from a special writing group of the Stroke Council, American Heart Association. Stroke 1994;25:2315.
5. de Rooij NK, Linn FH, van der Plas JA, et al. Incidence of subarachnoid haemorrhage: a systematic review with emphasis on region, age, gender and time trend. J Neurol Neurosurg Psychiatry 2007;78:1365.
6. Sarti C, Tuomilehto J, Salomaa V, et al. Epidemiology of subarachnoid hemorrhage in Finland from 1983 to 1985. Stroke 1991;22:848.
7. Ogungbo B, Gregson B, Blackburn A, et al. Aneurysmal subarachnoid hemorrhage in young adults. J Neurosurg 2003;98:43.
8. Horiuchi T, Tanaka Y, Hongo K, Kobayashi S. Aneurysmal subarachnoid hemorrhage in young adults: a comparison between patients in the third and fourth decades of life. J Neurosurg 2003;99:276.
9. Hop JW, Rinkel GJ, Algra A, van Gijn J. Case-fatality rates and functional outcome after subarachnoid hemorrhage: a systematic review. Stroke 1997; 28:660.
10. Broderick JP, Brott T, Tomsick T, et al. Intracerebral hemorrhage more than twice as common as subarachnoid hemorrhage. J Neurosurg 1993;78:188.
11. Feigin VL, Rinkel GJ, Lawes CM, et al. Risk factors for subarachnoid hemorrhage: an updated systematic review of epidemiological studies. Stroke 2005;36:2773.
12. Feigin V, Parag V, Lawes CM, et al. Asia Pacific Cohort Studies Collaboration. Smoking and elevated blood pressure are the most important risk factors for subarachnoid hemorrhage in the Asia-Pacific region: an overview of 26 cohorts involving 306,620 participants. Stroke 2005;36:1360.
13. Rosen D, Novakovic R, Goldenberg FD, et al. Racial differences in demographics, acute complications, and outcomes in patients with subarachnoid hemorrhage: a large patient series. J Neurosurg 2005;103:18.
14. Labovitz DL, Halim AX, Brent B, et al. Subarachnoid hemorrhage incidence among Whites, Blacks and Caribbean Hispanics: the Northern Manhattan Study. Neuroepidemiology 2006;26:147.
15. Juvela S, Siironen J, Kuhmonen J. Hyperglycemia, excess weight, and history of hypertension as risk factors for poor outcome and cerebral infarction after aneurysmal subarachnoid hemorrhage. J Neurosurg 2005;102:998.
16. Broderick JP, Viscoli CM, Brott T, et al. Hemorrhagic Stroke Project Investigators. Major risk factors for aneurysmal subarachnoid hemorrhage in the young are modifiable. Stroke 2003;34:1375.
17. Ballard J, Kreiter KT, Claassen J, et al. Risk factors for continued cigarette use after subarachnoid hemorrhage. Stroke 2003;34:1859.
18. Linn FH, Rinkel GJ, Algra A, van Gijn J. The notion of "warning leaks" in subarachnoid haemorrhage: are such patients in fact admitted with a rebleed? J Neurol Neurosurg Psychiatry 2000;68:332.
19. Verweij RD, Wijdicks EF, van Gijn J. Warning headache in aneurysmal subarachnoid hemorrhage: a case-control study. Arch Neurol 1988;45:1019.
20. Vermeulen MJ, Schull MJ. Missed diagnosis of subarachnoid hemorrhage in the emergency department. Stroke 2007;38:1216.
21. Adams HP, Jergensson DD, Kassell NF, Sahs ALP. Pitfalls in the recognition of subarachnoid hemorrhage. JAMA 1980;244:794.
22. Dodick DW, Brown RD Jr, Britton JW, Huston J 3rd. Nonaneurysmal thunderclap headache with diffuse, multifocal, segmental, and reversible vasospasm. Cephalalgia 1999;19:118.
23. Broner S, Lay C, Newman L, Swerdlow M. Thunderclap headache as the presenting symptom of myocardial infarction. Headache 2007;47:724.
24. Nagumo K, Nakamori A, Kojima S. Spontaneous intracranial internal carotid artery dissection: 6 case reports and a review of 39 cases in the literature. Rinsho Shinkeigaku 2003;43:313.
25. Yakushiji Y, Haraguchi Y, Soejima S, et al. A hyperdense artery sign and middle cerebral artery dissection. Intern Med 2006;45:1319.
26. Nager BJ, Lanska DJ, Daroff RB. Acute demyelination mimicking vascular hemicrania. Headache 1989;29:423.
27. van Gijn J, van Dongen KJ. Computerized tomography in the diagnosis of subarachnoid haemorrhage and ruptured aneurysm. Clin Neurol Neurosurg 1980;82:11.
28. Edlow JA, Caplan LR. Avoiding pitfalls in the diagnosis of subarachnoid hemorrhage. N Engl J Med 2000;342:29.
29. Boesiger BM, Shiber JR. Subarachnoid hemorrhage diagnosis by computed tomography and lumbar puncture: are fifth generation CT scanners better at identifying subarachnoid hemorrhage? J Emerg Med 2005;29:23.
30. Fisher CM, Kistler JP, Davis JM. Relation of cerebral vasospasm to subarachnoid hemorrhage visualized by computerized tomographic scanning. Neurosurgery 1980;6:1.
31. Kistler JP, Crowell RM, Davis KR, et al. The relation of cerebral vasospasm to the extent and location of subarachnoid blood visualized by CT scan: a prospective study. Neurology 1983;33:424.
32. Schievink WI, Maya MM, Tourje J, Moser FG. Pseudo-subarachnoid hemorrhage: a CT-finding

in spontaneous intracranial hypotension. Neurology 2005;65:135.

33. Jayaraman MV, Mayo-Smith WW, Tung GA, et al. Detection of intracranial aneurysms: multi-detector row CT angiography compared with DSA. Radiology 2004;230:510.

34. Karamessini MT, Kagadis GC, Petsas T, et al. CT angiography with three-dimensional techniques for the early diagnosis of intracranial aneurysms: comparison with intra-arterial DSA and the surgical findings. Eur J Radiol 2004;49:212.

35. Dehdashti AR, Rufenacht DA, Delavelle J, et al. Therapeutic decision and management of aneurysmal subarachnoid haemorrhage based on computed tomographic angiography. Br J Neurosurg 2003;17:46.

36. Uysal E, Yanbuloglu B, Erturk M, et al. Spiral CT angiography in diagnosis of cerebral aneurysms of cases with acute subarachnoid hemorrhage. Diagn Interv Radiol 2005;11:77.

37. Teksam M, McKinney A, Casey S, et al. Multi-section CT angiography for detection of cerebral aneurysms. AJNR Am J Neuroradiol 2004;25:1485.

38. Noguchi K, Seto H, Kamisaki Y, et al. Comparison of fluid-attenuated inversion-recovery MR imaging with CT in a simulated model of acute subarachnoid hemorrhage. AJNR Am J Neuroradiol 2000;21:923.

39. Ronkainen A, Puranen MI, Hernesniemi JA, et al. Intracranial aneurysms: MR angiographic screening in 400 asymptomatic individuals with increased familial risk. Radiology 1995;195:35.

40. Ida M, Kurisu Y, Yamashita M. MR angiography of ruptured aneurysms in acute subarachnoid hemorrhage. AJNR Am J Neuroradiol 1997;18:1025.

41. Raabe A, Beck J, Rohde S, et al. Three-dimensional rotational angiography guidance for aneurysm surgery. J Neurosurg 2006;105:406.

42. Earnest F, Forbes G, Sandok BA, et al. Complications of cerebral angiography: prospective assessment of risk. AJR Am J Roentgenol 1984;142:247.

43. Dion JE, Gates PC, Fox AJ, et al. Clinical events following neuroangiography: a prospective study. Stroke 1987;18:997.

44. Jung JY, Kim YB, Lee JW, et al. Spontaneous subarachnoid haemorrhage with negative initial angiography: a review of 143 cases. J Clin Neurosci 2006;13:1011.

45. Topcuoglu MA, Ogilvy CS, Carter BS, et al. Subarachnoid hemorrhage without evident cause on initial angiography studies: diagnostic yield of subsequent angiography and other neuroimaging tests. J Neurosurg 2003;98:1235.

46. Duong H, Melancon D, Tampieri D, Ethier R. The negative angiogram in subarachnoid haemorrhage. Neuroradiology 1996;38:15.

47. Ellamushi HE, Grieve JP, Jäger HR, Kitchen ND. Risk factors for the formation of multiple intracranial aneurysms. J Neurosurg 2001;94:728.

48. Kassell NF, Torner JC. Aneurysmal rebleeding: a preliminary report from the Cooperative Aneurysm Study. Neurosurgery 1983;13:479.

49. Rosenorn J, Eskesen V, Schmidt K, Ronde F. The risk of rebleeding from ruptured intracranial aneurysms. J Neurosurg 1987;67:329.

50. Jane JA, Winn HR, Richardson AE. The natural history of intracranial aneurysms: rebleeding rates during the acute and long term period and implication for surgical management. Clin Neurosurg 1977;24:176.

51. Thai QA, Raza SM, Pradilla G, Tamargo RJ. Aneurysmal rupture without subarachnoid hemorrhage: case series and literature review. Neurosurgery 2005;57:225.

52. Molyneux A, Kerr R, Stratton I, et al. International Subarachnoid Aneurysm Trial (ISAT) Collaborative Group. International Subarachnoid Aneurysm Trial (ISAT) of neurosurgical clipping versus endovascular coiling in 2143 patients with ruptured intracranial aneurysms: a randomised trial. Lancet 2002;360:1267.

53. Molyneux AJ, Kerr RS, Yu LM, et al. International Subarachnoid Aneurysm Trial (ISAT) Collaborative Group. International Subarachnoid Aneurysm Trial (ISAT) of neurosurgical clipping versus endovascular coiling in 2143 patients with ruptured intracranial aneurysms: a randomised comparison of effects on survival, dependency, seizures, rebleeding, subgroups, and aneurysm occlusion. Lancet 2005;366:809.

54. Origitano TC. Current options in clipping versus coiling of intracranial aneurysms: to clip, to coil, to wait and watch. Neurol Clin 2006;24:765.

55. Hacein-Bey L, Connolly ES, Mayer SA, et al. Complex intracranial aneurysms: combined operative and endovascular approaches. Neurosurgery 1998;43:1304.

56. Fraser JF, Riina H, Mitra N, et al. Treatment of ruptured intracranial aneurysms: looking to the past to register the future. Neurosurgery 2006;59:1157.

57. Minh T, Hwang PY, Nguyen KC, Ng I. Neurosurgical management of intracranial aneurysms following unsuccessful or incomplete endovascular therapy. Br J Neurosurg 2006;20:306.

58. Menghini VV, Brown RD, Sicks JD, et al. Incidence and prevalence of intracranial aneurysms and hemorrhage in Olmsted County, Minnesota, 1965 to 1995. Neurology 1998;51:405.

59. Meyers PM, Halbach VV, Barkovich AJ. Anomalies of cerebral vasculature: diagnostic and endovascular considerations. In Barkovich AJ, ed. Pediatric Neuroimaging, 4th ed. Philadelphia: Lippincott Williams & Wilkins, 2005.

60. Bromberg JE, Rinkel GJ, Algra A, et al. Familial subarachnoid hemorrhage: distinctive features and patterns of inheritance. Ann Neurol 1995;38:929.

61. Schievink WI, Parisi JE, Piepgras DG. Familial intracranial aneurysms: an autopsy study. Neurosurgery 1997;41:1247.

62. Olson JM, Vongpunsawad S, Kuivaniemi H, et al. Search for intracranial aneurysm susceptibility gene(s) using Finnish families. BMC Med Genet 2002;3:7.

63. Nahed BV, Seker A, Guclu B, et al. Mapping a Mendelian form of intracranial aneurysm to 1p34.3-p36.13. Am J Hum Genet 2005;76:172.

64. Broderick JP, Sauerbeck LR, Foroud T, et al. The Familial Intracranial Aneurysm (FIA) study protocol. BMC Med Genet 2005;6:17.

65. Takagi T, Takayasu M, Suzuki Y, Yoshida J. Prediction of rebleeding from angiographic features in vertebral artery dissecting aneurysms. Neurosurg Rev 2007;30:32.
66. Yamaura A, Watanabe Y, Saeki N. Dissecting aneurysms of the intracranial vertebral artery. J Neurosurg 1990;72:183.
67. Rabinov JD, Hellinger FR, Morris PP, et al. Endovascular management of vertebrobasilar dissecting aneurysms. AJNR Am J Neuroradiol 2003;24:1421.
68. Wollschlaeger G, Wollschlaeger PB, Lucas FV, Lopez VF. Experience and result with postmortem cerebral angiography performed as routine procedure of the autopsy. Am J Roentgenol Radium Ther Nucl Med 1967;101:68.
69. Teal JS, Rumbaugh CL, Bergeron RT, Segall HD. Angiographic demonstration of fenestrations of the intradural intracranial arteries. Radiology 1973;106:123.
70. Sanders WP, Sorek PA, Mehta BA. Fenestration of intracranial arteries with special attention to associated aneurysms and other anomalies. AJNR Am J Neuroradiol 1993;14:675.
71. Finlay HM, Canham PB. The layered fabric of cerebral artery fenestrations. Stroke 1994;25:1799.
72. Campos J, Fox AJ, Vinuela F, et al. Saccular aneurysms in basilar artery fenestration. AJNR Am J Neuroradiol 1987;8:233.
73. Hacein-Bey L, Muszynski CA, Varelas PN. Saccular aneurysm associated with posterior cerebral artery fenestration manifesting as a subarachnoid hemorrhage in a child. AJNR Am J Neuroradiol 2002;23:1291.
74. Sim SY, Shin YS, Cho KG, et al. Blood blister-like aneurysms at nonbranching sites of the internal carotid artery. J Neurosurg 2006;105:400.
75. Joo SP, Kim TS, Moon KS, et al. Arterial suturing followed by clip reinforcement with circumferential wrapping for blister-like aneurysms of the internal carotid artery. Surg Neurol 2006;66:424.
76. Nutik SL. Subclinoid aneurysms. J Neurosurg 2003;98:731.
77. Sekula RF Jr, Cohen DB, Quigley MR, Jannetta PJ. Primary treatment of a blister-like aneurysm with an encircling clip graft: technical case report. Neurosurgery 2006;59(1 Suppl 1):168.
78. McNeely PD, Clarke DB, Baxter B, et al. Endovascular treatment of a "blister-like" aneurysm of the internal carotid artery. Can J Neurol Sci 2000;27:247.
79. Larson PS, Reisner A, Morassutti DJ, et al. Traumatic intracranial aneurysms. Neurosurg Focus 2000;8:e4.
80. Uzan M, Cantasdemir M, Seckin MS, et al. Traumatic intracranial carotid tree aneurysms. Neurosurgery 1998;43:1314.
81. Fleischer AS, Patton JM, Tindall GT. Cerebral aneurysms of traumatic origin. Surg Neurol 1975;4:233.
82. Fleischer AS, Guthkelch AN. Management of high cervical-intracranial internal carotid artery traumatic aneurysms. J Trauma 1987;27:330.
83. Hunt WE, Hess RM. Surgical risk as related to time of intervention in the repair of intracranial aneurysms. J Neurosurg 1968;28:14.
84. Mullan S, Dawley J. Antifibrinolytic therapy for intracranial aneurysms. J Neurosurg 1968;28:21.
85. Crowell RM, Ogilvy CS, Gress DR, Kistler JP. General management of aneurysmal subarachnoid hemorrhage. In Ojemann RG, Heros RC, Crowell RM, Ogilvy CS, eds. Surgical Management of Cerebrovascular Disease, 2nd ed. Baltimore, Williams & Wilkins, 1995.
86. Sheehan JP, Polin RS, Sheehan JM, et al. Factors associated with hydrocephalus after aneurysmal subarachnoid hemorrhage. Neurosurgery 1999;45:1120.
87. Andaluz N, Zuccarello M. Fenestration of the lamina terminalis as a valuable adjunct in aneurysm surgery. Neurosurgery 2004;55:1050.
88. Kim JM, Jeon JY, Kim JH, et al. Influence of lamina terminalis fenestration on the occurrence of the shunt-dependent hydrocephalus in anterior communicating artery aneurysmal subarachnoid hemorrhage. J Korean Med Sci 2006;21:113.
89. Varelas P, Helms A, Sinson G, et al. Clipping or coiling of ruptured cerebral aneurysms and shunt-dependent hydrocephalus. Neurocrit Care 2006;4:223.
90. Shimoda M, Oda S, Shibata M, et al. Results of early surgical evacuation of packed intraventricular hemorrhage from aneurysm rupture in patients with poor-grade subarachnoid hemorrhage. J Neurosurg 1999;91:408.
91. Nakagawa T, Suga S, Mayanagi K, et al. Keio SAH Cooperative Study Group. Predicting the overall management outcome in patients with a subarachnoid hemorrhage accompanied by a massive intracerebral or full-packed intraventricular hemorrhage: a 15-year retrospective study. Surg Neurol 2005;63:329.
92. Claassen J, Bernardini GL, Kreiter K, et al. Effect of cisternal and ventricular blood on risk of delayed cerebral ischemia after subarachnoid hemorrhage: the Fisher scale revisited. Stroke 2001;32:2012.
93. Azmi-Ghadimi H, Heary RF, Farkas JE, Hunt CD. Use of intraventricular tissue plasminogen activator and Guglielmi detachable coiling for the acute treatment of casted ventricles from cerebral aneurysm hemorrhage: two technical case reports. Neurosurgery 2002;50:421.
94. Varelas PN, Rickert KL, Cusick J, et al. Intraventricular hemorrhage after aneurysmal subarachnoid hemorrhage: pilot study of treatment with intraventricular tissue plasminogen activator. Neurosurgery 2005;56:205.
95. Pluta RM, Afshar JK, Boock RJ, Oldfield EH. Temporal changes in perivascular concentrations of oxyhemoglobin, deoxyhemoglobin, and methemoglobin after subarachnoid hemorrhage. J Neurosurg 1998;88:557.
96. Takeuchi K, Miyata N, Renic M, et al. Hemoglobin, NO, and 20-HETE interactions in mediating cerebral vasoconstriction following SAH. Am J Physiol Regul Integr Comp Physiol 2006;290:R84.
97. Roman RJ, Renic M, Dunn KM, et al. Evidence that 20-HETE contributes to the development of acute

and delayed cerebral vasospasm. Neurol Res 2006;28:738.

98. Takeuchi K, Renic M, Bohman QC, et al. Reversal of delayed vasospasm by an inhibitor of the synthesis of 20-HETE. Am J Physiol Heart Circ Physiol 2005;289:H2203.

99. Hacein-Bey L, Harder DR, Meier HT, et al. Reversal of delayed vasospasm by TS-011 in the dual hemorrhage dog model of subarachnoid hemorrhage. AJNR Am J Neuroradiol 2006;27:1350.

100. Kwak R, Niizuma H, Ohi T, Suzuki J. Angiographic study of cerebral vasospasm following rupture of intracranial aneurysms, part I: time of the appearance. Surg Neurol 1979;11:257.

101. Niizuma H, Kwak R, Otabe K, Suzuki J. Angiography study of cerebral vasospasm following the rupture of intracranial aneurysms, part II: relation between the site of aneurysm and the occurrence of the vasospasm. Surg Neurol 1979;11:263.

102. Weyer GW, Nolan CP, Macdonald RL. Evidence-based cerebral vasospasm management. Neurosurg Focus 2006;21:E8.

103. Pickard JD, Walker V, Brandt L, et al. Effect of intraventricular haemorrhage and rebleeding following subarachnoid haemorrhage on CSF eicosanoids. Acta Neurochir (Wien) 1994;129(3-4):152.

104. Chyatte D, Fode NC, Nichols DA, Sundt TM. Preliminary report: effects of high dose methylprednisolone on delayed cerebral ischemia in patients at high risk for vasospasm after aneurysmal subarachnoid hemorrhage. Neurosurgery 1987;21:157.

105. Yasukawa K, Kamijou Y, Momose G, et al. The experiences of a large amount of steroid therapy for symptomatic vasospasm after subarachnoid hemorrhage: clinical analysis of 21 cases. No Shinkei Geka 1994;22:17.

106. Karnik R, Valentin A, Prainer C, et al. Steroid therapy in subarachnoid hemorrhage. Wien Klin Wochenschr 1990;102:1-4.

107. Schürkämper M, Medele R, Zausinger S, et al. Dexamethasone in the treatment of subarachnoid hemorrhage revisited: a comparative analysis of the effect of the total dose on complications and outcome. J Clin Neurosci 2004;11:20.

108. Hasan D, Lindsay KW, Wijdicks EF, et al. Effect of fludrocortisone acetate in patients with subarachnoid hemorrhage. Stroke 1989;20:1156.

109. Lynch JR, Wang H, McGirt MJ, et al. Simvastatin reduces vasospasm after aneurysmal subarachnoid hemorrhage: results of a pilot randomized clinical trial. Stroke 2005;36:2024.

110. Tseng MY, Czosnyka M, Richards H, et al. Effects of acute treatment with statins on cerebral autoregulation in patients after aneurysmal subarachnoid hemorrhage. Neurosurg Focus 2006;21:E10.

111. Origitano TC, Wascher TM, Reichman OH, Anderson DE. Sustained increased cerebral blood flow with prophylactic hypertensive hypervolemic hemodilution ("triple-H" therapy) after subarachnoid hemorrhage. Neurosurgery 1990;27:729.

112. Kassell NF, Peerless SJ, Durward QJ, et al. Treatment of ischemic deficits from vasospasm with intravascular volume expansion and induced arterial hypertension. Neurosurgery 1982;11:337.

113. Pinto AN, Canhao P, Ferro JM. Seizures at the onset of subarachnoid haemorrhage. J Neurol 1996;243:161.

114. Dennis LJ, Claassen J, Hirsch LJ, et al. Nonconvulsive status epilepticus after subarachnoid hemorrhage. Neurosurgery 2002;51:1136.

115. Naidech AM, Kreiter KT, Janjua N, et al. Phenytoin exposure is associated with functional and cognitive disability after subarachnoid hemorrhage. Stroke 2005;36:583.

116. Willmore LJ. Antiepileptic drugs and neuroprotection: current status and future roles. Epilepsy Behav 2005;7(Suppl 3):S25.

117. Wijdicks EF, Ropper AH, Hunnicutt EJ, et al. Atrial natriuretic factor and salt wasting after aneurysmal subarachnoid hemorrhage. Stroke 1991;22:1519.

118. Nguyen BN, Yablon SA, Chen CY. Hypodipsic hypernatremia and diabetes insipidus following anterior communicating artery aneurysm clipping: diagnostic and therapeutic challenges in the amnestic rehabilitation patient. Brain Inj 2001;15:975.

119. Urbaniak K, Merchant AI, Amin-Hanjani S, Roitberg B. Cardiac complications after aneurysmal subarachnoid hemorrhage. Surg Neurol 2007;67:21.

120. Donaldson JW, Pritz MB. Myocardial stunning secondary to aneurysmal subarachnoid hemorrhage. Surg Neurol 2001;55:12.

121. Lanzino G, Kongable GL, Kassell NF. Electrocardiographic abnormalities after nontraumatic subarachnoid hemorrhage. J Neurosurg Anesthesiol 1994;6:156.

122. Weir BK. Pulmonary edema following fatal aneurysm rupture. J Neurosurg 1978;49:502.

123. Wartenberg KE, Schmidt JM, Claassen J, et al. Impact of medical complications on outcome after subarachnoid hemorrhage. Crit Care Med 2006;34:617.

124. Wintermark M, Ko NU, Smith WS, et al. Vasospasm after subarachnoid hemorrhage: utility of perfusion CT and CT angiography on diagnosis and management. AJNR Am J Neuroradiol 2006;27:26.

125. Feng L, Fitzsimmons BF, Young WL, et al. Intraarterially administered verapamil as adjunct therapy for cerebral vasospasm: safety and 2-year experience. AJNR Am J Neuroradiol 2002;23:1284.

126. Andaluz N, Tomsick TA, Tew JM, et al. Indications for endovascular therapy for refractory vasospasm after aneurysmal subarachnoid hemorrhage: experience at the University of Cincinnati. Surg Neurol 2002;58:131.

127. Liu JK, Tenner MS, Gottfried ON, et al. Efficacy of multiple intraarterial papaverine infusions for improvement in cerebral circulation time in patients with recurrent cerebral vasospasm. J Neurosurg 2004;100:414.

128. Eskridge JM, McAuliffe W, Song JK, et al. Balloon angioplasty for the treatment of vasospasm: results of first 50 cases. Neurosurgery 1998;42:510.

129. Rosen CL, Sekhar LN, Duong DH. Use of intra-aortic balloon pump counterpulsation for refractory

symptomatic vasospasm. Acta Neurochir (Wien) 2000;142:25.

130. Rabinstein AA, Wijdicks EF. Cerebral vasospasm in subarachnoid hemorrhage. Curr Treat Options Neurol 2005;7:99.

131. van Gijn J, van Dongen KJ, Vermeulen M, Hijdra A. Perimesencephalic hemorrhage: a nonaneurysmal and benign form of subarachnoid hemorrhage. Neurology 1985;35:493.

132. Rinkel GJE, Wijdicks EFM, Vermeulen M, et al. Nonaneurysmal perimesencephalic subarachnoid hemorrhage: CT and MR patterns that differ from aneurysmal rupture. AJNR Am J Neuroradiol 1991;12:829.

133. Kershenovich A, Rappaport ZH, Maimon S. Brain computed tomography angiographic scans as the sole diagnostic examination for excluding aneurysms in patients with perimesencephalic subarachnoid hemorrhage. Neurosurgery 2006;59:798.

134. Canhão P, Ferro JM, Pinto AN, et al. Perimesencephalic and nonperimesencephalic subarachnoid haemorrhages with negative angiograms. Acta Neurochir (Wien) 1995;132(1-3):14.

135. van der Schaaf IC, Velthuis BK, Gouw A, Rinkel GJ. Venous drainage in perimesencephalic hemorrhage. Stroke 2004;35:1614.

136. Matsuyama T, Okuchi K, Seki T, et al. Perimesencephalic nonaneurysmal subarachnoid hemorrhage caused by physical exertion. Neurol Med Chir (Tokyo) 2006;46:277.

137. Huttner HB, Hartmann M, Kohrmann M, et al. Repeated digital substraction angiography after perimesencephalic subarachnoid hemorrhage? J Neuroradiol 2006;33:87.

138. Sert A, Aydin K, Pirgon O, et al. Arterial spasm following perimesencephalic nonaneurysmal subarachnoid hemorrhage in a pediatric patient. Pediatr Neurol 2005;32:275.

139. Greebe P, Rinkel GJ. Life expectancy after perimesencephalic subarachnoid hemorrhage. Stroke 2007;38:1222.

140. Levine SR, Brust JC, Futrell N, et al. Cerebrovascular complications of the use of the "crack" form of alkaloidal cocaine. N Engl J Med 1990;323:699.

141. Nanda A, Vannemreddy P, Willis B, Kelley R. Stroke in the young: relationship of active cocaine use with stroke mechanism and outcome. Acta Neurochir Suppl 2006;96:91.

142. Howington JU, Kutz SC, Wilding GE, Awasthi D. Cocaine use as a predictor of outcome in aneurysmal subarachnoid hemorrhage. J Neurosurg 2003;99:271.

143. Nanda A, Vannemreddy PS, Polin RS, Willis BK. Intracranial aneurysms and cocaine abuse: analysis of prognostic indicators. Neurosurgery 2000;46:1063.

144. Su J, Li J, Li W, et al. Cocaine induces apoptosis in cerebral vascular muscle cells: potential roles in strokes and brain damage. Eur J Pharmacol 2003;482(1-3):61.

145. Shin EH, Bian S, Shim YB, et al. Cocaine increases endoplasmic reticulum stress protein expression in striatal neurons. Neuroscience 2007;145:621.

146. Noël B. Vascular complications of cocaine use. Stroke 2002;33:1747.

147. Hillbom M, Kaste M. Alcohol intoxication: a risk factor for primary subarachnoid hemorrhage. Neurology 1982;32:706.

148. Arauz A, Velásquez L, Cantú C, et al. Phenylpropanolamine and intracranial hemorrhage risk in a Mexican population. Cerebrovasc Dis 2003;15:210.

149. Takahashi S, Sonobe M, Shirane R, et al. Computer tomography of ruptured intracranial arteriovenous malformations in the acute stage. Acta Neurochir (Wien) 1982;66(1-2):87.

150. Shephard RH. Spinal arteriovenous malformations and subarachnoid haemorrhage. Br J Neurosurg 1992;6:5.

151. Moussouttas M, Abubakr A, Grewal RP, Papamitsakis N. Eclamptic subarachnoid haemorrhage without hypertension. J Clin Neurosci 2006;13:474.

152. Ursell MR, Marras CL, Farb R, et al. Recurrent intracranial hemorrhage due to postpartum cerebral angiopathy: implications for management. Stroke 1998;29:1995.

153. Nagumo K, Nakamori A, Kojima S. Spontaneous intracranial internal carotid artery dissection: 6 case reports and a review of 39 cases in the literature. Rinsho Shinkeigaku 2003;43:313.

154. Yakushiji Y, Haraguchi Y, Soejima S, et al. A hyperdense artery sign and middle cerebral artery dissection. Intern Med 2006;45:1319.

155. Kim DS, Kim JK, Yoo DS, et al. Takayasu's arteritis presented with subarachnoid hemorrhage: report of two cases. J Korean Med Sci 2002;17:695.

156. Somarajan A, Ashalatha R, Syam K. Moya Moya disease: an unusual clinical presentation. J Assoc Physicians India 2005;53:49.

157. Yamamoto M, Fukushima T, Ikeda K, et al. Intracranial cavernous angioma manifesting as subarachnoid hemorrhage—case report. Neurol Med Chir (Tokyo) 1993;33:706.

158. Hentschel S, Toyota B. Intracranial malignant glioma presenting as subarachnoid hemorrhage. Can J Neurol Sci 2003;30:63.

159. Berlis A, Schumacher M, Spreer J, et al. Subarachnoid haemorrhage due to cervical spinal cord haemangioblastomas in a patient with von Hippel-Lindau disease. Acta Neurochir (Wien) 2003;145:1009.

160. Inci S, Bozkurt G, Gulsen S, et al. Rare cause of subarachnoid hemorrhage: spinal meningeal carcinomatosis: case report. J Neurosurg Spine 2005;2:79.

161. Chukwudelunzu FE, Brown RD, Wijdicks EF, Steckelberg JM. Subarachnoid haemorrhage associated with infectious endocarditis: case report and literature review. Eur J Neurol 2002;9:423.

162. Nakahara K, Oka H, Utsuki S, et al. Pituitary apoplexy manifesting as diffuse subarachnoid hemorrhage. Neurol Med Chir (Tokyo) 2006;46:594.

163. Mueller RF, Buckler J, Arthur R, et al. The 3–M syndrome: risk of intracerebral aneurysm? J Med Genet 1992;29(2):425.

CHAPTER 16

Pediatric Central Nervous System Vascular Malformations

Thomas J. Altstadt • Mitesh V. Shah

This chapter discusses the various central nervous system (CNS) vascular malformations that occur in childhood. These CNS vascular malformations consist of arteriovenous malformations (AVMs), vein of Galen malformations (VoGMs), cavernous malformations, capillary telangiectasias, and venous angiomas. The pathology, presentation, evaluation, and management of each of these lesions are discussed.

Arteriovenous Malformations

Pathology

Arteriovenous vascular malformations are the most common cause of nontraumatic intracerebral hemorrhage (ICH) in young adults.[1] An AVM is defined as a tightly woven tangle of thin-walled vessels that serve as a shunt from enlarged feeding arteries to its dilated draining vein with interposed abnormal, gliotic brain (Figs. 16-1 and 16-2).[2]

Incidence

The incidence of AVMs in the general population is estimated to be 0.6% with a slight male predominance.[2] In several series, it has been found that approximately 12% to 18% of AVMs occur in pediatric patients.[3-6]

Presentation

The most common presentation of an AVM is ICH, followed by seizures and headache or other neurologic signs resulting from cerebral steal. Infants with

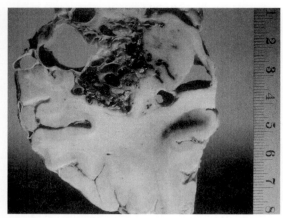

FIGURE 16-1   Gross pathologic specimen of large AVM.

AVMs may present with high-output heart failure owing to the large shunt and low blood volumes. ICH as the presenting symptom occurs in 69.5% to 79% of pediatric vascular malformations.[7,21] Most AVMs in children and adults are supratentorial, but in a comparison between a pediatric and adult population, Kondziolka and colleagues[7] found that there were significantly higher percentages of cerebellar (13%) and brainstem (11%) AVMs in the pediatric cohort than in the adult cohort (3.3% and 2%).[7]

Diagnostic Studies

The initial radiologic workup for any patient presenting with a new-onset seizure disorder, headache, or neurologic deficit is a non–contrast-enhanced computed tomography (CT) scan of the head. A non–contrast-enhanced CT scan of the head shows an area of hemorrhage or an area of calcification suspicious for AVM. Frequently, magnetic resonance imaging (MRI) and MR angiography are then employed to identify the lesion and provide information about the feeding vessels. Cerebral angiography remains the gold standard for treatment planning of AVMs (Fig. 16-3).

Familial Occurrence

Hereditary hemorrhagic telangiectasia (HHT), or Rendu-Osler-Weber syndrome, is a rare autosomal dominant disorder characterized by multiple mucocutaneous telangiectasias and associated vascular malformations in multiple organ systems.[8,9] Approximately 5% to 13% of patients with HHT have cerebrovascular malformations.[10,11] The cerebrovascular malformations found in patients with HHT consist of AVMs, venous angiomas, and telangiectasias.[9,10] HHT is associated with gene defects in the transforming growth factor-β binding protein endoglin on chromosome 9q and non–endoglin-related genes on chromosome 12q.[12-15]

Neurologic symptoms in HHT are most commonly secondary to pulmonary AVMs leading to ischemic strokes from paradoxical emboli or brain abscesses from septic emboli.[8] Patients with AVMs can present with ICH, seizures, and headache. In a study

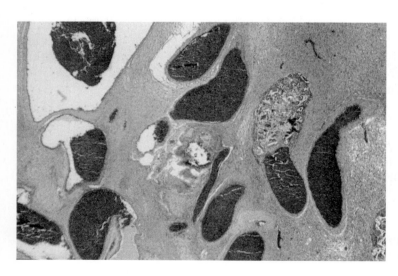

FIGURE 16-2   Pathologic specimen of AVM shows dilated sinusoidal vessels and surrounding gliotic parenchyma.

Natural History

The natural history of an AVM manifesting in childhood seems to have a more ominous course than AVMs manifesting in adulthood, although this question has not been adequately addressed because there are so few series of pediatric AVMs. AVMs are associated with a continued risk of ICH and progressive neurologic deficit secondary to vascular steal. The risk of hemorrhage of an adult AVM has been estimated at 2% to 4% per year.[17,18] So[21] reported a risk of repeat hemorrhage of 24% within 5 years of initial hemorrhage. Celli and coworkers[3] found that there was a statistically significant higher rate of hemorrhage in children studied compared with adults, although no specific rates were given. It also has been reported that the highest risk of hemorrhage occurred between the ages of 16 and 25.[19] To calculate the lifetime risk of AVM hemorrhage, the following formula is used: Risk of hemorrhage = 1−(risk of no hemorrhage) expected years of remaining life.[20] The fatality rate of the initial hemorrhage from an AVM in pediatric patients has been reported to be 5.4% to 8%.[5,21]

Treatment

The goals of therapy are to remove the risk of hemorrhage, control seizures, and relieve symptoms related to the vascular steal phenomenon. The treatment of AVMs requires a multidisciplinary approach between the neurosurgeon, the neurointerventionalist, and the radiation therapist.

When a child presents with an ICH from an AVM, emergent surgery is rarely necessary, unless the hematoma is life-threatening.[22] Typically, the surgeon waits several weeks after an ICH to allow the brain to relax and the child's condition to optimize. Under these conditions, surgery is undertaken with the goal of total extirpation to eliminate the risk of repeat hemorrhage. The risk of operative intervention is based on the classification scheme of Spetzler and Martin.[23] This scheme classifies AVMs in grades I through V based on the size of the AVM (1 to 3, from small to large), its pattern of venous drainage (0 for superficial, 1 for deep), and the eloquence of the

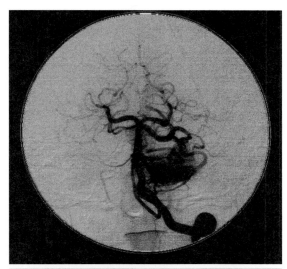

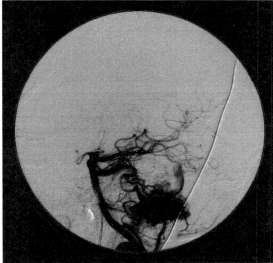

FIGURE 16-3   Anteroposterior (*top*) and lateral (*bottom*) views angiographic show large left cerebellar AVM in a 15-year-old boy.

of HHT patients, the cerebrovascular malformations consisted mostly of multiple low-grade AVMs, with females more often affected than males.[10] The risk of hemorrhage from these AVMs ranged from 0.41% to 0.72% per year, which is significantly less than the risk of hemorrhage from sporadic AVMs.[10]

AVMs also are seen in Klippel-Trénaunay-Weber syndrome.[16] This syndrome is characterized by varicose veins, cutaneous hemangioma, and hypertrophy of the involved limb. Spinal and cerebral AVMs have been reported with this syndrome (see Chapter 14, Fig. 14-4).

surrounding brain (0 for noneloquent, 1 for eloquent). The points are summed, and a grade is given from I to V (easiest to resect to most difficult to resect).

Before any surgical intervention is undertaken, the neurointerventionalist should embolize as much of the AVM as possible to reduce the surgical blood loss. In large AVMs, there is a considerable amount of vascular steal from the surrounding brain. The risk of edema and hemorrhage after surgery is increased because of normal perfusion breakthrough. Staged preoperative embolization is used to obliterate the arteriovenous shunt in stages to reduce the risk of normal perfusion breakthrough and its complications.

In some high-grade AVMs, the risks of surgical intervention are unacceptable. Stereotactically guided radiotherapy has been used in these cases. Several studies have documented the effectiveness and safety of gamma knife radiosurgery, stereotactic heavy-charged-particle Bragg peak radiosurgery, and stereotactic radiosurgery with a linear accelerator.[24-28] All systems use stereotactically guided assistance to direct radiotherapy. The most widely used form of stereotactic radiosurgery is the gamma knife. The advantage of radiosurgery is that it is typically done on an outpatient basis, and the complication rate is low. The disadvantages are that it takes approximately 2 years for obliteration of an AVM nidus, and there continues to be a risk of hemorrhage during that time. Results of radiosurgery of pediatric AVMs have shown the rate of angiographic obliteration at 2 years to be 75% to 94%.[24,26]

One feature unique to pediatric AVMs is that they have been reported to recur several years after documented angiographic obliteration.[29] Because of this fact, it has been proposed that pediatric AVMs be studied for 5 years after documented obliteration.[29]

Vein of Galen Malformations

Pathology

VoGMs encompass a diverse collection of AVMs all having in common a dilated venous pouch located in the velum interpositum and quadrigeminal cistern consisting of the persistence of the fetal medial prosencephalic

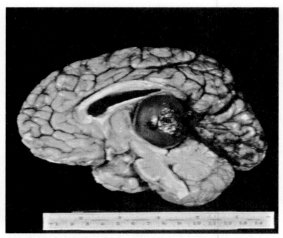

FIGURE 16-4   Gross pathologic specimen of VoGM.

vein of Markowski (Fig. 16-4).[30] The name is a misnomer.

Yasargil[31] classified VoGM into four categories. Type I is a pure fistula between arteries and the vein of Galen with the nidus being the ampulla of the vein of Galen. The lesion is entirely extrinsic to the brain parenchyma. Type II consists of thalamoperforators that travel through the brain parenchyma to form a fistula with the vein of Galen. The lesion is intrinsic and extrinsic to the CNS. Type III is a mixed form of types I and II. Type IV lesions consist of proximal AVMs that have draining veins that drain into the vein of Galen.

Another classification scheme proposed by Quisling and Mickle[32] divides VoGMs into three categories. Type I consist of true fistulas with direct arteriovenous communication via a single choroidal arterial trunk. Type II are deep AVMs drained by the galenic system. Type III malformations are similar to type I, but are fed by anterior and posterior choroidal arteries and the distal anterior cerebral artery. Type III malformations have the greatest arteriovenous shunt and are most likely to occur in the newborn period with high-output heart failure.

Incidence

VoGMs are rare clinical entities; they are estimated to represent approximately 1% of intracranial AVMs. The true incidence is unknown, but more than 300 cases are reported in the literature.[31,33-37]

Presentation

In a classification scheme proposed by Amacher and Shillito,[38] an attempt was made to categorize signs and symptoms of presentation with age. Group I consists of neonates presenting with severe high-output cardiac failure and cranial bruit. Group II consists of neonates with mild heart failure and craniomegaly. Group III consists of infants with craniomegaly and a cranial bruit. Group IV consists of children presenting after age 3.5 years with headaches, exercise syncope, and a calcified mass in the pineal region.

Severe high-output cardiac failure is the major cause of mortality in neonates with VoGMs.[39] The low-resistance arteriovenous shunt directs most of the neonate's cardiac output to the cerebrum. Heart failure typically manifests after birth as the placenta with its low vascular resistance competes with the VoGM for the cardiac output of the fetus. The typical signs of severe congestive heart failure with VoGM are tachycardia, tachypnea, hepatomegaly with distended jugular veins, and bounding pulses and precordium.

Hydrocephalus or ventriculomegaly in VoGM is multifactorial, and its cause is debated. Causes include obstruction of the sylvian aqueduct, resorptive blocks secondary to increased pressure within the superior sagittal sinus, and hydrocephalus ex vacuo secondary to cerebral atrophy.[33]

Developmental delay is a common finding in children with VoGM. Mechanisms for cerebral damage include arterial steal, venous hypertension leading to decreased arterial perfusion, and venous infarction.[33]

Evaluation

Ultrasound is an excellent noninvasive means for evaluating VoGMs in utero and in neonates.[40,41] Color Doppler ultrasound provides information about the feeding and draining vessels and assesses the patency of the VoGM. On CT, VoGMs appear as rounded masses in the quadrigeminal cistern lying behind and anteriorly displacing the third ventricle. With contrast administration, homogeneous opacification of the VoGM and the draining sinuses is seen (Fig. 16-5).

Angiography remains the gold standard for evaluating and classifying VoGMs. If other imaging studies suggest a VoGM, it is best to perform the diagnostic angiogram in conjunction with therapeutic intervention (Fig. 16-6).

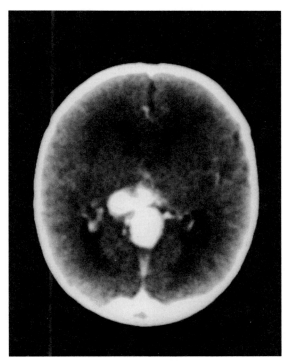

FIGURE 16-5 Contrast-enhanced head CT scan shows large enhancing mass in the pineal region consistent with VoGM.

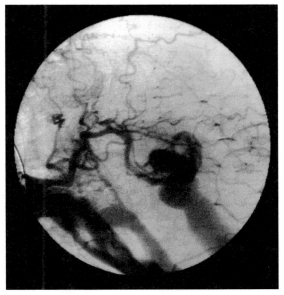

FIGURE 16-6 Lateral angiogram shows large venous pouch located in the quadrigeminal cistern.

Associated Syndromes

VoGMs are seen with Turner syndrome and blue rubber bleb nevus syndrome.[42,43] Turner syndrome is the absence of a single X chromosome in a female and is associated with amenorrhea and other vascular anomalies such as coarctation of the aorta. Blue rubber bleb nevus syndrome manifests with blue, nipple-like, compressible skin lesions composed of blood-filled venous and cavernous angiomas.

Treatment

The treatment of VoGM is best undertaken by a team consisting of a pediatric neurosurgeon and a neurointerventionalist able to employ a multidisciplinary approach to neurovascular disease.[44-46] It is ideal if the team is experienced in treating these complex vascular entities. A neonate with severe cardiac failure should be treated aggressively with staged embolization to avoid decompensation from the heart failure.[36,47,48] A patient who presents with hydrocephalus is best served by careful, staged embolization and surgical treatment of the hydrocephalus.[33] Surgery typically is reserved for lesions not amenable to neurointerventional techniques. Gamma knife radiosurgery has been used in the treatment of VoGMs in select clinically stable patients.[49]

Cavernous Malformations

Pathology

A cavernous malformation is a discrete, well-circumscribed lesion with a reddish purple, multilobulated appearance similar to a cluster of mulberries. Microscopically, a cavernous malformation comprises sinusoidal spaces lined by a single layer of endothelium and separated by a collagenous stroma devoid of elastin, smooth muscle, or mature vascular wall elements. A characteristic marker is the lack of intervening neural parenchyma (Fig. 16-7).[2] Venous malformations are commonly found in association with cavernous malformations.[50,51]

Cavernous malformations are found throughout the CNS, but are most common in the supratentorial compartment. They are frequently multiple and range in size from less than 0.1 to 9 cm.[52] The prevalence of cavernous malformations in the general population has been estimated to be 0.4% to 0.9%.[52] They are found equally in males and females.[52] Cavernous malformations are found sporadically and are inherited in an autosomal dominant fashion.[53]

Presentation

In young children, the most common presentation of a cavernous malformation is hemorrhage and acute neurologic deficit.[54,55]

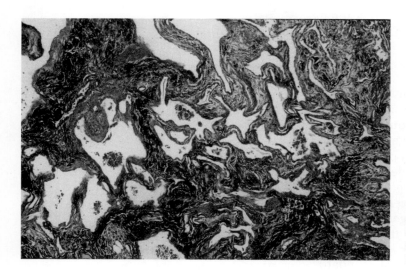

FIGURE 16-7 Trichrome-stained cavernous malformation shows dilated sinusoidal vessels with surrounding gliosis without intervening neural parenchyma.

Clinically significant intraparenchymal hemorrhage is heralded by an acute onset of headache, focal neurologic deficit based on the location of the lesion, and change in the level of consciousness. Subarachnoid hemorrhage is rare except when the cavernous malformation is located in the optic nerve, chiasm, or ventricle. Hemorrhage from a cavernous malformation is rarely life-threatening.

In older children and adults, the most common presentation of a cavernous malformation is epilepsy. The pathophysiology of epilepsy in cavernous malformations is postulated to be caused by irritation and compression from mass effect and multiple local hemorrhages with the exposure of the surrounding brain to blood breakdown products and subsequent local gliomatous reaction.

Acute or progressive focal neurologic deficit is another presentation of a cavernous malformation. Intralesional or perilesional hemorrhage is usually the culprit and can be documented with MRI. The neurologic deficit depends on the lesion location and size. The deficit may be fixed, transient, or recurrent.

Familial Occurrence

A familial form of cavernous malformations was first described in Mexican-Americans, but now has been documented in other nationalities as well.[53,56] In 54% of patients with cavernous malformations, the trait is inherited in an autosomal dominant fashion.[53] Three genetic loci have been identified that predispose a patient to cavernous malformations. The CCM1 locus resides on chromosome 7q21-q22. The CCM1 locus has been identified as the *KRIT1* gene. Many mutations in the *KRIT1* gene have been identified.[57-59] The *KRIT1* gene product interacts with *RAP1A*, which is a renin-angiotensin system guanosine triphosphatase hypothesized to function as a tumor suppressor gene.[59] The locus for CCM2 resides on chromosome 7p13-p15, and CCM3 resides on chromosome 3q25.2-q27.[60] The genes encoded by CCM2 and CCM3 have yet to be identified. It has been postulated that CCM1, CCM2, and CCM3 account for 40%, 20%, and 40% of the familial cases of cavernous malformations.[58]

In a study of the natural history of familial cavernous malformations, it was noted that those patients were more likely to have multiple lesions, and it was common for new cavernous malformations to develop on MRI with follow-up.[61,62] The calculated symptomatic spontaneous hemorrhage rate for familial cavernous malformations is 1.1% per lesion per year, which is higher than the hemorrhage rate seen with spontaneous cavernous malformations.[61]

Evaluation

The CT appearance of cavernous malformations is a well-circumscribed, nodular lesion of uniform or variegated mixed density reflecting the calcification, hemorrhage, and cystic components of the lesion. Cavernous malformations may enhance faintly with contrast administration. Frequently, recent hemorrhage is seen as a homogeneous hyperdensity and obscures the lesion.

The MRI appearance of cavernous malformations is the most sensitive diagnostic test for cavernous malformations, and it is characteristic.[63] A cavernous malformation appears as a well-defined, lobulated lesion with a central core of reticulated mixed signal surrounded by a rim of signal hypointensity. The typical low T2 signal surrounding cavernous malformations is due to the ferritin from erythrocyte breakdown that is a consequence of intralesional and perilesional hemorrhages. The reticulated low T2 signal within the cavernous malformation reflects intralesional calcification. Areas of signal hyperintensity within the lesion represent acute and subacute hemorrhage in various stages of thrombus organization and resolution (Fig. 16-8).

Natural History

The natural history of the cavernous malformation is still being elucidated. Cavernous malformations are dynamic lesions that have been shown to change in size and signal characteristics on neuroimaging studies. The appearance of new cavernous malformations has been documented in patients with existing lesions and patients with no

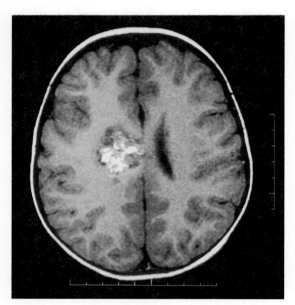

FIGURE 16-8   T1-weighted MR image shows mixed density lesion consistent with cavernous malformation.

history of cavernous malformations.[64] Cases of cavernous malformations forming de novo after radiation therapy for tumors have been reported in the literature.[65] The annual clinically significant hemorrhage risk has been estimated to be 0.6% to 1.1% per lesion per year, with the highest rates occurring with familial cavernous malformations.[61,66] Cavernous malformations that bleed are at increased risk of hemorrhage in the future, and there is an association between female hormones and hemorrhage.[67]

Treatment

The goals of therapy are to control epilepsy, prevent or evacuate hemorrhage, and treat focal neurologic deficit. The treatment of epilepsy is typically medical. A patient with medically intractable epilepsy may benefit, however, from surgical extirpation of the cavernous malformation.[68] Before this procedure is undertaken, the patient must be thoroughly evaluated to identify the epileptogenic focus. During surgery, the grossly abnormal adjacent brain should be resected as well to ensure removal of the seizure focus.[68]

Surgery also may be undertaken to extirpate the lesions that have shown repeated hemorrhage and focal neurologic problems.[52,55,69] This extirpation is particularly

important with brainstem cavernous malformations because the brainstem does not tolerate mass effect from recurrent hemorrhage.[70-72] The resection of brainstem cavernous malformations should not be undertaken until the malformation presents to the surface to avoid injury to eloquent areas.[71,72]

Radiosurgery for cavernous malformations is a topic that is still under debate. Conflicting results are reported in the literature regarding its effectiveness.[73-77] The success of radiosurgery is difficult to ascertain because cavernous malformations are not visualized on angiogram, and the lesions frequently regress in size on MRI. Radiosurgery of cavernous malformations has shown higher complication rates of edema and radiation necrosis than for AVMs.[77] It has been postulated that the blood breakdown products present in cavernous malformations act as a radiopotentiator.

Venous Angiomas

Pathology

Venous angiomas or venous malformations are the most common cerebrovascular malformation.[2] They are composed of radially arranged anomalous medullary veins that converge in a centrally located dilated trunk that is surrounded by normal neural parenchyma.[2] There is a well-known association between venous angiomas and cavernous malformations.[50]

Presentation

Most venous angiomas are discovered as incidental findings, but they have been associated with epilepsy, headaches, and various neurologic signs related to the location of the angioma.[78-83] Rarely, venous angiomas manifest with hemorrhage and its associated signs and symptoms.[84]

Evaluation

The CT appearance of venous angiomas is linear or curvilinear enhancement after contrast administration.[85,86] The MRI appearance consists of a prominent transcerebral

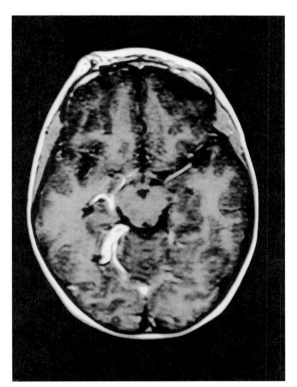

FIGURE 16-9 Gadolinium-enhanced MR image shows right parieto-occipital Developmental Venous Anomalies (DVAs).

draining vein frequently associated with an area of increased parenchymal signal on T2-weighted images and occasionally with decreased signal on T1-weighted images (Fig. 16-9).[87,88] The angiographic appearance of venous angiomas is multiple, dilated medullary veins appearing in the venous phase and converging toward a central, equally dilated, draining vein with a caput medusae appearance.[86]

Natural History

Venous angiomas generally are considered to be benign, indolent lesions. The overall risk of hemorrhage has been estimated to be 0.22% to 0.34% per year.[89] This rate may be falsely elevated, however, because the hemorrhage could be caused by an associated, unrecognized cavernous malformation.

Treatment

The current management strategy of a venous angioma consists of observation as the primary mode of therapy.[89] Surgery is recommended only for removal of clot causing significant neurologic deficit or mass effect. The venous angioma should not be resected because this may remove the venous drainage of the normal local parenchyma leading to morbidity and mortality. For the same reason, radiosurgery plays no role in the treatment of isolated venous angiomas.

Capillary Telangiectasias

Capillary telangiectasias are composed of capillaries whose walls are devoid of smooth muscle and elastic fibers with intervening brain parenchyma (Fig. 16-10).[2] Their size varies widely, ranging from saccular dilations of capillary vessels to frankly ectatic, dilated groups of capillaries that resemble cavernous spaces in some areas (Fig. 16-11).[90] The true incidence is unknown, but they are frequently seen in Rendu-Osler-Weber syndrome. The most common location of capillary telangiectasias is in the basis pontis. Capillary telangiectasias are typically asymptomatic. Hemorrhage from capillary telangiectasias is exceedingly rare.[91,92] Capillary telangiectasias typically are not visualized on CT. The MRI appearance is small, homogeneously enhancing lesions, hypointense to isointense on T1-weighted images and isointense to hyperintense on proton-weighted images and marked gradient echo signal loss.[93]

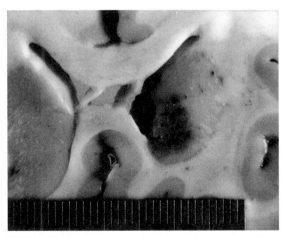

FIGURE 16-10 Gross pathologic specimen of capillary telangiectasia.

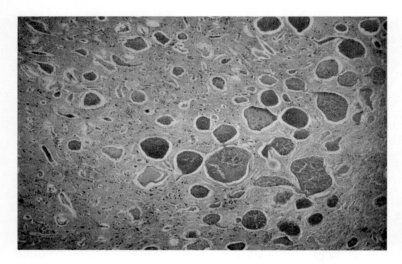

FIGURE 16-11   Pathologic specimen of a capillary telangiectasia shows dilated capillaries and sinuses.

Conclusion

Vascular malformations of the central nervous system (CNS), a group of focal networks of non-neoplastic disorders of the cerebral blood vessels, include: capillary telangiectasias, cavernous malformations (CM), developmental venous anomalies (DVAs), and arteriovenous malformations (AVMs), including varix of the great vein of Galen, and other vascular malformations. These malformations may occur in isolation or may be associated with other CNS malformations, or head and neck malformations. The natural history, potential complications, diagnostic strategies, and management options, are reviewed.

REFERENCES

1. Toffol GJ, Biller J, Adams HP. Non-traumatic intracerebral hemorrhage in young adults. Arch Neurol 1987;44:483.
2. McCormick WF. Classification, pathology, and natural history of angiomas of the central nervous system. Neurol Neurosurg Weekly Update 1978;1:3.
3. Celli P, Ferrante L, Palma L, Cavedon G. Cerebral arteriovenous malformations in children. Surg Neurol 1984;22:43.
4. Mazza C, Pasqualin A, Scienza R, et al. Intracranial arteriovenous malformations in the pediatric age: experience with 24 cases. Child Brain 1983;10:369.
5. Gerosa M, Cappellotto P, Iraci G, et al. Cerebral arteriovenous malformations in children (56 cases). Child Brain 1981;8:356-371.
6. Yasargil MG. Microneurosurgery IIIB. AVM of the Brain, Clinical Considerations, General and Special Operative Techniques, Surgical Results, Non-Operated Cases, Cavernous and Venous Angiomas, Neuroanesthesia. New York: Thieme Medical, 1988.
7. Kondziolka D, Humphreys RP, Hoffman HJ, et al. Arteriovenous malformations of the brain in children: a forty year experience. Can J Neurol Sci 1992; 19:40.
8. Adams HP, Subbiah B, Bosch EP. Neurologic aspects of hereditary hemorrhagic telangiectasia. Arch Neurol 1977;34:101.
9. Guttmacher AE, Marchuk DA, White RI. Hereditary hemorrhagic telangiectasia. N Engl J Med 1995; 333:918.
10. Willemse RB, Mager JJ, Westermann CJJ, et al. Bleeding risk of cerebrovascular malformations in hereditary hemorrhagic telangiectasia. J Neurosurg 2000;92:779.
11. Haitjema T, Disch F, Overtoom TTC, et al. Screening family members of patients with hereditary hemorrhagic telangiectasia. Am J Med 1995;99:519.
12. McAllister KA, Grogg KM, Johnson DW, et al. Endoglin, a TGF-beta binding protein of endothelial cells, is the gene for hereditary haemorrhagic telangiectasia type 1. Nat Genet 1994;8:345.
13. Berg JN, Gallione CJ, Stenzel TT, et al. The activin receptor-like kinase 1 gene: genomic structure and mutations in hereditary hemorrhagic telangiectasia type 2. Am J Hum Genet 1997;61:60.
14. Vincent P, Plauchu H, Hazan J, et al. A third locus for hereditary hemorrhagic telangiectasia maps to chromosome 12q. Hum Mol Genet 1995;4:945.
15. Johnson DW, Berg JN, Baldwin MA, et al. Mutations in the activin receptor-like kinase 1 gene in hereditary hemorrhagic telangiectasia type 2. Nat Genet 1996;13:189.
16. Benhaiem-Sigaux N, Zerah M, Gherardi R, et al. A retromedullary fistula associated with the Klippel-Trenaunay-Weber syndrome: a clinicopathologic study. Acta Neuropathol (Berl) 1985;66:318.
17. Brown RD, Wiebers DO, Forbes G, et al. The natural history of unruptured intracranial arteriovenous malformations. J Neurosurg 1988;68:352.

18. Fults D, Kelly DL. Natural history of arteriovenous malformations of the brain: a clinical study. Neurosurgery 1984;15:658.

19. Graf CJ, Perret GE, Torner JC. Bleeding from cerebral AVM's as part of their natural history. J Neurosurg 1983;58:331.

20. Kondziolka D, McLaughlin MR, Kestle JRW. Simple risk predictions for arteriovenous malformation hemorrhage. Neurosurgery 1995;37:851.

21. So SC. Cerebral arteriovenous malformations in children. Child Brain 1978;4:242.

22. Ogilvy CS, Stieg PE, Awad I, et al. Recommendations for the management of intracranial arteriovenous malformations. Stroke 2001;32:1458.

23. Spetzler RF, Martin NA. A proposed grading system for arteriovenous malformations. J Neurosurg 1986; 65:476.

24. Tanaka T, Kobayashi T, Kida Y, et al. Comparison between adult and pediatric arteriovenous malformations treated by gamma knife radiosurgery. Stereotact Funct Neurosurg 1996;66(Suppl 1):288.

25. Baumann GS, Wara WM, Larson DA, et al. Gamma knife radiosurgery in children. Pediatr Neurosurg 1996;24:193.

26. Kondziolka D, Lunsford LD, Flickinger JC. Stereotactic radiosurgery in children and adolescents. Pediatr Neurosurg 1990-1991;16:219.

27. Levy RP, Fabrikant JI, Frankel KA, et al. Stereotactic heavy-charged-particle Bragg peak radiosurgery for the treatment of intracranialarteriovenous malformations in childhood and adolescence. Neurosurgery 1989;24:841.

28. Loeffler JS, Rossitch E, Siddon R, et al. Role of stereotactic radiosurgery with a linear accelerator in treatment of intracranial arteriovenous malformations and tumors in children. Pediatrics 1990;85:774.

29. Ali MJ, Bendok BR, Rosenblatt S, et al. Recurrence of pediatric cerebral arteriovenous malformations after angiographically documented resection. Pediatr Neurosurg 2003;39:32.

30. Raybaud CA, Strother CM, Hald JK. Aneurysms of the vein of Galen: embryonic considerations and anatomical features relating to the pathogenesis of the malformation. Neuroradiology 1989;31:109.

31. Yasargil MG. Microneurosurgery IIIB. New York: Thieme Medical Publishers, 1988.

32. Quisling RG, Mickle JP. Venous pressure measurements in vein of Galen aneurysms. AJNR Am J Neuroradiol 1989;10:411.

33. Horowitz MB, Jungreis CA, Quisling RG, Pollack I. Vein of Galen aneurysms: a review and current concepts. AJNR Am J Neuroradiol 1994;15:1486.

34. Jones BV, Ball WS, Tomsick TA, et al. Vein of Galen malformation: diagnosis and treatment of 13 children with extended follow-up. AJNR Am J Neuroradiol 2002;23:1717.

35. Lasjaunias P, Rodesch G, Terbrugge K, et al. Vein of Galen aneurysmal malformations report of 36 cases between 1982 and 1988. Acta Neurochir (Wien) 1989;99:26.

36. Hamasaki T, Kai Y, Hamada J, et al. Successful treatment of a neonate with vein of Galen aneurismal malformation. Pediatr Neurosurg 2000;32:200.

37. Hoffman HJ, Chuang S, Hendrick EB, et al. Aneurysms of the vein of Galen experience at the hospital for sick children, Toronto. J Neurosurg 1982;57:316.

38. Amacher LA, Shillito J. The syndromes and surgical treatment of aneurysms of the great vein of Galen. J Neurosurg 1973;39:89.

39. Chevret L, Durand P, Alvarez H, et al. Severe cardiac failure in newborns with VGAM. Intensive Care Med 2002;28:1126.

40. Heiling KS, Chaoui R, Bollmann R. Prenatal diagnosis of an aneurysm of the vein of Galen with three-dimensional color power angiography. Ultrasound Obstet Gynecol 2000;15:333.

41. Lee TH, Shih JC, Peng SSF, et al. Prenatal depiction of angioarchitecture of an aneurysm of the vein of Galen with three-dimensional color power angiography. Ultrasound Obstet Gynecol 2000;15:337.

42. Jarrell HR, Schochet SS, Krous H, et al. Turner's syndrome and vein of Galen aneurysm: a previously unreported association. Acta Neuropathol 1981; 55:189.

43. Rosenblum WI, Nakoneczna I, Konderding HS, et al. Multiple vascular malformation in the "blue rubber bleb naevus" syndrome: a case with aneurysm of the vein of Galen and vascular lesions suggesting a link to the Weber-Osler-Rendu syndrome. Histopathology 1978;2:301.

44. Lasjaunais P, Rodesch G, Pruvost P, et al. Treatment of vein of Galen aneurismal malformation. J Neurosurg 1989;70:746.

45. Halbach VV, Dowd CF, Higashida RT, et al. Endovascular treatment of mural-type vein of Galen malformations. J Neurosurg 1998;88:74.

46. Mickle JP, Quisling RG. The transtorcular embolization of vein of Galen aneurysms. J Neurosurg 1986;64:731.

47. Ciricillo SF, Edwards MSB, Schmidt KG, et al. Interventional neuroradiological management of vein of Galen malformations in the neonate. Neurosurgery 1990;27:22.

48. Mitchell PJ, Rosenfeld JV, Dargaville P, et al. Endovascular management of vein of Galen aneurysmal malformations presenting in the neonatal period. AJNR Am J Neuroradiol 2001;22:1403.

49. Payne BR, Prasad D, Steiner M, et al. Gamma surgery for vein of Galen malformations. J Neurosurg 2000;93:229.

50. Rigamonti D, Spetzler RF. The association of venous and cavernous malformations. Acta Neurochir (Wien) 1988;92:100.

51. Abe T, Singer RJ, Marks MP, et al. Coexistence of occult vascular malformations and developmental venous anomalies in the central nervous system: MR evaluation. AJNR Am J Neuroradiol 1998;19:51.

52. Maraire JN, Awad IA. Intracranial cavernous malformations: lesion behavior and management strategies. Neurosurgery 1995;37:591.

53. Rigamonti D, Hadley MN, Drayer BP, et al. Cerebral cavernous malformations. N Engl J Med 1988; 319:343.

54. Scott RM, Barnes P, Kupsky W, et al. Cavernous angiomas of the central nervous system in children. J Neurosurg 1992;76:38.

55. Ciricillo SF, Cogen PH, Edwards MSB. Pediatric cryptic vascular malformations: presentation, diagnosis and treatment. Pediatr Neurosurg 1994;20:137.
56. Mason I, Aase JM, Orrison WW, et al. Familial cavernous angiomas of the brain in an Hispanic family. Neurology 1988;38:324.
57. Zhang J, Clatterbuck RE, Rigamonti D, et al. Mutations in KRIT1 in familial cerebral cavernous malformations. Neurosurgery 2000;46:1272.
58. Verlaan DJ, Davenport WJ, Stefan H, et al. Cerebral cavernous malformations. Neurology 2002;58:853.
59. Kehrer-sawatzki H, Wilda M, Braun VM, et al. Mutation and expression analysis of the KRIT1 gene associated with cerebral cavernous malformations. Acta Neuropathol 2002;104:231.
60. Craig HD, Guenel M, Cepeda O, et al. Multilocus linkage identifies two new loci for a Mendelian form of stroke, cerebral cavernous malformations at 7p 15-13 and 3q 25, 2-27. Hum Mol Genet 1998;7:1851.
61. Zabramski JM, Wascher TM, Spetzler RF, et al. The natural history of familial cavernous malformations: results of an ongoing study. J Neurosurg 1994;80:422.
62. Labauge P, Brunereau L, Laberge S, et al. Prospective follow-up of 33 asymptomatic patients with familial cerebral cavernous malformations. Neurology 2001;57:1825.
63. Rigamonti D, Drayer BP, Johnson PC, et al. The MRI appearance of cavernous malformations. J Neurosurg 1987;67:518.
64. Detwiler PW, Porter RW, Zabramski JM, et al. De novo formation of a central nervous system cavernous malformation: implications for predicting risk of hemorrhage. J Neurosurg 1997;87:629.
65. Larson JL, Ball WS, Bove KE, et al. Formation of intracerebral cavernous malformations after radiation treatment for central nervous system neoplasia in children. J Neurosurg 1998;88:51.
66. Kondziolka D, Lunsford LD, Kestle JRW. The natural history of cerebral cavernous malformations. J Neurosurg 1995;83:820.
67. Aiba T, Tanaka R, Koike T, et al. Natural history of intracranial cavernous malformations. J Neurosurg 1995;83:56.
68. Cohen DS, Zubay GP, Goodman RF. Seizure outcome after lesionectomy for cavernous malformations. J Neurosurg 1995;83:237.
69. Giulioni M, Acciarri N, Padovani R, et al. Surgical management of cavernous angiomas in children. Surg Neurol 1994;42:194.
70. Scott RM. Brain stem cavernous angiomas in children. Pediatr Neurosurg 1990-1991;16:281.
71. Porter RW, Detwiler PW, Spetzler RF, et al. Cavernous malformations of the brainstem: experience with 100 patients. J Neurosurg 1999;90:50.
72. Zimmerman RS, Spetzler RF, Lee KS, et al. Cavernous malformations of the brainstem. J Neurosurg 1991;75:32.
73. Pollock BE, Garces YI, Stafford SL, et al. Stereotactic radiosurgery for cavernous malformations. J Neurosurg 2000;93:987.
74. Kondziolka D, Lunsford LD, Flickinger JC, et al. Reduction of hemorrhage risk after stereotactic radiosurgery for cavernous malformations. J Neurosurg 1995;83:825.
75. Hasegawa T, McInerney J, Kondziolka D, et al. Long-term results after stereotactic radiosurgery for patients with cavernous malformations. Neurosurgery 2002;50:1190.
76. Amin-Hanjani S, Ogilvy CS, Candia GJ, et al. Stereotactic radiosurgery for cavernous malformations: Kjellberg's experience with proton beam therapy in 998 cases at the Harvard cyclotron. Neurosurgery 1998;42:1229.
77. Karlsson B, Kihlstrom L, Lindquist C, et al. Radiosurgery for cavernous malformations. J Neurosurg 1998;88:293.
78. Rigamonti D, Spetzler RF, Medina M, et al. Cerebral venous malformations. J Neurosurg 1990;73:560.
79. Truwit CL. Venous angioma of the brain: history, significance, and imaging findings. AJR Am J Roentgenol 1992;159:1299.
80. Biller J, Toffol GJ, Shea JF, et al. Cerebellar venous angiomas. Arch Neurol 1985;42:367.
81. Saito Y, Kobayashi N. Cerebral venous angiomas. Radiology 1981;139:87.
82. Moritake K, Handa H, Mori K, et al. Venous angiomas of the brain. Surg Neurol 1980;14:95.
83. Sarwar M, McCormick WF. Intracerebral venous angioma. Arch Neurol 1978;35:323.
84. McLaughlin MR, Kondziolka D, Flickinger JC, et al. The prospective natural history of cerebral venous malformations. Neurosurgery 1998;43:195.
85. Olson E, Gilmor RL, Richmond B. Cerebral venous angiomas. Radiology 1984;151:97.
86. Valvanis A, Wellauer J, Yasargil MG. The radiological diagnosis of cerebral venous angioma: cerebral angiography and computed tomography. Neuroradiology 1983;24:193.
87. Augustyn GT, Scott JA, Olson E, et al. Cerebral venous angiomas: MR imaging. Radiology 1985;156:391.
88. Cammarata C, Han JS, Haaga JR, et al. Cerebral venous angiomas imaged by MR. Radiology 1985;155:639.
89. Kondziolka D, Dempsey PK, Lunsford LD. The case for conservative management of venous angiomas. Can J Neurol Sci 1991;18:295.
90. Rigamonti D, Johnson PC, Spetzler RF, et al. Cavernous malformations and capillary telangiectasia: a spectrum within a single pathological entity. Neurosurgery 1991;1:60.
91. McCormick PW, Spetzler RF, Johnson PC, et al. Cerebellar hemorrhage associated with capillary telangiectasia and venous angioma: a case report. Surg Neurol 1993;39:451.
92. Bland LI, Laphma LW, Ketonen L, et al. Acute cerebellar hemorrhage secondary to capillary telangiectasia in an infant. Arch Neurol 1994;51:1151.
93. Lee RR, Becker MW, Benson ML, et al. Brain capillary telangiectasia: MR appearance and clinicohistopathologic findings. Radiology 1997;205:797.

CHAPTER 17

Vascular Disorders of the Spinal Cord in Children and Young Adults

Richard B. Rodgers • Michael B. Pritz

Various spinal cord vascular malformations occur in young individuals. These lesions are rare, but the clinical consequences of hemorrhage and ischemia can be devastating. Although spinal cord vascular malformations were first described more than 100 years ago,[1] the natural histories of the various types of malformations are poorly understood because they are so rare. Each type can cause severe neurologic sequelae with variable recovery. Treatment generally is based on the type of malformation. Some malformations are treated conservatively. Others are treated with surgery, endovascular occlusion, or often a combination of techniques. A team approach is often required. Advances in imaging and endovascular therapy have greatly influenced the management of these patients.[2]

Classification

Various classification schemes have existed since the first autopsy description in 1885.[1] Radiologic diagnosis historically was made by myelography. With the advent of spinal angiography in the 1960s and later magnetic resonance imaging (MRI), these lesions became better understood. Numerous schemes have been described. Regardless of the type of classification, all are based on the angioarchitecture of the malformation (Table 17-1). Intramedullary arteriovenous malformations (AVMs) classically have been subdivided into glomus AVMs and juvenile AVMs. Other categories of vascular malformations are perimedullary arteriovenous fistula (AVF), cavernous malformation, and complex vascular malformations. Dural AVMs or AVFs are considered acquired lesions of older adults and are not discussed further.[3,4]

TABLE 17-1 **Types of Spinal Cord Vascular Malformations**

Intramedullary
  Arteriovenous malformation
    Glomus
    Juvenile
  Cavernous malformation
Perimedullary
  Arteriovenous fistula
Complex
    Metameric lesions (Cobb syndrome)
Disseminated angiomatosis (Rendu-Osler-Weber syndrome)

Pathophysiology of Injury from Vascular Malformations

The spinal cord is susceptible to injury from various causes. The pathophysiology of injury secondary to a vascular malformation depends on the type of malformation. Usually, neurologic sequelae result from a combination of direct compression, hemorrhage, and ischemia.[5]

Compression of the spinal cord occurs because of the mass of the malformation. The spinal column is a rigid tube housing the spinal cord bathed in a thin layer of cerebrospinal fluid. Any additional contents, such as dilated veins or aneurysms, can compress and distort the spinal cord and its roots, resulting in temporary or permanent neurologic injury.[6]

Bleeding can occur with any category of vascular malformation. Its occurrence is more common in lesions with high flows and arterial or venous aneurysms.[3,4,7] Hemorrhage into the subarachnoid space results in meningeal irritation and its subsequent signs and potentially ends in arachnoiditis. If the bleeding is rapid or massive or both, a localized hematoma can occur outside of the cord, causing spinal cord and nerve root compression. Hemorrhage also can occur directly into the spinal cord parenchyma, typically causing acute neurologic deficits.[4,5]

Ischemia can result from steal or from venous hypertension. Ischemia caused by arterial steal most commonly occurs in large malformations, especially with high-flow states. It is due to shunting of oxygen-rich blood through the malformation instead of to the cord.[8] Venous hypertension occurs because veins of the spinal cord lack valves, which results in the spinal venous pressure reaching arterial pressures. This arterial pressure causes venous congestion and ultimately diminished perfusion of the cord.[4,9]

Arteriovenous Malformations

Intramedullary spinal AVMs, similar to their cerebral counterparts, are considered congenital. They have been subdivided into glomus and juvenile types based on their angioarchitecture.[4,5] Both groups are high-flow shunts, characterized by large blood volumes under arterialized pressures.[10] Arterial and venous aneurysms are common. Approximately half of patients present with chronic ischemic symptoms, whereas half have an apoplectic event prompting diagnosis.[3] It is exceedingly rare to find an incidental AVM in an asymptomatic patient. The true natural history is unknown.[5] Approximately 20% of patients with an intramedullary spinal AVM have an associated vascular anomaly, including Klippel-Trénaunay-Weber syndrome, Rendu-Osler-Weber syndrome, or other spinal or cerebral AVMs or aneurysms.[3,4]

Glomus Arteriovenous Malformation

A glomus AVM has a compact intramedullary nidus, or complex mass of arteriovenous channels, with no intervening spinal cord tissue (Fig. 17-1). These AVMs usually are located in the midline of the cervical spinal cord or at the cervicomedullary junction. They have been reported at all other sites of the spinal cord, however.[3,11,12] Patients typically present at a relatively young age (mean of around 25 years) with neurologic deficits.[4,13] The diagnosis is made by MRI and confirmed by spinal angiography.[5,10]

Management is directed at complete obliteration without compromise of the blood supply to the spinal cord. Usually this obliteration requires open operation. Multiple reports of good results have been documented, with the best outcomes occurring in patients with a compact, superficial nidus.

FIGURE 17-1 **AVM of the conus.**
A, Appearance of a ruptured AVM of the conus (*arrows*) is shown on sagittal T2-weighted MR image. **B,** Spinal angiography shows feeding vessel (*long arrow*), glomus (*short arrow*), and draining vein (*arrowheads*) on this anteroposterior view.

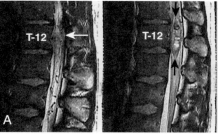
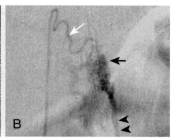

The risk of neurologic deterioration after surgery has been reported to be 20%, however, and residual malformation documented by spinal angiography is frequent. Endovascular embolization techniques have been used, alone and in combination with surgery. Decisions for embolization are based on the angioarchitecture of the AVM and the proximity of feeding vessels of the AVM to the normal arterial supply of the cord. Embolization is safer for cervical cord AVMs owing to increased collaterals to the cervical spinal cord.[12]

Juvenile Arteriovenous Malformation

Juvenile AVMs are extremely rare. Juvenile AVM is characterized by a large nidus with dilated channels and multiple feeding vessels over a long segment of cord. Functional spinal cord tissue is interspersed within the channels of the AVM.[11] These are more common in the cervical and upper thoracic spinal cord.[12]

Patient presentation is similar to glomus AVM, but even less is known about the natural history. These lesions usually are considered more dangerous because of multiple feeding vessels and functional nervous tissue within the nidus. Diagnosis is suggested by spinal MRI and confirmed by angiography.[5,12]

Because of extensive involvement of the spinal cord, juvenile AVM is often unable to be safely treated solely by an operation. Therapy often combines staged endovascular embolization with surgery reserved for small residual AVM or for a patient with an AVM whose features are considered high risk for hemorrhage (e.g., feeding artery aneurysm). A team approach is required to treat and care for these patients.[5,10,12]

Perimedullary Arteriovenous Fistula

Perimedullary AVF was first described in 1977. It is a direct fistula of intradural extramedullary vessels, usually a branch or branches of the anterior spinal artery and a tortuous and elongated paraspinal draining vein, without an intervening nidus (Fig. 17-2). The lesion lies on the pial surface and in the subarachnoid space.[14] The most common location is in the thoracolumbar area, with a propensity to involve the conus medullaris ventrally.[15] These have been subclassified further based on size, venous engorgement, and flow characteristics.[11]

FIGURE 17-2 **Perimedullary AVF.**
A, Sagittal T2-weighted MR images show venous pouch (*asterisk*) and several dilated vessels in more superior subarachnoid space. **B,** Spinal angiography, lateral view, shows feeding artery (*arrow*) and venous pouch (*asterisk*).

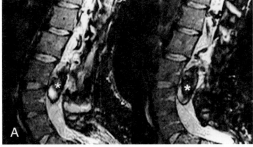
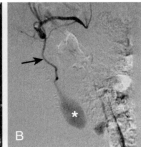

Perimedullary AVFs are rare. The natural history seems to be aggressive, with the largest lesions occurring in childhood or adolescence.[16] The average age at presentation is 25 years. Most patients experience a gradual onset of myelopathy secondary to ischemia. Acute symptoms from hemorrhage, either subarachnoid or intraparenchymal, have been reported, however.[5,7,17] The diagnosis of the malformation is usually suggested by MRI, but the exact site of the abnormal arteriovenous connection requires spinal angiography (see Fig. 17-2).[18]

Treatment is directed at obliteration of the fistula connection. A good-quality, superselective arteriogram is necessary. In a patient with a single abnormal connection, surgical occlusion is the treatment of choice and potentially curative. The more complex the fistula, the less likely it is to be treated with surgery alone. Endovascular embolization with coils or cyanoacrylate is recommended for giant high-flow AVFs.[7,16,18]

Cavernous Malformations

Spinal cord cavernous malformation (also referred to as cavernoma, cavernous angioma, occult vascular malformation, or cryptic angioma) is a well-circumscribed collection of sinusoidal venous channels, often described as "mulberry" or "popcorn-like," lacking intervening nervous system parenchyma (Fig. 17-3). It is identical to its cerebral counterpart, but much less common. Only 3% to 5% of all cavernous malformations occur in the spinal cord. The size of the malformation can range from a few millimeters to several centimeters. Although commonly considered congenital, the malformations can occur spontaneously and have been reported after radiation therapy. A familial syndrome has been described.[19] Cavernous malformations can be found throughout the cord, generally with a volume-based distribution (i.e., thoracic more common than cervical, which is more common than lumbar), and are usually intramedullary, but can be intradural extramedullary and even epidural.[3,20] A slight female predominance has been reported.[21]

Three classic patterns of presentation occur. The most dangerous is the acute neurologic sequelae from a hemorrhage. Clinical examination identifies the area of affected spinal cord. The second is the onset of

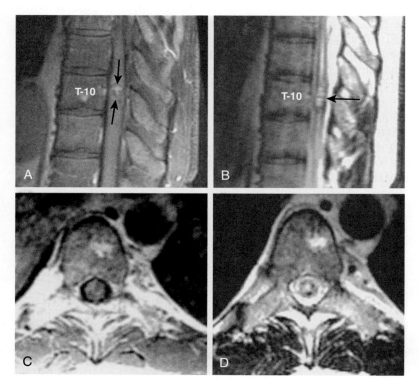

FIGURE 17-3 **Cavernous malformation. A-D,** Typical appearance of an intraspinal cavernous malformation is seen on sagittal (**A** and **B,** *arrows*) and axial MR images (**C** and **D**) on T1 (**A,** with contrast; **C,** without contrast) and T2 (**B** and **D**) sequences.

slowly progressive neurologic deficits owing to gradual enlargement of the malformation causing mass effect, or possibly from the toxic effects of hemosiderin following hemorrhage. The third and most common presentation is with episodic symptoms from which the patient may or may not completely recover.[19,22-24]

The diagnosis of a spinal cord cavernous malformation is usually made based on its pathognomonic appearance on MRI (see Fig. 17-3).[25] Typically, a popcorn-like lesion of mixed signal intensity on T1-weighted and T2-weighted images, with little to no enhancement with gadolinium contrast administration, and a characteristic hypointense ring of hemosiderin deposition are seen.[19] Although these lesions are vascular, they rarely appear on spinal angiography except for an occasional venous blush (hence the terms "cryptic" or "occult" vascular malformation) because the involved vessels are beyond the resolution of present-day angiography.[26]

The treatment for spinal cord cavernous malformations is almost exclusively surgical. There have been multiple reports of good outcomes and neurologic improvements after surgical resection for symptomatic lesions. The incidence of permanent neurologic worsening is about 5%.[13] A shorter duration of symptoms correlates with an improved postoperative course. Although some evidence for surgical treatment for the asymptomatic lesion has been advanced, this is controversial.[19] Endovascular embolization has no role in the treatment of these lesions. Radiosurgery seems to be of little use and is possibly detrimental.[13,27]

Complex Vascular Malformations

Complex or metameric vascular malformations are formidable but very rare lesions. By definition, the metameric vascular malformation is a spinal cord AVM in which the associated tissues surrounding the spinal column are involved (Fig. 17-4).[5] When the

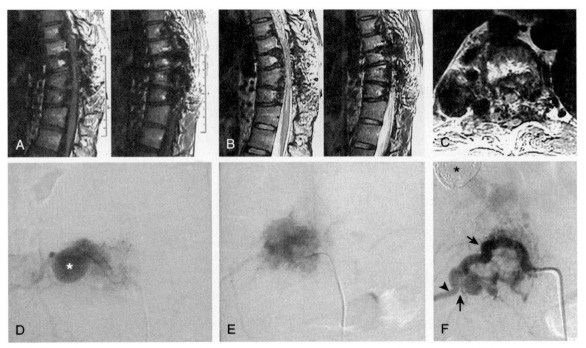

FIGURE 17-4 **Metameric AVM. A-C,** AVM involving the spinal cord and surrounding bone and soft tissue is shown on sagittal T1-weighted (**A**), sagittal T2-weighted (**B**), and axial T2-weighted (**C**) sequences. **D-F,** Subtracted angiographic appearance on anteroposterior views is seen after injection of the right T9 (**D**), right T10 (**E**), and right T11 (**F**) intercostal arteries. A large venous varix (*asterisk* in **D**) has been occluded with Guglielmi detachable coils (*asterisk* in **F**). A portion of the nidus is seen in **E**. In **F**, an enlarged feeding artery (*arrow*), a venous pouch (*short arrow*), and draining vein (*arrowhead*) are illustrated.

spinal cord, vertebrae, and skin are involved, the eponym Cobb syndrome is applied.[28] The abdominal viscera or thoracic organs also can be affected. These types of lesions also have been reported with Rendu-Osler-Weber syndrome. Patients typically present with symptoms from the spinal cord AVM. Occasionally, diagnosis is made after a thorough evaluation of the skin lesion. Identification is suggested by MRI and confirmed by angiography. Treatment is palliative, and typically combines endovascular embolization with percutaneous vertebroplasty. Surgery is reserved for areas thought to be at high risk for hemorrhage, similar to juvenile AVM. Complete cure is rare, even with multimodality therapy.[29]

Acknowledgments

The authors thank J. Corbitt, for manuscript preparation; J. Murphy, for help with the figures; and Drs. T. Horner and T. Leipzig, for providing some of the images used in the figures.

Conclusion

Spinal cord vascular malformations encompass a heterogeneous group of blood vessel disorders that affect the spinal cord either directly or indirectly. Most prevalent of these rare malformations are AVMs or dural arteriovenous fistulas (AVFs). A distinct entity is the conus medullaris AVM. Diagnostic delays continue to challenge clinicians. Pain may be a presenting feature; ischemic changes may account for a chronic progressive radiculomyelopathy (Foix-Alajouanine syndrome). Hemorrhagic complications include subarachnoid hemorrhage, hematomyelia, or epidural hematomas. Diagnostic evaluation of the angioarchitecture and hemodynamics of these malformations, and proper management strategies requires a collaborative effort and multidisciplinary expertise.

REFERENCES

1. Hebold O. Aneurysmen der kleisnten rucken marksgefass. Arch Psychiatr Nervnkr 1885;16:813.
2. Akopov SE, Schievink WI. History of spinal cord vascular malformations and their treatment. Semin Cerebrovasc Dis Stroke 2002;2:178.
3. Spetzler RF, Detwiler PW, Riina HA, et al. Modified classification of spinal cord vascular lesions. J Neurosurg 2002;96(2 Suppl):145.
4. Rosenblum B, Oldfield EH, Doppman JL, et al. Spinal arteriovenous malformations: a comparison of dural arteriovenous fistulas and intradural AVMs in 81 patients. J Neurosurg 1987;67:795.
5. Jahan R, Vinuela F. Vascular anatomy, pathophysiology, and classification of vascular malformations of the spinal cord. Semin Cerebrovasc Dis Stroke 2002;2:186.
6. El Mahdi MA, Rudwan MA, Khaffji SM, et al. A giant spinal aneurysm with cord and root compression. J Neurol Neurosurg Psychiatry 1989;52:532.
7. Mourier KL, Gobin YP, George B, et al. Intradural perimedullary arteriovenous fistulae: results of surgical and endovascular treatment in a series of 35 cases. Neurosurgery 1993;32:885.
8. Djindjian M, Djindjian R, Hurth M, et al. Steal phenomena in spinal arteriovenous malformations. J Neuroradiol 1978;5:187.
9. Aminoff MJ, Barnard RO, Logue V. The pathophysiology of spinal vascular malformations. J Neurol Sci 1974;23:255.
10. Oldfield E. Spinal vascular malformations. In Wilkins R, Rengachary S, eds. Neurosurgery, 2nd ed. New York: McGraw-Hill, 1996.
11. Anson JA, Spetzler RF. Classification of spinal arteriovenous malformations and implications for treatment. Barrow Neurological Institute Quarterly 1992; 8:2
12. Atkinson JLD, Piepgras DG. Surgical treatment of spinal cord arteriovenous malformations and arteriovenous fistulas. Semin Cerebrovasc Dis Stroke 2002;2:201.
13. Connolly ES Jr, McCormick PC. Intramedullary vascular malformations: type II glomus arteriovenous malformations and cavernous malformations. In Barrow DL, Awad IA, eds. Spinal Vascular Malformations. Park Ridge, IL: The American Association of Neurological Surgeons, 1999.
14. Djindjian M, Djindjian R, Rey A, et al. Intradural extramedullary spinal arterio-venous malformations fed by the anterior spinal artery. Surg Neurol 1977;8:85.
15. Hurst RW, Bagley LJ, Marcotte P, et al. Spinal cord arteriovenous fistulas involving the conus medullaris: presentation, management, and embryologic considerations. Surg Neurol 1999;52:95.
16. Gueguen B, Merland JS, Riche MC, et al. Vascular malformations of the spinal cord: intrathecal perimedullary arteriovenous fistulas fed by medullary arteries. Neurology 1987;37:969.
17. Tomlinson FH, Rufenacht DA, Sundt TM Jr, et al. Arteriovenous fistulas of the brain and spinal cord. J Neurosurg 1993;79:16.
18. Cawley CM, Barrow DL. Intradural perimedullary spinal cord arteriovenous fistulas. In Barrow DL, Awad IA, eds. Spinal Vascular Malformations. Park Ridge, IL: The American Association of Neurological Surgeons, 1999.
19. Lemole GM Jr, Henn JS, Riina HA, et al. Spinal cord cavernous malformations. Semin Cerebrovasc Dis Stroke 2002;2:227.

20. Harrison MJ, Eisenberg MB, Ullman JS, et al. Symptomatic cavernous malformations affecting the spine and spinal cord. Neurosurgery 1995; 37:195.
21. McCormick PC, Stein BM. Spinal cavernous malformations. In Awad IA, Barrow DL, eds. Cavernous Malformations. Park Ridge, IL: The American Association of Neurological Surgeons, 1993.
22. Canavero S, Pagni CA, Duca S, et al. Spinal intramedullary cavernous angiomas: a literature metaanalysis. Surg Neurol 1994;41:381.
23. McCormick PC, Michelson WJ, Post KD, et al. Cavernous malformations of the spinal cord. Neurosurgery 1988;23:459.
24. Deutsch H, Jallo GI, Faktorovich A, et al. Spinal intramedullary cavernoma: clinical presentation and surgical outcome. J Neurosurg 2000;93:65.
25. Barnwell SL, Dowd CF, Davis RL, et al. Cryptic vascular malformations of the spinal cord: diagnosis by magnetic resonance imaging and outcome of surgery. J Neurosurg 1990;72:403.
26. Furuya K, Sasaki T, Suzuki I, et al. Intramedullary angiographically occult vascular malformations of the spinal cord: clinical study. Neurosurgery 1998;42:1220.
27. Pollock BE, Garces YI, Stafford SL, et al. Stereotactic radiosurgery for cavernous malformations. J Neurosurg 2000;93:987.
28. Cobb S. Haemangioma of the spinal cord: associated with skin naevi of the same metamere. Ann Surg 1915;62:641.
29. Caragine LP Jr, Halbach VV, Ng PP, et al. Endovascular treatment of spinal cord vascular malformations. Semin Cerebrovasc Dis Stroke 2002;2:236.

INDEX

Note: Page numbers followed by *f* refer to figures; page number followed by *t* refer to tables.